A WELLNESS Way of life

third edition

of life

Gwen Robbins

Debbie Powers

Sharon Burgess

Ball State University

Brown & Benchmark
PUBLISHERS

Madison, WI Dubuque Guilford, CT Chicago Toronto London
Mexico City Caracas Buenos Aires Madrid Bogotá Sydney

Book Team

Acquisitions Editor *Ed Bartell*
Project Editor *Theresa Grutz*
Developmental Editor *Deborah Daniel*
Production Editor *Debra DeBord*
Proofreading Coordinator *Carrie Barker*
Designer *Jamie O'Neal*
Art Editor *Rita Hingtgen*
Photo Editor *Laura Fuller*
Production Manager *Beth Kundert*
Production/Costing Manager *Sherry Padden*
Production/Imaging and Media Development Manager *Linda Meehan Avenarius*
Marketing Manager *Pamela S. Cooper*
Copywriter *Jennifer Smith*
Proofreader *Mary Svetlik Anderson*

Basal Text *10/12 Goudy*
Display Type *Universe*
Typesetting System *Macintosh™ QuarkExpress™*
Paper Stock *50# Restorecote*

Brown & Benchmark
PUBLISHERS

Executive Vice President and General Manager *Bob McLaughlin*
Vice President, Business Manager *Russ Domeyer*
Vice President of Production and New Media Development *Victoria Putman*
National Sales Manager *Phil Rudder*
National Telesales Director *John Finn*

A Times Mirror Company

Cover image © Marc Romanelli/The Image Bank

Copyedited by Sarah Lane; proofread by Rose R. Kramer

Photo Credits: Chapter 1: pp. 6, 9, 12, 14, 19, 21 (all): Brenda Lewis, Westminster Colorado; Chapter 2: p. 28: Brenda Lewis, Westminster, Colorado; p. 29: Courtesy of Ball State University Photographic Services; 2.1, 2.2, p. 37: Brenda Lewis, Westminster, Colorado; p. 39: Paul Troxell; Chapter 4: 4.1, 4.2: Courtesy of Ball State University Photographic Services; 4.3, 4.4, 4.5, 4.6, 4.7, 4.8, 4.9, 4.10, 4.11, 4.12, 4.13, 4.14, 4.16, 4.17, 4.18, 4.19, 4.20: Brenda Lewis, Westminster, Colorado; Chapter 5: pp. 102, 109 (all), 110: Brenda Lewis, Westminster, Colorado; Chapter 6: p. 115: Gwen Robbins; p. 128: Courtesy of Ball State University Photographic Services; Chapter 7: p. 149: Brenda Lewis, Westminster, Colorado; p. 159: Reprinted with permission from *Hatha Yoga: Developing The Body, Mind and Inner Self* by Dee Ann Birkel, Eddie Bowers Publishing, Inc. Dubuque, Iowa; 7.3: Brenda Lewis, Westminster, Colorado; Chapter 8: pp. 167, 180: Courtesy of Ball State University Photographic Services; p. 182: Brenda Lewis, Westminster, Colorado; Chapter 9: pp. 187, 191: Brenda Lewis, Westminster, Colorado; Chapter 10: p. 221: Brenda Lewis, Westminster, Colorado; Chapter 11: p. 240: Paul Troxell; Chapter 12: p. 264: Brenda Lewis, Westminster, Colorado; p. 279: Paul Troxell; Chapter 13: p. 283: Brenda Lewis, Westminster, Colorado; p. 295: Paul Troxell; Chapter 14: pp. 302, 304 (all), 305, 306, 312: Brenda Lewis, Westminster, Colorado.

Library of Congress Catalog Card Number: 95–83871

ISBN 0–697–25915–3

Printed in the United States of America by Times Mirror Higher Education Group, Inc., 2460 Kerper Boulevard, Dubuque, IA 52001

10 9 8 7 6 5 4 3 2 1

contents

Chapter 7
Coping with Stress   139

Chapter 8
Special Exercise Considerations   165

Chapter 9
Nutrition   185

Chapter 13

Chapter 14

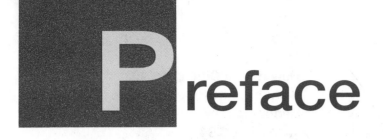

Preface

From the Authors

This book is about enjoying life—living it to your fullest potential. The purpose of *A Wellness Way of Life* is to help you pursue a wellness lifestyle. We wanted to provide a book that would present a body of knowledge that goes beyond fitness. This knowledge helps you make informed, responsible decisions affecting your wellness. However, we know it takes much more than knowledge. It takes personal commitment, self-management skills, and coping strategies to live a healthy lifestyle. Therefore, a primary focus of this book is identifying behavior changes that you can easily incorporate into your life. Our goal is not only to deliver fitness and health information but to motivate and guide you toward making positive choices.

Abraham Lincoln said, "We are about as happy as we make up our minds to be." We believe that one secret to happiness is having the competence and confidence to make informed decisions that affect your daily well-being. Self-responsibility and self-empowerment are means of increasing the quality and quantity of life. There is no better feeling than to know that you are doing something good for yourself! As you read each chapter, you will learn strategies for taking control of your life and discover the joy in traveling the wellness journey. This book will help you wade through the myriad of health and wellness information and ultimately make you an informed wellness consumer. The end result will be the indescribable joy in knowing you are attaining your highest potential for well-being.

Gwen Robbins
Debbie Powers
Sharon Burgess

About the Audience

This text is designed to meet the needs of a course that goes beyond the basics of physical fitness to encompass the broader scope of wellness. The content—covering all aspects of fitness, nutrition, weight management, stress management, heart health, and substance use and abuse—easily accommodates a variety of fitness, wellness, and health courses. It is a flexible book that fits nicely into a lecture/fitness activity format. The text has been classroom-tested since the late 1980s in a fitness/wellness program that started the current trend that is sweeping the nation.

New Features in This Edition

Based on the idea of self-responsibility, *A Wellness Way of Life* gives students practical information about how to make good decisions that will positively affect their well-being throughout their lives. It's an open, accessible resource that minimizes technical jargon and presents health as a positive, dynamic process. New features for this third edition include

➤ A seventh dimension of wellness—environmental wellness—has been added to help students understand that wellness extends to their impact on the environment.
➤ More information on people from diverse backgrounds broadens understanding for all readers.
➤ New American College of Sports Medicine Manual of Exercise Prescription Standards guidelines for health promotion and endurance provide realistic guidelines for the amount of exercise needed to stay healthy.

- New nutritional information on antioxidants, calcium, food labels, and fats keeps students and instructors up-to-date.
- New learning activities for each chapter help students apply to their own lives what they've learned through reading and lecture.
- New information on LSD, heroin, the Clock method for smoking cessation, the prevention of date rape, age-adjusted fitness norms, heart health, stress reduction, and fitness tests gives readers the most up-to-date facts available.
- The new book design, featuring a larger format and new activities tabs, improves readability and helps students more easily find activities related to chapters.
- A new glossary helps students master the language of wellness.
- Prochaska Stages of Change Model helps students make their behavioral change a successful reality.

What Is the Prochaska Stages of Change Model?

In order to help people be more effective in their attempts to change their behavior, psychologists James Prochaska, John Norcross, and Carlo DiClemente decided to study individuals who had successfully changed health-related behaviors on their own. Prochaska and his colleagues wanted to find out which behavior change techniques successful changers found to be most helpful. What these researchers discovered during their years of studying behavior change is that individuals progress through distinct stages of change on their way to improved well-being. Their initial research was done on people who quit smoking but has expanded to cover other health behaviors. The stages of change are

1. *Precontemplation*. People at this stage see no problem with their behavior and have no intention of changing it.
2. *Contemplation*. In this stage, people come to understand their problem and its causes, and they start to think about taking action to solve it.
3. *Preparation*. In the preparation stage, people are planning to take action within the next month and are putting together a plan of action.
4. *Action*. A person in the action stage has taken the leap and is actively making behavior changes.
5. *Maintenance*. Even after action has been taken successfully, it must be maintained to prevent relapse.

Prochaska and his colleagues noted that certain behavioral change techniques work better than others in some stages of change. This model has received a great deal of attention in both the popular press and among health educators. Prochaska et al. published a successful trade book called *Changing for Good* on how to use their model to change behavior successfully.

Pedagogical Highlights

A *Wellness Way of Life* includes a number of built-in resources that make learning easy:

Chapter Objectives   Found at the beginning of each chapter, the objectives provide a starting point and focus for readers.

Key Terms   Important terms are highlighted in boldface to catch students' attention, increase retention, and indicate glossary terms.

Chapter Summary   The key points from each chapter are summarized at the end to increase student comprehension and retention of vital information.

References   Accurate and current documentation is provided at the ends of the chapters.

Suggested Readings   A number of sources for additional reading and research are cited to provide students with a handy, useful reference.

Resources A listing of additional current resources is provided to encourage further exploration.

Appendices and Activities The appendices and chapter activities provide lab-like opportunities for students to apply to their own lives what they've learned and information on specific activities for the development of fitness, such as aerobic dance, bicycling, fitness swimming, indoor exercise equipment, jogging, walking, and water exercise/aqua aerobics.

Supplements

An *Instructor's Manual* provides everything instructors need to make the most of *A Wellness Way of Life*, from chapter overviews to teaching strategies.

A comprehensive *Test Item File* makes testing easier, with over 1,200 test questions.

Testing, quizzing, and grading are easy with the help of *MicroTest III Software* for Macintosh and IBM.

A set of 50 full-color *Brown & Benchmark Fitness & Wellness Transparencies* vividly illustrates important concepts.

Qualified adopters of *A Wellness Way of Life* may receive a free subscription to the *Berkeley Wellness Newsletter*.

For additional help on nutrition and diet, *Food Processor Software** helps students analyze their eating habits, as well as realize the impact of lifestyle changes on their nutritional needs.

To assist students in designing their own personal lifestyle changes, *Lifestyle Improvement Inventory Software** prompts users to answer a variety of questions and then recommends specific behavior modifications.

The *Health & Wellness Videodisc** encourages exploration and helps stimulate critical thinking.

Acknowledgments

We would like to thank the reviewers of this edition for their time and assistance:

➤ Thomas L. Dezelsky
Arizona State University

➤ Robert Koslow
James Madison University

➤ Rebecca R. Leas
Clarion University

➤ Patsy Livingston
Point Loma Nazarene College

➤ Jacqueline T. Poythress
DeKalb College

➤ Timothy Voss
Trinity College

We wish to express our gratitude to the following individuals for their assistance in the development of this book:

➤ Sam Minor II, Department of Art, College of Fine Arts, Ball State University, for artwork

➤ Brenda Lewis and Paul Troxell for the photographs

A special thank you goes to Dr. John Reno for his continued support of the fitness/wellness program at Ball State University.

We dedicate this third edition to the devoted fitness/wellness faculty at Ball State. Their support and suggestions have been invaluable.

*Available to qualified adopters.

chapter 1

Wellness

➤ Objectives

After reading this chapter, you will be able to:

1. Explain the focus of the publication *Healthy People 2000*.

2. List ten health habits that, when practiced, can reduce the risk of health problems.

3. Distinguish between health and wellness.

4. Define *wellness*.

5. Identify the seven dimensions of wellness, and give three examples within each dimension.

6. List and describe the six factors that influence growth in wellness, as shown on the wellness wheel.

7. Differentiate between self-managed behavior change and willpower.

8. Identify and describe Prochaska's nine behavior change processes and his five stages in behavior change.

9. Write a behavior change contract/plan.

10. Give four examples of ways society supports wellness, and four examples of ways society detracts from wellness.

Terms

- Emotional dimension
- Environmental dimension
- Health
- Health promotion
- Intellectual dimension
- Occupational dimension
- Physical dimension
- Self-management
- Social dimension
- Societal norm
- Spiritual dimension
- Wellness

Life is not merely to be alive, but to be well.

Martial

as Rob lay in the coronary care unit, his eyes surveyed various tubes and wires connected to his tired body. The nightmare of the last 24 hours was over, but the pain and confusion lingered.

"How can this be? I'm only 49 years old. How could I have had a heart attack? What if I die? What about my wife? My son? My daughter? I've just become a grandpa. I was given a big promotion at work. Why now?" Rob's mind drifted.

"But I'm an athlete! Well, I *was* an athlete, back in high school. Once I started college there was no time for sports or exercise. Started smoking, too. Figured I'd stop when the pressure was off, but the pressure never stopped. Drank too much, too; partied a lot. Still like several drinks to end the day. I always thought I'd lose those extra 30 pounds—always next year, always a New Year's resolution. Diet? Too busy. Vending machines, hot dog stands, snacks in front of the TV, fast food. No time. Too much to do. Money to make. A lot of stress. Can't stop now. There'll be time later."

Rob's mind drifted back to his room. He could hear his doctor's voice—"Stop smoking. Change in lifestyle. Low-fat diet. Start exercising. Cholesterol is 280. Break old habits." Rob thought, "How I wish I could turn back the clock!"

This scenario is all too common in the United States. In fact, more than half of all deaths in this country are attributed to coronary heart disease and stroke. Even though most heart attacks occur after middle age, many are a result of years of lifestyle abuse. One hundred years ago the leading causes of death were infectious diseases such as tuberculosis, polio, diphtheria, pneumonia, and influenza and various diseases of infancy. Advances in medicine, the discovery of antibiotics, and improved sanitation di-

The "good life"?

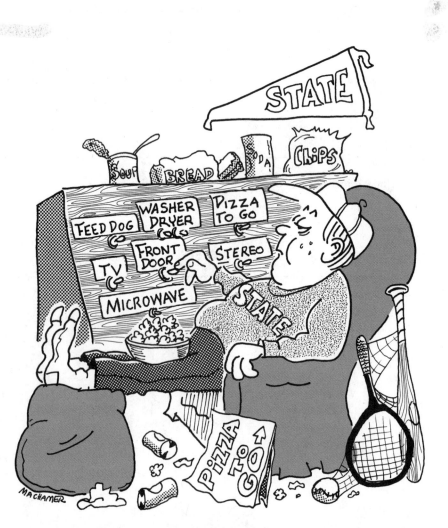

FIGURE 1.1 ➤

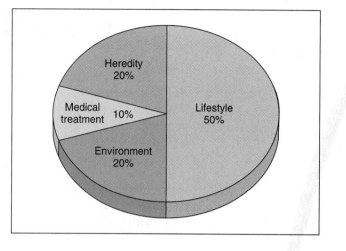

minished these ravaging diseases and increased the average life span. Through scientific discovery, technology, industrial growth, and automation, the entire American lifestyle has changed. We use remote controls to change television channels and to open garage doors. Appliances wash our clothes, dishes, and teeth. We ride vehicles to work, school, and even while playing golf! We allow ourselves to be bused and trucked, elevated, and escalated and then wonder why we grow fat and are out of shape. This so-called "good life" has created sedentary living, changes in eating habits (fast foods, increased fats and sweets, processed foods), stress, alcohol and drug abuse, and obesity.

The latest statistics released by the American Heart Association are startling. In a single year, diseases of the heart and blood vessels kill far more Americans than were killed in World Wars I and II, the Korean War, and the Vietnam War, *combined*. Those who survive a coronary incident are often faced with a restricted, less fulfilling life that causes an unnecessary, costly drain on the resources available for health care. Such horrendous figures should outrage the public and should cause a demand for reform, since carnage is normally the basis for alarm and legislation. Instead, apathy is the general response of many, and many of us do not even begin to worry about health until it is lost.

The harsh truth is that a high percentage of disease and disability affecting the American people is preventable, a consequence of unwise behavior and lifestyle choices. The decision to smoke, for instance, is responsible for one of every six deaths in the United States each year. Twenty-one percent of heart disease deaths, 87 percent of lung cancer deaths, and 30 percent of all cancer deaths are linked to smoking. Smoking costs our society over $52 billion annually.[1] Dr. William Foege at the Centers for Disease Control in Atlanta states that as much as *two-thirds* of all disability and death up to age 65 would be preventable in total or in part if we applied what we know about the effects of lifestyle on premature illness and death.[2] Figure 1.1 illustrates the extent to which our longevity is affected by a combination of our lifestyle decisions.

You may already possess some knowledge about these and other health topics. If you are like most, however, you generally underestimate your future risk of lifestyle diseases. This underestimation is of substantial concern, because action should be an outcome of knowledge. After all, the truly educated individual understands *cause* and *effect*. It is encouraging to know that the evidence is becoming more and more clear—health and longevity are not solely a result of genetics and luck but an outcome of personal behavior. This personal behavior involves responsible choices, self-discipline, and a commitment to excellence.

This chapter introduces the basic concept of health, the impact of lifestyle on well-being, and the dynamics of high-level wellness. It also explores the challenges and strategies involved in making self-managed behavior changes.

Basic Concepts of Health

Traditionally **health** has been viewed as the "lack of disease." If you show no signs or symptoms of illness, you are healthy. Health is seen as a state of being. You are either ill or healthy. Some health-care facilities still reflect this simplistic view. Many insurance companies pay for treatments and hospitalization when sickness occurs but pay nothing for preventive checkups or procedures. Employers allow "sick days," yet personal days or vacation days must be used for pursuing health-promoting activities. Because of this curative focus, a majority of our health-care dollars are spent on procedures for patching people up after the damage has been done. Billions of dollars are spent to treat the results of bad eating habits, stress, sedentary living, and smoking. This is a "sickness-care" system rather than a "health-care" system. Because of the medical procedures, drugs, and technologies presently available, many people have become complacent about their health habits. They think they can be "bailed out" by medical science (at the cost of billions of dollars a year to society).

Expanding the focus of health to include many different aspects of life (social, psychological, spiritual, and so on) as well as empowering individual responsibility involves health promotion.

Health promotion is "the science and art of helping people change their lifestyles to move toward a state of optimal health."[3] Health promotion involves systematic efforts by organizations to create healthy policies and supportive environments as well as the reorienting of health services to include more than clinical and curative care. Examples of health promotion programs are weight-loss workshops, smoking cessation clinics, and stress management seminars. Laws and policies such as those prohibiting drunk driving and those establishing smoke-free workplaces also assist in health promotion. More discussion of health promotion is found in Chapter 14.

Another trend in health care is renewed emphasis on medical self-care. Medical self-care includes all actions taken by an individual with respect to a medical problem. It accounts for 85 percent to 95 percent of all medical care.[4] Medical self-care promotes self-sufficiency in diagnosis and requires decision making as to whether a physician's services are needed. It is usually used for minor illnesses or injuries such as colds, flu, cuts, and sprains. Individual decision making becomes the focus. Do I need a physician for this problem? What can I do for myself? What can I expect from the health-care profession? However, medical self-care goes beyond minor illness. Individuals with diabetes, asthma, and allergies have a major responsibility for their own care. Even emergency procedures such as cardiopulmonary resuscitation (CPR) and the Heimlich maneuver fall into the realm of medical self-care. No longer are thermometers the only diagnostic tool in home medicine cabinets. It is now common to find blood pressure kits, home pregnancy tests, colon-rectal cancer detection kits, and blood sugar and cholesterol self-tests. The purpose of self-care is not to replace the physician but to promote personal responsibility for health, rather than total dependence on physicians.

Lifestyle and Health

The preventive aspects of health have become increasingly clear, and new research studies of scientists often become instant, sensationalized news headlines: *Yo-yo weight loss harmful. Vasectomy causes prostate cancer. Aspirin prevents heart attacks.* Sometimes the information is only partially reported, resulting in confusion and contradiction. Bewildered and wary, many Americans reject or ignore many health pronouncements: *Cut fat to under 30 percent of calories. Exercise aerobically 30 minutes five times per week. Eat five or more fruits and vegetables daily.* Unfortunately, a majority of present-day Americans continue to be sedentary and overweight. Stress levels and blood cholesterol readings continue to soar. The relationship between lifestyle and health is clear, but adopting healthy lifestyle habits has been difficult for many.

Healthy People 2000

Because of the concern for our nation's health and vitality, a vigorous national crusade for health promotion was initiated in 1990 with the publication of *Healthy People 2000: National Health Promotion and Disease Prevention Objectives.* Facilitated by the U.S. Public Health Service, *Healthy People 2000* is a statement of national opportunities, emphasizing individual control of our health destinies: "personal responsibility, which is to

table 1.1

A SAMPLE OF HEALTH OBJECTIVES FROM *HEALTHY PEOPLE 2000*

- Increase moderate daily physical activity to at least 30 percent of people (a 36 percent increase).
- Reduce overweight to a prevalence of no more than 20 percent of people (a 23 percent decrease).
- Reduce dietary fat intake to an average of 30 percent of calories (a 17 percent decrease).
- Reduce cigarette smoking prevalence to no more than 15 percent of adults (a 48 percent decrease).
- Reduce alcohol-related motor vehicle crash deaths to no more than 8.5 per 100,000 people (a 12 percent decrease).
- Reduce homicides to no more than 7.2 per 100,000 people (a 15 percent decrease).
- Reduce coronary heart disease deaths to no more than 100 per 100,000 people (a 26 percent decrease).
- Increase the daily consumption of fruits and vegetables to five or more servings per person (present average is 2½ servings).

say responsible and enlightened behavior by each and every individual, truly is the key to good health. . . . Our physical and emotional well-being is dependent upon measures that only we, ourselves, can affect."[5]

This document outlines specific health objectives for the nation targeted for the year 2000 in twenty-two priority areas (physical activity, nutrition, tobacco use, family planning, cancer, alcohol and drug use, sexually transmitted diseases, and heart disease to name a few). The document identifies three broad goals as the means of bringing about fuller human potential:[6]

1. Increase the span of healthy life for Americans.
2. Reduce health disparities among Americans.
3. Achieve access to preventive services for all Americans.

Table 1.1 lists just a few of the objectives found in *Healthy People 2000*. Because of the diversity and varying needs of Americans, reaching these goals is a challenge. Nevertheless, the federal government is playing a leadership role in cultivating a culture of healthier, life-enhancing habits for all Americans, regardless of income, race, sex, or other status. If we do not act now, the cost of health care in this country will reach $1.5 trillion by the end of the decade.[7]

Most of the proposals in *Healthy People 2000* to eliminate disease and create health are linked to everyday practices.[8] Not all of these lifestyle behaviors are easily undertaken. As you look through the following list of healthy habits, note that this book contains information to help you achieve many of them:

- ➤ Stop the use of all tobacco products (Chapter 12).
- ➤ Reduce blood pressure (Chapter 6).
- ➤ Consume little or no alcohol (Chapter 12).
- ➤ Manage stress (Chapter 7).
- ➤ Exercise in moderation three to five times per week (Chapter 2).
- ➤ Maintain an appropriate weight (Chapter 10).
- ➤ Reduce total blood cholesterol levels (Chapter 6).
- ➤ Eat more fresh fruit, vegetables, and fiber (Chapter 9).
- ➤ Practice safer sex (Chapter 13).
- ➤ Consume less red meat and poultry, substituting fish, lentils, and rice (Chapter 9).
- ➤ Participate in cancer self-exams and age-appropriate screenings (Chapter 11).
- ➤ Place smoke detectors in your home or apartment (Chapter 14).
- ➤ Drive within 5 miles per hour of the speed limit (Chapter 14).
- ➤ Wear seat belts in cars and helmets on bicycles and motorcycles (Chapter 14).

The typical American diet has become a serious health-risk factor.

There is nothing extreme or magical in this list. It does shift the main responsibility for health to the individual, rather than relegating the individual to a position of passivity amidst excessive surgeries, medications, and medical tests. One physician has appropriately summarized the issue by stating, "One of my frustrations in medicine was having people come to me expecting way too much of me and not expecting anything of themselves."[9] To evaluate your personal lifestyle habits, look to *Healthy Lifestyle: A Self-Assessment,* found in the Activities Section at the end of the book.

Understanding Risks

Often in this book we will talk about risks. In an effort to prevent disease and to promote health, it is important to identify the factors that cause disease and injury. From this, probabilities are determined as to the chances for occurrence. Like placing a bet at a race track, identifying risks is a way of quoting the odds. No one can honestly promise you that doing something or refraining from doing it will keep you safe or that doing one thing will positively kill you. You simply must draw your own conclusions from the evidence. Since there is no such thing as absolute safety, you only can choose to widen or narrow your risk margins with your habits.

One ongoing study has resulted in much of the information we know about the risk factors associated with coronary heart disease. The people of Framingham, Massachusetts, a community 18 miles west of Boston, have been studied and charted since 1950. The Framingham Study, as it has become known, has resulted in information about how heredity, environment, medical care, and lifestyle factors affect heart disease and general well-being. A comprehensive longitudinal study such as this, in contrast to a short-term, isolated study involving very few people, results in reputable data.

Heredity Is Not Destiny

For some, familial tendencies constitute a psychological trap. If your father died young of a heart attack or your mother has diabetes, your chances for following in their footsteps are greater than those of someone whose parents are healthy at 75 years of age. However, this is only the case if your parents' health problems were an actual result of genetics rather than environment or lifestyle habits. If you have inherited a genetic liability, this knowledge should give you additional motivation to live in such a way as to fight it. In the case of a family history of heart disease, you can lower your genetic odds significantly by controlling your blood pressure, blood cholesterol, weight, and stress level, and by getting regular exercise. On the other hand, having a father like Winston Churchill (who habitually smoked, drank, and ate rich food, and was obese, sedentary, and lived to 90) does not mean you are indestructible. Heredity is only one factor in the link to health and well-being. Even though our biological inheritance predisposes us to certain illnesses and protects us from others, it is the interaction of genetics, culture, environment, and habits that counts. Your environment and personal health habits can either magnify or inhibit the tendencies with which you were born. Of course, we hope you are thinking beyond mere "risk avoidance" to a life full of enrichment, self-fulfillment, and satisfaction. This dramatic shift in emphasis toward self-responsibility and an expanded quality of life has evolved into a concept called *wellness*.

High-Level Wellness

It is reassuring to know that we have a considerable amount of control over our health destiny. However, what are the upper limits of health? What is the ultimate in health? In the late 1950s, Dr. Halbert Dunn first used the term *wellness* in his writings about the pursuit of optimal well-being. He talked about the interrelated and interdependent whole person, a positive energy and vitality for living, personal growth and satisfaction, and the importance of viewing and promoting health as an *elevated* state of superb well-being, or high-level wellness.[10] Today, **wellness** is defined as an integrated and dynamic level of functioning oriented toward maximizing potential, dependent upon self-responsibility. Wellness involves not only preventive health behaviors, but a shift in *thinking* and *attitude*. Wellness is a mind-set of lifelong growth and achievement in the emotional, spiritual, physical, occupational, intellectual, environmental, and social dimensions. "Wellness is that continual process of evolution through life whereby the individual increases awareness, purpose, quality of life, and uniqueness in all areas of human potential."[11]

High-level wellness is applicable to all ages (old and young), all socioeconomic groups (poor and wealthy), and all types of people (able-bodied and disabled). It means working toward becoming the best you can be without accepting "traditional" limitations (i.e., age, race, gender, genetics). Wellness is a way of living in which growth and improvement are sought in all areas. It involves a lifestyle of deliberate choices and self-responsibility, requiring conscientious management and planning. Living a wellness lifestyle does not come about by accident or luck. It also involves much more than curing sickness, counting fat grams, jogging, or measuring body fat. It is a *mind-set* of personal empowerment. It means approaching life with optimism, confidence, and energy. Unlike sickness-care, which involves treatment, wellness is a lifelong quest toward optimal functioning in which you take charge. It involves accepting the changes in life while seeking the positive payoffs of change. This quest has rewards of high self-esteem, commitment to excellence, positive health, productivity, and a zest for living. Much like Maslow's self-actualizing person, individuals who strive for wellness have an exceptional openness to experience. Rather than fear new experiences and different ideas, they welcome them as a way to grow. They do not allow prejudices or stereotypes to distort their perceptions. They are autonomous in thought and action. They take control of life and face it with creativity and freshness. Living a wellness lifestyle has good potential for increasing longevity. However, this is not the sole purpose of wellness living. Wellness advocate Donald Ardell agrees. He states, "Wellness is not a goal to be attained but a process to be maintained."[12] Wellness is a fun, satisfying existence! Figure 1.2 shows a wellness/illness continuum. In which direction are you traveling?

FIGURE 1.2 ➤
Wellness/illness continuum. In
which direction are you traveling?

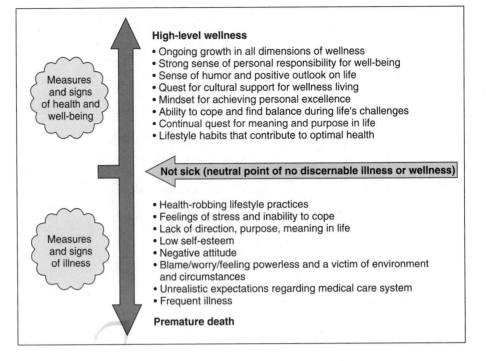

The following are listed in the figure:

High-level wellness
- Ongoing growth in all dimensions of wellness
- Strong sense of personal responsibility for well-being
- Sense of humor and positive outlook on life
- Quest for cultural support for wellness living
- Mindset for achieving personal excellence
- Ability to cope and find balance during life's challenges
- Continual quest for meaning and purpose in life
- Lifestyle habits that contribute to optimal health

Measures and signs of health and well-being

Not sick (neutral point of no discernable illness or wellness)

- Health-robbing lifestyle practices
- Feelings of stress and inability to cope
- Lack of direction, purpose, meaning in life
- Low self-esteem
- Negative attitude
- Blame/worry/feeling powerless and a victim of environment and circumstances
- Unrealistic expectations regarding medical care system
- Frequent illness

Premature death

Measures and signs of illness

The Dimensions of Wellness

The wellness lifestyle is a coordinated and integrated living pattern involving seven dimensions: physical, intellectual, emotional, social, spiritual, environmental, and occupational. There is a strong interdependence between dimensions, even though they function separately. For example, joining an exercise class in your community most notably enhances your physical well-being. But it can also be socially enriching and intellectually stimulating as you learn more about the functional capacity of the human body. It can also help relieve emotional stress. Attending the class with coworkers after work may improve your occupational wellness. In each dimension there is opportunity for personal growth, and, due to the dimensions' interrelationships, growth in one area often sparks interest in another. *Balancing* these dimensions, however, is an important factor in pursuing wellness. For example, being an avid reader yet not being able to get along with anyone is not an example of balanced wellness.

Physical Dimension

The **physical dimension** deals with the functional operation of the body. Ask yourself if your body is the best machine possible. The physical dimension involves the health-related components of physical fitness—muscular strength, muscular endurance, cardiorespiratory endurance, flexibility, and body composition. Dietary habits have a significant effect on physical well-being. Your sexual, drinking, and drug behaviors also play a role in physical health. Do you smoke? Do you get an adequate amount of sleep? Do you catch many colds? These questions deal with physical health.

The physical dimension also includes medical self-care—regular self-tests, checkups, proper use of medications, taking necessary steps when you are ill, and appropriate use of the medical system. Managing your environment also affects physical well-being. For example, do you try to minimize your exposure to tobacco smoke and harmful pollutants? Obviously, positive health habits are critical to physical well-being.

Intellectual Dimension

The **intellectual dimension** involves the use of your mind. Maintaining an active mind contributes to total well-being. Intellectual growth is not restricted to formal education—that is, school learning. It involves a continuous acquisition of knowledge throughout life, engaging your mind in creative and stimulating mental activities. Curiosity and learning should never stop. Reading, writing, and keeping abreast of cur-

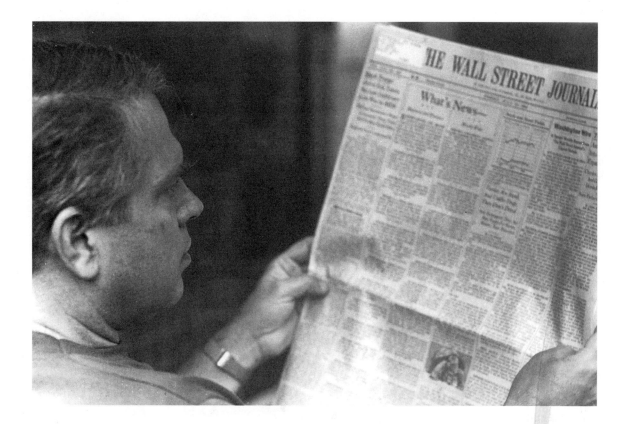

Learning should continue throughout life.

rent events are intellectual pursuits. Being able to think critically and analyze, evaluate, and apply knowledge are also associated with this dimension. The link between intellectual stimulation and healthy living is undeniable.

Emotional Dimension

Having a positive mental state is directly linked to wellness. Emotional wellness includes three areas: awareness, acceptance, and management. Emotional awareness involves recognizing your own feelings, as well as the feelings of others. Emotional acceptance means understanding the normality of human emotion, in addition to realistically assessing your own personal abilities and limitations. Emotional management is the ability to control or cope with personal feelings and knowing how to seek interpersonal support when necessary. The ability to maintain emotional stability at some mid-range between the highs and the lows is essential. The abilities to laugh, to enjoy life, to adjust to change, to cope with stress, and to maintain intimate relationships are examples of the **emotional dimension** of wellness.

Social Dimension

Everyone, with the possible exception of a hermit, must interact with people. Social wellness involves the ability to get along with others, as well as to appreciate the uniqueness of others. It means exhibiting concern for the welfare of your community and fairness and justice toward others. The **social dimension** of wellness also includes concern for humanity as a whole. You have achieved social wellness when you feel a genuine sense of belonging to a large social unit. Good friends, close family ties, community involvement, and trusting relationships go hand in hand with high-level wellness. Whereas feelings of isolation and loneliness are linked to ill health, feeling "connected" to a person, group, cause, or even a pet is a health strengthener.

Spiritual Dimension

Spiritual wellness is not always synonymous with religion. The **spiritual dimension** may not identify a creator, a god, or a theology. Instead, it involves the development of the inner self and one's soul. Spiritual wellness involves experiencing life and reflecting on that experience in order to discover a personal meaning and purpose in life. Why am I here? What path will lead to fulfillment in my life? What is life about? These questions are most often answered within the context of a larger reality beyond the physical and material aspects of existence. Selflessness, compassion, honesty, and the development of a clear, comfortable sense of right and wrong are components of spiritual wellness.

There is a strong connection between spirituality and self-esteem because of the internal feelings of self-worth that occur when a sense of hope, optimism, and morality are developed. Attempts to achieve long-term self-esteem by external constructs of power, socioeconomic status, or physical appearance fail.[13] Like all dimensions of wellness, spirituality does not "happen." It is a process of growth requiring time and attention.

Environmental Dimension

The **environmental dimension** of wellness deals with the preservation of natural resources and the protection of plant and animal wildlife. We all have basic biological needs that include adequate air, water, and food. Our dependence on the automobile, as well as the general industrialization of our world, have created worldwide pollution and changes in the atmosphere. Habits such as recycling, limiting the use of pesticides, carpooling, and conserving electricity show positive involvement in the environmental dimension of wellness. Demonstrating a commitment to the protection of wildlife and plants is also a component of environmental wellness. We must *all* take part and encourage others to do the same for the benefit of future generations.

Occupational Dimension

The **occupational dimension** involves deriving personal satisfaction from your vocation. Much of your life will be spent at work. Therefore, it is important that your chosen career provide the internal and external rewards you value. Do you want a job that allows for creativity, interaction with others, daily challenge, autonomy? Do you prefer opportunities for advancement, personal entrepreneurship, leadership, or helping others? How do you feel about mobility? Is salary your major motivation? Answering these questions may help you with career selection. Occupational wellness also involves maintaining a satisfying balance between work time and leisure time. It involves a work environment that minimizes stress and exposure to physical health hazards. A majority of your college life is spent analyzing and integrating your skills and interests with career choices. It is vital that your vocational choice be personally enriching and stimulating. If you are not happy with your occupation, you will find that your entire well-being suffers.

Wellness is a combination of all seven dimensions. It means striving for growth in each dimension, as well as appreciating the interconnectedness between all of them. Is there one dimension in which you are strongest? Which dimension is your weakest? Neglecting any dimension destroys the balance critical to high-level wellness. Certain dimensions may take on a greater importance at different times throughout your life. Nevertheless, striving for balance contributes to your wholeness. To evaluate your wellness in the seven dimensions, you are encouraged to take the wellness assessment in the activities section at the end of the book. Taking this assessment will also help you understand the broad array of choices within each dimension.

Growth in Wellness

We have described wellness as a dynamic course of action based on self-responsibility. The goal is to assume greater responsibility for your quality of life by making positive lifestyle decisions. How do you begin making positive lifestyle choices? How do you know the options available to you? How do you grow in wellness? As Figure 1.3 shows, growth in wellness is influenced by many factors. Since wellness living is an *active* process, understanding how each of the factors contributes to your growth in each dimension is important.

FIGURE 1.3 ➤
Factors affecting growth in
wellness. Growth in wellness is
influenced by many factors.

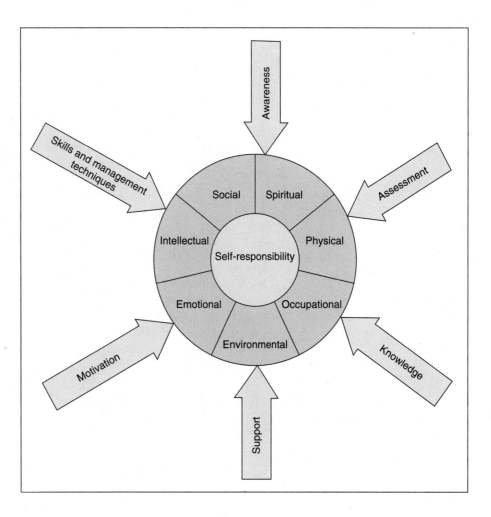

Awareness

Before you can grow in wellness you must have an awareness of the wellness option. It is an exciting alternative! This chapter differentiates between the state of wellness and "treatment" health. You are now aware that your health, happiness, and quality of life are strongly affected by your willingness to make wellness choices. The increasing general interest in wellness has made it easier for an individual to adopt a wellness lifestyle, because wellness choices now are not only available, but valued.

Assessment

Once you are aware of the wellness option, you should assess your lifestyle. Assessment allows you to see how you are presently conducting your life and identify where changes should occur. An assessment can be anything from medical tests (blood lipid profile, blood pressure, etc.) to physical fitness tests. They can be stress inventories, health risk appraisals, dietary logs, or even attitude questionnaires. Even personality assessments can help you understand your social and professional relationships. Assessment offers an opportunity to begin the process of self-observation as you confront a wellness issue.

Knowledge

Having knowledge in the lifestyle areas helps you make decisions. For example, suppose from an assessment you learn what your blood cholesterol level is. First of all, what level constitutes a high blood cholesterol? What does this mean? How do you go about reducing the fat in your diet? Knowledge can help you to understand your risk and can guide you in accomplishing your goal.

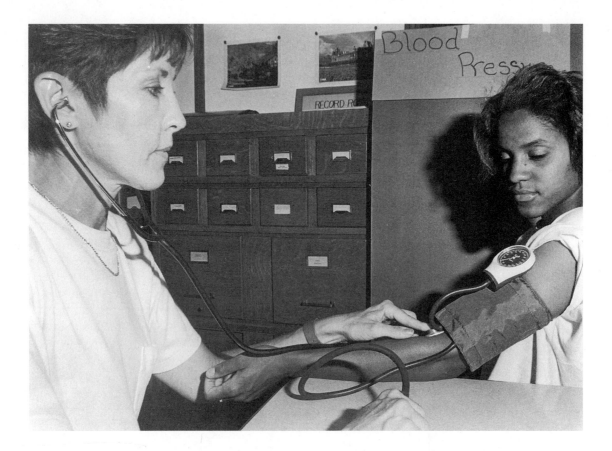

Having your blood pressure checked is an example of a wellness assessment.

Skills and Management Techniques

Skills and management techniques help you try some of the options. Skills in goal setting, behavior modification, and personal strategy building enable you to make the necessary lifestyle changes. How do I go about managing stress? Eating nutritiously in the residence hall or on a budget? Fitting regular exercise into my busy schedule? Skills and management techniques help you incorporate strategies of self-change into your life so that daily lifestyle choices are habitually "wellness choices." Realize that it takes time and practice to develop these skills into lifetime habits.

Motivation

Motivation is a powerful force in the wellness lifestyle. Motivation gets you started and keeps you going as you strive for continued wellness growth. Motivation is personal and complex. It changes throughout life and is specific to each person. At age 19 you may want to lose weight to look better. The 65-year-old may want to lose weight to help reduce high blood pressure.

Human behavior is purposeful and goal directed. External forces, including extrinsic rewards such as certificates, trophies, recognition, and T-shirts often stimulate one to action. However, intrinsic or internal motivation is more sustaining. Feelings of satisfaction, accomplishment, and enjoyment are the factors that motivate us to *persist* in the attainment of our goals.

A powerful factor affecting motivation is how much you value what it is you wish to change. We usually value things we believe make life worth living or satisfying. Whether the goal is to lose weight, to manage stress, or to get along better with your parents, a variety of complex factors affect your ability to sustain motivation.

Support

Maintaining positive lifestyle choices is best achieved when there is support and encouragement from the organizations and environments surrounding you. For example, suppose during one of your vacations you attend a smoking cessation class and quit smoking. You are starting your climb toward permanent behavior change. If you face returning to a roommate who smokes or to a workplace where coworkers smoke, your chances of maintaining your new behavior are considerably lower. Your family, friends, and group affiliations have a strong influence on your behavior. In fact, it has been found that there are significant correlations among self-esteem, social support, and a healthy lifestyle.[14] Choosing a living or working environment where others strive for wellness can assist you in wellness growth. Do you feel your roommates, friends, and family are supportive of wellness? How about your campus? Why or why not?

Self-Responsibility

At the center of wellness growth is self-responsibility. The goal is to assume greater responsibility for your quality of life by making positive lifestyle decisions. Understandably, for every decision to be made, there are alternatives and consequences. Your challenge is to make thoughtful decisions that direct you toward high-level wellness. It is a satisfying feeling to work toward being the best you can be. You know what you can and cannot control. Some circumstances are beyond your control. Part of self-responsibility is recognizing this and adjusting in order to continually strive toward full potential. Heredity is an example of something you cannot control. You had no voice in selecting your genetic tendencies. A physical disability is another uncontrollable life situation. Self-responsibility in wellness is making the best of the "hand you are dealt" regardless of your stage in life or your circumstances.

Self-responsibility in wellness means active involvement. It means understanding how choices affect the daily quality of your life, rather than looking at longevity as the primary payoff. The joy of wellness is the journey—the attempt to reach your potential in all seven dimensions. In a pure sense, the state of high-level wellness can never be reached. Everyone has setbacks or weaknesses. For you it could be a quick temper, chocolate chip cookies, or impatience with your younger brother. We sometimes let our lives become unbalanced. Having realistic expectations, a sense of personal accountability, and a sense of humor will help you see wellness living as a joyful experience. Self-responsibility involves self-control as opposed to going along with the crowd or merely reacting to what seems to happen. Just because everyone else is eating a triple order of french fries does not mean you must. When everyone else is grumbling about the weather, why not find something positive about it? Wellness is about personal empowerment—having a sense of ownership and control of the decision-making process.

As you make the decision to change your lifestyle, understand that such change does not need to be drastic. You are not doomed to a life without pleasure or to an existence full of rigid self-denial! It is not necessary that you jog 5 miles a day or become a vegetarian. On the contrary, the journey should be full of stimulation and satisfaction. It is exciting to realize that a few commonsense changes can make a big difference in the way you look and feel. With that in mind, how do you make lifestyle changes? To make any permanent behavior change, you need a distinct, systematic plan of action.

Self-Management

Even though there is evidence linking lifestyle abuse and lack of well-being, many still smoke cigarettes, drink excessive amounts of alcohol and caffeine, never exercise, burn out due to stress, eat vast amounts of high-fat foods, and refuse to fasten their seat belts. What a dilemma it is that "information does not equal prevention. . . . Information is necessary but not sufficient for creating meaningful change."[15] Traditional educational messages devised to arouse fear (antismoking brochures showing blackened lungs, seatbelt campaigns exhibiting crumpled cars, "this is your brain on drugs") have eliminated high risk behaviors in some people, but not in the majority of the population. Fear of a heart attack or cancer has not kept many Americans involved in ongoing programs of

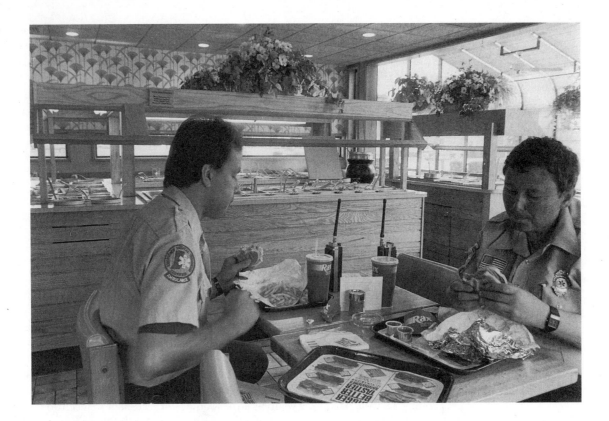

Do you make wise choices when eating out? Wise choices are a result of combining knowledge and behavioral skills.

exercise and dietary change. Even when the information is positive or inspirational, many still have difficulty making lifestyle behavior changes. What is missing in the link between knowledge and action is a systematic strategy called **self-management.**

More Than Willpower

Changing a behavior or breaking an unhealthy habit involves *learning new behavior.* Notice we used the word *learn.* Just as in learning anything else, you must understand and practice the basic principles and techniques of self-management. Many people are already excellent managers of their lives. They can study when they need to, exercise regularly, turn down an offer of chocolate creme pie, and refuse a beer at a party. These are powerful choices, choices that are linked to wellness. Do these people just have a lot of good old willpower? Is that what it takes? Willpower is an ambiguous entity. Others believe that merely *wanting* to change is enough. Certainly desire for change is important, but it has no strategy to follow through. The key to permanent change is having a plan. Self-management involves choosing goals and designing strategies to meet them. Self-management is actually a combination of specific skills and behaviors where *knowledge* and *action* are linked for the purpose of controlling behavior.

Self-Managed Behavior Change

Changing a behavior is a complex process. It has puzzled behavioral scientists for years how some people can successfully self-initiate and maintain major lifestyle changes (stop smoking, lose weight, conquer shyness, etc.), while others fail to even make moderate changes, even after participating in professional group programs (exercise groups, smoking cessation classes, low-fat cooking seminars, etc.). After studying this dilemma for many years, Prochaska, Norcross, and DiClemente[16] have revolutionized behavior-change theory by identifying nine major *processes* that, when integrated at appropriate stages of change, maximize the chances that the change will become permanent. These processes "are covert and overt activities and experiences that individuals engage in when they attempt to modify problem behaviors."[17] These processes and the behavior change techniques that they incorporate have been shown to be the *best* predictors of permanent lifestyle change.[18]

The nine processes (and example techniques) follow:[19]

1. *Consciousness-raising:* learning about the problem
   - asking, "Where is the fat in my diet?"
   - asking, "How many calories will I burn when I jog?"
   - investigating, "What actually triggers my angry outbursts?"
   - investigating, "What do I spend too much money on?"
   - asking, "What excuses am I using to rationalize not changing?"
2. *Social liberation:* incorporating new alternatives provided by the external environment
   - creating alternative atmospheres (community sponsored post-prom parties; no-smoking buildings, etc.)
   - using self-help groups
   - identifying advocacy groups
   - utilizing low-fat menu choices in restaurants and designated driver programs
   - empowering policy changes
3. *Emotional arousal:* experiencing emotions related to the problem
   - watching a dramatic movie pertaining to the situation or problem
   - using mental imagery to construct a scene (for example, imagining everyone alienating you because of your stubbornness)
   - blowing cigarette smoke into a handkerchief
   - utilizing mirrors (for weight loss)
4. *Self-reevaluation:* seeing how the problem behavior conflicts with personal values; balancing the pros and cons
   - asking, "Do I really want this beer?"
   - reflecting, "Is tanning really that important to me?"
   - analyzing, "Will being more assertive be threatening to my boyfriend?"
5. *Commitment:* accepting responsibility for changing and believing it can be done
   - publicly announcing your intentions
   - creating a plan of action and taking small steps
   - setting a specific date
6. *Reward:* rewarding one's self or receiving rewards from others for positive changes
   - utilizing self-talk ("way to go," "it feels good to be in control," "you can handle it")
   - making bets, pacts; using money, gifts
   - incorporating a step-by-step approach with reinforcements at each step
7. *Countering:* substituting alternative behaviors for problem behaviors
   - walking with your spouse rather than watching TV
   - practicing relaxation rather than arguing/retaliating
   - thinking positive, self-supporting thoughts
8. *Environment control:* restructuring the environment to reduce the temptation
   - removing ashtrays from the house
   - never shopping at the grocery when hungry
   - not buying high-fat foods
   - posting signs and reminders
   - planning ahead by visualizing your action when confronted with a temptation/trigger
9. *Helping relationships:* enlisting the help of someone who cares
   - discussing your plans with others
   - writing a contract with goals, countering techniques, and helpers' commitments
   - enlisting someone else to "buddy up" and change with you
   - utilizing support groups

After looking over these techniques you may say, "But I tried many of these techniques and *still* went back to my old habits!" The most dramatic implication of this behavior change research is "that efficient self-change depends on doing the right things

FIGURE 1.4 ➤

Five stages of change.

P. 54 from *Changing for Good* by
James Prochaska, John C. Norcross
and Carlo C. DiClemente. Copyright
© 1994 by James Prochaska, John
C. Norcross and Carlo C.
DiClemente. By permission of
William Morrow and Company, Inc.

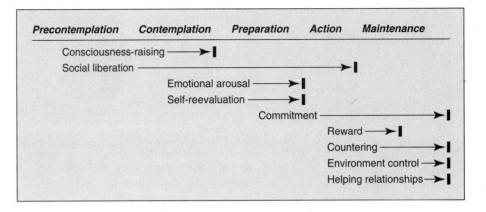

(processes) at the right time (stages)."[20] Prochaska, Norcross, and DiClemente identified five *specific* stages that occur in the process of permanently changing a behavior:[21]

1. *Precontemplation:* The individual resists changing a behavior, denies having a problem. ("I don't have a problem." "Smoking doesn't cause heart disease." "Obesity runs in the family.")
2. *Contemplation:* The individual acknowledges the problem and begins to think seriously about solving it but may not be quite ready. ("I know drinking is bad, and someday I'll quit." "Exercise would be good for me, but I don't want to do it.")
3. *Preparation:* The individual intends to take action and may even begin making some small behavioral changes/plans. ("Monday I start my diet." "I signed up for the parenting class." "I got a calendar to mark my spiritual-reading schedule.")
4. *Action:* The individual visibly begins taking action, requiring considerable commitment of time and energy (just doing it).
5. *Maintenance:* The individual stabilizes behavior change and works to prevent relapse (use of ongoing strategies, coping techniques).

In this way, the key to successful change is *knowing* what stage you are in and matching the change processes in order to maximize the problem-solving efforts. Figure 1.4 identifies the five stages of change and the nine processes that work best within each stage.

Many people join traditional action-oriented group programs designed to conquer smoking, achieve weight loss, control stress, initiate exercise, develop public speaking confidence, or practice self-assertiveness. The fact is that these programs often do not recognize that not everyone is in the "action stage." The result is often failure, guilt, or blame for the lack of willpower or motivation.

Making a Plan

One specific way to initiate a lifestyle change is to write a personal behavior-change contract or plan incorporating the processes for the change. Writing it out makes you think through your plan in its entirety, rather than letting things happen as they may. It specifies the *details* for carrying out your plan. Figure 1.5 shows a sample behavior-change contract. Remember: The changes you choose to make can pertain to any dimension of wellness—anything from improving study skills to losing weight to reducing stress to controlling anger. The most important outcomes of writing a contract are the self-evaluating and planning involved. Having a *plan* is what differentiates between successful change and a fleeting New Year's resolution. A blank contract is provided in the activities section at the end of the book for your use.

Identifying Your Goal

Being able to identify your goal is an important first step. Some make the mistake of selecting too broad a goal or trying to change too many things at once. There are a few key points to remember in goal identification:

FIGURE 1.5 ➤
Behavior change contract.

Behavior Change Contract

Name __Kate Christopher__
Date __February 10__

Goal: To keep my dietary fat grams under 50 per day

Motivation (What's in it for me?): Lose weight; feel less sluggish; protect my arteries; reduce future risk of cancer

Identify stage of change currently in:
____ Precontemplation ____ Contemplation __X__ Preparation
____ Action ____ Maintenance

Processes and techniques

1. Consciousness-raising
   —record the foods I typically eat and calculate the fat grams consumed
   —make a list of foods high in fat/low in fat
   —research the long-term health benefits of low-fat eating

2. Social liberation
   —take a low-fat cooking class
   —read the brochures provided in restaurants to see what foods are low in fat
   —investigate low-fat/no-fat alternative products at the grocery store

3. Emotional arousal
   —visualize my coronary arteries clogging
   —visit the hospital coronary care unit
   —watch a "beach movie"—all those thin people in bikinis!
   —think about my overweight uncle with a 320 cholesterol

4. Self-reevaluation
   —reflect on how eating fatty foods is not really that important to me—only a moment's pleasure!
   —I really want to be healthier and know this is what I need to do.

5. Commitment
   —keep a daily log of fat grams eaten
   —write out possible menus for a day
   —keep a chart of healthy food substitutes
   —when planning to eat out (or "pig out") watch the fat grams carefully early in the day, and during the previous day

6. Reward
   —$1.00 per day in a jar . . . eventually a new outfit
   —use self-talk

7. Countering
   —use low-fat substitutes (non-fat sour cream, salsa on potatoes, no-fat salad dressings)
   —eat bagels rather than donuts, etc.

8. Environment control
   —don't even buy junk food
   —take my own lunch to school
   —have veggies and low-fat foods ready in the refrigerator
   —post a sign in the kitchen with fat grams in a donut, cheese, potato chips, etc.

9. Helping relationships
   —discuss with nutrition professor
   —ask roommate to do this with me
   —tell Mom about my plan (prepare her for my summer eating)

1. *Prioritize your goals.* Do not attempt to change everything at once. You may fail if you try all at once to lose weight, stop smoking, get along better with your mother-in-law, and make the dean's list every semester. Start with only one goal.

2. *Make your goal realistic.* For example, if your goal is to lose 30 pounds in three weeks, study every Friday night, go to church every Sunday, jog 4 miles every day, never lose your temper, or make straight A's every semester, your plan is probably doomed!

3. *Specify the situation.* Goal identification is easier if you can specify the situation in which the behavior occurs. For example, instead of saying, "I eat too much," you might say, "I can't resist desserts." Or, instead of saying, "I'm self-centered," you might pinpoint, "I talk about myself too much." When you are identifying a goal, it is important to be truthful with yourself. It is not a time for denial: "But I'm not a big eater!" (spoken as you devour an entire sausage pizza!).

There are many ways to avoid temptations.

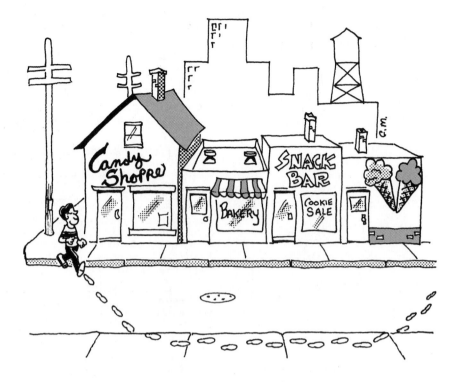

4. *Make your goal specific and measurable.* Not "lose some weight," but "lose 10 pounds in 16 weeks." Not "eat more nutritiously," but "eat four fruits/vegetables daily." Not "smoke less," but "cut down to three cigarettes per day." Not "get along with my roommate better," but "sincerely compliment my roommate in some way every day." Not "study more," but "study every Monday, Tuesday, and Wednesday, from 7:00 to 10:00 P.M. for the remainder of the semester." Self-management strategies are more effective when goals are stated in behavioral terms and quantified. Also, try to express your goals in positive terms. If a goal is to start doing something that you are not presently doing (for example, fastening your seat belt), state the goal in terms of what you want to do and in what situation you will do it.

Listing Motivations

Be able to truthfully answer the question, "What's in it for me?" List the reasons you want to change. Make a list of the pros and cons. Ask yourself how your life will be affected by your changed behavior. Changing behavior brings consequences to yourself and, most likely, others. (By quitting drinking I will have better health and less likelihood of suffering from an alcohol-related accident. However, I will lose some social friends and my "mood medication.") Honestly assessing the costs of changing will help you face yourself and your true motivations. This will help you anticipate the obstacles asked of you. To increase your motivation, you might talk to acquaintances who have successfully made the change you are attempting.

Preventing Relapse

In the first line of his best-selling book *The Road Less Traveled*, Dr. M. Scott Peck writes, "Life is difficult."[22] He further adds, "life is always difficult and is full of pain as well as joy."[23] Changing a habit takes *effort*; but the joy in the growth and self-empowerment is the wellness journey. In our society we have become accustomed to the quick fix: instant cash at the ATM machine, fast food, 24-hour shopping, FAX machines. Setbacks may occur when you are trying to change a behavior. In fact, they are quite common.[24] Instead of throwing in the towel, try to learn from these experiences. Maintaining your plan will require flexibility, particularly if the plan is not working properly, if unexpected obstacles arise, or if a support system is failing. Reevaluation is a necessary com-

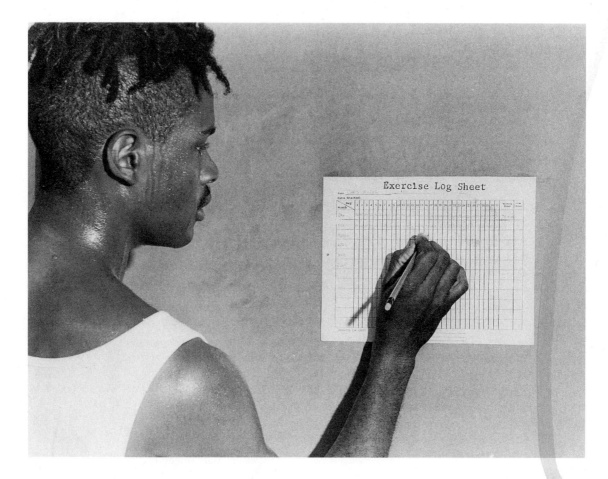

Keeping an exercise log helps you stick with your program.

ponent in making a permanent lifestyle change. The first line of defense against relapse is *planning*. If chocolate chip cookies are your downfall, don't buy any. (They'll just keep calling your name from the cupboard.) If you've tried and just can't get up 45 minutes earlier in the mornings to exercise, what about using your lunch hour? Take your walking shoes to work with you and invite a colleague to exercise with you. Plan so you'll succeed.

Remember that high-level wellness is a process involving growth and pursuit of a fuller life. The process of self-managing behavior means reassessing goals, monitoring behavior, reviewing strategies, learning from setbacks, and acknowledging the joy in the effort to be the best you can be. As you become the *cause* rather than the *effect* of actions, your confidence and self-esteem are enhanced. Emphasize the positive. Value your successes and your worth as a human being. Most of us do not realize that the majority of our supportive messages come from our own internal thought processes rather than from external sources. We carry on continual dialogue with ourselves each day.[25] Called *self-talk*, our inner voice can be a positive source of motivation. Self-talk that encourages us and reminds us of our achievements helps increase our self-esteem. Self-talk can also be negative, and, as a result, a source of discouragement. Suppose your goal is to become less verbally critical of your mother. For ten days you successfully avoid any confrontation. On the eleventh day, while riding with her in a car, you find yourself sharply criticizing her driving. An example of the resulting negative self-talk would be, "I am so awful. I have failed miserably in my goal. This just proves again what a rotten daughter I am." In contrast, a positive self-talk statement would be, "I didn't handle this situation very well. What can I learn from this so I'll do better next time?"

As you travel this wellness path, you will probably become more aware of how society can help and hinder your trip. One challenge we all face in attempting to pursue a wellness lifestyle is societal norms.

table 1.2

SOCIETAL NORMS THAT PROMOTE "UNWELLNESS"

- The idea that everyone must be extremely thin (especially women)
- The assumption that alcohol abuse is an acceptable rite of passage into college
- The media's portrayal of sex as being glamorous, without commitment or consequences
- Social events, parties, celebrations where alcohol and food abuse is expected (New Year's Eve, wedding receptions, Super Bowl parties, etc.)
- The number of high-sugar and high-fat gifts associated with holidays such as Halloween, Easter, Christmas, and Valentine's Day
- The habit of driving a car to go very short distances
- Equating tanned skin with beauty, wealth, power, and sex appeal (thus, the emergence of thousands of tanning salons)
- Convenient placement of ashtrays on restaurant tables
- Miles and miles of roads built *without* sidewalks
- The elimination of daily physical education in the schools coupled with the parental push for private sports lessons and competitive Little League football, baseball, soccer, etc. (often servicing only the best athletes and emphasizing "winning" rather than lifetime participation)
- Access to television 24 hours a day, with a choice of 100 cable stations—all changed by remote control
- Meals built around a red meat entree
- The notion that as you grow older it is okay to be inactive and fat

Societal Norms

We are constantly bombarded by subtle yet extremely powerful messages that are often obstacles to wellness. Our behavioral choices are strongly affected by unwritten codes that permeate our daily lives and can actually contradict and sabotage a wellness lifestyle. **Societal norms** are those behaviors or practices that are expected in a culture and that are accepted and supported by its members.

These unwritten rules are carried on from generation to generation. Table 1.2 lists circumstances and norms you have probably grown up with. As you look at them, consider the messages they give. Do they promote wellness as you know it? You can probably think of more examples than those listed. Why is it considered inappropriate for a woman to reapply her makeup after dinner at a restaurant table but acceptable for her to pull a cigarette from her purse, light it, inhale, and then blow carcinogens into the air?

Many of our norms encourage a sedentary lifestyle. Somehow we've absorbed the notion that minimal exertion is better. Heaven forbid if, when operating your car, you have to roll down your own windows, walk around the car to unlock the doors, or keep constant pressure on the accelerator while driving on the interstate. You can go to the bank, a fast food restaurant, a dry cleaners, and a milk store without ever leaving the comfort of your car. What kind of message is this sending?

The advertising industry is especially effective at mesmerizing us with messages. After all, we are told, "It's doctor recommended." We see former athletes guzzling beer that is "less filling." Every Saturday morning high-sugar snacks that are fun to eat and that "your mother trusts" are displayed on television. If the thin, attractive models on billboards enjoy smoking, perhaps you will, too.

In traveling the road to optimum well-being, be aware of these pitfalls and obstacles present in our society. Remember, it is you who will make the daily choices as to how to live your life. Self-responsibility is the key.

Are these messages in your best interest?

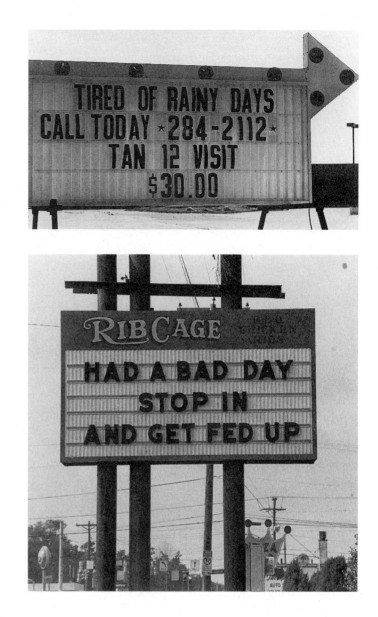

Changing Times: Making Wellness the Norm

Now that the wellness concept has begun to invade the health-care profession and society as a whole, we can see some norms already changing. Fifteen years ago the only people jogging were athletes in training or fitness "nuts." Now no one takes a second look even at senior citizens trudging along roads. Businesspeople pack their workout gear next to their business reports. Hotels hand out jogging maps to guests. Stress management, parenting, addictive behavior management, smoking cessation, and a multitude of other wellness topics are offered in community classes and workshops. As wellness permeates our society, there are more and more resources that support this lifestyle. There are positive choices available in grocery stores—more whole wheat breads and cereals, low-sugar and low-salt products, low-fat dairy items, even take-out salad and fruit bars. Restaurants are also responding to the consumer demand for more nutritious food selections. These are just a few of the positive changes that reflect wellness awareness. Only by drawing together all available resources (individual, community, media, school, corporate, government) will we fix current health problems. This multilevel approach is necessary to bring about changes in societal norms.

Beyond the physical, health-related factors of wellness, it is important to change people's attitudes. It should not be considered bizarre for people to arrive at work or at a class full of enthusiasm rather than full of complaints. It is also not weird to take a few moments to stretch or close your eyes to relax during the day, congratulate another person for doing well on an exam, adhere to the speed limit, have a fruit juice rather than a beer at a party, give someone a hug, or have fun in life. These are behaviors that reflect wellness and are brought about by awareness, education, and growth in wellness.

As we know, not everyone has responded to this trend of positive lifestyle choices. It will take time. You can do your part by encouraging those around you to make wellness a lifetime pursuit. Pass these attitudes and behaviors on to your children. Help continue to make wellness and self-responsibility society's norm.

SUMMARY

Many adults in the United States die prematurely from diseases that are primarily a result of lifestyle abuse. Health promoters stress the importance of healthy behaviors in deterring the ravaging effects of these "diseases of choice." With the cost of health care increasing so rapidly, *Healthy People 2000* was published by the federal government in an effort to spark a national commitment to self-responsibility for well-being and acknowledge the need for support systems to help those pursuing wellness lifestyles. Whereas health is often viewed as a neutral state of nonsickness, high-level wellness is a dynamic level of functioning that is oriented toward maximizing potential. It is an integrated living pattern involving seven dimensions—physical, intellectual, emotional, social, spiritual, environmental, and occupational. It is a lifelong journey that involves a conscientious effort to reach full potential. The cornerstone of wellness living is self-responsibility. Wellness growth involves a multifaceted approach of awareness, assessment, motivation, knowledge, support, and self-management skills. It includes intelligent deciphering of societal norms, recognizing your own power, making choices, interpreting risks, and understanding personal limitations.

Self-management is the use of a conscious, systematic plan for making a permanent change in behavior. To successfully change a behavior takes more than mere willpower. Permanent behavior change involves passing through five distinct transitional stages, while utilizing problem-solving processes and techniques within each stage. Even though setbacks may occur, a mind-set of commitment and self-empowerment can help continue the wellness journey.

The objective of wellness is a richer, satisfying life. Wellness is an attitude, not an end in itself. Our time on this earth is too short to be drawn toward complacency and futility. In their book *Changing for Good*, Prochaska, Norcross, and DiClemente state, "Our fullest freedom emerges when we have the opportunity to choose that which would enhance our life, our sense of self, and our society."[26] We should all consider and absorb the wisdom of W. Mitchell, mayor of Crested Butte, Colorado, who, though paralyzed from an airplane crash, maintains an active schedule. He writes, "The way I look at it, before I was paralyzed, there were ten thousand things I could do; ten thousand things I was capable of doing. Now there are nine thousand. I can dwell on the one thousand, or concentrate on the nine thousand I have left. And, of course, the joke is that none of us in our lifetime is going to do more than two or three thousand of these things in any event."[27]

REFERENCES

1. Sullivan, Louis W., M.D. "Creating a National Culture of Character: Personal Responsibility and Public Health." *Vital Speeches* 57 (January 15, 1991): 202–5.
2. Pelletier, Kenneth R. *Sound Mind, Sound Body: A New Model for Lifelong Health.* New York: Simon and Schuster, 1994.
3. O'Donnell, Michael P. "Definition of Health Promotion: Part III: Expanding the Definition." *American Journal of Health Promotion* 3 (winter 1989): 5.
4. Vickery, Donald M., M.D. "Medical Self-Care: A Review of the Concept and Program Models." *American Journal of Health Promotion* 1 (summer 1986): 23–28.
5. Department of Health and Human Services, Public Health Service.

Healthy People 2000: National Health Promotion and Disease Prevention Objectives. Washington, D.C.: Department of Health and Human Services, 1990.

6. *Healthy People 2000.*
7. Sullivan, Louis W., M.D. "Sounding Board: Healthy People 2000." *The New England Journal of Medicine* 323 (October 11, 1990): 1065–67.
8. Pelletier. *Sound Mind, Sound Body.*
9. Hettler, Bill, M.D. "Presenting the Wellness Concept to the Uninitiated." *Wellness Promotion Strategies.* Selected Proceedings of the Eighth Annual National Wellness Conference, Joseph P. Opatz, ed. Dubuque, Iowa: Kendall/Hunt Publishing Co., 1984, 28–38.
10. Dunn, Halbert L. "High-Level Wellness for Man and Society." *American Journal of Public Health* 49 (June 1959): 786–92.
11. Dossey, Barbara Montgomery, Lynn Keegan, Leslie Gooding Kolkmeier,

and Cathie E. Guzzetta. *Holistic Health Promotion: A Guide for Practice.* Rockville, Md.: Aspen Publishers, Inc.

12. Ardell, Donald B. "Definition of Wellness." *Ardell Wellness Report* 37 (winter 1995): 1.
13. Hawks, Steven. "Spiritual Health: Definition and Theory." *Wellness Perspectives: Research, Theory, and Practice* 10 (summer 1994): 3–13.
14. Bishop, George D. *Health Psychology: Integrating Mind and Body.* Boston: Allyn and Bacon, 1994.
15. Atkin, Charles, and Lawrence Wallack, eds. *Mass Communication and Public Health.* Newbury Park, Calif.: Sage Publications, 1990.
16. Prochaska, James O., John C. Norcross, and Carlo C. DiClemente. *Changing for Good.* New York: William Morrow and Co., 1994.
17. Prochaska, James O., Carlo C. DiClemente, and John C. Norcross.

"In Search of How People Change." *American Psychologist* 47 (September 1992): 1102–14.

18. Prochaska et al. "In Search of How People Change."
19. Prochaska et al. *Changing for Good.*
20. Prochaska et al. "In Search of How People Change."
21. Prochaska et al. *Changing for Good.*
22. Peck, M. Scott, M.D. *The Road Less Traveled.* New York: Simon and Schuster, 1978.
23. Peck. *The Road Less Traveled.*
24. Prochaska et al. "In Search of How People Change."
25. Brammer, Lawrence M. *How to Cope with Life Transitions: The Challenge of Personal Change.* New York: Hemisphere Publishing Corporation, 1991.
26. Prochaska et al. *Changing for Good.*
27. Corbet, Barry. *Options: Spinal Cord Injury and the Future.* Denver: A. B. Hirschfeld Press, 1980.

SUGGESTED READINGS

Ardell, Donald B. *Die Healthy: 16 Steps to a Wellness Lifestyle.* Western Australia: Wellness Australia, 1989.

Ardell, Donald B. *The History and Future of Wellness.* Dubuque, Iowa: Kendall/ Hunt Publishing Co., 1985.

Ardell, Donald B., and John G. Langdon, M.D. *Wellness: The Body Mind and Spirit.* Dubuque, Iowa: Kendall/Hunt Publishing Co., 1989.

Beasley, Joseph D., M.D. *The Betrayal of Health: The Impact of Nutrition, Environment, and Life-style on Illness in America.* New York: Times Books, 1991.

Bellingham, Richard, Barry Cohen, Todd James, and Leroy Spaniol. "Connectedness: Some Skills for Spiritual Health." *American Journal of Health Promotion* 1 (September/October 1989): 18–24, 31.

Bishop, George D. *Health Psychology: Integrating Mind and Body.* Boston: Allyn and Bacon, 1994.

Brammer, Lawrence M. *How to Cope with Life Transitions: The Challenge of Personal Change.* New York: Hemisphere Publishing Corporation, 1991.

Brehm, Barbara A. *Essays on Wellness.* New York: HarperCollins College Publishers, 1993.

Brownell, Kelly D., G. Alan Marlatt, Edward Lichtenstein, and G. Terence Wilson. "Understanding and Preventing Relapse." *American Psychologist* 41 (July 1986): 765–82

Dawber, Thomas Royle. *The Framingham Study: The Epidemiology of Atherosclerotic Disease.* Cambridge, Mass.: Harvard University Press, 1980.

Department of Health and Human Services, Public Health Service. *Healthy People 2000: National Health Promotion and Disease Prevention Objectives.* Washington, D.C.: Department of Health and Human Services, 1990.

Depken, Diane. "Wellness Through the Lens of Gender: A Paradigm Shift." *Wellness Perspectives: Research, Theory and Practice* 10 (winter 1994): 54–69.

Friedman, Myles I., and George H. Lackey, Jr., *The Psychology of Human Control: A General Theory of Purposeful Behavior.* New York: Praeger Publishers, 1991.

Glanz, Karen, Francis Marcus Lewis, and Barbara K. Riner, eds. *Health Behavior and Health Education.* San Francisco: Jossey-Bass Publishers, 1990.

Green, Judith, and Robert Shellenberger. *The Dynamics of Health and Wellness: A Biopsychosocial Approach.* Fort Worth, Tex.: Holt, Rinehart and Winston, Inc., 1991.

Harris, Jeffrey E. *Deadly Choices: Coping with Health Risks in Everyday Life.* New York: Basic Books, 1993.

Kabat-Zinn, Jon. *Full Catastrophe Living.* New York: Delta Books, 1990.

O'Brien, Justin. *The Wellness Tree: The Dynamic Six-Step Program for Rejuvenating Health and Creating Optimal Wellness.* St. Paul, Minn.: Yes International, 1993.

Pelletier, Kenneth R. *Sound Mind, Sound Body: A New Model for Lifelong Health.* New York: Simon and Schuster, 1994.

Prochaska, James O. "Strong and Weak Principles for Progressing from Precontemplation to Action on the Basis of Twelve Problem Behaviors." *Health Psychology* 13 (January 1994): 47–51.

Prochaska, James O., John C. Norcross, and Carlo C. DiClemente. *Changing for Good*. New York: William Morrow and Co., 1994.

Rosenfield, Mark S. *Wellness and Lifestyle Renewal: A Manual for Personal Change*. Rockville, Md.: American Occupational Therapy Association, 1993.

Ryan, Regina Sara, and John W. Travis. *Wellness: Small Changes You Use to Make a Big Difference*. Berkeley, Calif.: Ten Speed Press, 1991.

Shumaker, Sally A., Eleanor B. Schron, and Judith K. Ockene, eds. *The Handbook of Health Behavior Change*. New York: Springer, 1990.

Travis, John W., and Regina Sara Ryan. *The Wellness Workbook*, 2d ed. Berkeley, Calif.: Ten Speed Press, 1988.

University of California, Berkeley. *The Wellness Encyclopedia: The Comprehensive Resource to Safeguarding Health and Preventing Illness*. Boston: Houghton Mifflin Co., 1990.

Vierck, Elizabeth. *Health Smart: Your Personal Plan to Living Longer and Healthier*. Englewood Cliffs, N.J.: Prentice-Hall, 1995.

chapter 2

Physical Fitness

➤ Objectives

After reading this chapter, you will be able to:

1. Define *physical fitness*.
2. Identify and define the five health-related fitness components.
3. Identify five benefits of fitness.
4. Define and apply the FITT prescription factors for developing cardiorespiratory endurance.
5. Calculate training heart rate using the Karvonen formula.
6. Explain how to use the Rate of Perceived Exertion scale.
7. Identify the amount of time necessary for the results of a fitness program to become apparent.
8. Describe the purpose, content, and time of the three parts of a workout.
9. Define and correctly apply the principle of overload.
10. Define the principle of specificity.
11. Discriminate between aerobic and anaerobic exercise.
12. Define *cross training*.
13. Describe the ACSM/CDC recommendations for the amounts and types of physical activity that are needed for maintenance and promotion of health.
14. Explain the different quality and quantity requirements of exercising for maintenance and promotion of health and of exercising for cardiorespiratory endurance fitness.

Terms

- Aerobic
- Anaerobic
- Atrophy
- Ballistic stretching
- Body composition
- Cardiorespiratory endurance (CRE)
- Conditioning bout
- Cool-down
- Cross training

- FITT prescription factors
- Flexibility
- Hypertrophy
- Hypokinetic disease
- Karvonen equation
- Maximal heart rate (Max.HR)
- Maximal oxygen uptake (max VO_2)
- Muscular endurance
- Muscular strength

- Physical fitness
- Principle of overload
- Principle of specificity
- Rate of perceived exertion (RPE)
- Static stretching
- Target heart rate range (THR)
- Task specific activity
- Three-segment workout
- Training effect
- Warm-up

Those who think they have no time for bodily exercise will sooner or later have to find time for illness.

Edward Stanley, *The Conduct of Life*

to live a wellness lifestyle, you must be physically active. As you will learn later in this chapter, even moderate levels of activity produce improvements in health and well-being. Physical fitness, though, requires a higher level of activity and produces life-enhancing benefits at an accelerated rate. You will discover in this chapter, that there are differences among exercising for performance, as in athletics or running a 26.2–mile marathon; exercising for health; and exercising for fitness. Physical fitness is possibly the most important spoke in the wellness wheel. It is the foundation upon which the other wellness spokes are developed. Remember, also, that the mind and body are a whole; they cannot be separated to act independently. What affects one, ultimately affects the other. Unless the body is in good physical condition, the mind, in addition to other aspects of wellness, cannot function at optimal level. This is not to say that physical fitness is the only answer to living well in a complex world, but it is certainly a major step in the right direction.

So, you want to become more physically fit. How do you begin? This chapter will provide all the information you need to begin a fitness program—one you can live with.

Importance of Exercise

Human beings were designed for physical activity. The sedentary lifestyle produced by most occupations does not provide adequate physical labor. The homemaker, secretary, teacher, salesperson, and attorney have hectic, stressful lives but they fail to engage in the vigorous activity needed to be physically fit. Regular physical activity is a positive health habit and is vital to the overall wellness of the individual. We must learn to make intelligent decisions about lifetime health and physical fitness that include planning for daily vigorous exercise.

The decrease in the amount of physical labor required for survival has not reduced the body's need for physical activity. On the contrary, it has increased the need to obtain it from other sources. Yet, Americans desperately lack adequate physical fitness and suffer from lifestyle diseases called **hypokinetic diseases.** These conditions, caused by underactivity, include coronary heart disease, cancer, osteoporosis, diabetes, and obesity. Approximately 250,000 premature deaths every year in the United States can be attributed to lack of exercise.[1] According to Dr. Steven Blair, epidemiologist for the Cooper Institute for Aerobics Research, a sedentary lifestyle is as much a risk factor for disease as is high blood pressure, obesity, and smoking.[2] The college student shows early symptoms of hypokinetic disease through low levels of energy and creeping obesity. Can you relate to any of these warning signs? It is known that you reach the peak of your natural fitness during the late teens to early twenties and, unless you maintain physical activity, the body deteriorates and ages even more quickly.

Alarming headlines such as "Americans are fatter than ever," "The number of expanding Americans is expanding," and "Are Americans the fattest people in the world?" are cause for concern. Apparently, American waistlines are growing. In the last ten years, American adults have shown an average weight gain of nearly eight pounds per person.[3] Some studies show that a third of Americans are overweight.[4] What is the cause of this national problem? Experts place the blame on too many calories consumed and, more significantly, on not enough calories expended in exercise. The situation is compounded by the number of energy-saving devices Americans use—and the list grows yearly (electric garage door openers, TV remotes, computers, riding lawn mowers, electric car windows, snowblowers, leaf blowers). The amount of energy the average American expended even a decade ago is enormous compared to what we expend today.

Even more appalling, ongoing research shows there is a youth fitness crisis. Our nation's children have increased risk of heart disease—too much body fat, elevated blood pressure, high cholesterol, and poor fitness—caused by lack of exercise. Several

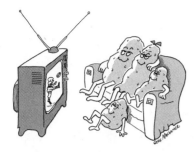

We have become a nation of spectators.

studies have shown that a full third of our nation's youth are not physically active enough for aerobic benefit.[5,6] They also weigh more and have more body fat than twenty years ago.[7,8] Although some experts disagree, the implication is that our children are going soft.[9,10] If things don't change, our nation's most precious asset, the adults of tomorrow, will likely contribute to future heart disease and cancer statistics. U.S. parents are surprised, and often apathetic, about the state of our children's health. We have become a nation accustomed to olympic dominance, professional sports superiority, and college athletic prominence. Other studies indicate that current school programs do little to promote lifetime fitness. To make matters worse, many physical education programs face elimination because they are considered a "frill" when educational budgets are crunched. Youngsters are losing the use of their arms and legs, for little opportunity exists today for running, throwing, and climbing. Playtime, nowadays, consists of low exercise activities such as video games or sports lessons, where standing, sitting, or listening consumes the major portion of the time. This type of play does not promote fitness since it does not involve regular participation in vigorous heart-stimulating activities. Children *and* adults must "get off their duffs" and start moving. The old saying—"Use it or lose it"—has never been more true.

What Is Physical Fitness?

While there is no universally accepted definition, most experts in the field of exercise would agree that **physical fitness** is the capacity of the heart, lungs, blood vessels, and muscles to function at optimal efficiency. The fit individual is able to complete the normal routine for the day and still have ample reserve energy to meet the other demands of daily life—recreational sports, rewarding relationships, and other leisure activities. Plus, the fit have adequate energy to handle life's emergency or crisis situations whenever they arise.

Physical fitness is multifaceted and involves skill-related and health-related components. The *skill-related components* of fitness are speed, power, agility, balance, reaction time, and coordination. These are primarily important in achieving success in athletics and are not as crucial for the development of better health. The five *health-related components* of physical fitness are cardiorespiratory endurance, muscular strength, muscular endurance, flexibility, and body composition.

No single activity or sport develops all five health-related fitness components. For example, joggers develop high levels of cardiorespiratory endurance but often have low levels of flexibility and upper body strength. For this reason, cross training has become a popular conditioning method that emphasizes the development of balanced fitness. You can read more about cross training later in this chapter.

Cardiorespiratory Endurance

Probably the most important fitness component is **cardiorespiratory endurance (CRE)**. It is the ability to deliver essential nutrients, especially oxygen, to the working muscles of the body and to remove waste products during prolonged physical exertion. It involves the efficient functioning of the heart, blood vessels, and lungs. Cardiorespiratory endurance is often expressed in terms of your **maximal oxygen uptake (max VO$_2$)**, which is the greatest amount of oxygen that can be utilized by the body during intense exercise. Vigorous exercise improves the functioning of the cardiorespiratory system and is directly related to reduced coronary risk. The American Medical Association states that exercise is the most significant factor contributing to the health of the individual.[11] This does not imply that if you exercise you will not have a heart attack. Other genetic and lifestyle factors may be involved. The heart attack death of Jim Fixx, marathon runner and author of *The Complete Book of Running*, in 1984 at age 52, is a case in point. Before he wrote *The Complete Book of Running*, he weighed over 200 pounds, he smoked three packs of cigarettes a day, and his brother died at an early age from a heart attack. Even though Fixx changed his lifestyle, the accumulation of risk factors took its toll. If you smoke cigarettes, have high blood pressure, or other coronary risk factors, you may still be at risk of coronary accident even though you exercise.

It's more fun to be a participant than a spectator.

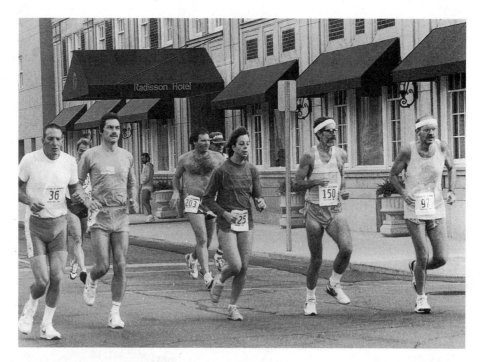

Muscular Strength and Muscular Endurance

Muscular strength is the ability of a muscle to exert one maximal force against resistance. It is characterized by activities of short duration at high intensity. Lifting a heavy object such as a suitcase or 100-pound weight one time are examples. **Muscular endurance** is the ability of the muscle to exert a submaximal force against resistance repeatedly or to sustain muscular contraction continuously over time. It is characterized by activities of long duration but low intensity. Examples of muscular endurance are performing repetitions of push-ups, sit-ups, or chin-ups. Strength and endurance are essential in everyday activities such as housework, yard work, and recreational sports.

Increase in muscle size is called **hypertrophy** and is due to an enlargement of the existing muscle fibers (the actual number of fibers, an inherited characteristic, does not increase). Muscles hypertrophy when exercised and they look firm and toned. Because females have lower levels of the male hormone (testosterone), their muscles do not become as bulky as the muscles of males. **Atrophy** is the opposite condition, when muscle size and strength have diminished through lack of use (when an arm or leg is immobilized in a cast, when you have not worked out for a couple of years). Muscular strength and endurance tend to decline with age. This loss can be delayed and strength can be maintained by participating in a strength program. Many people have joined health clubs and are enjoying the benefits of using weight equipment such as Universal, Nautilus, and Cybex. The result is a better physical appearance and greater efficiency in both everyday activities and sudden emergencies. For more information about muscular strength and endurance see Chapter 3.

Flexibility

Flexibility refers to the movement of a joint through a full range of motion. Flexibility is essential to smooth, efficient movement and may help prevent injuries to ligaments and joints. Being able to sit and touch your toes without bending your knees is an example of hamstring flexibility. You need arm and shoulder flexibility to scratch your back. Women usually have more joint flexibility than do men because men have bulkier skeletal muscles. Older adults may have trouble performing routine tasks such as getting in and out of an automobile, turning to watch traffic while driving, and fastening buttons or zippers at the back since flexibility diminishes with age. You can counter this loss by making stretching part of your lifetime exercise program. Chapter 3 has more information about flexibility.

Body Composition

Body composition refers to the amount of body fat in proportion to fat-free weight. The ratio between body fat and fat-free weight is a better gauge of fatness than is body weight. There are various ways to measure body composition (body mass index—see Chapter 10, skinfold calipers, bioelectrical impedance, hydrostatic underwater weighing technique), and all are superior to the height/weight chart method. For instance, a height/weight chart may label a 6-foot, 210-pound football player as overweight, when in reality he has only 10 percent body fat, as measured with skinfold calipers. On the other hand, someone who looks good in her size eight jeans may have 32 percent body fat. The best advice is to have your body composition analyzed by a professional. Obesity is not only unhealthy and uncomfortable, it is associated with increased risk for heart disease, diabetes, high blood pressure, and joint and lower back problems.

Physical Fitness and Wellness

Becoming physically fit is a positive health habit that has a major impact on your wellness. It is one area where you can assume control of your lifestyle. It is the golden thread that penetrates all the dimensions of wellness (Table 2.1 on page 30).

There now is strong scientific evidence linking fitness not only to better health but also to decreased medical costs and to improved job productivity. Do you want an edge on the future job market? Employers who must absorb medical care costs of their employees are fast realizing it costs less to keep an employee healthy than it does to treat workers once sick. Many employers are now looking to hire the "fit employee," one who has already adopted a wellness lifestyle. Decide now to be more than half-well. Climb up the wellness ladder to become more physically fit and exert greater control over your wellness destiny.

Everybody benefits from physical activity.

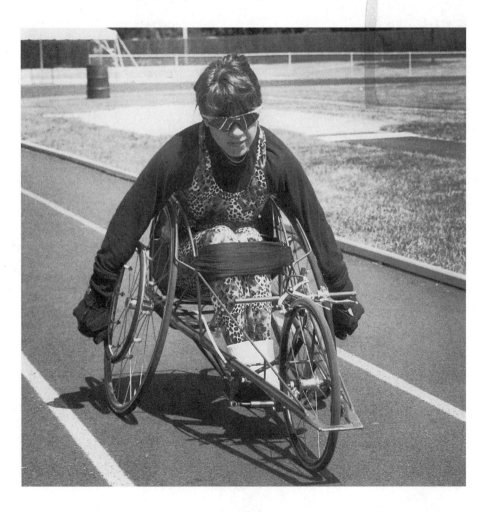

table 2.1

BENEFITS OF PHYSICAL FITNESS ON WELLNESS DIMENSIONS

Physical	Slows down the aging process; increases energy; improves posture and physical appearance; helps control weight; improves flexibility; improves muscular strength and endurance; strengthens bones, reducing osteoporosis; reduces risk for coronary heart disease.
Emotional	Relieves tension; aids in stress management; improves self-image; evens out emotional swings; provides time for adult play.
Social	Enhances relationships with family and friends; increases opportunity for social contacts.
Intellectual	Develops concepts of mind and body oneness; increases alertness; enhances concentration; motivates toward improved personal habits (smoking cessation, reducing drug and alcohol use, better nutrition); stimulates creative thoughts.
Occupational	Decreases absenteeism; increases productivity; decreases disability days; lowers medical care costs; lowers job turnover rate; increases networking possibilities.
Spiritual	Develops appreciation of body/mind connection; enhances appreciation for healthy environment; builds compassion for those less able.
Environmental	Develops appreciation for healthy air and water; increases concern for recycling and preservation of our natural resources; increases interest in eliminating toxins and chemicals from food chain.

Benefits of Physical Fitness

The number-one reason people begin exercising is to improve their physical appearance. Certainly, physical appearance will be enhanced because of decreased body fat and firmer, well-toned muscles. These are not the only benefits, though. There are a number of physiological (cardiorespiratory, body composition, and metabolic) and psychological (mental and emotional) health benefits. As individuals age, less attention is directed toward physical fitness benefits and more emphasis is directed to the total health benefits. Exercise has both short- and long-term effects. The immediate effects of vigorous exercise, regardless of the fitness level, are an increase in the respiration rate, an increase in the heart rate, and some sweating. After a few weeks of regular, vigorous exercise, the body begins to adapt. It becomes better suited to meeting the demands of regular exercise. These physiological adaptations (the total beneficial changes) are called the **training effect.**

Cardiorespiratory Benefits

1. consistent reduction in resting heart rate;
2. increase in stroke volume (the amount of blood pumped out of the heart with each beat), improving heart efficiency;
3. increased rest for the heart between beats due to slower resting heart rate and increased stroke volume;
4. increased oxygen-carrying capacity of the blood, due to the greater supply of red blood cells and hemoglobin, and greater endurance in exercising muscles due to increased energy and improved elimination of waste products;
5. improved exercise performance on timed tests, due to more efficient utilization of oxygen;
6. possible reduction in blood pressure;
7. improved blood lipid profile by increasing the number of protective high-density lipoproteins;
8. quicker recovery to resting heart rate after vigourous exercise, due to improved cardiac efficiency;
9. possible regression of atherosclerosis; and
10. fewer illnesses and deaths due to coronary heart disease.

Body Composition/Physical Appearance Benefits

1. reduced body fat percentage;
2. increased lean body mass; and
3. firmer, more toned muscles.

Psychological Benefits

1. enhanced sense of well-being and self-esteem, resulting in increased energy, alterness, and vitality;
2. increased sense of self-discipline, due to the determination needed to stick to an exercise program;
3. reduced state of anxiety and mental tension, resulting in increased stress-coping ability;
4. improved quality of sleep, resulting in the ability to fall asleep faster and with less tossing and turning during sleeping time;
5. decreased level of mild to moderate depression; and
6. increased release of endorphins (brain chemicals), producing a relaxed state.

The psychological benefits can be the most rewarding and are often the main reason people keep exercising. These mental and emotional benefits are real and can be measured.[12] Fitness produces other benefits that are also important to your health and well-being. You burn extra calories while exercising, which helps to promote weight loss and reverse obesity. Exercise and weight management helps prevent and manage diabetes.[13,14] Fit people can exercise longer at the same level of intensity, and their perception of how hard they are working decreases. This is due to increased muscular strength and endurance. Tendons, ligaments, and joints may also be strengthened through exercise. Additionally, exercise stimulates bone strengthening and may help counteract and reverse osteoporosis.[15]

The FITT Prescription for Fitness

Many studies have been conducted in exercise physiology laboratories to determine the best prescription for developing CRE. These studies confirm that CRE fitness development involves four **FITT prescription factors**: Frequency, Intensity, Time, and Type of exercise.

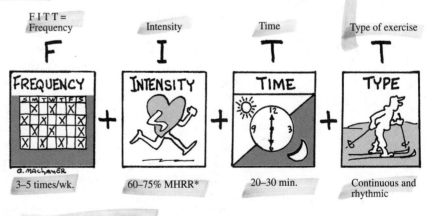

FITT =
Frequency   Intensity   Time   Type of exercise

F   I   T   T

FREQUENCY   INTENSITY   TIME   TYPE

3–5 times/wk.   60–75% MHRR*   20–30 min.   Continuous and rhythmic

*MHRR = Maximal heart rate reserve

This prescription is recommended for the individual who wishes to develop a high level of quality CRE fitness. It is not the recommended training regime for performance in intercollegiate athletics or for the individual who wishes to run a 26.2-mile marathon, bike 100 miles, or swim a 2-mile event. However, many athletes of all ages apply the FITT prescription to their exercise programs to maintain their CRE fitness in the off-season.

Attaining and maintaining CRE fitness requires a vigorous, total-body effort. Exercising for health purposes (reduction and/or prevention of coronary heart disease, diabetes, cancer, and improved quality of life) may be less demanding in terms of intensity and quality of exercise. Se the section titled "Relationship Between Activity and Health" later in this chapter.

"F" Equals Frequency

How often should you exercise? Exercise three to five times per week with no more than 48 hours between workouts is necessary to maintain CRE fitness. After 48 hours, the body starts to decondition or lose some of the benefits gained in the last workout. It is not necessary to exercise every day of the week in order to develop fitness, although five-day-a-week programs produce greater improvements than do three-day-a-week programs. However, since fitness exercise is vigorous, time for recovery is necessary. This is especially true if you are just beginning a fitness program. The body needs time to adapt to this new activity. So start slowly at first, working out three days per week, every other day, gradually increasing the frequency as your body can handle it.

"I" Equals Intensity

How hard should you exercise? The level of intensity of the workout needs to be between 60 percent and 75 percent of the maximal heart rate reserve. This allows for a range of intensity that assures adequate stimulation of the cardiorespiratory system (providing training effect benefits) yet is not so strenuous that symptoms of overtraining develop (Table 2.2).

Karvonen Equation

To determine the **target heart rate range (THR)** for exercise, we will use a formula, the **Karvonen equation** (Table 2.3), that takes into account your current fitness level based on your resting heart rate (RHR). Karvonen, a Finnish researcher, discovered in 1957 that the heart rate during exercise must be raised by at least 60 percent of the difference between resting and maximal heart rates (called the *Maximal heart rate reserve*, MHRR) to produce cardiorespiratory fitness.[16] Subsequent research has revealed that an adequate upper intensity level is 75 percent of the difference between resting and maximal heart rate.

It is necessary to know your **maximal heart rate (Max.HR)** in order to calculate your target heart rate range. Max.HR is your highest possible heart rate. It can be determined during a treadmill exercise tolerance test in a laboratory or hospital while you exercise to exhaustion. The maximal heart rate ranges from 180 to 200 beats per minute (bpm) in young people and decreases with age. For most people, it is easier and safer to estimate their Max.HR by subtracting their age from 220. For example, if you are 21 years old, your estimated Max.HR is 199 (220 − 21 = 199).

Next, you will need to know your resting heart rate (RHR) for one minute. Check it now, using a stopwatch or a watch with a second hand. You can find the pulse by placing your fingertips (not your thumb) over your heart, at the carotid artery in your neck, or on the thumb side of your wrist (Figs. 2.1 and 2.2). Count the number of beats for 30 seconds and multiply by two to calculate your 1-minute pulse.

By using your age and your own RHR, you can calculate your personalized target heart rate range (Table 2.3 and target heart rate worksheet in the Chapter 2 activities).

Now that you know your target heart rate range, you will be able to measure the intensity of every workout. Count your pulse during exercise and immediately upon finishing the conditioning bout. Rather than counting your pulse for a full minute, you may find it easier to count for 6 or 10 seconds only. For a 6-second count, add a zero to the number of heartbeats and, for a 10-second count, multiply the heartbeats by 6. Either method gives you a quick, 1-minute heart rate count. It will take some practice, but in time you will become accurate at checking your heart rate.

Examining the chart for the target heart rate range (Fig. 2.3), you can see that exercise heart rates differ by age. If your exercise heart rate is above the upper range (higher than 75 percent MHRR), you may be exercising more intensely than is necessary for fitness. The American College of Sports Medicine (ACSM) recommends an exercise intensity range of 60 percent to 90 percent during exercise. Ninety percent may be too

table 2.2

SYMPTOMS OF OVERTRAINING, OVERSTRESS, OVERUSE, AND CHRONIC FATIGUE

1. Persistent soreness and stiffness in joints, tendons, or muscles
2. Increases of six to eight beats per minute in resting pulse, checked regularly, first thing in the morning
3. Labored breathing during a workout of normal intensity, a sudden drop in performance, or inability to finish a workout
4. Persistent lethargy, fatigue, and unusual disinterest in exercise
5. Lowered general resistance: frequent mild colds, sniffles, cold sores
6. Lack of enthusiasm, depression, inability to relax, irritability
7. Poor coordination (general clumsiness, tripping, poor auto driving)
8. Difficulty in getting to sleep or staying asleep
9. Swelling or aching lymph glands in the neck, underarm, or groin area
10. Skin eruptions in nonadolescents
11. Loss of appetite
12. Chronic thirst
13. Morning weight 3 percent less than normal
14. Sudden diarrhea or constipation
15. Anemia or amenorrhea (in women)

table 2.3

CALCULATING THE TARGET HEART RATE RANGE USING THE KARVONEN FORMULA

THR = [maximal heart rate − resting heart rate] × intensity factor + resting heart rate

This example shows a 22-year-old with a resting rate of 78 bpm:

- Estimation of maximal heart rate = 220 minus age 22
- Resting heart rate = pulse at complete rest for one minute
- Intensity = range of 60% to 75%

THR at 60% = [(220 − 22) − 78] × 0.60 + 78
           = [198 − 78] × 0.60 + 78
           = 120 × 0.60 + 78
           = 72 + 78
           = 150

THR at 75% = [(220 − 22) − 78] × 0.75 + 78
           = [198 − 78] × 0.75 + 78
           = 120 × 0.75 + 78
           = 90 + 78
           = 168

Target heart rate range = 150 to 168.

FIGURE 2.1 ➤
Pulse at carotid artery.

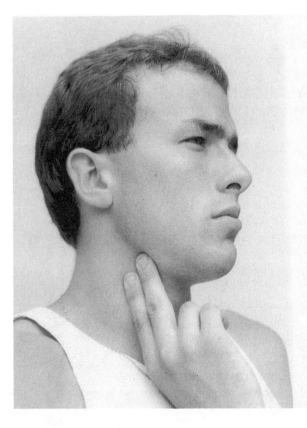

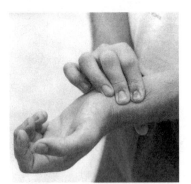

FIGURE 2.2 ➤
Pulse at the thumb side of wrist.

intense for many exercisers, especially on a regular basis. A general rule of thumb is to apply the *talk test*. You should be able to comfortably carry on a conversation with a companion while exercising. If you are too breathless to talk, you are exercising too hard.

Use caution when using your running or walking THR to measure the intensity of your exercise when you swim, bike, or water run. If you try to reach your running/walking THR during nonweight-bearing activities, you may feel uncomfortably stressed and, more importantly, risk injury by working out too hard.[17] As a general rule of thumb, reduce cycling THR by 5 percent and swimming THR by 10 percent. In any case, you should still be able to pass the "talk test." Consider the following two examples:

A. If your THR for running/walking is 150 to 170 bpm, your *cycling* THR would be approximately 142 to 161 bpm.
   1. $150 \times 0.05 = 7.5$ (or 8); $170 \times .05 = 8.5$ (or 9)
   2. $150 - 8 = 142$; $170 - 9 = 161$
   3. THR = 142 to 161 bpm

B. If your THR for running/walking is 150 to 170 bpm, your *swimming* THR would be approximately 135 to 153 bpm.
   1. $150 \times 0.10 = 15$; $170 \times 0.10 = 17$
   2. $150 - 15 = 135$; $170 - 17 = 153$
   3. THR = 135 to 153 bpm

Also, remember to set different heart rate goals for cross training. When switching sports for cross training, a good way to achieve an effective workout is to monitor your rate of perceived exertion and not worry about your THR.[18] This means paying attention to how hard or how easy your exercise feels.

Rate of Perceived Exertion (RPE)

Many people do not check their heart rate during exercise, and an alternate method of assessing intensity of exercise has become popular in recent years. This method uses a **rate of perceived exertion (RPE)** scale developed by Gunnar Borg (Table 2.4). Borg discovered that exercisers are able to "sense" (or perceive) their own exercise intensity

FIGURE 2.3 ►
Estimated target heart rate range (based on RHR of 72 bpm).

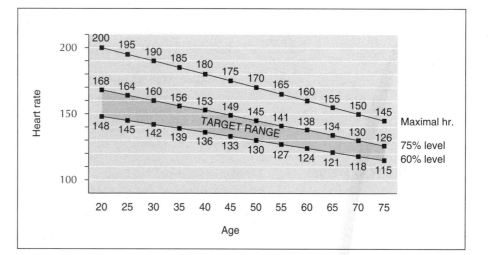

table 2.4

BORG'S RATE OF PERCEIVED EXERTION (RPE)

(RPE) CHART

6		
7	Very, very light	Warm-up/cool-down zone
8		
9	Very light	
10		
11	Fairly light	
12		Target zone
13	Somewhat hard	
14		
15	Hard	
16		
17	Very hard	Working too hard zone
18		
19	Very, very hard	
20		

G. Borg, "Psychophysical Bases of Physical Exertion—Perceived Rate of Exertion," *Medicine and Science in Sport & Exercise,* 14, 344–86, 1982, © by The American College of Sports Medicine.

levels. He found that the RPE scale correlated very highly with heart rate, ventilation, oxygen consumption, and blood lactate concentrates.[19] These items are commonly assessed in a laboratory setting to measure exercise intensity. Borg found that the descriptive words in the right column of the table closely paralleled the actual heart rate of the exerciser, which is illustrated by the numbers in the left column.

Most exercisers should be working in the target zone which is the "Fairly light" to "Somewhat hard" to "Hard" zone—(RPE 10–15). "Very, very light" describes feelings of exertion at rest; and "Very, very hard" describes feelings just before collapsing from exhaustion. Notice the descriptors used for the warm-up and cool-down zone.

It is important to cross-check your heart rate with your perceived rating when first beginning to use this method. After several weeks, you should be able to predict your exercise heart rate by your own perceived exertion of the exercise session. When exercising, ask, "How do I feel?" Describe how you feel using the descriptors on the Borg scale. Adjust the intensity of your workout accordingly. This is a safe and accurate way to monitor exercise intensity anywhere, anytime, without using a stopwatch or pace clock.

Whether you monitor the intensity of exercise by checking your pulse or through rate of perceived exertion, listen to your body and make adjustments in the intensity of your exercise when necessary.

"T" Equals Time

How long should each workout be? Research points out that the conditioning bout should be 20 or (preferably) 30 minutes in duration to provide the desired training effects. This does not include the warm-up and cool-down segments but refers only to the actual conditioning bout when the intensity level is sustained at 60 percent to 75 percent maximal heart rate reserve. The time duration recommended by the ACSM is 20 minutes to 60 minutes. If time permits and the exercise session is enjoyable, or if you are training for a long distance event (i.e., minimarathon), exercising for longer than 30 minutes is permissable but not necessary for basic fitness. A typical workout would be as follows:

| warm-up 5–15 min. | conditioning 20–30 min. | cool-down 5–15 min. |

When beginning a CRE fitness program, it is best to limit your conditioning periods to 20 minutes or less and then progress slowly until you can comfortably work out for 20 to 30 minutes in your target heart rate range.

"T" Equals Type

What type of exercise promotes aerobic fitness? The activity should be vigorous, rhythmic, and continuous. This includes activities that accelerate respiration and maintain a heart rate in the target range. Aerobic dance, lap swimming, bicycling, cross-country skiing, jogging, and fitness walking are activities that come to mind. Riding a bike across campus does not get the job done. This is not CRE fitness riding. Ask yourself, "Did my heart rate reach the prescribed target heart rate range? Did I keep my heart rate in that range for 20 to 30 minutes or more?" Rope jumping or even stair climbing can be aerobic activities, providing the CRE FITT prescription factors are met. Tennis, bowling, golf, weight training, and softball, although enjoyable and health-promoting activities, are not considered to be aerobic. (See the section titled "The Relationship Between Activity and Health" later in this chapter.) Can you name other sports or activities that meet the FITT prescription?

How Long Before Results Become Apparent?

It varies with the individual, but CRE fitness results can occur within 8 to 12 weeks. The key is staying with the exercise program. Studies indicate that over 50 percent of all adults who start an exercise program drop out within the first three to six months.[20] Most people recognize the benefits of being physically fit but few make fitness a habit. People generally fall into three exercise categories: nonexercisers (the true couch potatoes), start-and-stop exercisers (the wannabe's who try exercising but keep relapsing into periods of inactivity), and regular exercisers. Nonexercisers and start-and-stop exercisers are less convinced of the benefits of being active than are the regular exercisers. Regular exercisers use more cognitive and behavioral strategies to sustain the exercise habit. They focus on the positive benefits of exercise, reminding themselves of how good they feel after a good workout, and pat themselves on the back for progress.

So if you're a couch potato or a start-and-stopper, how can you begin and stay with an exercise program long enough to experience the benefits of the training effect? First, review in Chapter 1 the series of stages that people who want to engage in a new behavior go through. Then use the helpful strategies that follow:

1. *Make up a contract.* People who sign a contract for a definite period of time are more likely to reach their goals.[21] A contract for 12 weeks is ideal. At the end of the contract, reward yourself—you've earned it. Immediately, renegotiate your contract for another 12-week period.

Recording workouts helps you
see progress.

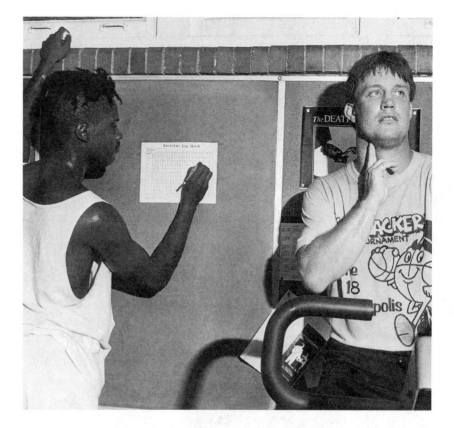

2. *Make exercise social and fun.* Exercising with a partner or group of friends is more fun than is working out alone. Friends rely on each other for moral support and help each other stay committed to their fitness program.

3. *Take lessons.* Join an aerobic dance class or a health club. Work with a personal trainer. Try different activities until you find one you enjoy. Start slowly and progress gradually to avoid injuries. If exercise is too difficult or too intense, you will be unlikely to stay on your program.

4. *Make it convenient* by developing your own home gym or purchase an exercise video or two. Keep your exercise gear available at all times, so that you can squeeze in a quick workout.

5. *Treat exercise like an appointment.* Schedule a time that works best for you; whether that be morning, noon, or evening. Table 2.5 gives the advantages and disadvantages of various times.

6. *Keep a chart to monitor your progress.* It's rewarding to see how much you have progressed.

7. *Finally, don't stop!* It's difficult to get going again. Remember to plan for changes in your schedule (for example, pack your exercise equipment when you travel). However, don't feel guilty if you miss an exercise session. Consider this a lifetime commitment and resume exercising as soon as possible.

Three-Segment Workout

A **three-segment workout** includes a warm-up, a conditioning bout, and a cool-down.

Warm-Up

The **warm-up** is an important beginning to a workout session. Two important physiological changes occur during the warm-up. The internal temperature of the muscles increases, enhancing their elasticity. Heart rate and respiration increase, providing greater blood flow to the exercising muscles. The warm-up prepares the body physically and mentally

table 2.5

BEST TIME TO EXERCISE

There is no perfect time of day for exercise. What works best for one individual may not fit the life of another. Find the time that works best for your individual needs, preferences, and schedule. You may want to experiment with several exercise times before you are able to determine what feels best for you. The key is to commit to a lifestyle that includes a definite time for daily physical activity and to stick with this commitment for life.

TIME	ADVANTAGE	DISADVANTAGE
Morning	• Less chance other activities will conflict with exercise • Wakes you up and energizes you for the day's activities • Usually the coolest time on hot summer days • Fewer problems with ozone and other air pollutants • Gets your showering over with for the day • Good time to mentally organize a "to do" list for the day	• Some people like to "sleep in" • Energy reserves may be low because of the long span of time between the evening meal and breakfast • May need longer warm-up because muscles are colder and stiffer than later in the day • May be colder during winter months • May rush you to be on time for work or school • Dangerous to exercise outside before daylight
Noon	• Allows for a refreshing tension-relieving break during the middle of the day • Can help curb lunch appetite • Energizes you for the remainder of the day • Generally, more people are around to share the workout • Good time to "network" and make business and social contacts • May be warmest time of the day during cold months	• Workout time, exercise facilities, and shower less likely to be available • Conflicts more likely to arise • Difficult if you have frequent business lunches • May be too hot during warm months • May feel rushed to combine workout with lunch
Evening	• Works off the accumulated stress of the day • May help you sleep more soundly • Can help curb dinner appetite • Works as a "pick-me-up" for the rest of the evening (if you plan to study late or have other activities) • May be cooler than midday during summer • Exercising at a fitness facility on the way home from school or work is convenient	• Easy to postpone exercise due to other activities, coming home late, feeling too tired, etc. • Easy to say "I'll get up early tomorrow and work out" • May stimulate you too much so that falling asleep is difficult • It is recommended that you wait an hour or two before exercising after a heavy meal

for the conditioning bout and may reduce the chance of injury while exercising. There is no set length of time for the warm-up, although 5 to 15 minutes is adequate. On cold days, or at times when you feel sluggish, the warm-up may take longer. When you're feeling energetic or when the temperature is warm, the warm-up period may be shorter. A good method of gauging whether you have had an adequate warm-up is to pay attention to how you feel. Do you feel ready to exercise vigorously? If you still feel stiff and sluggish, you need a longer warm-up. A slight sweat is a good indication of an adequate warm-up.

Three activities may be included in the warm-up. They are simple calisthenics (such as jumping jacks), mild stretching exercises, and **task specific activity**. The task specific activity is a short period of exercise that uses the same muscles that will be used in the conditioning bout. It specifically prepares those muscles that will be used. **Static stretching**, in which a stretch is held for 15 to 30 seconds, is recommended. **Ballistic stretching,** with jerking and bouncing movements, is *not* recommended. Stretching during warm-up is mainly preparation for the activity, not for flexibility. Most experts agree that the best time to stretch for flexibility is during the cool-down phase because the muscles are warmer and more elastic.

The final portion of the warm-up should lead into the actual activity you will be doing in the conditioning bout but at a lowered intensity level (lower heart rate). For example, joggers should include a short period of walking or slow jogging before beginning the intensity of the conditioning bout. Aerobic dancers should do routines of lowered intensity before proceeding into the main body of the workout (conditioning bout) where the heart rate should reach target heart rate intensity. See Chapter 3 for exercises that can be used for warm-up and cool-down.

Conditioning Bout

The **conditioning bout** consists of vigorous aerobic exercise that stimulates the cardiorespiratory system. It should follow the FITT formula. Progress slowly and listen to your body. Gradually increase the intensity and frequency of your workouts. You do not want to be sidelined by illness or injury because of overtraining. Your goal is a lifetime of exercise. Select an aerobic activity you will enjoy; do not be influenced into participating in an activity simply because it is in vogue. Depending on your age, current fitness level, or physical limitations, you can enjoy walking, jogging, aerobic dance, water exercise, fitness swimming, bicycling, cross-country skiing, or any other vigorous activity.

Cool-Down

The **cool-down** is the final segment of the workout. The purpose of the cool-down is to safely ease your body back to its resting state. You should gradually reduce the intensity of exercise to enhance your recovery. Failure to cool down may allow the muscles to further tighten, potentially causing pain, soreness, and stiffness. Another problem with inadequate cool-down is the possibility of blood pooling in the lower extremities, resulting in faintness and dizziness. This is called *venous pooling*. Again, there is no set length of time for a cool-down period, but it will usually take 5 to 15 minutes. It should begin with the same activity performed in the conditioning bout but at a lowered intensity.

Flexibility gains are greatest during cool-down stretching.

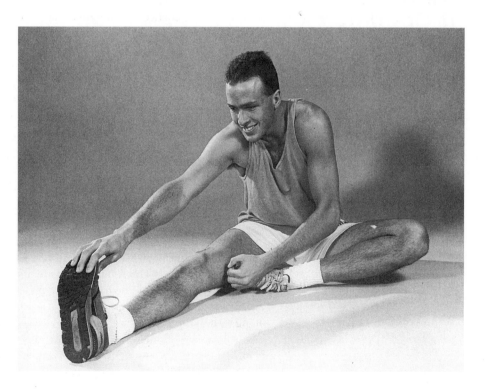

For example, if you jog, reduce the pace and end with a period of walking. Likewise, the aerobic dancer should reduce dance intensity. Cool-down should continue until the heart rate is approximately 100 to 110 beats per minute or less. In the cool-down, spend a few minutes stretching while the muscles are thoroughly warm and elastic. Use the stretching exercises illustrated in Chapter 3. Greater flexibility is achieved when stretching occurs in the cool-down segment of the workout.

Principle of Overload

Overload is a gradual increase in physical activity, stressing a muscle group or body system beyond accustomed levels. The muscle group or system, such as the cardiorespiratory system, gradually adapts, resulting in improved physiological functioning. In addition, a decrease in the severity and a delay in the onset of fatigue occur. The overload doesn't have to be punishing or exhaustive for cardiorespiratory training effects to occur. The key to gradual overloading for CRE fitness is to follow the FITT formula but in the order of FTI: Frequency, Time, Intensity.

First, there should be a gradual increase in the *frequency* of workouts, starting with three and progressing to five workouts per week. Second, *time* or (duration) should be introduced. Start with workouts of 20 minutes (or less, if you are in poor condition) and gradually lengthen the workouts to 30 minutes each. The rate of increase should be no more than 10 percent per week. For example, if one week each conditioning bout is 20 minutes, the next week's workouts can be 22 minutes. Third, alter the *intensity* of workouts. Workouts should begin at 60 percent intensity and progress to the 75 percent range. By following the FTI order of overloading, you will make your normal activity a physiological pushover, since you will have trained to perform beyond normal levels.

We have learned that the old saying, "No pain, no gain!" is inappropriate advice. Simply follow the prescription factors in the correct order and listen to your own body. Check your heart rate and stay within your target heart rate range. Watch for any signs of overtraining (shown in Table 2.2). Remember, exercise is for a lifetime.

Principle of Specificity

The **principle of specificity** is that only the muscles or body systems being exercised will show beneficial changes. To improve the cardiorespiratory system, exercise the heart and lungs through aerobic activities; to improve flexibility, do stretching exercises; and to improve muscular strength, lift weights.

You cannot strengthen the muscles of the arms by jogging, nor can you increase cardiorespiratory fitness by doing yoga. This principle also helps to explain why you are wiped out after a fitness swim workout when your usual mode of training is jogging.

Aerobic and Anaerobic Exercise

The term **aerobic** literally means "with oxygen." Aerobic activities are those that demand large amounts of oxygen and follow the FITT prescription. They are vigorous, continuous, and rhythmic. The outcome of aerobic exercise is improved cardiorespiratory endurance, which produces the many physiological and psychological benefits (training effect) that come from improved fitness.

Anaerobic exercise means "without oxygen." Anaerobic activities are start and stop, such as sprinting, where the heart rate is not kept at a rhythmic, continuous level. Anaerobic exercise is a high-intensity effort of short duration. This type of activity demands more oxygen than the body can supply during exertion, causing an oxygen debt. Anaerobic exercise causes waste products (lactic acid) to accumulate in muscles, which, along with the depletion of stored energy, leads to exhaustion. Many activities—tennis, baseball, basketball, and weight training—are anaerobic. They aid in the development of agility, eye-hand coordination, and muscular strength and endurance, as well as flexibility, but they are not aerobic.

Cross Training

Cross training involves developing all five health-related components of fitness. It is a method of exercise programming that achieves balanced fitness by emphasizing comprehensive conditioning in the major muscle groups. Traditionally, of the five components of fitness, cardiorespiratory endurance has received the most emphasis. Certainly, this component is essential to high-level health, but the other four health-related components are also important. No single type of exercise can offer complete conditioning for all parts of the body.

Originally, *cross training* referred to a conditioning regimen used by triathletes to train in three events—running, biking, and swimming. However, in the strictest sense, training for a triathlon is not cross training. It is triple, task-specific training for three separate events in which the main emphasis is cardiorespiratory endurance. Today, the purpose of cross training is to enhance several fitness components, not athletic performance, although performance may improve due to increased strength and flexibility. An example of cross training (for a 20-year-old) would be one swimming session and two weight training workouts in combination with three jogging workouts per week. Add some stretching exercises after each workout and you have a balanced fitness program. (See Table 2.6 for other cross training activities.)

It's not only the elite athlete who profits from muscular strength and endurance, flexibility, a lean body, and high-level cardiorespiratory endurance. These ingredients of balanced fitness are needed by people from all walks of life, including college students. Expand your fitness program to include cross training activities. The time and energy you invest will give big payoffs. Look at the advantages:

1. Cross training builds overall fitness. This occurs because all five fitness components are emphasized. Cross training entices the exerciser to apply the overload principle in workouts, thus improving fitness gains in every component.
2. Cross training develops high levels of fitness. Participating in a variety of activities recruits new muscle fibers and develops neuromuscular pathways, formerly left untapped. Higher levels of cardiorespiratory endurance can result.[22]

table 2.6

CROSS TRAINING ACTIVITIES FOR THE FIVE COMPONENTS OF FITNESS

FLEXIBILITY

Yoga, stretching, swimming, water exercise, or other activities that allow muscles to move through a full range of motion are excellent methods of developing flexibility.

CARDIORESPIRATORY ENDURANCE

Running, fitness walking, aerobic dance, bench and stair stepping, rope jumping, cross-country skiing, swimming, cycling, rowing, and water exercise (aqua-aerobics) are recommended for developing cardiorespiratory endurance.

MUSCLE STRENGTH

Weight machines, free weights, rubberbands, gymnastics, calisthenics (push-ups, abdominal curls, etc.) provide ways to enhance muscle strength.

MUSCLE ENDURANCE

Lighter weights or resistance with increased repetitions of the exercises used to develop muscle strength are advised.

BODY COMPOSITION

Minute for minute, activities that develop cardiorespiratory endurance expend the most calories. Muscular strength and endurance activities also help maintain the appropriate lean-to-fat ratio.

3. Cross training reduces risk of overtraining and injury. A single type of activity used to develop cardiorespiratory endurance will continually stress the same body parts. This is especially true in weight-bearing activities such as running. Repetitive impact injuries (such as shin splints) can result. Because the stress imposed by cross training is spread around the body to different muscle groups, a high volume of training can be performed without overtraining and injury.
4. Cross training develops muscle symmetry. Muscle symmetry involves the balance of both strength and flexibility in opposing muscle groups. Without the appropriate ratio, selected sites of muscles can become strong and their opposing muscles disproportionately weak. Well-balanced muscle pairs working in concert allow for more effective and efficient movement and eliminate some of the risk for injury.
5. Cross training reduces boredom and provides motivation. Because a variety of activities are used in cross training, interest in exercise remains high and adherence is greater.
6. Cross training aids in weight loss. Changing activities helps reduce muscle soreness and fatigue, which can result in an increased ability to exercise longer and more frequently—therefore, more total calories are expended.

The Relationship Between Activity and Health

The proof is in. We can no longer ignore the scientific evidence that documents how a sedentary lifestyle is killing us (Fig. 2.4). Stop for a moment to think about the impact exercise has on heart disease, cancer, and other causes of death. Americans worry about cholesterol in their diets and are giving up cigarettes, yet they continue to get more obese every year. Why do Americans ignore the reports on the relationship of exercise to health and weight control? The thought of not brushing our teeth every day seems ridiculous to most of us. After all, our teeth have to last a lifetime. But exercise every day? Even though mortality statistics overwhelmingly point to the health value of activity, most people still do not include exercise in their daily schedule.[23,24] Approximately 12 percent of all deaths every year in the United States can be attributed to a lack of exercise.[25] That is more than 250,000 deaths! Doesn't your heart have to last a lifetime, too? How sad it is that we pay more attention to our teeth than to our hearts.

We all understand the value of exercise. The problem is few of us make it a priority in our lives. Only 22 percent of Americans engage in leisure activity at the level recommended for health benefits. Only 12 percent of this group can be labeled vigorously active—that is, as following the FITT prescription factors. That's the good news. The bad news is that over one-fourth of adult Americans are *completely sedentary* and are badly in need of more physical activity. Another one-half of our population is *inadequately active* and would also benefit from increased physical activity. In essence, nearly three-fourths of American adults need more physical activity to merely improve their health.[26] The fitness boom of the 1960s and 1970s has ended and now appears to be declining. The exercise objective in *Healthy People 2000: Objectives for a Nation*, calling for "50 percent of all Americans to participate in fitness activities by year 2000" and "for most Americans to participate in regular activity as a part of their daily lifestyle," will never be met.[27] Among ethnic minority populations, older adults, and those with lower incomes or educational levels, participation in regular physical activity has remained consistently low. Every American must realize that sedentary living affects life and death as much as does cigarette smoking, high blood pressure, high cholesterol, and obesity. What is the cause of this seriously low level of physical activity in America? Is it because we don't know what is involved in getting fit? Or could it be that most people perceive that fitness takes too much time, energy, and money and requires athletic ability?

An important study conducted at the Institute for Aerobics Research in Dallas by Steven Blair and colleagues provides evidence that physical fitness is associated with longevity (Fig. 2.5). In this eight-year study, physical fitness was quantified using an exercise tolerance test on a treadmill. The subjects were categorized into five levels of physi-

FIGURE 2.4 ➤

Exercise and health. An eight-year study of 13,344 people (10,224 men, 3,120 women) shows that physical activity reduces the risk of death from virtually all causes. Charts compare death rates.

source: Institute for Aerobics Research, "Physical Fitness and All-Cause Mortality." *Journal of the American Medical Association* 262, no. 17 (Nov. 3, 1989).

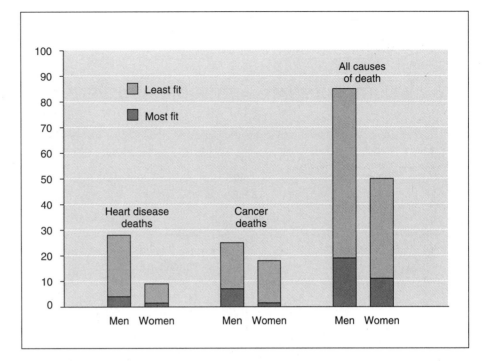

FIGURE 2.5 ➤

Comparison of fitness levels and risk of death. Notice that the death rates for the least fit men (level 1) were 3.4 times higher than for the most fit men (level 5). Death rates for the least fit women (level 1) were 4.6 times higher than for the most fit women (level 5). The most dramatic drop in risk of death occurs between levels 1 and 2 (from 3.4 to 1.4 for men; from 4.6 to 2.4 for women).

source: Blair, Steven, et al. "Physical Fitness and All-Cause Mortality: A Prospective Study of Healthy Men and Women." *Journal of the American Medical Association* 262 (Nov. 3, 1989): 2395–401.

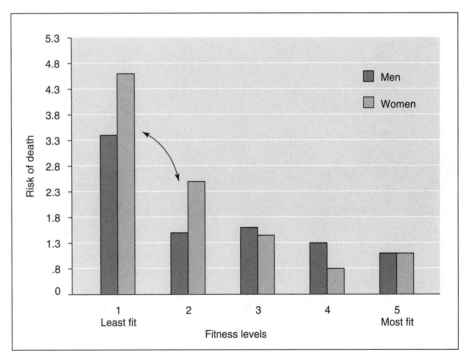

cal fitness based on the treadmill test. As Figure 2.5 shows, the greatest reduction in risk of death occurs between the lowest level of fitness and the next lowest level. In other words, the least active people who modestly increase their activity stand to gain the most.

The scientific study by Dr. Blair clearly demonstrates that regular, *moderate-intensity* physical activity is an important component of improving the quality of life. In response to Dr. Blair's findings and the fact that most Americans fall into the sedentary category, representatives from the American College of Sports Medicine (ACSM) and the U.S. Centers for Disease Control (CDC) collaborated to recommend the type and amount of physical activity that is needed for maintenance and promotion of health.[28] The key phrase here is "promotion of health," not development of fitness. Remember,

A New Recommendation for Physical Activity and Health

table 2.7

LIGHT, MODERATE, AND VIGOROUS LEVELS OF ACTIVITY/EXERCISE

The role of exercise and the improvement of health and quality of life have recently gained national attention. Sedentary living increases the risk for coronary heart disease, cancer, and diabetes, not to mention stroke, osteoporosis, and depression.

Exercise/activity in the moderate-intensity range (3 to 6 METs) is recommended for enhancing health benefits. CRE fitness gains and lower mortality rates occur when exercise/activity is in the vigorous-intensity range (6+ METs).

	METs*	EXAMPLE
Light	< 3	• strolling <3 mph • archery • bowling • golf (with a foursome)
Moderate	3 < 6	• walking briskly 3–4 mph • heavy gardening and jobs around the house • raking leaves • dancing
Vigorous	6+	• fast walking (>4 mph) • fitness activities that follow the FITT prescription • racket sports • hill climbing • rope skipping • snow shoveling • mowing lawn with hand mower • splitting wood

*METs (metabolic equivalents) is a measure of calorie intensity and a method of classifying various activities and exercises. It represents the rate of energy (calories) expended at rest and used to rate activities in multiples above rest. One MET represents the energy expended at rest (approximately 1.25 calories per minute or 3.5 ml of oxygen per kg (2.2 pounds) of body weight per minute). Six METs, for instance, simply means that the activity requires six times more energy than required at rest (about 8 calories per minute).

CRE fitness requires a vigorous, total-body effort and adherence to the FITT prescription factors. The ACSM/CDC recommendations are as follows:

➤ *Every* American should accumulate *30 minutes* or more of *moderate-intensity* physical activity over the course of most days of the week.

➤ The recommended 30 minutes of physical activity may also come from planned exercise and recreation such as jogging, playing tennis, swimming, and cycling.

➤ Activities that can contribute to the 30-minutes total include walking briskly, climbing the stairs (instead of using escalators and elevators), gardening, raking leaves, playing with the children, cleaning the house, dancing, and walking the dog. For example, walking briskly at moderate intensity would be equivalent to walking two miles at a 15- to 20-minute mile pace (Table 2.7).

The activity does not have to be all in one bout. Incorporationg bits of activity every day, whenever and wherever you can is okay. The idea is to *pulse* activity into our daily lives. Also, realize physical activity does not have be punishing to be beneficial, nor do you have to be soaked with sweat for improvements in health to occur. The key is to get enough activity at the *moderate-intensity level* every day. Look for opportunities to add daily activity: Get up earlier, utilize TV commercial time, walk the dog after dinner, walk to the grocery when you only need a few items, ride your bike to mail a letter, go to the mall before the stores open and walk a few laps inside.

The advice to "exercise lite," as some have called it, is not telling the physically fit segment of our population (the 12 percent who apply the FITT formula) to slow down (Table 2.7). On the contrary, this new advice is aimed at convincing the sedentary group that they do not have to run marathons or swim the English Channel to reap the benefits of physical exercise. The real issue is getting people moving again; to convince American couch potatoes that exercise is a normal human need. There is no longer any question that increased physical activity at the moderate intensity level improves health and quality of life. In addition, for those Americans who exercise at higher intensity levels (FITT), these same benefits are reaped and more—increased longevity.[29,30]

Sedentary lifestyle habits of Americans will not change overnight. Mark Twain said it best: "Habits are habits. You can't throw them out the window. You have to coax them downstairs one step at a time." This is exactly the intent of the ACSM/CDC exercise guidelines: to encourage Americans to change their sedentary lifestyles . . . one step at a time. With small, moderate increases in physical activity, perhaps people will begin to enjoy their new active lifestyle and begin to "see and feel" the benefits of exercise. Eventually then, they may wish to invest additional time and energy in exercise, which will in turn increase their potential to acquire the even greater health benefits that come from being physically fit.

To enhance the appeal of participating in moderate-intensity activity, it is time we deemphasize the medical/scientific approach. Although medical screening and precise exercise prescription (exact THR) is recommended, it is more important to get moving. In the past, the scientific approach to exercise may have turned some people off to exercise. They may have had the impression that exericse was too complicated, took too much time, involved special equipment, and wasn't convenient. Our society is at a point where the best advice is, "Don't measure it; just do it!"

How Can Society Help?

Our high-tech society entices people to be inactive. Cars, television, and labor-saving devices have profoundly changed the way many people perform their everyday tasks. Furthermore, their surroundings often present barriers to participation in physical activity. Americans are not likely to change their lifestyles until environmental and social barriers to physical activity are reduced or eliminated, which can happen. Society can promote more physical activity by taking such steps as putting attractive staircases at easy-to-use locations in buildings instead of tucking them away in hard-to-find, dimly lit places. Communities must support in schools, worksites, and community organizations programs that emphasize lifelong physical activity. Efforts should be made to develop walking, biking, and hiking trails and other exercise facilities and to encourage walking and biking for transportation. Physicians and other health professionals should be encouraged to routinely counsel all patients to adopt and maintain regular physical activity. Special efforts need to be made to increase the amount of activity in target populations—namely, minority ethnic groups, the less educated, and older adults. Physical activity promotions targeted to people with disabilities and chronic diseases should be supported. These promotions should stress the importance of carrying out daily living with a minimum of assistance.

Schools are fundamental starting points for changing future physical activity patterns. However, many school systems facing financial cutbacks are eliminating physical education and fitness programs. This definitely is not in the best interest of American youth. Comprehensive wellness programs that promote physical activity should be supported. Physical education curricula should provide experiences that are enjoyable and promote lifelong participation in physical activity.

You are faced with a tremendous challenge. As our nation's future homemakers, parents, and leaders, you hold in your hands the responsibility for the health and well-being of the next generation. Each one of you can make an enormous impact on the activity patterns of your own children, family, friends, and neighbors by setting a good example. So go to it: Get up off the sofa, turn off the TV, put away the video games. Accept the challenge today to make exercise a daily habit, one as important as brushing your teeth.

Encourage your friends and neighbors to get out and work in the garden, walk around the block, mow the lawn, walk the dog, participate in recreational sports (bowling, tennis, golf, softball), and go dancing. Anyone can begin the journey toward wellness with a single step and begin reaping health benefits immediately.

SUMMARY

The sedentary lifestyle of most Americans is seriously undermining the health and welfare of our nation. We are fast becoming overfat and under-fit, resulting in reduced levels of well-being. From the information you have acquired in this chapter, you now have the tools necessary to confidently develop a personalized physical fitness program, based on sound scientific principles and your age, resting heart rate, interests, and abilities. You also realize there is a difference among exercising for athletic performance, for health, and for CRE fitness. You have gained a better understanding of the health benefits that can be achieved by incorporating moderate activity into your daily life. By applying the FITT prescription factors and the concept of a three-segment workout and by finding ways to increase daily activity, you can be on your way to a lifetime of improved health, fitness, and wellness.

REFERENCES

1. Pate, Russell R., et al. "Physical Activity and Public Health. A Recommendation from the Centers for Disease Control and Prevention and the American College of Sports Medicine." *Journal of American Medical Association* 273, no. 5 (February 1, 1995): 402.

2. Powell, Kenneth E., and Steven N. Blair. "The Public Health Burdens of Sedentary Living Habits: Theoretical but Realistic Estimates." *Medicine and Science in Sports and Exercise* 26, no. 7 (1994): 851–56.

3. Kuczmarski, Robert J., et al. "Increasing Prevalence of Overweight Among U.S. Adults." *Journal of American Medical Association* 272, no. 3 (July 20, 1994): 315.

4. Kuczmarski. "Increasing Prevalence of Overweight Among U.S. Adults."

5. Bar-Or, O. "A Commentary to Children and Fitness: A Public Health Perspective." *Research Quarterly for Exercise and Sport* 58 (1987): 304.

6. Ignico, Arlene. "A Comparison of Fitness Levels of Children Enrolled in Daily and Weekly Physical Education Programs." *Journal of Human Movement Studies* 18 (1990): 129–39.

7. "The National Children and Youth Fitness Study II." *Journal of Health, Physical Education, Recreation and Dance* (November–December 1987): 50.

8. Bar-Or, O. "A Commentary to Children and Fitness: A Public Health Perspective."

9. Blair, Steven N. "Are American Children and Youth Fit? The Need for Better Data." *Research Quarterly for Exercise and Sport* 63 (1992): 120–23.

10. Corbin, C. B., and Pangrazi, R. P. "Are American Children and Youth Fit? The Need for Better Data." *Research Quarterly for Exercise and Sport* 63 (1992): 96–106.

11. Blair, S., H. Kohl, R. Paffenbarger, D. Clark, K. Cooper, L. Gibbons. "Physical Fitness and All-Cause Mortality: A Prospective Study of Healthy Men and Women." *JAMA* 66, no. 17 (November 3, 1989): 2,395.

12. "The Health Benefits of Exercise (Part I): A Round Table." *The Physician and Sports Medicine* 15, no. 10 (1987): 131.

13. Hoeger, Werner. *Principles and Labs for Physical Fitness and Wellness*. Englewood, Colo.: Morton Publishing Co., 1988.

14. "1992 Health Guide, Fitness, No Pain and Lots of Gain." *U.S. News and World Report* (May 4, 1992): 30.

15. "1992 Health Guide, Fitness, No Pain and Lots of Gain."

16. Karvonen, M., K. Kentala, and O. Mustala. "The Effects of Training on Heart Rate: A Longitudinal Study." *Annals of Medicine and Experimental Biology* 35 (1957): 307–15.

17. American Running and Fitness Association. *Running and Fitness* 10, no. 6 (June 1992): 3.

18. Svedenhag, Jan, and Jan Seger. "Running on Land and in Water: Comparative Exercise Physiology." *Medicine and Science in Sports and Exercise* 24, no. 10 (1992): 1155–69.

19. Borg, G. "Psychophysical Bases of Physical Exertion." *Medicine and Science in Sport and Exercise* 14 (1982): 707.

20. Nash, Joyce D. "Why Exercise Isn't a Habit." *Healthline* (December 1994): 2.

21. Dishman, Rod K. "Prescribing Exercise Intensity for Healthy Adults Using Perceived Exertion." *Medicine and Science in Sports and Exercise* 26, no. 9 (1994): 1087–94.

22. Cooper Institute for Aerobics Research, ed. *Reebok Instructors News* 5, no. 2 (1992): 8.

23. Powel and Blair. "The Public Health Burdens of Sedentary Living Habits: Theoretical But Realistic Estimates," 851.

24. Paffenbarger, Ralph S., et al. "The Association of Changes in Physical Activity Level and Other Lifestyle Characteristics with Mortality Among Men." *The New England Journal of Medicine* (February 25, 1993): 887.

25. Pate. "Physical Activity and Public Health. A Recommendation from the Centers for Disease Control and Prevention and the American College of Sports Medicine," 402.

26. Blair, Steven N. "Physical Activity, Physical Fitness and Health" (C. H. McCoy Research Lecture). *Research Quarterly for Exercise and Sport* 64, no. 4 (December 1993): 365.

27. U.S. Department of Health and Human Services Public Health Services. *Healthy People 2000: National Health Promotion and Disease Prevention Objectives.* D.H.H.S. Publication No. 19–50212 (1991).

28. Pate. "Physical Activity and Public Health. A Recommendation from the Centers for Disease Control and Prevention and the American College of Sports Medicine," 402.

29. Kohl, H. W., III, Steven N. Blair, et al. "Changes in Physical Fitness and All-Cause Mortality; A Perspective Study of Healthy and Unhealthy Men." *Journal of American Medical Association* 273, no. 14 (April 12, 1995): 1,093.

30. Lee, I-M., C. Hsieh, R. S. Paffenbarger. "Exercise Intensity and Longevity in Men: The Harvard Alumni Health Study." *Journal of American Medical Association* 273, no. 15 (April 19, 1995): 1,179.

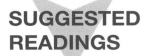

SUGGESTED READINGS

American College of Sports Medicine. *ACSM Fitness Book.* Champaign, Ill.: Human Kinetics Publishers, 1992.

Baechle, Thomas R., and Roger Earle. *Fitness Weight Training.* Champaign, Ill.: Human Kinetics Publishers, 1995.

Blair, S. N. *Living with Exercise.* Dallas, Tex.: American Health Publishing Company, 1991.

Brooks, Christine. "Active Lifestyle Motivation." *Fitness Management* (May 1992).

Corbin, Charles, and Ruth Lindsey. *Concepts of Physical Fitness with Laboratories.* Dubuque, Iowa: Wm. C. Brown Communications, 1991.

Dawber, T. R. *The Framingham Study.* Cambridge, Mass.: Harvard University Press, 1980.

Dishman, Rod. *Advances in Exercise Adherence.* Champaign, Ill.: Human Kinetics Publishers, 1994.

Dishman, Rod. "Exercise Adherence Research: Future Directions." *American Journal of Health Promotion* 3, no. 1 (summer 1988): 53–56.

Gaines, Mary Beth Pappas. *Fantastic Water Workouts.* Champaign, Ill.: Human Kinetics Publishers, 1993.

Gavin, James. *The Exercise Habit.* Champaign, Ill.: Human Kinetics Publishers, 1992.

Golding, Lawrence, and Clayton Myers. *Y's Way to Physical Fitness. The Complete Guide to Fitness Testing and Instruction.* Champaign, Ill.: Human Kinetics Publishers, 1989.

American College of Sportsmedicine. *Guidelines for Graded Exercise Testing and Exercise Prescription.* Philadelphia: Lea and Febiger, 1991.

Haywood, K. M. 1991. "The Role of Physical Education in the Development of Active Lifestyle" *Research Quarterly for Exercise and Sport* 62 (1991): 151–56.

Howley, Edward, and Don Franks. *Health Fitness Instructor's Handbook.* Champaign, Ill.: Human Kinetics Publishers, 1992.

Klug, Gary, and Janice Lettunich. *Exercise and Physical Fitness.* Guilford, Conn.: The Dushkin Publishing Group, Inc., 1992.

McNickle, R. G. *Cross Training: Combining Sports for Exciting Balanced Total-Body Workouts.* Stamford, Conn.: Longmeadow Press, 1994.

Mackinnon, Laurel. *Exercise and Immunology.* Champaign, Ill.: Human Kinetics Publishers, Inc., 1992.

Paffenbarger, R. S., Jr., A. L. Wing, and R. T. Hyde. "Physical Activity as an Index of Heart Attack Risk in College Alumni." *American Journal of Epidemiology* 108 (September 1978): 161–75.

Paffenbarger, R. S., Jr., R. T. Hyde, A. L. Wing, et al. "Physical Activity, All Cause Mortality, and Longevity of College Alumni," *New England Journal of Medicine* 314 (March 10, 1988): 605–13.

Roberts, Glyn. *Motivation in Sport and Exercise.* Champaign, Ill.: Human Kinetics Publishers, 1992.

Seaman, Janet, ed. *Physical Best and Individuals with Disabilities: A Handbook for Inclusion in Fitness Programs.* Reston, Va.: American Association for Active Lifestyles and Fitness of American Alliance for Health, Physical Education, Recreation and Dance (1900 Association Drive, Reston, VA 22091–1599), 1995.

Safran, M. R., W. E. Garrett, A. V. Seaber, et al. "The Role of Warm-up in Muscular Injury Prevention." *American Journal of Sportsmedicine* 16, no. 2 (1988): 123–29.

Samuelson, Joan. *Running for Women.* Emmaus, Penn.: Rodale Press, 1995.

Summary of Findings from National Children and Youth Fitness Study II. *Journal of Health, Physical Education, Recreation and Dance* (November/December 1988): 49–96.

"The Health Benefits of Exercise (Part II): A Round Table." *The Physician and Sportsmedicine* 15, no. 11 (November 1987): 120–31.

U.S. Department of Health and Human Services, Public Health Service. *Healthy People 2000: National Health Promotion and Disease Prevention Objectives.* H.H.S. Publication No. 19-50212 (1991).

Van Camp. S. P. "The Fixx Tragedy: A Cardiologist's Perspective." *The Physician and Sportsmedicine* 12, no. 9 (1984): 153–55.

Weinberg, Robert. *Foundations of Sport Psychology.* Champaign, Ill.: Human Kinetics Publishers, 1995.

Yacenda, John. *Fitness Cross-Training.* Champaign, Ill.: Human Kinetics Publishers, 1995.

chapter 3

Strength and Flexibility

➤ Objectives

After reading this chapter, you will be able to:

1. Identify five benefits of strength training.

2. List five cautions for strength training.

3. Identify two differences between training programs for strength and programs for muscular endurance.

4. Describe three types of muscle contraction and give an example of each.

5. Define three principles of strength training.

6. Identify correct safety guidelines for weight training.

7. List four out of five types of strength programs.

8. List and define two types of stretching.

9. Identify correct guidelines for flexibility development.

10. Define the chapter terms.

Terms

- Agonist
- Antagonist
- Circuit
- Concentric contraction
- Dynamic flexibility
- Eccentric contraction
- Isokinetic

- Isometric
- Isotonic
- Muscular power
- Plyometrics
- Progressive overload
- Proprioceptive neuromuscular facilitation (PNF)

- Repetition (rep)
- Repetition maximum (1 RM)
- Set
- Static flexibility
- Stretch reflex
- Valsalva maneuver

Exercise is a gift you give yourself.

Anonymous

a t one time, physical fitness programs consisted almost entirely of strength and flexibility exercises. Then, in the 1970s, aerobic activities rose to prominence. As a result, strength and flexibility exercises were swept into the role of supplemental activities and added to the main workout only if time permitted. As people flocked to gyms for aerobics, they were exposed to weight training and began to value the benefits of muscular fitness. Today, as the emphasis on balanced fitness grows, strength and flexibility assume new importance. They can enhance ability to perform daily tasks as well as athletic performance. Muscular strength and endurance make it easier to perform routine activities such as carrying groceries upstairs, lifting a child, or moving the couch. Flexibility enables us to reach, bend, twist, and perform movements without excessive tightness or stiffness. Enhanced strength and flexibility allow us to perform vigorous activity with less risk of straining muscles or connective tissue, so they are important in the prevention and rehabilitation of injuries.

Muscular Fitness

Many people start muscular fitness programs in order to look better, feel better, shape and tone muscles, or increase lean muscle mass. At the same time, they increase muscular strength and endurance. In this section, we will first examine benefits, muscle structure and function, general principles, safety, and specific exercise programs for muscular strength and endurance. Flexibility development will be covered in the second part of the chapter.

Strength Training: Benefits and Cautions

An advantage of aerobic activities is their cardiorespiratory benefits. Strength training can offer additional benefits, whether your goal is health-related fitness or improved athletic performance.

Weight Control. The more muscle a person has, the higher his or her metabolism and the more calories he or she burns, even at rest. This is one reason men can consume more calories without gaining weight than can women of equal size—the average male has roughly twice the muscle mass of the average female. Muscle is active, high-metabolic tissue, while fat is storage tissue. Weight training increases muscle mass, so it makes weight control easier. While women do not appear to gain as much muscle as men do from weight training, when differences in body size are taken into account, gains are comparable. Over a four- to six-month period, a man may gain 4 to 6 pounds of muscle and a woman 2 to 3 pounds. Muscle is denser than fat and pound for pound takes up less space, so as muscle is gained, if fat is lost, the result is a loss of unwanted inches. While aerobic exercise and a nutritious low-fat diet are the quickest ways to reduce body fat, weight training does offer advantages in long-term weight control.

Weight Gain. For those who wish to gain weight, increasing lean muscle mass, not fat, is a desirable goal, and there is no better way than weight training. However, rate and quantity of muscle tissue gains vary from person to person because they are partially genetically determined. Those with a naturally tall, lean build tend to gain muscle slower than do those with a stockier build, and men gain faster than women. A weight-gain program is outlined in the weight-training section for those who wish to increase lean weight.

Appearance. Developing a lean, well-toned body is the main reason many people exercise. If you feel that you need to lose weight, but your body fat percentage is in the average range, reevaluate. Weight loss alone does not give a firm, well-toned appearance to flabby thighs or abdominals. Weight training is the most effective way to shape and tone muscles, resulting in a trimmer appearance. Posture improves when agonist/antagonist muscles are in balance. Strengthening weak muscles and stretching tight, inflexible muscles helps develop good body alignment so that you move more fluidly and feel and look better.

Time Economy. Instead of doing 50 leg lifts without weights, you can cut your workout time by adding resistance. Lift a weight heavy enough to produce fatigue in 8 to 12 repetitions, and you will get more benefit in fewer lifts. For basic strength fitness, a balanced weight-training workout of 10 to 12 exercises takes approximately 30 minutes to complete. Despite what you may observe in the gym, more is not necessary. While body builders, competitive weightlifters, or other strength-event athletes will work out much more than this, keep in mind that they have different goals. Health-related fitness levels can be developed and maintained in much less training time than is needed for competition.

Energy. Performance and efficiency improve with strength training—more work can be done with less effort as muscular strength and endurance increase.

Athletic Performance. All other things being equal, a strong person can run faster, jump higher, and throw a ball farther than can a weaker individual.[1]

Injury Prevention. Aerobic exercises such as jogging and aerobic dance have the potential to cause injury through repetitive, forceful impact against unyielding surfaces. Strong, flexible muscles and connective tissue can better withstand the stress of many forceful landings during a workout. When ligaments, tendons, muscle, and bone are strengthened through muscular exercise, risk of injury is decreased.[2] Many aerobic activities tend to develop strength in only a few groups of muscles, leaving others weak. For example, jogging strengthens quadriceps but leaves the hamstrings weak. Weak muscle groups are more susceptible to strains or pulls. A well-designed strength-training program develops balanced, proportional strength in both agonists (prime movers) and antagonists (opposing muscle groups). If injury does occur, it may be less severe and may heal more quickly if the muscle is well-conditioned. A carefully designed program can also rehabilitate injuries to regain normal (or better) strength levels. For more detailed information on injury prevention, see Chapter 5.

Bone Strength. Resistance exercises decrease the risk of osteoporosis.[3] The pull of muscles on bone in weight-bearing exercise stimulates development of increased bone density and preserves existing bone. Lifting heavy weights in a few repetitions may be more effective in increasing bone mass than is lifting a light weight many times.

Flexibility. Moving weights through a full range of motion, from full extension to full contraction, both stretches and strengthens muscles. This is an important training technique to master in order to maintain flexibility. Muscles become shortened if exercises are performed repeatedly through only a partial range of motion.

Cholesterol. Although little significant change in max VO_2 occurs in strength training, studies have shown a significant reduction in total cholesterol and total cholesterol/HDL ratios after three to four months of weight training. The studies suggest that strength training may lower cardiovascular disease risk.

Psychological Benefits. While many people begin an exercise program in order to improve appearance, many other less visible but equally important effects may result. Benefits in the emotional dimension of wellness from regular exercise include feeling better, decreased stress, decreased depression, and enhanced self-esteem and self-confidence.

Social Benefits. In addition to offering physical and psychological benefits, lifting with a partner or friend offers social benefits. There are many more opportunities for conversation and interaction when you work out with someone than when you watch a movie.

Benefits at Any Age. Regardless of your age, you can benefit from strength training. It is untrue that loss of strength is inevitable with age or that older people cannot gain strength. While the typical sedentary individual can lose up to 30 percent of his or her muscle mass between the ages of 20 and 70, this loss is more from atrophy due to disuse rather than to aging alone. Recent studies including people in their 70s, 80s, and 90s participating in weight training have shown that they increased muscle mass, more than doubled their strength, and improved their functional mobility and ability to perform daily living activities.[4,5,6,7]

Disadvantages and Cautions. Although strength training has many benefits, it does have disadvantages. Strength training is not a complete exercise program since it does not develop cardiorespiratory endurance. As in any physical activity, injury is possible if you are careless or ignore safety procedures. You may have trouble accessing equipment. Also, you can expect some mild muscle soreness during the first week of your program.

Individuals with cardiovascular problems or high blood pressure should seek medical guidance due to the tendency of blood pressure to increase during strength training.[8] Those who have hernias, arthritis, or lower back problems should also seek medical clearance. Individuals with these health concerns may benefit from strength training but should be aware that they may need special exercise modifications.

Avoid use of hand and ankle weights during jogging, high-impact aerobic dance workouts, or other activities involving running and jumping. Ankle weights particularly distort proper form, increase stress to legs and feet, and increase risk of strains and sprains. While small increases in oxygen consumption and caloric expenditure do result from using light weights, the same effect can be produced with less risk by exercising longer or harder.

When used with controlled form and rhythm in a muscle toning or walking program, however, light weights are beneficial for increasing heart rate and upper body strength. All in all, strength training offers few drawbacks and many major advantages for the time invested.

Muscle Function

Muscles are made of individual muscle fibers bound together and sheathed in connective tissue. They end in a tendon that connects the muscle to a bone. An example is the Achilles tendon, which you can feel above your heel, connecting your calf to your foot. Muscle fibers can contract to shorten the muscle or relax and return to their resting length. They are also elastic. They can be stretched and will spring back to their resting length.

Muscles cannot expand and push. Movement is produced as muscle contracts, shortens, and pulls on bones across a joint. As a muscle on one side of a bone contracts, a muscle on the other side must relax to allow movement to occur. The contracting muscle that initiates movement is called the **agonist.** The opposing muscle is called the **antagonist.** In a biceps curl (Fig. 3.1), the agonist is the biceps, and the antagonist is the triceps. In a triceps extension, the roles reverse.

Determinants of Muscular Strength

Strength gains result from neurologic and muscular adaptations. Dramatic strength gains early in a program are often due to a "learning effect"—that is, you learn how to lift weights more efficiently. Your body both represses its self-protective reflexes and increases its ability to fully recruit muscle fibers when needed.[9]

Your overall potential for development of muscular strength is determined by the number and size of muscle fibers you possess and how well your muscular system can recruit them during muscular effort. The more muscle fibers you have, the larger they are, and the better your system is at activating them during muscular effort, the greater your strength. While the number of muscle fibers you possess is genetically determined, size and muscle fiber recruitment are a product of training.

Muscle Fiber Recruitment

When a muscle contracts, only the number of muscle fibers required for that momentary effort will shorten. Individual muscle fibers cannot contract partially. They either are working as hard as possible or not at all. This is called the *all-or-nothing principle*. For example, when a biceps curl calls for a 50 percent effort, all fibers in the muscle do not contract at 50 percent effort; rather, a portion of the muscle's fibers contract fully while the remainder rest. After these first muscle fibers contract, fatigue slightly decreases their ability to apply force. On each subsequent contraction, more fibers must be recruited to continue to lift the same

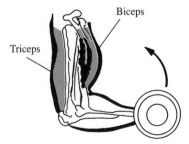

Biceps

Triceps

FIGURE 3.1 ➤
Biceps curl demonstrating muscle function.

weight. After several muscle contractions, enough fibers are fatigued that the muscle temporarily can no longer generate the same effort in what is called *temporary muscular failure*. Muscle fibers increase strength only if they are stimulated by intensity of effort. If your goal is to develop maximal muscular strength, try to recruit, or activate, as many muscle fibers as possible by working a muscle to a state of temporary muscular failure. If you are working for health-related fitness levels, a less intense effort is adequate.

Muscle Hypertrophy

When muscles grow stronger, muscle fibers hypertrophy or increase in size. This increase occurs in both men and women and is proportional to muscle mass. Since the average man has about twice the muscle mass of the average woman, hypertrophy in men is more pronounced.

Some women worry that they will develop big shoulders or massive, masculine musculature by weight training, and this myth is reinforced by televised images of women's bodybuilding competitions. Be assured that shoulder width, like hip width, is strongly influenced by genetics and that significant muscle gains require years of strenuous daily effort. They don't occur by accident, nor with a 30-minute muscle toning workout three times a week.

Muscular Strength, Muscular Endurance, and Muscular Power

In increasing muscular strength, endurance, or power, the key variables are resistance, repetitions, and speed. The purest example of strength is one maximal lift, and the closer a program comes to this, the greater the strength gains. However, risk of injury is high when working at or near maximal levels. Athletes working to develop strength often exercise at 80 percent to 95 percent or higher effort a few (three to six) times. Muscular endurance is enhanced by contracting repeatedly (i.e., one to two sets of 15 to 20 reps) with moderate (50 percent to 60 percent) effort.

There is some crossover effect between muscular strength and muscular endurance. Development of muscular strength also produces some increase in muscular endurance; for example, if you can lift a 100-pound weight five times, you can probably lift a 5-pound weight 20 times. However, muscular endurance does not enhance strength. If you can lift a 5-pound weight 20 times, you may not be able to lift a 100-pound weight even once. If you want to develop both muscular strength and endurance, a muscular strength program can pay double benefits.

Muscular power, a function of strength and speed, is the ability to apply force rapidly. Power is increased by performing a muscle contraction quickly, as in plyometric exercises, discussed later in this chapter. While muscular power is not necessary for health-related physical fitness, it is an asset in many sports.

Types of Strength Training Programs

Three basic types of muscle contraction are isometric, isotonic, and isokinetic. Different strength programs have been developed for each type.

Isometric

Iso means "equal or constant" and *meter* refers to length. In **isometric** exercise, the muscle contracts but does not change length, and no movement occurs. If you pushed your palms together hard, your pectoral muscles would contract and try to shorten, but your arms would not move (Fig. 3.2). An advantage of isometric exercise is that it requires little or no equipment and can be done almost anywhere—for instance, while sitting at a desk. However, because resistance is applied at only one point in your range of motion, strength development is limited. Also, it is difficult to know how much force is being exerted, so strength gains are not as easy to observe as when equipment is being used. Three isometric exercises are illustrated in Figure 3.2. For additional exercises, consult the suggested readings at the end of this chapter. Caution: For these and other strength exercises, breathe throughout the exercise. Do not hold your breath during exertion, as this can produce a potentially harmful elevation in blood pressure.

FIGURE 3.2 ➤
Isometric exercises.

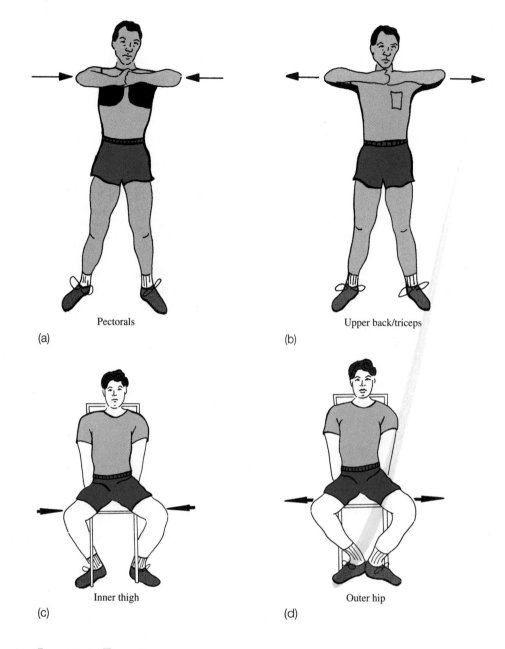

Pectorals
(a)

Upper back/triceps
(b)

Inner thigh
(c)

Outer hip
(d)

Isometric Exercises

A. *Pectorals:* Press palms together at chest level for a count of five. Repeat five times.

B. *Upper back/triceps:* Clasp hands together at chest level. Pull outward for a count of five. Repeat 10 to 15 times.

C. *Inner thigh:* Sitting, place your knees outside the chair legs. Squeeze your thighs together for a count of five. Repeat 10 to 15 times.

D. *Outer hip:* Sitting, place your feet inside the chair legs. Press out for a count of five. Repeat 10 to 15 times.

Isotonic

Tonic refers to tone or tension, so in **isotonic** exercise as the muscle contracts, tension, or force, is controlled throughout the motion. Isotonic contractions may be either concentric or eccentric.

In a **concentric contraction,** a muscle shortens as it overcomes resistance. For example, a weight is lifted as the biceps contract during the lifting phase of a biceps curl. **Eccentric contraction** occurs when a muscle lengthens and contracts at the same time, gradually allowing a force to overcome muscular resistance; for example, the biceps contracts eccentrically during the lowering phase of a biceps curl. Eccentric contraction is an important component of strength development because it makes up half of the muscular effort.

Advantages of isotonic exercise are that it strengthens through a full range of motion, the load is measurable, and a variety of isotonic programs are available. Calisthenics, free weights, or machines such as Universal or Nautilus use isotonic exercise.

Isokinetic

Kinetic means "motion," and in **isokinetic** exercise, speed of movement is controlled. If you apply great force or a light force, the resistance is adjusted to maintain a constant rate of contraction. The advantage of isokinetic work is that the load is totally controlled by the efforts of the user. The disadvantage is that it requires special machinery, such as Cybex or Orthotron, often used by athletic trainers for injury rehabilitation. You can get a sense of isokinetic movement by sweeping an arm through water. The harder you press, the more resistance you create.

Principles of Strength Training

Principles of strength development include progressive overload, specificity, and recovery.

Progressive Overload

Progressive overload is the most important principle of strength development. To stimulate a muscle to increase strength, it must gradually be overloaded or forced to work at a higher than normal effort. Either the number of lifts performed or the amount of weight must gradually be increased. Increasing the number of repetitions increases muscular endurance. Increasing the weight lifted increases strength. General programs increase both until a desired maintenance goal is reached.

You must exercise three times per week to improve muscular fitness. To maintain strength, two intense workouts are adequate.

Specificity

The speed of contraction, range of motion, amount and type of resistance, and number and type of exercise are a few of the variables that determine the results of strength training. If you desire a specific result, such as an increase in muscle mass, your program must be designed and executed to produce that result.

Recovery

Exercise stimulates the muscle to take in more protein and nutrients and undergo changes that increase its ability to forcefully contract. After a workout, you will be weaker, not stronger, due to fatigue. Improvement occurs during recovery, which gives the muscle fibers time to repair and grow. Strength workouts are best done every other day (48 hours rest) to allow recovery and improvement to occur.

Guidelines for Strength Development

Optimal results can be obtained from any strength-training program and risk of injury can be minimized if you follow the guidelines in Table 3.1.

Sequence

Ideally, work large muscle groups first, ending with small muscle groups. It is difficult to adequately exercise large muscle groups if you have already fatigued the smaller supporting muscles. The suggested order of exercises is hips/legs, torso, arms, abdominals (see the sample weight-training program).

Form

Never sacrifice form for weight. After progressive overload, correct exercise form is the most important (and most neglected) factor in maximizing strength gains and mini-

table 3.1

SAFETY GUIDELINES FOR STRENGTH TRAINING

1. Warm up before each workout and stretch afterward.
2. Use good technique—keep your abdominals tight, back straight, hips tucked under, knees relaxed.
3. Work each exercise through a full range of motion from full extension without lockout to full contraction.
4. Perform each exercise smoothly, with control. Do not swing the limbs or use momentum. Faster is not better.
5. Before you lift, inhale. Exhale on the exertion. Do not hold your breath.

mizing risk of injury. Improvement is more rapid if correct technique, not just quantity of weight, is emphasized. Always work through a complete range of motion for flexibility and maximum strength gains. Move from full extension without lockout to full flexion. Keep your back straight and abdominals tight to protect your lower back. In addition, when doing standing exercises, keep your knees slightly bent and your hips tucked under to support your back. Avoid "cheating," a breakdown in exercise form that occurs when extra muscles are utilized to complete the exercise, decreasing the load to the prime mover. Cheating generally occurs when the load is too heavy or you are fatigued. Remember: Quality of work is more important than the amount of repetitions or weight lifted.

Rest Between Sets

A rest period between sets of an exercise should allow sufficient recovery so that good form can be maintained. This time will vary, depending on the intensity of lifting, with 1 to 2 minutes rest recommended between sets of a general program, and 2 to 4 minutes between sets of a strength program. To make efficient use of time, you may alternate exercises on different body parts—for example, legs, then arms—so that one muscle group is recovering while you are working another.

Muscle Balance

Since muscles work in pairs, it is important to strengthen muscles on both sides of a bone so that they pull evenly across joints and maintain body alignment. For example, if pectorals are stronger than upper back muscles, rounded shoulders result. When upper back muscles are strengthened, shoulders are naturally held erect. Tight lower back muscles opposed by weak, sagging abdominals pull the back into an exaggerated curve. This stresses lumbar vertebrae, increasing back fatigue and risk of lower back pain. Well-toned abdominals support the back, improve appearance, and prevent back problems. Strength programs must be planned to develop proportional strength in the following muscle pairs: biceps/triceps, pectorals/trapezius-rhomboids, abdominals/lower back, hamstrings/quadriceps, gastrocnemius/anterior tibialis, and deltoids/latissimus dorsi (Figure 3.3).

Breathing

Exhale on the exertion; inhale on the release. Holding your breath while you strain against a closed epiglottis is called the **Valsalva maneuver** and can elevate blood pressure dangerously.

Speed of Movement

Exercising in a smooth, controlled manner maximizes strength gains and reduces injuries. Take two seconds to lift (concentric or shortening contraction) and two to four seconds to lower (eccentric or lengthening contraction). Control the movement; do

FIGURE 3.3 ➤
Major muscles of the body.
Front.

From John W. Hole, Jr., Human
Anatomy and Physiology, *4th ed.
Copyright © 1987 Wm. C. Brown
Publishers, Dubuque, Iowa. All
Rights Reserved. Reprinted by
permission.*

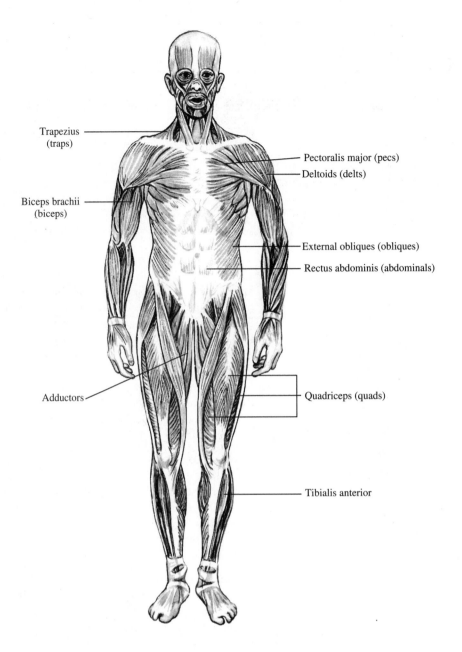

Trapezius (traps)

Pectoralis major (pecs)

Deltoids (delts)

Biceps brachii (biceps)

External obliques (obliques)

Rectus abdominis (abdominals)

Quadriceps (quads)

Adductors

Tibialis anterior

not fling, swing, or kick. Jerky movements will cause excessive wear and tear on your joints. Also, when you use momentum to perform an exercise, you apply force and develop strength only through the first part of the movement. Lower a limb with the same control used to lift it. Do not drop weights with a crash. You are stronger lowering a weight than lifting it.

Strength-Training Programs

There are many different kinds of strength-training programs. The type of program you select will depend on your goals and the type of equipment (if any) you plan to use. Regardless of the type of program you select, you can keep track of your progress with the Strength-Training Log in the Activities (p. 371).

Weight Training

Weight training is a noncompetitive exercise program used to develop several health-related physical fitness components: muscular strength, muscular endurance, flexibility, and body composition. It differs significantly in its goals from the competitive sports of weight lifting and bodybuilding. Male, female, young, old, athlete, or fitness exerciser—

FIGURE 3.3 ➤
Major muscles of the body. Back.

From John W. Hole, Jr., Human Anatomy and Physiology, 4th ed. Copyright © 1987 Wm. C. Brown Publishers, Dubuque, Iowa. All Rights Reserved. Reprinted by permission.

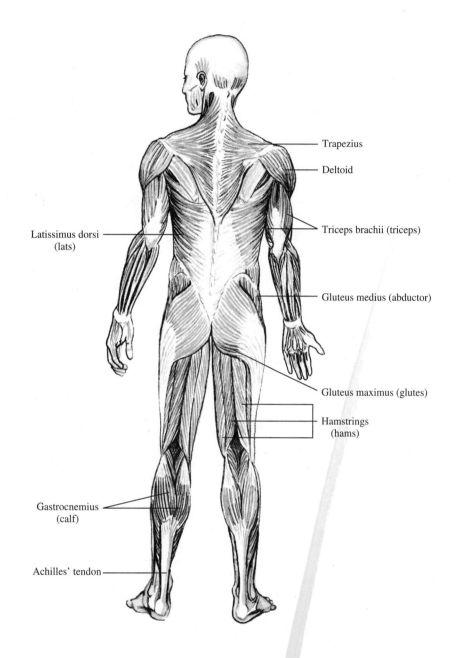

Trapezius

Deltoid

Triceps brachii (triceps)

Latissimus dorsi (lats)

Gluteus medius (abductor)

Gluteus maximus (glutes)

Hamstrings (hams)

Gastrocnemius (calf)

Achilles' tendon

all benefit from weight training. Beginners with low levels of muscular fitness benefit the most and will notice results more quickly than will experienced lifters. Weight training can build strength levels so that recreational, competitive, or daily activities are accomplished more easily, with less strain and fatigue.

What to Wear
Any comfortable workout gear will do. Shorts, T-shirt, and nonslip rubber-soled shoes are appropriate. A towel is useful for wiping sweat off your hands to prevent a slippery grip. Lifting gloves, which improve your grip, and a lifting belt to support your lower back and abdominals are not essential, though some lifters prefer to use them.

Equipment
For beginners, it really doesn't matter what type of equipment is used. A beginner will improve on almost any type of program as long as an adequate overload is provided. Two major types of equipment used in weight training are free weights and machines. Both have advantages and disadvantages.

table 3.2

SAFETY USING WEIGHTS

1. Never attempt to lift more than you know you can handle. Work out—don't show off.
2. Always make sure that the weight pins, bars, or collars are secure.
3. Don't lift weights alone. Always work with someone else.
4. Keep sweat wiped off your hands; it makes weights slippery.
5. When using free weights, work with a trained spotter.
6. Return all equipment to the proper place. Don't leave it lying around for someone to trip over.

Free weights are far less expensive than machines, so you can have your own set at home. Free weights cost about $100 on sale, double that if you add a padded bench and rack. Machines can cost upward of $500 to $5,000. You have more variety of exercises on free weights than on machines because you have the freedom to lift in so many different positions. Lifting with proper technique is crucial. A wrong move can cause injury with any lifting but particularly with free weights. To lift free weights safely, you must have a skilled spotting partner who can handle the weight in case you start to lose control. For strength development, free weights have an advantage over machines since they develop strength not only in the prime movers, but also in muscles required to balance and control the weight. Follow the guidelines in Table 3.2.

Machines such as Nautilus and Universal are easy to use and safer than free weights because they guide your movements and control the weights. An advantage of Nautilus equipment is that it prestretches the muscle and takes the joint through the full range of motion. Also, it provides variable resistance, adjusting the load for strength variations throughout a lift. Universal gives the exerciser more control over range of motion and allows people to work more closely together. Because of the cost of machines, it is best to start your machine-workout program at a health club or gym. Proper lifting technique is easier to learn on machines, and you won't need a spotting partner. Loads can be changed quickly, so the workout may take less time than with free weights. For safety, convenience, and time, machines have the edge.

Weight Room Etiquette

Be aware of and follow common weight room etiquette guidelines while working out:

➤ Wipe sweat off benches after use.
➤ Rerack weights when you are done.
➤ Don't lay around on the equipment chatting between sets if someone else is waiting to use the machine. Let them work in between sets while you are resting.
➤ Don't drop or bang the weights together. This can damage the equipment and increases the noise level unnecessarily.

Program for General Conditioning

A conditioning program should develop balanced strength. Many muscle strains occur because of weakness in the pulled muscle or its opposing muscle. A general strength program prevents strength imbalances. If you exercised only problem areas, you would increase imbalances. The following exercises, listed in the order of large to small muscle groups, may be done on Universal (Figure 3.4). Alternate free weight exercises are listed in parentheses. These may be done with a set of barbells or hand weights. If you plan to use Nautilus equipment, your first workouts should include learning how to adjust and efficiently use the equipment.

FIGURE 3.4 ➤
Weight training exercises.

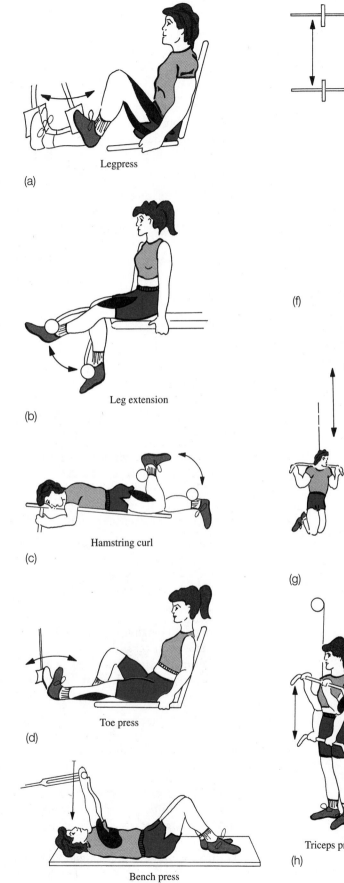

(a) Legpress

(b) Leg extension

(c) Hamstring curl

(d) Toe press

(e) Bench press

(f) Military press

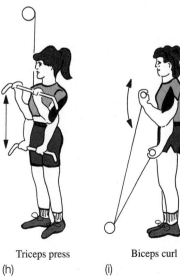

(g) Lat pull

(h) Triceps press

(i) Biceps curl

Weight Training Exercises

A. Leg press (squats on free weights)
Prime movers: quadriceps, hamstrings, and gluteus maximus
On leg press, sit on seat, adjust position to last slot or to a 90 degree knee angle. Place feet squarely on pedals, press out smoothly (do not lock knees), and return to starting position.

B. Leg extension (lunge on free weights)
Prime movers: quadriceps
Sit on bench with both feet under the rollers. Toe in slightly. Do not lie back. Extend your legs, hold 1 second, and return to starting position.

C. Hamstring curl (squats)
Prime movers: hamstrings and gluteus maximus
Lie face down on the bench, hook both heels under the rollers. Position knees at the pivot point where the rollers attach to the bench. Pull up to 90 degrees, hold for one second, and return to starting position.

D. Toe press (calf raise with free weights)
Prime mover: gastrocnemius
On leg press station, place feet squarely on pedals, press out to full leg extension without knee lockout. Press with toes from flat-footed position to foot extension and return.

E. Bench press (same with free weights)
Prime movers: pectorals and triceps
Lie on bench, head next to the machine. The grips should be lined up approximately with the shoulders. Place your feet flat on the bench with knees bent and back flat. Press to extension and return.

F. Military press (same with free weights)
Prime movers: deltoids and triceps
Sit on the stool or stand with abdominals tight, back flat, and knees slightly bent. With shoulders close to handles, extend upward with arms until they are straight but not locked and return.

G. Lat pull (pull-ups or rowing with free weights)
Prime movers: latissimus dorsi
Grip bar directly above shoulders or at handles. Pull down until you are kneeling or sitting. From this position, pull down to chest or touch the back of shoulders and return.

H. Triceps press (standing tricep press)
Prime movers: triceps
Stand facing lat bar. With palms facing down, grasp the bar so that hands are shoulder-width apart. Keep elbows at waist. Press down to extension and return.

I. Biceps curl (same)
Prime movers: biceps
Stand facing the weights, hold bar with both hands, palms up. Flex arms until the bar meets shoulders. Return to starting position. Keep back straight, abdominals firm.

How to Begin and Progress

A good general conditioning program would involve lifting one to two sets of 8 to 12 repetitions three times per week (for instance, M-W-F). A **repetition (rep)** is one lift; a **set** is a group of lifts.

The first week, a beginner should lift one set of 8 to 12 repetitions under the supervision of a trained professional. The first workouts should use light weights and concentrate on form, rhythm, and breathing. This will also minimize muscular soreness. The second week, an additional set can be added, and the third week, a starting load can be established.

Establishing Your Workload

To establish your workload, for each exercise find the maximum amount of weight you can lift once with good form (one **repetition maximum** or **1 RM**). Seventy-five percent of that weight will be your workload. In the workout, lift to fatigue at each station. If you can do fewer than six reps, the weight is too heavy. If you can do 12 or more reps at that load, the weight is too light. Increase or decrease the load the next workout, if necessary. At the correct workload, the last two reps of each exercise should be difficult for you to do, and you should reach temporary muscular failure between 8 and 12 reps.

Increasing Your Workload

When you can do 12 reps, increase the amount of weight. If you can do at least six reps at the new weight, stay with that weight until you can do 12 reps. If, when you increase the weight you cannot do at least six reps, drop back to your old weight and increase the number of reps each time until you can do 15. You should then be able to increase the weight and do at least six reps.

Variety

You can incorporate variety into your workout by changing the workload, recovery period, number of sets, reps, rhythm, and number or order of lifts. Here are a few examples of different programs:

1. *General:* two sets of 8 to 12 reps at 70% to 75% 1 RM. Rest 1 to 2 minutes between sets.
2. *Strength:* three sets of four to six reps at 80% to 90% 1 RM. Rest 2 to 4 minutes between sets.
3. *Endurance:* one to two sets of 20 reps at 50% to 60% 1 RM. Rest 30 to 60 seconds between sets.
4. *Eccentric emphasis (negatives):* Lift for two counts, lower for eight. Some experts say that lowering the weight is more important to strength development than lifting it. This does tend to promote more muscle soreness. Strength increases occur with eccentric lifting alone, and because you can lower more weight than you can lift, you may need to increase resistance.
5. *Supersets:* Work opposite muscle groups immediately (triceps/biceps, hams/quads).
6. *Continuous set:* Lift to muscular exhaustion at your regular weight, lower one plate and lift to exhaustion, and continue to lower weight as you fatigue. This is a type of muscular endurance program. It is supposed to increase muscular definition. It can be done with machines, but it is difficult with free weights.
7. *Pyramid:* Lift six reps at 70% 1 RM; four reps at 80%, 1 RM; two reps at 90%, 1 RM; one rep at 100%, 1 RM. This program emphasizes strength.
8. *Split routine:* Work upper body one day and lower body the next day; or do pushers (i.e., quads, triceps) one day, pullers (i.e., hams, biceps) the next. You must work 6 days per week. This reduces total body fatigue but requires more time.
9. *Aerobic circuit:* A circuit is a group of exercises performed with very little rest between each. Lighten weight to 40% to 60% of 1 RM. Lift quickly 30 seconds (20 lifts), recover for 30 seconds, while switching to the next station and setting the weight. Alternate a leg station with an arm station as you proceed through the circuit. As the goal is aerobic conditioning, you may also include a jump rope, bench step, jumping jacks, or jogging in place station. Begin with one set of 10 to 12 exercises and work up to three sets, maintaining a target pulse. This is designed to strengthen the heart as well as develop muscular endurance. Be very careful to maintain good form—it is easy to get sloppy and hurt yourself in this workout because the lifting rhythm is so quick.

10. *Weight gain program:* A bulk-up of three to five sets of five, gradually increasing to 10 reps at 70% to 80% effort should be performed for several months to increase lean weight.

Common Discomforts

After lifting for a few weeks, you may notice a buildup of callus on your palms. If it bothers you, lifting gloves will offer some protection. If you experience nausea or lightheadedness, stop and figure out the cause. Did you allow enough time since your last meal? Are you exhaling on the effort? Are you trying to progress too quickly? If you experience pain, particularly joint pain, pay attention. It could be an early warning sign of injury. You may be lifting too heavy a weight or stressing your joints with poor form. Have a professional check your form periodically to make sure you are not falling into bad habits.

How to Shape and Tone Without Weights

There are many different ways to develop muscular strength and endurance. While weight training is an excellent program, it is not always convenient. The programs described next can be done at home. The abdominal, hip and thigh, or upper body programs require no special equipment. Partner exercises add a social dimension to a workout. Elastic resistance produces results without bulky equipment. Finally, for those who enjoy a special challenge, add plyometrics to one or two workouts a week.

Abdominals, Hips, and Thighs

While weights add intensity to a workout, they are not always necessary when the goal is to shape and tone. Muscles develop firmness by working against a resistance, and that resistance can be your own body weight. This program emphasizes muscular endurance rather than strength by increasing reps. Abdominals, in particular, benefit from a muscular endurance routine because their function is one of endurance—sustained contraction. If you would like a total body program, combine this with the upper body routine that follows it.

These exercises (Fig. 3.5) will not burn calories like aerobic work will, so if you want to remove inches, diet and aerobic exercise are still important. Also, fat will not burn off just in the area exercised. While you can't spot reduce fat, say, in the thighs by doing leg lifts, you can spot tone flabby muscles. Be patient, and you may begin to see a difference in 8 to 12 weeks. You do not need to count repetitions. Select one exercise for each body area, and perform it for one minute. Start with one set and build up to two or three sets, three days a week. Variations are given to add variety to your program. If you wish to add intensity without purchasing weights, a sand-filled sock can be tied on as an ankle weight. You will want a mat or carpeted surface to work on.

Workout for Abdominals, Hips, and Thighs

A. Rectus abdominis

1. Abdominal curl
   Abdominal curl "crunch"
   Lie on back with knees bent, heels next to buttocks. Keep lower back on the ground, curl shoulders up 3 inches and return.
   Variations: Place one hand behind shoulders to support head, and reach other hand through knees. Do with feet raised or resting on a chair. Add resistance by moving hands from across chest to behind shoulders or by holding a 2-pound weight on each shoulder or behind neck. Do not pull or jerk on head.

2. Reverse abdominal curls
   From the starting position in number 1, hold trunk steady and curl hips 1 to 2 inches off the ground; then lower slowly.

FIGURE 3.5 ➤
Abdominals, hips, and thighs.

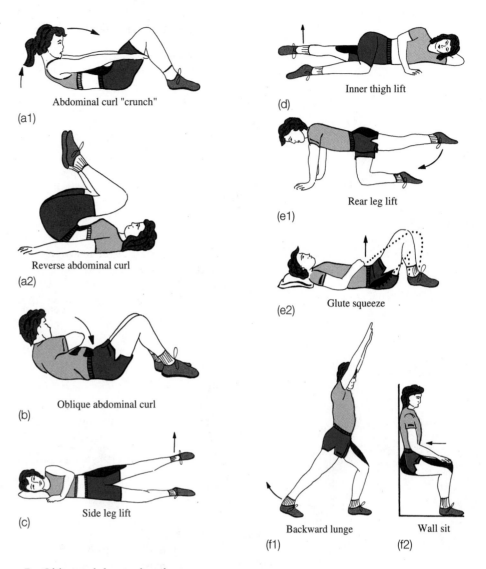

Abdominal curl "crunch"
(a1)

Reverse abdominal curl
(a2)

Oblique abdominal curl
(b)

Side leg lift
(c)

Inner thigh lift
(d)

Rear leg lift
(e1)

Glute squeeze
(e2)

Backward lunge
(f1)

Wall sit
(f2)

B. Oblique abdominal curls

Start in the same position as for abdominal curls, but add a twist, first bringing right shoulder toward left knee and then left shoulder toward right knee.

Variations: Cross right foot over left knee and twist right and then switch. Cross ankles, raise feet, and twist right and then left. Lay both knees to left, curl toward right hip, and then switch. To increase resistance, hold a 2-pound weight on each shoulder.

C. Outer hip (hip abductors)

1. Lying side leg lift

Lying on one side, head resting on arm and lower leg bent for balance, slowly raise and lower top leg.

Variations: This can be done standing. Keep foot level and leg lifting directly to side, not toward front.

2. Kneeling side leg lift

Take a hands and knees position with one leg extended to side.

Tighten abdominals, and round back to protect it. You may also support weight on one forearm if desired. Tense hip and raise and lower leg slowly no higher than 6 inches.

Variations: Circle leg forward, then reverse.

Strength and Flexibility

D. Inner thigh (thigh adductors)

1. Inner thigh lift

    Lying on left side, raise and lower leg, keeping foot turned to side (not upward). Repeat right. To increase resistance, press gently on left calf with right foot as you raise and lower leg, or add an ankle weight.

2. Plié

    Standing with feet 3 feet apart and knees bent, place hands lightly on inner thighs. Press thighs against hands, pulling in hard for a count of five. Repeat.

E. Gluteus exercises

1. Rear leg left

    On hands and knees, hollow abdomen and round back to protect it. Extend right leg to the rear. Tense gluteus. Raise and lower leg slowly six to eight counts. Repeat left.

2. Glute squeeze

    Lying on back with knees bent, squeeze gluteus hard, raising hips no more than 3 inches from floor. Do not arch back. Hold for a count of five, relax, repeat.

F. Quadriceps, hamstrings

1. Backward lunge

    Keeping shoulders erect and weight centered over right foot, step back and touch lightly with left foot and then return to starting position. Repeat. Switch legs after 1 minute of reps.

2. Wall sit

    Hold a sitting position with back against a wall for balance. Keep hips above knee level.

Upper Body

Upper body exercises can improve appearance by straightening rounded shoulders, firming upper arm muscles, and toning pectorals that underlie and support the breasts. You do not need to count repetitions. Select one exercise for each body area and repeat for one minute. If you wish to increase resistance, bricks, books, or cans of food can serve as hand weights. Upper body exercises are illustrated in Figure 3.6.

Workout for Upper Body

A. Push-ups (pectorals/triceps)

    These may be done standing, with hands against a wall and feet placed about 3 feet away from the wall (easiest), on the floor with knees bent (medium), or with weight supported on hands and feet (hardest). Keep abdominals firm and hips slightly flexed to support back. Lower to right angles of arms and then press back to arm extension.

    Variations: Keeping hands close emphasizes triceps. Keeping hands wide increases pectoral strengthening.

B. Dips (pectorals/triceps)

    Dips are an alternative way to tone the same muscle groups as push-ups do. They may be done on a dip bar or using chairs. With weight evenly distributed between bars or two sturdy chairs, place a hand on each. Bend knees or extend legs so that weight is on arms, not feet. Bend arms to right angles and return to extension.

FIGURE 3.6 ➤
Upper body exercises.

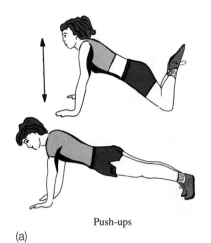

Push-ups

(a)

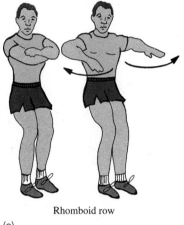

Dips

(b)

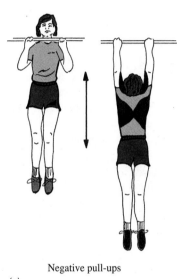

Negative pull-ups

(c)

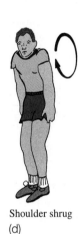

Shoulder shrug

(d)

Rhomboid row

(e)

C. Negative pull-ups (latissimus dorsi/biceps)

Negative pull-ups offer the same benefits as full pull-ups for upper back and arms. Stand on a chair if necessary to grasp a pull-up bar with arms flexed. SLOWLY lower yourself to a count of five. As you gain strength over several weeks, try to start with a few full pull-ups and finish with negatives.

D. Shoulder shrugs (trapezius)

Shoulder shrugs can tighten upper back muscles to reduce rounded shoulders. Combine this with pectoral stretches for best results. Rotate shoulders in full circles—up-back-down—working to pull shoulder blades together.

Variations: Add resistance by holding a weight in each hand.

E. Rhomboid row (rhomboids)

Rhomboids are muscles that pull the shoulder blades back, down, and together. These also need to be strengthened to reduce rounded shoulders. With arms slightly below shoulder level, elbows bent, pull elbows fully back, squeezing shoulder blades together, and hold for a count of five. Rest two counts. Repeat.

table 3.3

SAFETY TIPS FOR ELASTIC RESISTANCE EXERCISE

1. Check the band for tears before every workout. Do not use it if it shows cracks or tears because it may break.
2. Point the band away from your face.
3. Sweat makes the band slippery—keep sweat wiped off.
4. Keep the wrist in line with the forearm—flexion against resistance stresses the carpal joints of the wrist.
5. Stretch the band slowly and release slowly, leaving light tension in the band. Do not let the band go slack.
6. Wearing socks can prevent the band biting into the ankles in the leg exercises.
7. Begin with 30 seconds of repetitions, and work up to 1 minute for each. Completing two sets is a good goal.

Elastic Resistance

Elastic resistance exercise was developed in the 1950s. It was originally used by physical therapists who gave patients surgical rubber tubing to add resistance to rehabilitative exercise programs. Elastic bands and tubing are lightweight, portable, and readily available at fitness centers and medical supply companies. They are inexpensive but do not last forever and need to be replaced as they wear out. Safety tips are listed in Table 3.3. They come in different strengths, based on thickness of the elastic. Thin bands are best for beginners and upper body work. Thicker bands are useful for lower body work. Two thin bands can be used in place of one thick band. All principles of form, rhythm, and breathing apply here as for any strength training program. Elastic resistance exercises are illustrated in Figure 3.7.

Elastic Resistance Exercises

A. Leg extension (quadriceps)
   Step on one end of band with right foot and hook other end around left foot. Lie back, knees bent and feet on floor. Keeping knees and thighs together, straighten knee, lifting left foot as high as possible. Release and repeat. Change legs.

B. Hamstring curl (hamstrings and gluteus)
   Place the band around right ankle and arch of left foot. Lie face down with arms under chin or hands under hips. Bending knee, slowly lift left foot. Release slowly, maintaining some tension in band. Repeat. Change legs.

C. Side leg lift (hip abductors)
   Place band one inch above both knees. Lying on right side, torso supported by arms, slightly bend lower leg. Keep hips facing forward and lift left leg. Lower, keeping tension on the band and repeat. Change sides.

D. Inner thigh lift (thigh adductors)
   Place band around right arch and left leg. Lie on left side, with trunk supported by arms. Lift left leg slowly, hold briefly, lower slowly, repeat. Switch legs.

E. Chest crossover (pectorals)
   Standing with back straight and abdominals tight, hold band in both hands, cross forearms in front, palms facing down, and press across chest. Keep arms slightly below shoulder level.

F. Deltoid raise (deltoids and triceps)
   Standing with good posture, hold one end of band under armpit and press other arm directly upward.

FIGURE 3.7 ➤
Elastic resistance exercises.

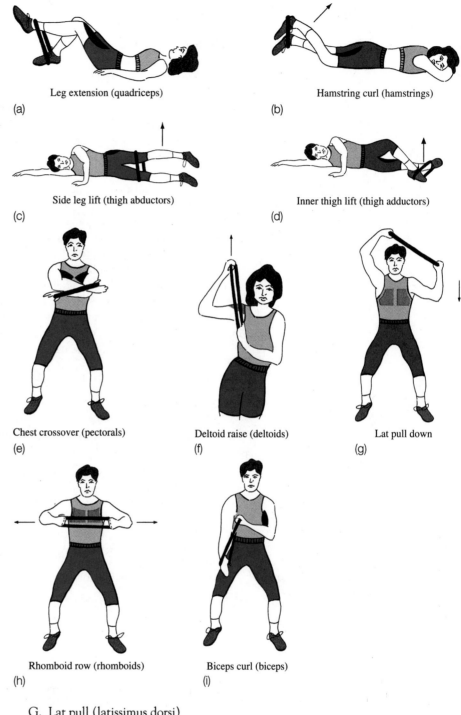

Leg extension (quadriceps)
(a)

Hamstring curl (hamstrings)
(b)

Side leg lift (thigh abductors)
(c)

Inner thigh lift (thigh adductors)
(d)

Chest crossover (pectorals)
(e)

Deltoid raise (deltoids)
(f)

Lat pull down
(g)

Rhomboid row (rhomboids)
(h)

Biceps curl (biceps)
(i)

G. Lat pull (latissimus dorsi)

Hold band overhead, elbow extended but not locked. Pull down behind head to shoulder level with other hand. Be careful not to get hair caught.

H. Rhomboid row (rhomboids)

Hold band in front of body. Pull elbows back, pulling shoulder blades together. Release with control and repeat.

I. Biceps curl (biceps)

Hold band in both hands, placing left hand on hip, palm down, and turning right hand palm up. Keeping elbow at your side, curl right arm to shoulder and slowly release.

Plyometrics

Plyometrics became popular in the 1960s when athletes in the Soviet Union and Eastern Block countries began using bounding and jumping drills to increase explosive power. **Plyometrics** use the stretch reflex to convert the rapid stretching of a muscle into a forceful contraction.

For the experienced strength trainer, plyometrics can offer variety and additional challenge. Plyometrics are not for everyone, however. They are an intense high-impact activity that can injure joints not prepared for repetitive landings at three to six times body weight. A thorough warm-up beforehand is imperative. The safest application for plyometrics is as part of a water exercise program. Jumping, skipping, and bounding exercises can be done in waist- to chest-deep water safely with minimal impact stress.

Plyometrics should comprise no more than 10 percent to 15 percent of a program and should be done no more than twice a week. The landing surface should be resilient—mats, wood floor, grass, not concrete. It is best to do plyometrics at the beginning of a workout, before fatigue affects coordination. Do not do these exercises if you are overweight, have leg or back problems, or are not in good fitness. The stress on muscles and joints is very high. With these precautions in mind, you might wish to work one to two of the following exercises below into a circuit training program to increase lower body strength and power. A **circuit** is a group of exercises, each performed a certain number of reps or amount of time, generally at different exercise stations. Once all exercises have been completed, the circuit may be repeated. The plyometric exercises shown in Figure 3.8 progress from elementary to advanced.

Plyometric Exercises

A. Lunge walk

   Step into a forward lunge, with trunk erect and front leg forming a 90 degree angle. Continue for 10 feet to 30 feet.

B. Lunge jump

   Start in a lunge, dip slightly, and explode upward, switching legs to land with the other leg forward. Continue for 10 to 30 feet. To increase difficulty, keep hands on hips.

C. Bounding run

   Leap into the air, leading with right leg and left arm. Land on right leg and immediately drive left leg and right arm into the air. There should be maximum hang time. Height, not forward momentum, is the object.

D. Bounding skip

   Skip into the air, driving right knee and left arm high. Take off and land on same leg and then switch. Again, aim for air time.

E. Tuck jump

   From a standing position, bend at knees and waist as you swing arms behind you. Swinging arms forward, jump vertically and grasp knees briefly with both hands. Land in place.

F. Vertical squat jump

   With hands on hips, squat, explode up, and land, flexing knees. Avoid flexing knees deeper than 90 degrees (thighs parallel to floor).

G. Long jump

   Using arms to add momentum and balance, perform a series of standing long jumps over a 10- to 30-foot distance.

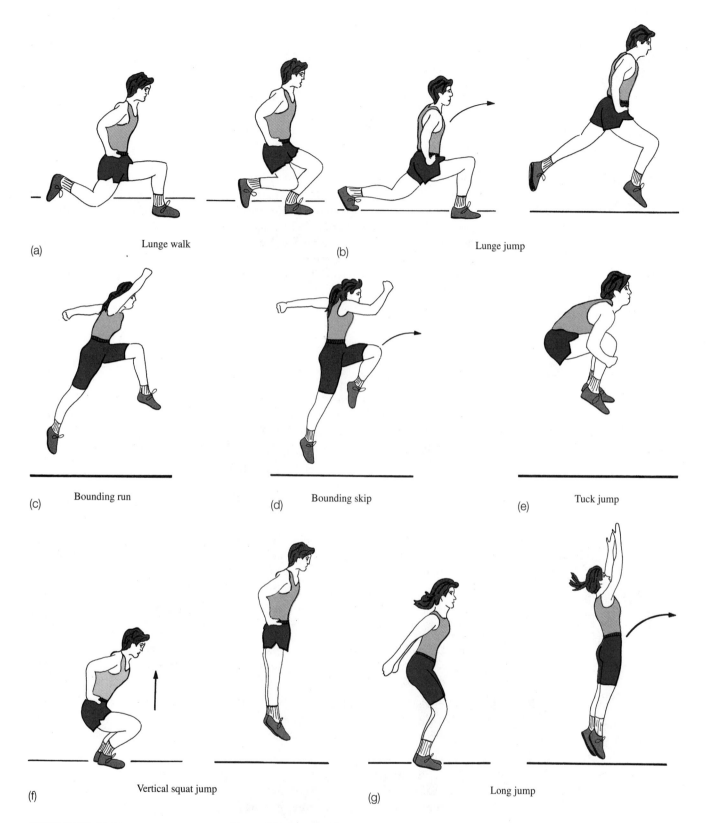

(a) Lunge walk

(b) Lunge jump

(c) Bounding run

(d) Bounding skip

(e) Tuck jump

(f) Vertical squat jump

(g) Long jump

FIGURE 3.8 ➤
Plyometrics.

Box Plyometrics

Box routines are excellent for building explosive leaping power. If you do not have a sturdy box, you can use a bench or stair.

Use an 8-inch to 18-inch box or set of boxes placed 2 feet to 3 feet apart.

1. Jump with two feet on, off, on, off.
2. Jump with left foot on, off, on, off. Repeat with right.
3. Jump with two feet, over, over, over.
4. Step off box forward/backward and rebound as high as possible.

Stair Plyometrics

Keep a hand on a rail for balance and use sets of 10 to 15 steps. Walk down.

1. With feet together, jump up one step at a time.
2. Jump up using only left foot. Repeat with right.
3. Jump with two feet, touching every other step.
4. Jump with one foot, touching every other step.
5. Sprint as quickly up stairs as possible, hitting every step.
6. Sprint, hitting every other step.

Partner Exercises

Exercising with a partner can be both challenging and enjoyable. Partner communication and sensitivity to your levels of strength and fatigue are important. The partner must vary resistance for different muscle groups and increase resistance during the eccentric part of each contraction. While many of these exercises can be done without equipment, to add variety, you may wish to try them using a towel to pull on (bicep curls) or a broomstick (overhead press). This is a balanced program of four lower-body and five upper-body exercises. Do not count reps. Perform each exercise for a minute and work up to two to three sets (Fig. 3.9).

Partner Strength Exercises

A. Leg extension (quadriceps)

Sit on a bench or chair. Move one leg from flexion to full extension and back as partner resists by pressing on front of lower leg.

B. Hamstring curl (hamstrings, gluteus)

Lie face down while partner straddles your thighs and places a hand on each ankle. Bend knees and curl calves toward buttocks as your partner resists. Continue the resistance as you return to the starting position.

C. Inner/outer thigh press (thigh adductors and abductors)

Sit, facing each other, legs forward, hands behind hips for balance. One partner places both feet inside the other's feet and presses outward as the other partner resists by pressing inward. Switch positions after six to eight reps.

D. Foot flexion (anterior tibialis)

Sit with legs extended. Partner kneels and presses down on top of both feet as you flex them and then return to extension.

E. Overhead press (deltoids, triceps)

Sit with hands at shoulder level, palms up. As partner resists, press up toward ceiling and then return to starting position.

F. Lat pull (latissimus dorsi)

Sit and reach high overhead to grasp partner's hands. As partner resists, pull down to shoulder level and slowly return to starting position.

G. Elbow press forward (pectorals)

Sit with elbows out and hands touching shoulders. As partner resists at the elbows, pull them in toward your midline and return to starting position.

H. Elbow press backward (rhomboids)

Sit with elbows out or with arms crossed. Partner sits behind, pressing on your elbows as you press back, pulling shoulder blades together. As partner continues resistance, return to starting position.

I. Biceps curl (biceps)

Stand, palms facing upward. Partner resists on your palms as you curl arm from extension to flexion and back. This may also be done holding a towel in one hand in front of body. Partner sits or kneels facing you, resisting on other end of towel as you curl your arm.

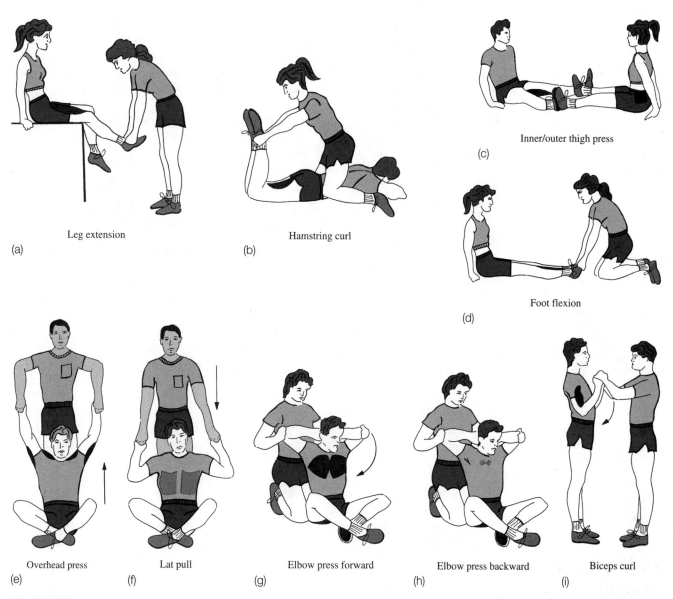

(a) Leg extension

(b) Hamstring curl

(c) Inner/outer thigh press

(d) Foot flexion

(e) Overhead press

(f) Lat pull

(g) Elbow press forward

(h) Elbow press backward

(i) Biceps curl

FIGURE 3.9 ➤
Partner strength exercises.

Flexibility

The ability to move your joints through their full range is an asset that can be maintained throughout life. As children, we are naturally flexible, but as we age, flexibility tends to decrease. Disuse, injury, excessive body fat, and muscle imbalances are common factors in this loss of range of motion. You can maintain youthful flexibility by incorporating stretching into your regular workouts.

The flexibility exercises in this section are grouped as follows: a basic fitness flexibility program with exercises for joggers, walkers, aerobic dancers, cyclists, swimmers, and water exercisers and examples of PNF partner-assisted stretches.

Benefits and Cautions

There are five main benefits to be gained from flexibility development:

➤ *It may decrease risk of injury.*[10,11,12,13,14] When tight muscles restrict the natural range of motion of a joint, the slightest unusual twist can cause a strain or pull, such as a strained hamstring. Inflexibility also is a precipitating factor in overuse injuries such as tendinitis, because inelastic muscles transfer excessive stress to even less pliable connective tissue.

> *It decreases aches and pains.* Tight, inflexible muscles pull unevenly across joints, causing skeletal misalignment, poor posture, unnecessary fatigue, and muscle and joint pain. Stretching can alleviate these problems.
> *It increases the ability to move freely and easily* and to perform activities such as bending down to tie your shoes, scratching your back, or turning to look back as you are driving.
> *It enhances athletic performance.* In racquetball, golf, tennis, volleyball, or swimming, greater range of motion and ability to apply force through that range of motion can give a winning edge.
> *It feels good.* Stretching reduces muscular tension, promoting relaxation.

If carelessly done, however, stretching can cause injury. You must be careful not to overstretch, particularly when muscles are cold and tight. Stretching is not a competitive activity, so don't try to imitate the most flexible person in your class. Injured areas should be stretched with great care and not into pain, which risks reinjury. If you feel pain during stretching, particularly joint pain, stop!

Types of Flexibility

There are two basic types of flexibility: static and dynamic. **Static flexibility** refers to the range of motion you can achieve through a slow, controlled stretch. **Dynamic flexibility** is the range of motion achieved by quickly moving a limb to its limits.

Static stretching techniques are those in which you slowly stretch a muscle to the point of tension and hold, such as in holding a sitting hamstring stretch. The stretching force is provided by gravity or the force of one limb pulling on another. When a muscle is stretched and held at a constant length, after a period of time there is a gradual loss of tension and muscle lengthening.

Dynamic stretching programs employ swinging or ballistic moves, such as a high forward kick. Ballistic exercises may be useful in preparation for athletic activities requiring such moves, but they do carry increased risk that a muscle or joint could be overstretched, resulting in muscle or tendon tears and joint injury. Also, ballistic exercises initiate the **stretch reflex,** a natural response that causes the stretched muscle to contract. This contraction is designed to protect the muscle from being overstretched, but it also limits flexibility gains. While both types of stretching can increase flexibility, static stretching is preferred in health-related fitness programs because it is highly effective and carries little risk of muscle or joint strain.

Principles of Flexibility Development

Both types of flexibility are specific to the joint; that is, flexibility in one leg does not guarantee identical flexibility in the other leg, and flexibility in the shoulders does not ensure flexibility in the lower back.

An individual's flexibility range for any particular joint is not only specific, but also partially genetically determined. You may have observed that some people seem to be naturally more flexible than others, even "double jointed" (they aren't really). Flexibility is determined by joint structure and elasticity of muscle and connective tissue. While you may not be able to change your genetics, you can improve your degree of flexibility within your genetically determined range of motion. People who have never been able to touch their toes may, for example, be able to get inches closer with practice but may never be able to wrap their palms around their feet without bending their knees.

Flexibility gains are proportional to the overload applied: to the frequency, intensity, and time (duration) of stretching. *Frequency:* Stretch at least three to four days a week and daily if possible. Greater flexibility is produced by more frequent stretching. *Intensity:* Low-intensity stretching is best. Progress at your own speed. Stretching is not competitive. Flexibility changes from day to day, and some days you might not be able to stretch as far as you did the day before. Stretch just slightly beyond the normal range of motion, to the point of tension, and hold. Do not force a stretch. *Time:* Many programs recommend a 10- to 30-second stretch, though holding up to 60 seconds in a cooldown stretch can increase flexibility retention. The optimal number of repetitions has not been determined, but one 10- to 30-second sustained stretch for each muscle group should be considered a minimum; repeat once or twice if time permits.

While less flexible individuals may envy those who can do splits with ease, keep in mind that, with flexibility, more is better only up to a point. There is concern (though no hard evidence) that excessive flexibility, unless accompanied by muscular strength, may increase joint laxity and susceptibility to injury.[15] For this reason, it is wise to combine stretching with muscle strengthening for optimal fitness benefits.

Guidelines for Flexibility Development

Everyone can benefit from flexibility. To maximize results from the time invested, implement the following guidelines into your next stretching session:

➤ *Warm up before stretching.* An increase in muscle temperature produced by fast walking, slow jogging, jumping jacks, or other large muscle exercise will make stretching safer and more productive. You are sufficiently warmed up when you begin to sweat.

➤ *After warm-up, use stretching as preparation for activity.* While some feel that stretching during warm-up decreases risk of injury in the activity that follows, there is no evidence that this is true. Warm-up stretching is different from a planned program of stretching for general flexibility. Warm-up stretching can be limited to what is essential, avoiding overstretching. Stretch muscle groups used in the activity, hold at the point of tension for 5 to 10 seconds, and do not push for flexibility increases. Any gains will be minimal due to the tightening effect of the workout that follows.[16]

➤ *Stretch for flexibility during cool-down.* Muscles are warmest and most elastic at this point. Stretching is easier. More permanent changes in muscle lengthening occur with low-force, long-duration stretching if muscles are allowed to cool in a stretched position. Cooling muscles before releasing tension apparently causes muscle collagen (connective tissue), like stretched taffy, to stabilize toward its new stretched length.[17]

➤ *Stop at the point of tension, not pain.* Stretching to the point of pain, or until muscles quiver, can risk overstretching injury.

➤ *Don't bounce.* A sustained stretch is more effective.

➤ *Incorporate 8 to 12 stretches into your program.* Since flexibility is specific to a joint, a well-planned program for general flexibility will contain one stretch for each major muscle group. Warm-up or cool-down stretching may contain fewer exercises because such stretching is activity specific and has different goals. Pay particular attention to body areas that are least flexible and stretch them more often.

➤ *Strive for muscle balance.* When stretching muscle on one side of a joint, stretch those on the other side as well; for example, if you stretch hamstrings, stretch quadriceps, too.

Flexibility Exercises for Basic Fitness

As part of a warm-up or cool-down, exercises A through F are important for runners, walkers, and aerobic dancers. Cyclists, swimmers, and water exercisers should add upper body stretches G through I. If time is limited, save stretching for the cool-down. For basic fitness flexibility, perform the full program of exercises in Figure 3.10. Hold each 10 to 30 seconds and repeat once or twice.

A. Hamstring stretch
   Keeping shoulders erect, press abdomen forward. Hold. Repeat with other leg.

B. Lower back/hip flexor stretch
   With hands behind thigh, press thigh toward chest. Keep extended leg straight. Repeat left.

C. Spinal twist (lower back and hip abductors)
   Sit with right leg extended, step left leg over right, and turn upper body toward left. Repeat on other side.

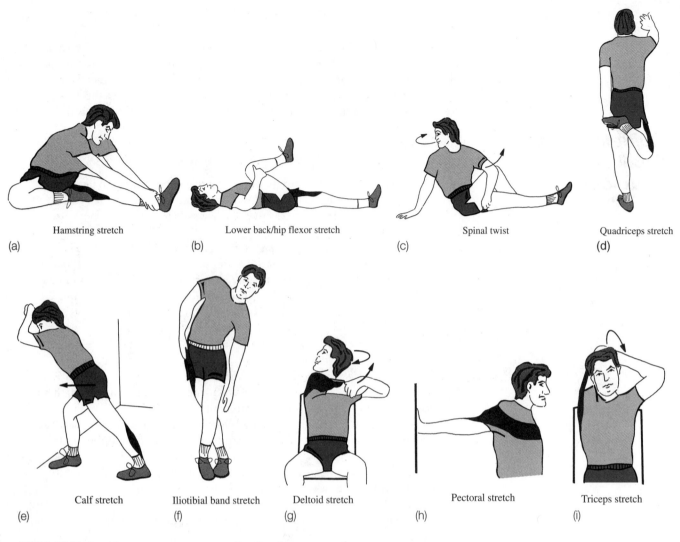

FIGURE 3.10 ➤
Flexibility exercises.

D. Quadriceps stretch

With left hand, pull right heel toward buttocks. Keep shoulders up, abdominals tight, and hips tucked under to prevent back hyperextension. Omit if you have knee problems.

E. Calf stretch

Standing in forward lunge position, toes pointing forward, press heel toward floor. Repeat with other leg.

F. Iliotibial band stretch

Cross left foot over right, press hips to left. Repeat with other side.

G. Deltoid stretch

Cross right arm in front of body and pull it in toward midline with left hand.

H. Pectoral stretch

Place right hand on wall, elbow extended but not locked. Twist shoulders left. Repeat with left arm.

I. Triceps stretch

Pull left elbow behind head. Repeat right.

PNF Partner-Assisted Stretches

A type of static stretching called **proprioceptive neuromuscular facilitation (PNF),** a partner-assisted stretch often used by athletic trainers, is one of the most effective methods known for increasing flexibility. To perform a PNF stretch, you first perform a 20- to 30-second static stretch, then contract the muscle 10 to 20 seconds to produce fatigue, and then relax while a partner stretches your limb 20 to 30 seconds.

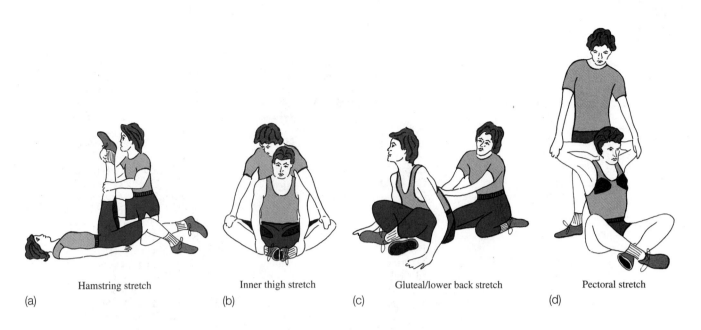

Hamstring stretch (a) Inner thigh stretch (b) Gluteal/lower back stretch (c) Pectoral stretch (d)

FIGURE 3.11 ➤
PNF partner-assisted stretches.

It is important to be sensitive to your partner's needs and flexibility levels. Be sure to communicate when more/less resistance or pressure is needed throughout each exercise. Work with the same partner throughout the series. Switching partners can lead to injury because of unfamiliarity with the flexibility limits of the person being stretched. Some examples of PNF stretches are illustrated in Figure 3.11. Consult the suggested readings for more ideas.

A. Hamstring stretch

Lie on your back and lift one leg into the air. Partner supports ankle and knee in a static stretch. Next, keeping knee extended but not locked, push against your partner as he or she resists. Stretch and then relax, as partner eases leg into a new stretch.

B. Inner thigh stretch

Sit with knees out and bottoms of feet together. Press down on knees in a static stretch. Next, partner kneels behind and resists on knees as you press them upward. Finally, relax as partner gently presses them toward the floor in a stretch.

C. Gluteal/lower back stretch

Sit cross-legged and stretch forward. Partner kneels behind you with hands on your upper back. Next, resist back against partner. Then, stretch forward as partner assists.

D. Pectoral stretch

Sit cross-legged with fingers interlaced behind your head and back supported by partner's thigh. Partner gently pulls your elbows back for 10 seconds and then resists as you attempt to pull them forward. Next, relax as partner gently stretches them back.

SUMMARY

Muscular strength, muscular endurance, and flexibility exercises are a vital supplement to a regular program of aerobic exercise. They can enhance appearance by improving the shape, firmness, and tone of muscles. Enhanced posture, decreased risk of lower back pain, greater ease of movement, improved athletic performance, and more energy are benefits. While injury is possible in any exercise program if safety guidelines are ignored, sensible strengthening and stretching programs generally decrease risk of injury for those who participate in health-related fitness programs or athletics.[18,19]

REFERENCES

1. Tanner, Suzanne. "Weighing the Risks." *The Physician and Sportsmedicine* 21 (June 1993): 105.
2. Tanner, Suzanne. "Weighing the Risks."
3. Thigpen, L. Kay. "Building Strength." *Sports Medicine Secrets*, Morris B. Mellion, ed. Philadelphia: Hanley & Belfus, Inc., 1995.
4. "Never Too Late to Build Up Your Muscle." *Tufts University Newsletter* 12 (September 1994): 6–7.
5. Young, A., and D. A. Skelton. "Applied Physiology of Strength and Power in Old Age." *International Journal of Sports Medicine* 15 (April 1994): 149–51.
6. Treuth, M., et al. "Effects of Strength Training on Total and Regional Body Composition in Older Men." *Journal of Applied Physiology* 77 (August 1994): 614–20.
7. Drought, J. H. "Resistance Training and Strength Benefits for Elderly Individuals." *Journal of Strength and Conditioning Research* 16 (June 1994): 26–30.
8. Williams, Mark A. "Cardiovascular and Respiratory Anatomy and Physiology: Responses to Exercise." *Essentials of Strength Training and Conditioning*, T. R. Baechle, ed. Champaign, Ill.: Human Kinetics, 1994.
9. Thigpen, L. Kay. "Building Strength."
10. Blanke, Daniel. "Flexibility." *Sports Medicine Secrets*, Morris B. Mellion, ed. Philadelphia: Hanley & Belfus, Inc., 1995.
11. Allerheiligen, William B. "Stretching and Warm-up." *Essentials of Strength Training and Conditioning*, T. R. Baechle, ed. Champaign, Ill.: Human Kinetics, 1994.
12. Mechelen, et al. "Prevention of Running Injuries by Warm-up, Cool-down, and Stretching Exercises." *The American Journal of Sports Medicine* 21 (September–October 1993): 711.
13. Pina, et al. "Are Warm-up and Cool-down Exercises Important?" *The Physician and Sportsmedicine* 21 (July/August 1993): 144j.
14. Bowyer, Brian, M.D., et al. "Preventing Common Runners' Injuries." *Patient Care* 28, no. 12 (July 15, 1994): 72–86.
15. Alter, Michael J. *Science of Stretching*. Human Kinetics Books, Champaign, Ill.: 1988.
16. Alter, Michael J. *Science of Stretching*.
17. Alter, Michael J. *Science of Stretching*.
18. Blanke, Daniel. "Flexibility."
19. Thigpen, L. Kay. "Building Strength."

SUGGESTED READINGS

Baechle, T. R., ed. *Essentials of Strength Training and Conditioning*. Champaign, Ill.: Human Kinetics, 1994.

Chu, Donald A. *Jumping into Plyometrics*. Champaign, Ill.: Leisure Press, 1992.

Fahey, T. D. *Basic Weight Training for Men and Women*, 2d ed. Mountain View, Calif.: Mayfield Pub. Co., 1994.

Institute for Aerobics Research Staff & Kenneth H. Cooper. *The Strength Connection: How to Build Strength and Improve the Quality of Your Life with Strength Training Exercises*. New York: Bantam Books, 1993.

Kurz, Thomas. *Stretching Scientifically: A Guide to Flexibility Training*, 3d ed. Island Pond, N.Y.: Stadion Pub. Co., 1994.

Mellion, M. B., ed. *Sports Medicine Secrets*. Philadelphia: Hanley & Belfus, Inc., 1994.

Robinson, Jerry. *The Weightless Workout*. Los Angeles, Calif.: Health for Life, 1993.

Rothenberg, Beth, and Oscar Rothenberg. *Touch Training for Strength*. Champaign, Ill.: Human Kinetics, 1994.

Shazryl, Eskay, and Jarrod Hanks. *Sports and Stress Therapy: Athletic Rehabilitation on Massage, Stretching, and Strengthening*. Oklahoma City, Okla.: Eskay, Inc., 1994.

Sprague, Kim. *The Gold's Gym Book of Strength Training for Athletes*. New York: Perigee Books, 1994.

Tobias, Maxine. *New Stretching Book*. New York: David McKay Co, Inc., 1993.

chapter 4

Fitness Assessment

4 q's

➤ Objectives

After reading this chapter, you will be able to:

1. Identify one or more tests for each component of health-related fitness.
2. Calculate body fat percentage using a nomogram.
3. Use textbook norms to identify fitness levels in four fitness components, based on the results of fitness assessments.
4. Determine an appropriate fitness program using workout charts for specific aerobic activities in the Appendix and the results of a cardiorespiratory fitness assessment.

Terms

- Exercise tolerance test
- Fat-free tissue
- Lean body mass
- Skinfold calipers
- Subcutaneous fat

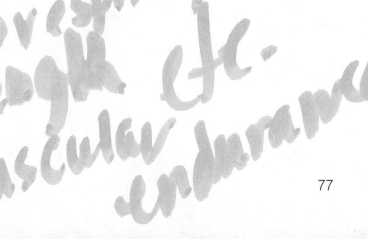

Purpose for fitness assessment

Health related components

↓ flexibility, cardiorespiratory Strength etc. muscular endurance

All our dreams can come true if we have the courage to pursue them.

Anonymous

physical fitness tests are often divided into two categories: health related and skill related. Skill-related tests, such as a vertical jump or shuttle run, are performance based and are related to athletic ability. Health-related tests are related to functional well-being in the areas of cardiorespiratory endurance, muscular strength and endurance, flexibility, and body composition. These areas of physiological functioning can be improved or maintained through regular exercise and offer protection from the negative effects of a sedentary lifestyle.

Do you know how fit you are? We all seem to have a natural curiosity about how we compare to others. The main purpose of fitness testing is to help you identify your current fitness levels in several health-related categories. Such an evaluation should tell you whether your current lifestyle is effective in developing and maintaining a level of fitness conducive to optimal wellness. Your results can be used as a basis for setting personal fitness goals, for developing an appropriate individualized exercise prescription, and finally, for measuring the effectiveness of your fitness program in reaching your goals.

This chapter gives norms that enable you to compare your fitness levels with those of other students. Norms reflect achievements of people who have completed a 12- to 15-week fitness course.[1] When evaluating your fitness and setting goals, keep in mind that scoring in the "low" category does not reflect negatively on you as a person. While "excellent" is an attainable goal for some, relatively few people achieve this level in one or more areas of fitness. Bodies are different. Your current fitness level does not indicate your potential. Physical capacity to achieve any particular level of fitness is partially genetically determined. You may find that you gain strength easily but must constantly work on flexibility or vice versa. Health-related fitness benefits can be experienced at the "average" fitness level. Also keep in mind that all tests are subject to some measurement variability. Use these norms as guidelines. Finally, testing should not dominate your program but help you measure its effectiveness. You may wish to measure at the beginning of your program and remeasure eight to twelve weeks into the program to see how you are progressing.

A *Personal Fitness Profile* is located in the Activities section at the back of the book. When completed, it will indicate areas of fitness you can maintain and areas needing improvement. It will help you decide where to begin in your fitness program.

Guidelines for Medical Clearance

According to American College of Sports Medicine guidelines,[2] it is generally safe to begin a vigorous exercise program if you are under 40 years of age for men and under 50 for women, are healthy, and have had a satisfactory medical checkup in the past two years. Also, if you have been exercising regularly, it is probably safe to continue progressing gradually from your current activity level. Prior to participation, you should complete the *Health/Exercise Assessment Form* found in the Activities section to identify any potential health concerns.

If you are over these age guidelines or if, regardless of age, you have had health concerns noted on the *Health/Exercise Assessment Form*, it is important to check with your personal physician before taking a cardiorespiratory fitness test or participating in vigorous exercise. The *Exercise Clearance Form* in the Activities section is designed to assist your instructor in individualizing your fitness program according to your physician's recommendations. You may need to have a medical checkup and diagnostic exercise test. If you smoke cigarettes, have been sedentary over the past several months, have diabetes, are 20 or more pounds overweight, or have family members who have positive risk factors for heart disease, it is particularly important that you see your physician. Also, check with your physician if you are unsure or have concerns about your health.

Cardio-respiratory Endurance

A person with a high level of cardiorespiratory fitness can do more work with less fatigue than can a person with low cardiorespiratory fitness. Increased cardiorespiratory fitness can enhance quality of life by increasing the rate of energy production during physical activity. Low levels of cardiorespiratory fitness may result in a limited lifestyle due to low energy reserves, quick exhaustion with moderate exertion, and resulting inability to participate in vigorous, oxygen-demanding activities. High-level wellness is inextricably tied to a physically active lifestyle. If you want to be an active participant in life—not just a spectator—cardiorespiratory fitness is essential. The ability of your heart and lungs to supply oxygen during activity is one of the best indicators of overall physical fitness. There are several ways to measure your body's ability to use oxygen. The most accurate method is an **exercise tolerance test** on a treadmill or on a bicycle ergometer in a laboratory (Fig. 4.1). In an exercise tolerance test, a person exercises strenuously while heart rate and oxygen consumption are measured. This, however, is complex, expensive, and time consuming and requires elaborate equipment and trained personnel. It is impractical for testing large numbers of people.

Cardiorespiratory fitness can also be measured in field tests conducted out of the laboratory setting. What they lose in accuracy they make up in the practicality of self-testing or testing many people at the same time. Field tests of cardiorespiratory endurance are generally based on physiological performance (distance or time tests) or a parameter such as pulse rate (step test).

A field test used to estimate oxygen consumption measures the time it takes you to jog 1.5 miles. Studies have shown that time on the 1.5-mile run correlates well with maximal oxygen uptake. The faster you cover the distance, the more efficient your heart and lungs are at their job of supplying oxygenated blood and nutrients to the working muscles and in carrying away waste products. Field tests make it easy for you to measure your own fitness and to detect progress as you train. Keep in mind that if you retest within a few weeks, early improvements may be due to a "learning effect" rather than true cardiovascular changes. That is, you will learn to pace yourself better throughout the distance. It will take eight to twelve weeks for significant cardiovascular improvement to occur. You should only take the *1.5-Mile Run Test* if you are conditioned for it. It is best if you have been building up to the distance gradually for several weeks prior to taking the test. Other field tests that measure cardiorespiratory endurance are the *1-Mile Walk Test*, the *5-Mile Bicycling Test*, the *500-Yard Swim Test*, the *500-Yard Water Run Test*, and the *Step Test*. You can choose the test most appropriate for your chosen physical conditioning activity.

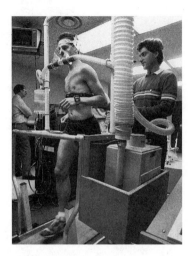

FIGURE 4.1 ➤
Treadmill exercise tolerance test.

General Instructions

For any of the cardiorespiratory endurance tests, you will need comfortable clothes appropriate for the activity and a stopwatch or a watch with a second hand.

➤ If possible, avoid taking the test under conditions of extreme heat or cold, particularly if you are not accustomed to exercising under those conditions.
➤ Do not eat a heavy meal or smoke for up to three hours prior to the test.
➤ Rest from vigorous exercise at least one day prior to taking the test.
➤ Warm up and stretch before taking the test and then cool down and restretch afterward.
➤ If at any point during the test you begin to feel ill, dizzy, faint, or extremely short of breath, stop! Your body is telling you that you are not yet ready for this level of exertion.

Do not be ashamed of stopping before completing the test, especially if you are unfit. Test performance may be limited by local muscular endurance or by aerobic capacity. You may record the amount of time in the test you were able to complete and work toward a fitness level that will enable you to complete the test.

1.5-Mile Run Test

The *1.5-Mile Run Test* requires six laps around a standard quarter-mile track, or it can be done on a measured section of road. You should consider taking this test only if you have been exercising previously. The *1-Mile Walk Test* may be more appropriate for you

table 4.1

1.5-MILE RUN NORMS

MEN

Age	18–29	30–39	40–49	50–59	60+
Excellent	<8:26	<9:10	<9:55	<10:40	<11:25
Good	8:26–10:21	9:10–11:10	9:55–12:00	10:40–12:50	11:25–13:40
Average	10:22–12:17	11:11–13:30	12:01–14:40	12:51–15:50	13:41–17:00
Low	12:18–14:14	13:31–15:35	14:16–16:50	15:31–18:05	16:45–19:20
Very Low	>14:14	>15:35	>16:50	>18:05	>19:20

WOMEN

Age	18–29	30–39	40–49	50–59	60+
Excellent	<10:52	<12:15	<13:35	<14:55	<16:15
Good	10:52–13:40	12:15–14:40	13:35–15:40	14:55–16:40	16:15–17:40
Average	13:41–16:28	14:41–17:13	15:41–17:58	16:41–18:43	17:41–19:28
Low	16:29–19:16	17:14–19:46	17:59–20:16	18:44–20:46	19:29–21:16
Very Low	>19:16	>19:46	>20:16	>20:46	>21:16

if you are over 35 years of age or 20 or more pounds overweight or if you have been out of shape for quite some time but are otherwise in good health.

Goal: To run 1.5 miles as quickly as you can.

Directions:

1. Locate a standard quarter-mile track or measure a section of road that has few stoplights.
2. Have a stopwatch or a watch with a second hand.
3. Warm up before taking the test.
4. This is a test of your maximum capacity, so do the best you can. Push yourself to cover the distance as fast as possible without overdoing. Try to maintain a continuous, even pace. Run as long as you can and then walk when necessary. In a group of runners, it is helpful for runners to be given the right-of-way on the inner lanes and people who need to walk to move to the outer lanes.
5. When you complete the 1.5-mile distance, record your time and cool down with walking and stretching.
6. Check Table 4.1 for your fitness level.

1-Mile Walk Test

For those starting a walking program or for whom the *1.5-Mile Run Test* may be too vigorous, the *1-Mile Walk Test* is an option. You will need a 1-mile measured course (four laps of a quarter-mile track), your walking shoes, and a watch with a second hand.

Goal: To walk one mile as quickly as you can.

Directions:

1. Warm up and stretch before beginning.
2. Walk 1 mile as quickly as you can.
3. Record your time to the nearest second.
4. Cool down and stretch.
5. Locate your fitness level in Table 4.2.

table 4.2

1-MILE WALK NORMS

MEN

Age	18–29	30–39	40–49	50–59	60+
Excellent	<11:07	<12:07	<13:07	<13:37	<14:37
Good	11:07–12:31	12:07–13:31	13:07–14:07	13:37–14:50	14:37–15:37
Average	12:32–13:56	13:32–14:56	14:08–15:19	14:51–16:00	15:38–16:40
Low	13:57–15:20	14:57–15:50	15:20–16:19	16:01–17:00	16:41–17:40
Very Low	>15:20	>15:50	>16:20	>17:00	>17:40

WOMEN

Age	18–29	30–39	40–49	50–59	60+
Excellent	<12:02	<13:02	<14:02	<15:02	<16:02
Good	12:02–13:05	13:02–14:05	14:02–15:05	15:02–16:05	16:02–17:05
Average	13:06–14:10	14:06–15:10	15:06–16:10	16:06–17:10	17:06–18:10
Low	14:11–15:14	15:11–16:14	16:11–17:14	17:11–18:14	18:10–19:14
Very Low	>15:14	>16:14	>17:14	>18:14	>19:14

5-Mile Bicycling Test

If your main fitness activity is bicycling, you can test your cardiorespiratory fitness with a timed 5-mile bicycle ride. This test can be done on a bike track or on a measured section of road with few stoplights or stop signs.

Goal: To bicycle five miles as quickly as possible.
Directions:
1. Warm up by riding for a few minutes and stretching.
2. Cycle the 5 miles as quickly as you can. If you are doing this on the road, be careful to obey all traffic rules.
3. Try to pace evenly. Time the ride with a stopwatch or a watch with a second hand. Record the time.
4. Cool down and stretch.
5. Check your results in Table 4.3 on page 82.

500-Yard Swim Test

If your fitness program primarily involves swimming, you will find a swimming endurance test useful. A regulation 25-yard pool is recommended, and you will need a friend to time you. You may swim any stroke, although best results will be obtained with the front crawl.

Goal: To swim 500 yards as quickly as you can.
Directions:
1. Warm up.
2. Have a friend time you and count lengths. In a 25-yard pool, 500 yards is 20 lengths.
3. Record your time, cool down, and stretch.
4. Check Table 4.4 on page 82 for your fitness level.

500-Yard Water Run Test

The *500-Yard Water Run Test* (Fig. 4.2) was designed for those involved in aerobic water exercise programs in which swimming skills are not required. It can be done lengthwise in a pool of constant depth or widthwise across the shallow end of a pool of variable

table 4.3

5-MILE BICYCLING NORMS

MEN

Age	18–29	30–39	40–49	50–59	60+
Excellent	<14:00	<15:00	<16:00	<17:00	<18:00
Good	14:00–15:20	15:00–16:10	16:00–17:00	17:00–17:50	18:00–18:40
Average	15:21–17:00	16:11–18:00	17:01–19:00	17:51–20:00	18:41–21:00
Low	17:01–18:30	18:01–19:20	19:01–20:10	20:00–21::20	21:00–22:10
Very Low	>18:30	>19:20	>20:10	>21:20	>22:10

WOMEN

Age	18–29	30–39	40–49	50–59	60+
Excellent	<15:30	<16:30	<17:30	<18:30	<19:30
Good	15:30–16:50	16:30–17:40	17:30–18:30	18:30–19:20	19:30–20:10
Average	16:51–18:30	17:41–19:30	18:31–20:30	19:21–21:30	20:11–22:30
Low	18:31–20:00	19:31–20:50	20:31–21:40	21:31–22:30	22:31–23:20
Very Low	>20:00	>20:50	>21:40	>22:30	>23:20

table 4.4

500-YARD SWIM NORMS

MEN

Age	18–29	30–39	40–49	50–59	60+
Excellent	<6:12	<6:30	<7:00	<7:30	<8:00
Good	6:12–7:44	6:30–8:14	7:00–8:44	7:30–9:14	8:00–9:44
Average	7:45–9:19	8:15–9:49	8:45–10:19	9:15–10:49	9:45–11:19
Low	9:20–10:52	9:50–11:22	10:20–11:52	10:50–11:22	11:20–12:52
Very Low	>10:52	>11:22	>11:52	>11:22	>12:52

WOMEN

Age	18–29	30–39	40–49	50–59	60+
Excellent	<7:05	<7:35	<8:05	<8:35	<9:05
Good	7:05–8:49	7:35–9:19	8:05–9:49	8:35–10:19	9:05–10:49
Average	8:50–10:34	9:20–11:04	9:50–11:34	10:20–12:04	10:50–12:34
Low	10:35–12:19	11:05–12:49	11:35–13:19	12:05–13:49	12:35–14:49
Very Low	>12:19	>12:49	>13:19	>13:49	>14:49

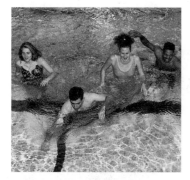

FIGURE 4.2 ➤
500-yard water run test. This is a valid field test for nonswimmers. (Note: The water level should be midpoint between navel and nipple.)

3-Minute Step Test

depth. It helps to work in pairs, with one partner on deck counting completed laps for the other. For most accurate results, runners should carve their own paths through the water and avoid drafting in the wake of other runners. Runners should use their arms to pull as they run but must maintain a vertical body position. No swimming is allowed.

Goal: To run 500 yards in the water as quickly as possible.
Directions:
1. Measure pool width and calculate the number of lengths required to cover 500 yards.
2. Have a partner on deck count laps and keep the time.
3. Warm up with a couple minutes of easy jogging in the water.
4. To give runners of different heights a similar level of water resistance in a variable depth pool, select a starting point along the pool wall where the water level is at a midpoint between the runner's navel and nipple. Shorter runners will start in shallower water, taller runners in deeper water.
5. Take a position in the water, note your starting time, and run the necessary number of widths. Record your time to the nearest second.
6. Cool down and stretch.
7. Check Table 4.5 for your fitness level

There are a variety of step tests useful for testing cardiorespiratory fitness indoors. They involve stepping on and off a bench for a 3- to 5-minute period and measuring the heart rate recovery. The step test is based on the fact that the heart rate of a person who is physically fit is lower at any work load and recovers faster than does the heart rate of a person who is unfit. Although it is not the best measure of cardiorespiratory fitness, it is a quick and simple way to evaluate the heart's response to exercise. It is easy to

table 4.5

500-YARD WATER RUN NORMS

MEN

Age	18–29	30–39	40–49	50–59	60+
Excellent	<6:50	<7:20	<7:50	<8:20	<9:50
Good	6:50–7:32	7:20–8:02	7:50–8:32	8:20–9:02	9:50–10:32
Average	7:33–8:15	8:03–8:45	8:33–9:15	9:03–9:45	10:33–10:45
Low	8:16–8:58	8:46–9:28	9:16–9:58	9:46–10:28	10:45–10:58
Very Low	>8:58	>9:28	>9:58	>10:28	>10:58

WOMEN

Age	18–29	30–39	40–49	50–59	60+
Excellent	<7:59	<8:30	<9:00	<9:30	<10:00
Good	7:59–8:38	8:30–9:08	9:00–9:38	9:30–10:08	10:00–10:38
Average	8:39–9:18	9:09–9:48	9:39–10:18	10:09–10:48	10:39–11:18
Low	9:19–9:58	9:49–10:28	10:19–10:58	10:49–11:28	11:19–11:58
Very Low	>9:58	>10:28	>10:58	>11:28	>11:58

table 4.6

3-MINUTE STEP TEST NORMS

	MEN	WOMEN
Excellent	<31	<37
Good	31–37	37–41
Average	38–41	42–44
Low	42–45	45–49
Very Low	>45	>49

administer to an individual or to large groups, requires no special skill to perform, and requires little equipment (Fig. 4.3).

Goal: To step on and off a bench for three minutes.

Directions:

1. Locate a 15-inch bench or a 16-inch roll-out bleacher step.
2. Warm up.
3. Work with a partner. While your partner is stepping on and off the bench, stand in front of him or her to prevent falling. Then switch.
4. You will need to step up and down at 96 counts per minute. A metronome or recorded music at a tempo of 96 beats per minute will help you keep cadence, or your instructor will call the cadence: "Up-up-down-down." At the signal "Begin," step up with your right foot and then your left foot and then step down with your right and then your left. Continue for 3 minutes. Straighten your knees as you step up on the bench. To prevent leg soreness, you may want to switch lead legs about halfway through the test.
5. Stop at the end of 3 minutes and sit down. Five seconds after completing the test, the tester should count the partner's pulse for 15 seconds. The tester can check the partner's carotid pulse by lightly pressing against the neck under the jawbone. The partner being tested can double-check his or her own pulse at the radial artery, located on the thumb side of the wrist. The partners' pulse counts should not vary more than one or two beats if counting is accurate.
6. Record the pulse.
7. Cool down and stretch.
8. Compare your pulse with the norms given in Table 4.6 to assess your cardiorespiratory fitness. If you are unable to keep the cadence for the full 3 minutes, consider yourself to have very low cardiorespiratory endurance.

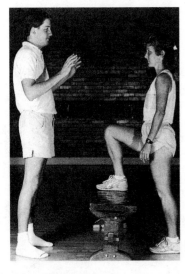

FIGURE 4.3 ➤
Step test.

Muscular Strength and Endurance

Muscular strength and endurance are assets in the ability to perform daily activities—lifting, carrying, pushing, pulling—without strain or undue fatigue. Strength and endurance of the abdominal muscles are particularly important for good posture and lower back health. Muscular fitness activities add shape and firmness to muscles, resulting in a trim, well-toned appearance.

Muscular strength and muscular endurance tests have been used as a measure of physical fitness for years. Physical conditioning activities require and can develop both components. Strength is best developed by weight training and is often measured by one maximal lift with weights (see Chapter 3). Muscular endurance can be measured without special equipment, using tests provided here. Abdominal curls are perhaps the best way to assess the endurance of the abdominal muscles. The traditional *Bent-Knee Sit-up*

FIGURE 4.4 ➤
Abdominal curls. Fingertips
move forward 3 inches.

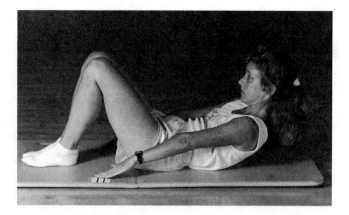

Test requires use of the thighs and hip flexors as well as abdominals and may put the back at risk. Abdominal curls isolate and test only abdominal muscles, decreasing risk to the lower back. Directions and norms for abdominal curls are given. To test the muscular endurance of the arms and upper body muscles, norms are also given for push-ups.

Abdominal Curls

Goal: To complete as many abdominal curls as possible in one minute.

Directions:

1. Tape a 3-inch wide strip on the floor and lie on your back on the floor with your fingertips at the edge of the strip. Bend your knees and bring your heels as close as possible toward your buttocks.
2. Curl forward until your fingertips have moved forward across the 3-inch strip and then curl back until your shoulder blades touch the floor. Your shoulders should lift from the floor with each curl, but the lower back should stay on the ground. If you are working with a partner who is counting your curls, your partner should not hold your feet down, nor should your feet lift off the ground—if they do, you are curling too high (Fig. 4.4).
3. Complete as many curls as possible in 1 minute; then check the results in Table 4.7.

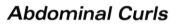

table 4.7

1-MINUTE ABDOMINAL CURL NORMS

MEN

Age	18–29	30–39	40–49	50–59	60+
Excellent	>95	>80	>65	>49	>44
Good	82–95	65–80	53–65	42–49	33–44
Average	68–81	55–64	45–52	35–41	27–32
Low	54–67	44–54	36–44	28–34	22–25
Very Low	<54	<44	<36	<28	<22

WOMEN

Age	18–29	30–39	40–49	50–59	60+
Excellent	>88	>70	>56	>45	>36
Good	76–88	61–70	49–56	39–45	31–36
Average	63–75	50–60	40–48	32–38	24–30
Low	49–62	39–49	31–39	25–31	18–23
Very Low	<49	<39	<31	<25	<18

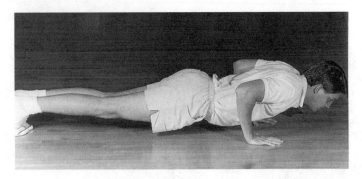

FIGURE 4.5 ➤
Push-up—standard position. Note the 90° elbow angle.

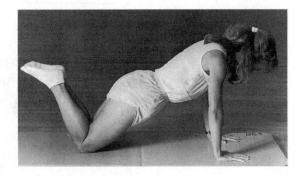

FIGURE 4.6 ➤
Push-up—modified position.

Push-Ups

Goal: To complete as many push-ups as possible in one minute.

Directions:

1. Start in an "up" position with your weight on your toes (men) or knees (women) and hands (Figs. 4.5 and 4.6).
2. Lower yourself until your elbows form a right angle and your upper arm is parallel to the floor.
3. Complete as many full push-ups as you can in 1 minute. Be sure to keep your abdominals tight, hips slightly piked, and your back straight to protect your lower back. Record, and check your score in Table 4.8.

table 4.8

1-MINUTE PUSH-UP NORMS

STANDARD POSITION

Age	18–29	30–39	40–49	50–59	60+
Excellent	>64	>54	>43	>33	>23
Good	51–64	41–54	31–43	26–33	18–23
Average	37–50	27–40	22–31	17–25	11–17
Low	23–36	18–26	13–21	8–16	6–10
Very Low	<23	<18	<13	<8	<6

MODIFIED POSITION

Age	18–29	30–39	40–49	50–59	60+
Excellent	>54	>43	>33	>23	>17
Good	44–54	31–43	26–33	18–23	15–17
Average	32–43	22–31	17–25	11–17	10–14
Low	20–31	13–21	8–16	6–10	4–9
Very Low	<20	<13	<8	<6	<4

Flexibility

Flexibility is a valuable asset in daily activities or in any type of vigorous exercise program. The ability to move joints through a full range of motion without stiffness or tightness makes exercise more comfortable and decreases risk of injuries. The tests included in this section will indicate whether you have a normal range of motion in the lower back and other important areas.

Quick Checks for Flexibility

The quick checks for flexibility shown in Figures 4.7 to 4.12 are easy ways of measuring flexibility of major muscle groups often shortened and tightened in daily activities. Each quick check is also a stretch, so if your range of motion is limited or if you feel excessive tightness in a joint or muscle group, use the same position to improve flexibility in that area (see Chapter 3 for basic fitness flexibility guidelines).

Sit and Reach Test

The *Sit and Reach Test*, which measures hamstring flexibility, can be done with a flex box. If you do not have a flex box, the test can be performed with a ruler on a bench or on the ground with feet flexed (Fig. 4.13). Norms are given using the soles of the feet as the 0 inches mark.

Goal: To measure flexibility of the hamstrings.
Directions:
1. Warm up.
2. Sit with your feet flat against the flex box about 5 inches apart. Keep your legs straight.
3. Place your hands together. Without bending your knees, reach as far forward as possible, extending fingertips along the box. Hold the position for 3 seconds.
4. Find your flexibility in Table 4.9.

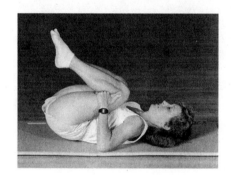

FIGURE 4.7 ➤
Lower back flexibility test.

Muscle: Erector spinae (lower back)

Test: Lying on your back, pull both thighs to chest.

Passing: Thighs should touch chest.

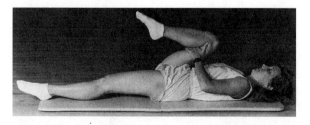

FIGURE 4.8 ➤
Hip flexor flexibility test.

Muscle: Iliopsoas (hip flexor)

Test: Lying on your back, pull one knee to chest, keeping other leg fully extended on the floor.

Passing: Calf of extended leg must remain on the floor; knee must not bend.

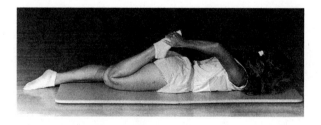

FIGURE 4.9 ➤
Quadriceps flexibility test. Caution: Avoid if you have or experience knee problems.

Muscle: Quadriceps (front of thigh)

Test: Lying face down with knees together, pull heel toward buttocks.

Passing: Heel should comfortably touch buttocks.

FIGURE 4.10 ➤

Hamstring flexibility test.

Muscle: Hamstrings (back of thigh)

Test: Lying on your back, lift one leg, keeping other leg flat on floor without bending either knee.

Passing: The raised leg must reach vertical (90°).

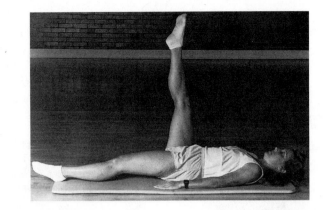

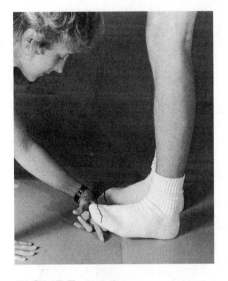

FIGURE 4.11 ➤

Calf flexibility test.

Muscle: Gastrocnemius (calf)

Test: Standing without shoes, raise one forefoot off floor, keeping knees relaxed and heels down.

Passing: Ball of foot should clear floor by height equal to width of two fingers.

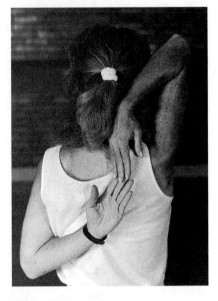

FIGURE 4.12 ➤

Shoulder girdle flexibility test.

Muscle: Shoulder girdle

Test: Try to touch fingertips behind back both ways.

Passing: Fingertips touch.

FIGURE 4.13 ➤

Sit and reach test.

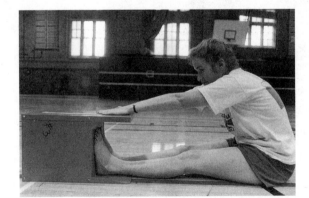

table 4.9

SIT AND REACH NORMS (INCHES)

	MEN	WOMEN
Excellent	>7.0	>8.5
Good	4.0–7.0	6.5–8.5
Average	1.0–3.9	4.0–6.4
Low	−2.0–0.9	1.0–3.9
Very Low	<−2.0	<1.0

FIGURE 4.14 ➤
Sit and reach wall test.

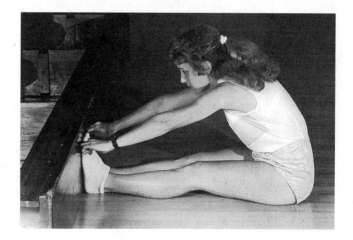

Sit and Reach Wall Test

The *Sit and Reach Wall Test* is a self-check for flexibility and can quickly be performed by a large number of people. All you need is a wall! (Fig. 4.14).

Goal: To measure flexibility of the hamstrings.
Directions:
1. Warm up by walking and static stretching.
2. Remove shoes, sit facing a wall, and keep your feet flat against the wall and your knees straight.
3. Reach forward as far as possible to touch your fingertips, knuckles, or palms to the wall and hold the position for 3 seconds (Fig. 4.14).
4. Check your flexibility evaluations in Table 4.10.

Body Girth Measures

One reason many people begin a fitness program is that they are concerned about their physical appearance. Basic body build is an inherited characteristic, and only about 5 percent of the population can aspire to the current cultural "ideal" of model-like proportions. Take a look at your parents and grandparents to get an idea of your genetic endowment and what is realistic for you. While your basic structure cannot be altered, as fitness improves, fat may be lost from deposit areas and muscles will become firmer, enhancing body contours. You may notice a loss of unwanted inches from the waist, hips,

table 4.10

SIT AND REACH WALL TEST SCORES

RESULT	FLEXIBILITY
Cannot touch wall	Low
Fingertips touch wall	Average
Knuckles touch wall	Good
Palms touch wall	Excellent

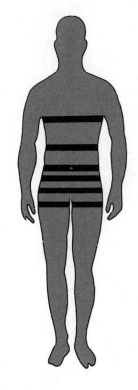

FIGURE 4.15 ➤
Body girth measurement sites.

or thighs or a desirable reshaping of body contours before noticing any weight change. Body girth measures will help you set goals to work for a trim, healthy body shape.

Goal: To measure body girths.
Directions:

Recruit a partner to measure you. You will need a measuring tape. For each measurement, pull the tape snugly, but do not indent the flesh. Take the measurements at the following sites (Fig. 4.15):

➤ *Chest:* across the nipple line at the midpoint of a normal breath
➤ *Abdominal 1:* across the floating ribs, halfway between the chest and waist, at the midpoint of a normal breath
➤ *Waist:* the narrowest point, across the navel
➤ *Abdominal 2:* across the iliac crest (hip bones), midway between waist and hips
➤ *Hips:* with feet together, across the pubic bone in front and across the widest part in back
➤ *Thigh:* right side, widest part, 1 inch below the crotch
➤ *Calf:* widest part
➤ *Wrist:* narrow part, above the bone, with palm up

Body Composition

A certain amount of body fat is essential to good health. Fat acts as an insulator, conserving body heat. It pads bones and cushions internal organs, and it stores and supplies energy for later use.

In a diet-obsessed society in which both obesity and eating disorders abound, few people realize that excessive leanness can be as unhealthy as excessive fatness. Note that, for adults, an average range of body fat for women is 21 percent to 24 percent and for men it is 14 percent to 17 percent (Table 4.11 on page 94). Keep in mind that each of us has inherited a certain body build and fat distribution; it is natural for some bodies to carry more fat than others. Should body fat levels increase with age? While it may be common for people to gain weight with age, creeping weight gain is not desirable. A gain of only 1 pound per year, over 20 years, can leave a person 20 pounds overweight in their 40s, causing a significant health risk. A good rule of thumb is to maintain your weight and fat percentage from your 20s, if they were healthy.

While weight scales can tell you how much you weigh, they cannot tell you how much of your body is composed of fat or lean tissue. A sedentary individual may maintain a normal weight for height but increase fat and lose **lean body mass** (muscle tissue) over time. A body builder may be "overweight" according to height-weight charts, but this is due to development of muscle and bone rather than fat. Being overweight due to having a substantial amount of lean muscle tissue is not the same as being overweight due to excess fat tissue. A person who has a muscular build may think she is too heavy when the weight is mainly lean tissue. She could jeopardize her health trying to lose weight unnecessarily. On the other hand, a sedentary person who is satisfied with her weight may be shocked to discover her body fat percentage is over 30 percent, high enough to pose a health risk. In the early stages of a fitness program, excess fat will often be lost and lean muscle weight will increase as fitness improves. Even if no significant weight change occurs, the exerciser is leaner and appears trimmer because a pound of muscle is denser than a pound of fat.

Body fat is most accurately measured by underwater weighing in a laboratory. Because fat is more buoyant than muscle tissue, underwater weighing can estimate body composition within plus or minus 2 percent to 3 percent. However, this requires elaborate equipment, trained personnel, and considerable time to test each individual. Other laboratory tests of body composition currently being researched include bioelectrical impedance, near-infrared spectrophotometry, ultrasound, and photon absorptiometry.

Bioelectrical impedance is based on the fact that an electrical current travels through **fat-free tissue** (all parts of the body except fat) with its high water and electrolyte content more readily than it does through fat. The current is not harmful since it is too mild to be felt. Results vary with differences in hydration, placement of electrodes, skin temperature, and type of machine used. The validity of this technique has not been determined, and studies have found both over- and underestimation of body fat when compared to other criterion measures.[3,4,5]

Infrared technology traditionally has been used to determine the moisture, protein, and fat composition of food. When used to measure body composition, it tends to underestimate body fat, though some feel it is more accurate than other methods for very lean or obese individuals.[6]

Ultrasound devices measure the variation in diffusion rates of ultrasound waves through fat and lean tissue. Accuracy varies with the pressure exerted on the skin, body fluid balance, and the number of sites measured.

Photon absorptiometry is based on the variations in the rate of photon emissions from bone, lean, and fat tissue after the body is exposed to low-dose radiation. It is not commonly used due to its limited availability, expense, and complexity and due to concern over radiation exposure.[7,8]

A practical technique for measuring body composition involves the use of **skinfold calipers.** A caliper is a device that compresses the skin at a pressure determined by a spring. Skinfold measurements can be used to assess your proportion of fat to lean tissue because about 50 percent of your fat is **subcutaneous fat**—located directly under the skin. The amount of subcutaneous fat you have correlates highly with total body fat. An experienced measurer can assess body fat with skinfold calipers to within a range of plus or minus 2 percent to 5 percent. Two or more body sites may be measured, and accuracy increases with the number of sites sampled. Accuracy diminishes at the ends of the scale—for the very obese and the very lean—but for the average individual, skinfolds are quite reliable.

Self tests of body composition, though considerably less accurate than skinfold caliper measurements, involve body girth measures of body fat and the pinch test. Keep in mind that greater fitness is not guaranteed by low body fat, and that what constitutes a healthy fat percentage for you is an individual matter.

Body Composition Assessment Using Skinfold Calipers[9,10]

Goal: To accurately measure subcutaneous body fat.
Directions: Have a person trained in the use of skinfold calipers perform the following steps.
1. Measure skinfolds on the right side of the body using a skinfold caliper.
2. Grasp a fold of skin between thumb and forefinger, pulling it away from the underlying muscle.

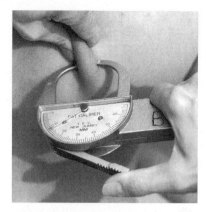

FIGURE 4.16 ➤
Skinfold measuring technique.

3. Apply the calipers about 0.25 inch below the fingers holding the skinfold (Fig. 4.16).
4. Take triceps and thigh measurements on a vertical skinfold. Take subscapular and suprailiac measures on a slight lateral slant along the natural fold of the skin.
5. Measure twice. Take readings to the nearest half millimeter. If the readings do not match, take a third measurement and average the closest two measurements.
6. Skinfold sites for women are the following:
   a. Triceps. Measure a vertical skinfold on the back of the arm midway between the shoulder and the elbow (Fig. 4.17).
   b. Suprailiac. Measure a slightly lateral fold at the middle of the side of the body just above the hip bone (iliac crest) (Fig. 4.18).
7. Skinfold sites for men are the following:
   a. Thigh. Measure a vertical fold on the front of the thigh midway between the inguinal fold (where the hip bends in front) and the top of the patella (knee cap) (Fig. 4.19).
   b. Subscapular. Measure a diagonal fold just under the right shoulder blade (scapula) (Fig. 4.20).
8. Mark your two skinfold measurements on the *Percent of Body Fat Chart* (Fig. 4.21) and connect the marks with a straight line. Read your percent of fat on the center scale (see Table 4.11).

FIGURE 4.17 ➤
Triceps.

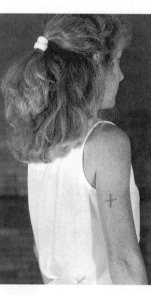

FIGURE 4.18 ➤
Suprailiac.

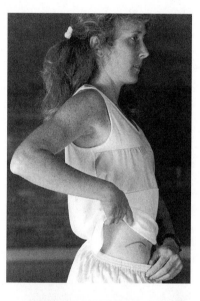

FIGURE 4.19 ➤
Thigh.

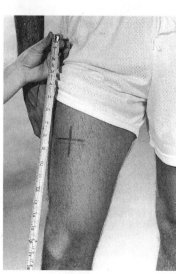

FIGURE 4.20 ➤
Subscapular.

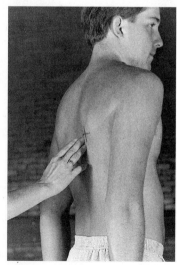

How to Determine Desirable Weight

Once you have measured your body fat percentage, it is useful to determine your desirable weight based on your present fat-free mass. For young adults, a reasonable body fat level in the trim range for women is 17 percent to 20 percent fat, and for men it is 10 percent to 13 percent fat (Table 4.11). The following steps use an example of a person who has 26 percent body fat and weighs 140 pounds to illustrate how to determine desirable weight at 18 percent body fat for females and 12 percent fat for males.

Goal: To calculate desirable weight at 18 percent fat for women and 12 percent fat for men.

Directions: Perform the calculations that follow using your own measurements:

➤ Body fat percentage = 26%.
➤ Weight = 140 lbs.

1. Body fat percentage × body weight = fat 0.26 × 140 lbs. = 36.4 lbs.
2. Body weight − fat = fat-free mass 140 lbs. − 36.4 lbs. = 103.6 lbs.
3. Fat-free mass ÷ 0.82 = desired weight for women at 18% fat.
   103.6 lbs. ÷ 0.82 = 126 lbs.
   Fat-free mass ÷ 0.88 = desired weight for men at 12% fat.
   103.6 lbs. ÷ 0.88 = 117 lbs.

Body Girth Measures of Body Fat

Body girth measures of fatness are considerably less accurate than other measures of body fat such as skinfolds. However, their advantage is that they do not require special equipment nor training, and they can be done with a measuring tape at home.

Directions:
1. Men should measure waist girth at the navel and women should measure hips at the widest point. Pull the tape so it is snug but does not indent the skin (Fig. 4.15).
2. Remove shoes. Men should measure their weight without clothing. Women should measure their height.
3. Mark the measurements on the appropriate circumference chart and connect them with a straight line (Fig. 4.22).

Waist-to-Hip Ratio

Recent investigations have begun pointing to the *location* of excess fat as a risk factor for heart disease and certain cancers. Fat distributed in the abdominal area is linked to increased health risks; hip/thigh fat is not as risky. As a result, the waist-to-hip ratio has become a common assessment for health-risk identification. To compute this ratio, divide the wait measurement by the hip measurement.

$$\frac{29 \text{ in. waist}}{38 \text{ in. hip}} = 0.76 \qquad \frac{42 \text{ in. waist}}{36 \text{ in. hip}} = 1.17$$

Studies indicate that health problems are increased for women whose ratio is 0.80 or higher and for men whose ratio is 0.95 or higher. (See Chapter 10 for more information on waist-to-hip ratio as a health-risk factor.)

Pinch Test

Another simple measure of body fatness is the pinch test. Grasp a skinfold at the midpoint of your side, just above your hip bone (iliac crest). More than a 1-inch skinfold thickness may indicate excessive body fat.

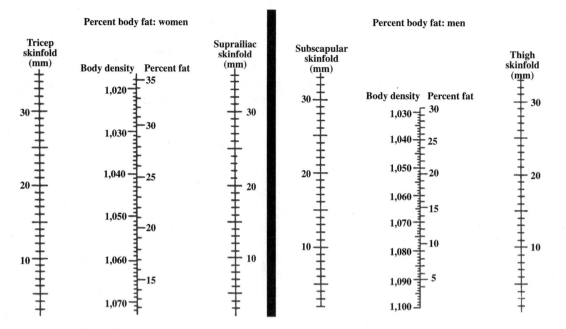

FIGURE 4.21 ➤

Percent body fat nomogram.

source: A. W. Sloan and J. Weir. "Nomograms for Prediction of Body Density and Total Body Fat from Skinfold Measurements." *Journal of Applied Physiology* 28:2 (1970): 221–22. Reprinted by permission of the American Physiological Society.

table 4.11

BODY FAT NORMS

	MEN	WOMEN
Very low fat	<10	<17
Low fat (trim)	10–13	17–20
Average	14–17	21–24
Above average (fat)	18–20	25–27
High fat	21–25	28–30
Obese	>25	>30

Circumference chart for women

Circumference chart for men

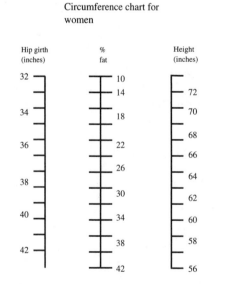

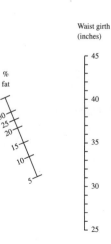

FIGURE 4.22 ➤

Circumference charts.

Nomograms developed by Jack Wilmore, University of Texas. Used by permission.

Assessment is a critical tool in developing any dimension of wellness. It helps you to understand your own strengths and weaknesses and to decide whether your current levels of cardiorespiratory endurance, muscular endurance, flexibility, and body fat are conducive to optimal wellness. With this knowledge, you can set reasonable fitness goals, establish a starting point for a fitness program, and develop a plan of action. Specific workout programs for different aerobic activities can be found in the Appendix. A *Health/Exercise Assessment Form* and a *Personal Fitness Profile* are also available in the Activities section.

As you progress in your fitness program, it may be useful to retest occasionally. While testing should not dominate your program, it will allow you to monitor your progress and can give additional motivation to continue regular exercise.

REFERENCES

1. Keener, E., D. Powers, G. Robbins, and J. Ruston. Undergraduate Student Physical Fitness Assessment, Ball State University, Muncie, Ind. (Spring 1989).
2. The American College of Sports Medicine. *Guidelines for Exercise Testing and Prescription*, 5th ed. Philadelphia: Lea & Febiger, 1995.
3. Chumlea, W. C., and R. N. Baumgartner. "Bioelectrical Impedance Methods for the Estimation of Body Composition." *Canadian Journal of Sport Sciences* 15 (September 1990): 172–79.
4. Kaminsky, L. A., and M. H. Whaley. "Variability in Predicting Body Composition Using Bioelectrical Impedance and Skinfold Measurements." *Medicine and Science in Sports and Exercise* 21 (April 1989): S74.
5. Lukaski, H. C., et al. "Body Composition Assessment of Athletes Using Bioelectrical Impedance Measurements." *Journal of Sports Medicine and Physical Fitness* 30 (December 1990): 434–40.
6. Israel, R. G., et al. "Validity of a Near-Infrared Spectrophotometry Device for Estimating Human Body Composition." *Research Quarterly for Exercise and Sport* 60 (1989): 379–83.
7. Clark, R. R., et al. "Prediction of Percent Body Fat in Adult Males Using Dual Energy X-ray Absorptiometry, Skinfolds, and Hydrostatic Weighing." *Medicine and Science in Sports and Exercise* 25 (April 1993): 528–35.
8. Shephard, R. J. "Human Body Composition." *Canadian Journal of Sport Science* 15 (June 1990): 88.
9. Lohman, Timothy G. *New Dimensions in Body Composition.* Champaign, Ill.: Human Kinetics, 1992.
10. Sloan, A. W., and J. Weir. "Nomograms for Prediction of Body Density and Total Body Fat from Skinfold Measurements." *Journal of Applied Physiology* 28 (1970): 221–22.

SUGGESTED READINGS

American College of Sports Medicine. *Guidelines for Exercise Testing and Prescription*, 5th ed. Philadelphia: Lea & Febiger, 1995.

Skinner, J. S., et al. "Assessment of Fitness." In C. Buchard et al., eds. *Exercise, Fitness and Health.* Champaign, Ill.: Human Kinetics, 1990.

Corbin, C. B., and R. Lindsey. *Concepts of Physical Fitness with Laboratories.* Dubuque, Iowa: Wm. C. Brown Publishers, 1991.

Francis, Peter, and Lorna Francis. "Flexibility Screening." *Dance-Exercise Today* (September 1987).

Heyward, V. H. *Advanced Fitness Assessment and Exercise Prescription*, 2d ed. Champaign, Ill.: Human Kinetics, 1991.

Kravitz, Len, and Vivian Heyward. "Getting a Grip on Body Composition." *IDEA Today* (April 1992): 34–39.

Lohman, Timothy G., et al. *Anthropometric Standardization Reference Manual.* Champaign, Ill.: Human Kinetics, 1991.

Lohman, Timothy G. *New Dimensions in Body Composition.* Champaign, Ill.: Human Kinetics, 1992.

Shephard, Roy J. *Aerobic Fitness & Health.* Champaign, Ill.: Human Kinetics, 1994.

chapter 5

Common Injuries and Care of the Lower Back

➤ Objectives

After reading this chapter, you will be able to:

1. Identify four main reasons injuries occur.

2. Give three tips for avoiding an overuse injury.

3. Explain how muscle weakness and inflexibility contribute to injuries.

4. Identify four common muscle imbalances.

5. List and explain the general recommended treatment for common injuries (R.I.C.E.).

6. Describe the basic causes and treatment of blisters, chafing, muscle soreness, side stitch, muscle cramp, muscle strain, tendinitis, plantar fasciitis, heel spur syndrome, shin splints, stress fracture, chondromalacia, and ankle sprain.

7. Identify the four symptoms of injury that indicate the need for medical attention.

8. Explain two vital components of rehabilitation needed in order to resume activity safely without injury.

9. Identify the two most important keys to preventing lower back pain.

10. List and describe six of the eight exercises recommended to reduce the risk of lower back pain.

Terms

- Blisters
- Chondromalacia
- Cramp
- Heel spur
- Intervertebral disc
- Ischemia
- Ligament

- Orthotics
- Overpronation
- Overuse
- Plantar fasciitis
- Pronation
- R.I.C.E.
- Shin splint

- Side stitch
- Sprain
- Strain
- Stress fracture
- Supination
- Tendinitis
- Tendons

An ounce of prevention is worth a ton of cure.

Anonymous

You walk into your first jogging class, eager to improve your fitness. You have not exercised regularly and you hope this class will help you get into shape. Your instructor begins with a warm-up and an easy jog around campus. After your run, you feel great and invigorated. The next morning, you wake up and your whole body aches. You don't remember having been run over by a truck. "What should I do now? Withdraw from class? Stay in bed? Buy stock in Ben-Gay? When will I be able to move again?"

Participation in fitness activities offers many benefits. These benefits far exceed the risk of injury. When you exercise, you intentionally use certain muscles to increase their strength and endurance. As your body adapts to these efforts, you may experience minor aches and soreness. Physical activity also carries some risk of overuse or injury. Fortunately, many of these discomforts are minor, and you will be able to continue or quickly resume your workouts. This chapter discusses how to prevent injuries, in addition to how to recognize their signs and symptoms and what treatments are recommended. It also examines how to maintain a healthy back, since chronic back pain is a common problem. Finally, factors that affect the musculature of the spine and how to avoid lower back injury are covered.

Injury Prevention

Prevention is the key to reducing the frequency of injuries. Understanding the cause of injury allows you to stop minor problems before they turn you into the "walking wounded." Prevention is far more conducive to wellness than any patch and repair job. There are four main reasons injuries occur:[1]

1. *Overuse*: doing too much too soon or too often, causing a breakdown at the weakest point—ankle, Achilles tendon, shin, knee, or back.
2. *Footwear*: wearing improper or worn-out shoes.
3. *Weakness and inflexibility*: muscles so weak or tight that the slightest unusual twist strains them.
4. *Mechanical problems*: the result of anatomical problems (the way the foot hits the ground, body build, etc.) or using poor form while exercising.

An individually adjusted workload, well-made and well-kept shoes, supplemental toning and stretching exercises, and mechanical improvements will prevent the majority of injuries.

Overuse

In order to improve or maintain fitness, you must overload, or push, beyond normal demands. Overload is necessary and good up to a point, but you must be able to recover between workouts. The goal is to exercise so that you improve but not so much that you cause **overuse,** excessive overload leading to injury or illness (Fig. 5.1). Overuse problems commonly occur at the beginning of a new exercise program and account for the majority of injuries. It is estimated that between 25 percent and 50 percent of athletes visiting sports medicine clinics have sustained overuse injuries.[2] The first four months of a new program are the most critical. The body and muscles must be given time to gradually adapt to the new demands.

Set realistic goals early in a fitness program. Your instructor will help you determine an appropriate entry-level conditioning program and progression. Gradually increase your exercise intensity and duration to attain your personal goals. For example, if you have never participated in aerobics, your first goal may be to perform 10 minutes of continuous aerobic exercise, although other members of the class may work out 25 or 30 minutes. Try not to compete or compare yourself with your friends who may be able to exercise for a longer duration or at higher intensity. You will be able to catch up in time, but if you attempt to keep up with them before your body is ready, you risk an overuse problem.

FIGURE 5.1►

Overload and overuse. Overload is good up to a point; overuse can cause injury.

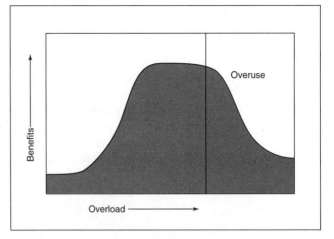

A good rule of thumb to follow is to increase the duration of the workout no more than 10 percent weekly. A beginner should not jump from a 20-minute workout up to 40 minutes. This principle holds true in aerobics, lap swimming, water exercise, bicycling, fitness walking, and jogging. Studies show an increasing injury rate with increasing weekly jogging distance beyond 20 miles per week.[3] Many fitness buffs and athletes have a feeling of invulnerability. They think their bodies can adapt to increased exercise workloads without any problem. Realize that more is not always better. By allowing your body to gradually adjust to new exercise demands, you will greatly reduce the risk of suffering an overuse injury.

Consider alternating an impact activity with a low impact or nonimpact activity. This alternation allows the muscles a period of rest and recovery and switches the demands to a new muscle group. It is repetitive stress on the body that causes problems. Some people enjoy alternating activities because it adds variety and develops total body fitness better than any single activity. It also allows specific muscles and joints a chance to rest and recover. For example, water exercise or bicycling is a good supplement to an impact exercise such as jogging.

It is crucial that you listen to your body during and after exercise. After a great workout, if you feel a little soreness, it should gradually decrease over the next couple of hours. However, if you develop excessive soreness or pain, cut back in your next workout, try a different activity, or take a day off. The importance of rest is often overlooked. It is when you are in a state of fatigue that you are most susceptible to developing a problem.

If you are getting the right amount of exercise, you should look good, feel good, and be alert and productive. Too much exercise, like too little, can be unhealthy. After a workout, you should get enough rest to be fully recovered by the next workout. Rest is probably the most neglected aspect of fitness. Your body does not improve during the exercise itself but during recovery. Exercise provides the overload that stimulates that improvement. During the rest period between workouts, the body makes adaptations to the demands made upon it. When the recovery is adequate, you will begin the next workout feeling strong and energetic. If you feel tired and washed out, rest will do you more good than exercise. Also keep in mind that exercise isn't the only source of overstress. Other aspects of daily life such as poor nutrition; emotional tension; job, social, or family problems; and lack of sleep can contribute to chronic fatigue.

The concept of "no pain, no gain" and "going for the burn" are outdated. Pain is the body's natural way of informing you that something is wrong. Pain may be localized in a specific spot or generalized over a broad area. However, pain is a subjective response, and each individual will tolerate it differently. Do not try to exercise through pain or injury. Almost every study shows that previous injury is a risk factor for future injuries.[4] Therefore, it is important to allow for complete healing and to correct mechanical problems before resuming activity.

Footwear

While many injuries are due to overuse, it is only part of the problem. Wearing improper or worn-out shoes places added stress on your hips, knees, ankles, and feet—the sites of up to 90 percent of all sports injuries.[5] The feet are the most abused and neglected part of the body. Good footwear is the best investment you can make in an exercise program. Each time your foot hits the ground when jogging, the force of impact is approximately three times your body weight. Your feet, ankles, shins, knees, hips, and lower back must absorb a tremendous amount of stress. If the stress is too great, breakdown occurs at the weakest link in the chain. A well-fitted pair of shoes is the first line of defense against impact injuries.

Shoes should provide good shock absorption, support, and stability yet maintain a reasonable degree of flexibility.[6] Your foot will naturally roll inward when you jog; therefore, the heel counter (the rigid plastic insert in the shoe's heel) must be firm to prevent excessive heel movement. The bottom of the shoe must have good traction to prevent slipping. Shoes are manufactured to be used for a certain number of miles, and they can lose their cushioning ability even if the uppers still look good. Each step compresses the sole, causing it to flatten and gradually lose shock absorbability. Exercise shoes typically lose about one-third of their ability to absorb shock after 500 miles of use.[7] The upper part of the shoe stretches and weakens, decreasing lateral support. This happens so gradually you may not notice it until you try on a new pair of shoes. With less cushioning and support, there is a greater chance of injury. If you wear the shoes five to ten hours a week during exercise (walking, jogging, aerobics, etc.), you should probably replace them every six months to retain adequate cushioning. Runners would be well-advised to keep a log of their mileage as a reminder of when to buy new shoes.

Weakness and Inflexibility

Sit down with your feet extended in front. Slowly reach toward your toes. Can you touch them without bending your knees? Many exercisers who neglect flexibility exercises cannot pass this test for minimal flexibility. Their legs are too tight, and this increases susceptibility to muscle and tendon injuries. Aerobic activities are great for the cardiorespiratory system, but they alone do not develop balanced fitness. They tend to shorten and tighten muscles that are used repetitively, leaving opposing, relatively unused muscles weak. This can lead to muscle imbalance. If some muscles are too tight, joint movement is restricted. Table 5.1 lists some common muscle imbalances. The solution to this problem is to stretch the tight muscles and strengthen the weak ones. Flexibility is one of the most important factors in injury prevention.

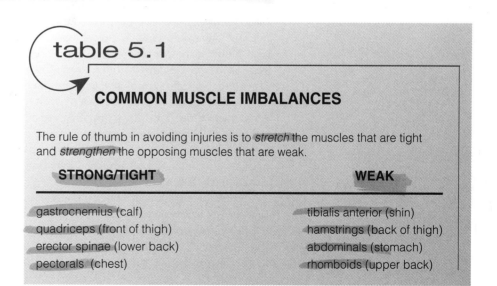

table 5.1

COMMON MUSCLE IMBALANCES

The rule of thumb in avoiding injuries is to *stretch* the muscles that are tight and *strengthen* the opposing muscles that are weak.

STRONG/TIGHT	WEAK
gastrocnemius (calf)	tibialis anterior (shin)
quadriceps (front of thigh)	hamstrings (back of thigh)
erector spinae (lower back)	abdominals (stomach)
pectorals (chest)	rhomboids (upper back)

FIGURE 5.2 ➤
Supination and overpronation.

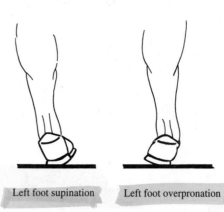

Left foot supination   Left foot overpronation

Incorporate a basic stretching routine into each workout, preferably during the cool-down. (See Chapter 3 for recommended strength and flexibility exercises.) Stretch gently, placing only slight tension on the muscles. Hard stretching or bouncy movements may activate the stretch reflex. This causes the muscle to involuntarily contract and shorten—exactly the opposite of what you're trying to do—to protect itself from injury. Concentrate on event-specific exercises. For example, if you are a swimmer, you will want to spend additional time stretching the shoulders and arms. If jogging or aerobics is your activity, concentrate on stretching the hamstrings, quadriceps, lower back, and calf. Abdominal curls are an important supplement to any fitness workout. Strong abdominals and a flexible lower back are critical in preventing lower-back problems.

Mechanics

Structural weaknesses, mainly affecting the legs, knees, ankles, and feet, are often revealed when a beginner starts a new exercise program or when overuse occurs. Biomechanical difficulties often arise in the feet. The foot is a marvelous structure of 26 bones, with almost double that number of ligaments and muscles. It strikes the ground about 80 to 90 times a minute during exercise. When a weak foot pounds the ground several thousand times a day, the potential for injury is great. Slight **pronation** of your foot is natural—that is, your foot will roll inward slightly after the outer edge of the heel strikes the ground. Since all bodies are not created equal, different foot types, gait styles, and body mechanics vary in susceptibility to injury. For example, flat feet may cause **overpronation**—too much inward rotation (Fig. 5.2). This can cause tendinitis, plantar fasciitis, or knee strain. Overpronation can be detected by excessive shoe wear on the inside of the forefoot. **Supination,** on the other hand, is the rolling outward of the foot upon contact. People with high arches tend to supinate. When the foot hits the ground, it does not roll inward enough to absorb the shock of impact, increasing the risk of shin splints, stress fractures, and medial knee and hip problems. Supination causes excessive wear on the outside of the shoe sole.

Moderate pronation problems can be corrected by wise shoe selection. Most exercise shoes are designed to limit overpronation, not eliminate all inward rotation. Observing the wear pattern on your shoes can help you select a shoe designed for your specific mechanics. Employees in many sports shoe stores are trained to help you select a proper shoe. If discomfort persists, you may want to consult a physician or podiatrist who will check your foot mechanics. He or she may prescribe **orthotics,** shoe inserts molded to your foot, to correct abnormalities. These allow the foot to operate mechanically efficiently. They are highly effective for alleviating excessive ankle pronation/supination.

Regardless of your body type, it is important for you to pay attention to form when participating in any aerobic activity. Participants in aerobic dance, water exercise, bicycling, and step aerobics and even those using stair climbing and cross country skiing machines need to understand the proper mechanics of each activity. In this way, many injuries and discomforts can be avoided. You will find technique and safety tips for a variety of aerobic activities in the Appendix. You may also want to refer to the "Contraindicated Exercises" listed in Chapter 8.

The body is a marvelous mechanism. Considering its complexity, it is a wonder it doesn't break down more often. Exercise is vital to maintain wellness. Illness and injury are less common in those who maintain peak performance through regular exercise than it is in those who exercise sporadically. Even when injuries do occur, few are debilitating. Many simply cause some inconvenience. The recommended treatment for many injuries, whether mild or severe, is rest, ice, compression, and elevation or **R.I.C.E.**

R.I.C.E.

Acute injuries to muscles, joints, and tendons are often accompanied by swelling. Rapid recovery requires keeping the swelling to a minimum. The aim of treatment is to assist the healing process.

R = Rest

The classic advice of old-time coaches was, "Run it off." On the contrary, the injured area should be rested for 24 hours to 72 hours, depending on the severity of the injury.[8] Using crutches, a plastic or fiberglass cast, or a sling are examples of ways to "rest" injured limbs. A minor complaint can become a major problem if you keep aggravating the situation. Healing progresses more rapidly when stress to the area is reduced. Frequently, people will start back into full activity before they are ready, and they reinjure the area. Once you return to your usual workout routine, reduce your duration, frequency, and/or intensity by 25 percent.[9] Do not resume your normal workout level until you are free of pain both during and after exercise.

I = Ice

Apply ice to the injured part immediately. A convenient way to apply ice is to put ice cubes in a plastic freezer bag and place it on the injured area. Reusable gel ice packs and chemical cold packs also work well. Do not apply the ice directly to the skin. A layer of wet towelling between the ice and skin transmits the cold to the area quite effectively without risking freezing the skin. Apply the ice for 15 to 20 minutes but for no more than 20 minutes at a time. The ice may make the injured part ache for the first 5 to 10 minutes. Keep it on! After 10 minutes, the part will become numb. This will give immediate pain relief by decreasing blood flow to the superficial tissues. It also reduces swelling, inflammation, and tissue damage. In deeper blood vessels, circulation increases, bringing blood, nutrients, and healing cells to the injured area. Ice the injured area every three to four waking hours for at least the first 48 to 72 hours. Icing should be continued after that time if swelling persists.

If you feel mild discomfort when exercising and suspect an overuse injury, such as tendinitis, you should apply ice to the tender areas right after you work out and reapply it several times a day for the next 48 hours. Remember: You can never go wrong with ice. Sportsmedicine physician Francis G. O'Connor states, "Ice is indicated as long as inflammation persists—from the onset of the injury, through rehabilitation, and into sports return."[10]

C = Compression

When not icing the injury, wrap the part with an elastic wrap to prevent fluid buildup in the injured area. Wrap it snugly but not tightly enough to interfere with circulation. If the part starts throbbing, the wrap may be on too tight. Remove the wrap and reapply it more loosely. Do not sleep with the wrap on.

E = Elevation

Raise the injured area above the level of the heart. This will reduce the swelling by combatting the effect of gravity pulling blood and fluids down to the injured area. Most people with an injured ankle or knee will place it on a pillow for elevation when going to sleep. However, you may move during the night and lose the elevation. Instead, place three or four books under your mattress to raise it approximately 6 to 8 inches.

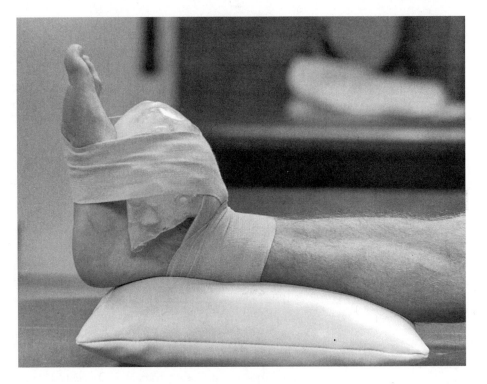

Heat and Pain Relievers

Many people mistakenly apply heat to an acute injury. Heat actually stimulates blood flow and increases inflammation. You should stick with ice for at least the first 48 to 72 hours after an injury and only then, *after swelling has completely subsided*, should heat be applied. At that point, heat may speed the healing and help relieve pain, relax muscles, and reduce stiffness. Either dry heat (heating pad or lamp) or moist heat (a hot bath, whirlpool, hot-water bottle, damp heat pack) will do. Apply the heat for 20 to 30 minutes, two or three times a day. You can also use it for 5 to 10 minutes before exercising to reduce stiffness.

Over-the-counter liniments and balms are popular methods for producing a warm feeling in muscles. The effect of these much-advertised products is only superficial—the active ingredients stimulate sensory nerve endings in the skin to produce a sensation of heat. This does little or nothing to promote healing and may actually mask the pain.

Aspirin or ibuprofen (such as Motrin or Advil) can reduce the pain and inflammation of minor sprains, strains, and tendinitis. Acetaminophen (such as Tylenol) is less helpful because it has no anti-inflammatory effect. Consult your doctor before using any drugs.

Common Injuries

In pursuit of wellness, you may occasionally push yourself beyond the current capabilities of your structure. Finding your peak and keeping it is a challenge and part of a process of learning about your body's own unique strengths and weaknesses. If, in your zeal to experience peak performance, you develop an athletic ailment, it will generally be minor and you will be able to resume activity within a few days. Here we will discuss the potential causes of, symptoms of, and treatments for the most common injuries.

Blisters

Blisters are a common problem, especially for beginning exercisers. They are, essentially, burns caused by the friction of a foot rubbing against a shoe. They are usually only a problem if they become infected or if they cause you to limp. The most common areas for blisters are the bottom of the foot, the sides of the big and little toes, and the back of the heel. A blister is a hot, red, and inflamed area, occasionally containing water or blood. Blisters can be prevented by eliminating the friction that causes them. Wear 100 percent acrylic (orlon) socks. Acrylic is best at dissipating moisture and preventing blisters from forming. Cotton socks produce twice as many blisters that are three times as large, and even worse is a cotton-acrylic blend.[11] Never wear new shoes for a workout without first breaking them in by walking around in them at home for a few days. Should a blister be opened? Some say no, let the fluid reabsorb into the system since an open blister invites infection. Others say to pop the blister if it is painful and causes you to limp. The best treatment is to apply a donut pad and lubricant to the blister to reduce friction and pressure. Some runners wear their socks inside out to avoid the abrasion of the rough interior seam. It may also help to wear two socks on the affected foot—a thin nylon sock inside an acrylic sock. If the blister is lanced, keep the area clean to prevent infection. Consult your physician if you think it may be infected.

Chafing

When skin rubs against skin or against clothing, it becomes irritated and can crack and bleed. The most common problem areas are between the thighs, under the armpits, and on the nipples (runner's nipples). While chafing can happen to anyone, frequency increases with body fat percentage. To prevent chafing, select clothing of smooth, nonabrasive material with few or well-covered seams. Avoid clothing that is tight or that bunches under the arms or between the legs. Treat chafing by applying petroleum jelly to the affected area. Wearing tights or knee-length exercise shorts can protect chafed thighs. Nipple chafing can be decreased by going shirtless in warm weather or by applying petroleum jelly and adhesive bandages to the nipples. Women should select a good exercise bra that has no seams across the nipple area.

Muscle Soreness

Muscle soreness may be fairly mild and usually is just a reminder that you had a good workout. Other than following a sensible progression, there is no real prevention for muscle soreness. It indicates that some muscles that were out of shape have been stimulated to tone up, usually occurring at the beginning of any new exercise program. For example, a person who has not recently lifted weights will develop muscle soreness following the first workout. Duration of activity and eccentric (lengthening) contractions are highly correlated to muscle soreness. For example, running downhill repeatedly will produce more quadricep soreness than will an equal amount of flat or uphill running. Muscle soreness is thought to be caused by microscopic tears or spasms of the connective tissue. There is no long-term damage from this. Muscle soreness may develop immediately or over a 24- to 36-hour period following unaccustomed exercise and will usually disappear within one to three days. There is no real pain but rather a mild achiness when you move the major muscle groups used in the activity. After several sessions of the same activity, soreness will diminish or disappear entirely. There is little or nothing that can be done for mild muscle soreness. While stretching is beneficial for flexibility, it has little effect on reducing soreness.[12]

Side Stitch

A **side stitch** may result from participating in vigorous activity before the body has had sufficient warm-up. It may be related to a lack of conditioning, weak abdominals, shallow breathing, consuming a meal before exercise, dehydration, excessive exercise intensity, or **ischemia** (inadequate oxygen) to the diaphragm or intercostal muscles between the ribs. A side stitch is basically a diaphragm spasm. It can be treated by stopping activity and stretching or holding the side. After cessation of the activity for a few minutes, the pain and spasm should subside. Taking a deep breath may also break the spasm. Once the pain has dissipated, activity may resume.

Muscle Cramp

A **cramp** is a sharp, involuntary muscle contraction. It may occur during exercise or at rest. The calf is the most common area for a muscle cramp to occur, but cramps may occur anywhere in the body. Muscle cramps may be caused by fatigue. This is a protective mechanism, your body telling you to quit or you will do yourself damage. Cramps may also be related to a strength imbalance, an electrolyte imbalance, or dehydration. Occasionally, low levels of circulating calcium and potassium in the blood can contribute to cramps. A muscle cramp will occur frequently in the summer when the weather is hot and humid. Nighttime calf cramps can happen in bed when you suddenly stretch your toes downward, causing the calf muscle to contract. Cramps can be treated with fluid intake and with gradual stretching of the muscle. A calf cramp may be treated by flexing the foot to a 90 degree angle. Occasionally, gentle massage may help.

Muscle cramps may be prevented by taking precautions when exercising in the heat. Wear light, loose clothing; drink water freely; gradually acclimatize yourself to the heat; and exercise during the cooler hours of the day. Extra salt is not needed. A regular program of stretching may also help prevent muscle cramps.

Muscle Strain

A muscle **strain** is a partial or complete tear of muscle fibers or a tendon and is sometimes referred to as a *pull*. There are many different causes, but it most often results from a violent contraction of the muscle. A strain may be caused by fatigue, overexertion, muscle imbalance or weakness, or electrolyte or water imbalance.

A strain may range from mild (more painful than just soreness) to a complete rupture of the muscle. Muscles most likely to be affected are the hamstrings, gastrocnemius, Achilles tendon, quadriceps, hip flexors, groin, and the rotator cuff muscles of the shoulder. Generally, symptoms include sharp pain, weakness with possible loss of function, spasm or extreme tightness, and tenderness to the touch. R.I.C.E. is used to treat muscle strain. Reduce or eliminate activity until the injury starts to heal. The severity of the injury and which muscle is injured will affect the recovery time. The hamstrings usually take the longest to heal and rehabilitate, while the quadriceps and hip flexors heal more quickly. If the strain is severe, it will heal with a significant amount of scar tissue. Scar tissue is not elastic like muscle, so stretching and strengthening exercises are important to return to normal function. To prevent strains, complete a full-body warm-up before working out, take care not to overdo, and work toward balancing the strength and flexibility in opposing muscles.

Tendinitis

Anytime you see *-itis*, think inflammation. **Tendinitis** is the inflammation of a tendon from repetitive stress. **Tendons** are the fibrous cords that connect muscles to bones. The most commonly known is the Achilles tendon, which can be felt at the back of the ankle. Tendons are vulnerable to inflammation because the force of muscle contractions is transmitted through them. When inflamed, the tendon may become hot, red, and swollen in moderate to severe cases. There will be pain on movement and activity. Normal daily activities, such as opening a door or walking up the stairs, can be painful. The most common areas to suffer tendinitis are the Achilles tendon, knee, shoulder, and elbow ("tennis elbow"). Tendinitis often affects participants in swimming, tennis, baseball, and volleyball. Achilles tendon problems, common to runners, fitness walkers, and aerobic dancers, are almost always due to tight calf muscles. When the foot flexes to push off, the powerful Achilles pulls the heel up. If the calf is too tight, it yanks the heel up prematurely, stressing the Achilles tendon. Rest from the activity that caused the injury and stretching to alleviate excessive tightness are recommended. Over-the-counter anti-flammatory medications (ibuprofen, aspirin) may also help. It may take two to three weeks to completely heal and rehabilitate. Continuing activity will only delay healing. Meanwhile, you may include alternate activities to maintain fitness. A regular program incorporating stretching and strengthening can help prevent tendinitis.

Plantar Fasciitis

The plantar fascia is a long thick band of connective tissue on the undersurface of the foot that attaches the base of the calcaneus (heel bone) to the base of the toes. An inflammation of the plantar fascia, **plantar fasciitis,** is usually felt as heel or arch pain before, during, or after activity. Injury to the fascia may result from excessive impact, worn shoes, or poor foot mechanics. Anatomical problems frequently cause plantar fasciitis—high arches, tight Achilles tendon, flat feet, excessive pronation. Also, with age and repeated weight-bearing stress, the fat pad under the heel becomes flattened and less shock absorbent. Rest, ice, and elimination of causal factors are the recommended treatments. Orthotics will reduce symptoms in 95 percent of cases of plantar fasciitis.[13]

Heel Spur Syndrome

A **heel spur** is a bony growth found on the underside of the calcaneus, behind the insertion of the plantar fascia. A heel spur is caused by chronic irritation of the plantar fascia at its insertion. Not all heel spurs cause pain. Heel spur syndrome is generally attributable to heel trauma from overuse, excessive impact, or a continuous pull on the plantar fascia, which strains the arch. It is most painful when a person first steps down on the foot in the morning, but pain may continue throughout the day. Treatment involves rest, anti-inflammatory medication, and insertion of a heel pad in the shoe to alleviate inflammation of the plantar fascia.[14]

Shin Splints

A **shin splint** refers to any pain in the front of the lower leg (shin). Early signs are acute burning pain or irritation in the lower third of the anterior tibialis. This may progress to slight swelling, redness, warmth, and inflammation. A variety of factors contribute to shin splints. They often come early in an exercise program and are particularly common in those who are out of shape, overweight, wide hipped, knock-kneed, or duck footed. Working out on very hard or very soft surfaces can bring on shin splints, even if a person is well-conditioned. Switching from a hard to a soft surface or vice versa, excessive mileage, improper footwear, poor foot mechanics, running on a road slope, and running the same direction all the time on an indoor track may cause them. Women, particularly those who wear high heels, are affected nearly three times more often than are men.[15]

Shin splints may be a sign of a long arch problem in the foot. As the long arch begins to sag, it stretches lower leg muscles and causes pain. Another cause is a muscle imbalance between the strong calf muscle and the weak anterior tibialis, which may lead to inflammation of the membrane between the tibia and the fibula. This imbalance can be corrected by flexion exercises to strengthen the anterior tibialis and by stretching the calf. These should be done each workout. If mechanical problems are not corrected, shin splints tend to recur.

To treat shin splints, rub ice on the affected area for 15 to 20 minutes three to four times a day. Occasionally, aspirin therapy may be indicated for a few days to reduce inflammation. If the pain is persistent, reduce your activity level and consult a physician to rule out a stress fracture.

Stress Fracture

A **stress fracture** is a microscopic break in a bone caused by overuse. Unlike a broken bone, which occurs with a distinct traumatic event, a stress fracture is the result of cumulative overload that occurs over many days or weeks. Doing too much too soon (overuse) is the major cause. Bone is living tissue that adjusts to exercise force demands placed on it. As force is applied, bone will remodel itself to better handle the force. If too much force is applied, the bone may fracture before it can successfully remodel. Running extreme mileage, doing impact aerobics, wearing worn-out shoes, exercising on hard surfaces such as asphalt or concrete, and having poor foot mechanics may cause a stress fracture. While it can occur anywhere in the lower legs and feet, it is most common at the end of the tibia near the ankle. Because they have smaller, lighter bones, women are more susceptible to stress fractures than are men. A stress fracture may be debilitating if not treated correctly. Frequently, a stress fracture may be confused with a case of severe shin splints. Stress fractures are difficult to detect clinically. Frequently, they will not show up on X ray until three to four weeks after the onset of symptoms. A bone scan can detect a stress fracture much earlier in the injury because it reveals the active bone formation that occurs while the fracture is healing.[16] The pain of a stress fracture will not go away with conventional treatments (ice, ultrasound) or medication. Only rest will decrease the pain.

Stages in the progression of a stress fracture include (1) pain during activity that subsides after the completion of exercise; (2) pain during activity that continues during the rest of the day into the evening; and (3) continuous pain throughout the day and night.

The best treatment for a stress fracture is rest from the activity that caused it. This does not mean elimination of exercise altogether. Riding a bicycle or swimming are good alternatives during the healing phase. Depending on the severity of the stress fracture, activity may be resumed within two to six weeks of diagnosis. "Running through the injury" is not recommended. This may lead to a nonunion fracture of the bone and a six- to eight-week recovery period in a cast.

Chondromalacia

Chondromalacia, knee cap pain, is a condition in which the cartilage on the underside of the patella is being irritated and worn away. Symptoms include pain when walking up and down stairs, pain when sitting with knees flexed, grating or roughness behind the kneecaps, the knee "locking up" or "giving away," and joint swelling, commonly called "water on the knee." It can be caused by excessive mileage, always running the same direction on the track, bouncing, and rapid ballistic movements such as those done in aerobics. One common cause is structural. Wide hips tend to make the quadriceps pull the kneecap out against the femur, producing inflammation. Loose kneecaps or a quadriceps muscle not strong enough to keep the patella in its groove also may lead to chondromalacia. The knee will not get better if you continue your activity during the injury. Rest and ice are the conventional treatments for this injury. To prevent recurrence, the knee must be rehabilitated. To stabilize the knee and to assist in correcting the tracking mechanism of the patella, strengthen the quadriceps with leg extension exercises. Stretching should increase hamstring and iliotibial band flexibility. In severe cases, surgery may be indicated.

Ankle Sprain

A **sprain** is a partial or complete tear of a **ligament,** the fibrous connective tissue that binds bones together to form a joint. A sprain is most often a result of a sudden force, typically a twisting motion that surrounding muscles are not strong enough to control. Both ankles and knees are vulnerable to sprains. An ankle sprain will typically exhibit signs of swelling and tenderness on the outside of the ankle. The amount of swelling depends upon the severity of the injury. In severe cases, discoloration or bruising will develop. Range of motion in the ankle may be decreased by swelling and pain. R.I.C.E. for the first 72 hours is the best treatment for sprains. It is extremely important to control the amount of swelling in the joint in order to return to activity quickly. Strong, flexible muscles help protect against sprains. For example, to prevent ankle sprain, strengthen ankles with flexion, inversion, and eversion exercises. High-top shoes or a commercial ankle wrap may also be worn to provide additional support to the joint.

When to Seek Medical Help

Whereas many fitness injuries can be self-treated with R.I.C.E., some injuries require professional medical treatment. You should seek medical assistance for an injury if you experience any of the following symptoms:

1. The injury is extremely painful or the pain has not decreased in intensity over the course of several days.
2. You heard a distinct "pop" or a "snap" when the injury occurred.
3. You are unable to bear complete weight on the part, or there is a loss of strength and the ability to do normal tasks.
4. The body part is not in its natural anatomical position.

Once injured, who should you see? Your family doctor will be able to treat common sprains and strains. However, there are other sports injury specialists who can help. Table 5.2 describes some of these specialists.

table 5.2

INJURY SPECIALISTS

Orthopedists: These M.D.s with specialized surgical training treat injuries to any part of the musculoskeletal system. Many specialize in athletic injuries.

Podiatrist: These D.P.M.s (doctors of podiatric medicine) treat foot-related problems that are common to fitness-related injuries. Though not M.D.s, they receive special training and are state licensed. They can prescribe medications, design orthotics, and perform some surgeries.

Physical Therapists: These therapists are licensed by the state to administer rehabilitative techniques—from massage to strength and flexibility exercises. Most states require you to obtain a doctor's referral before visiting a registered physical therapist.

Chiropractors: These D.C.s (doctors of chiropractic), believing that the alignment of the spine and proper nerve function are essential to body functioning, use manual manipulation and other physical therapy techniques to relieve pain and structural disorders.

Sports Medicine Clinics: Because sports medicine is a rapidly growing field, many communities and medical centers have specialized sports medicine clinics. Many clinics have "walk-in" hours and are likely to include some of the specialists already mentioned as part of their staffs.

Athletic Trainers: Many colleges, universities, and sports medicine clinics have athletic trainers who have extensive knowledge of and experience in dealing with injuries. They are highly trained and must pass rigorous written and practical examinations to become certified.

Communicating with a doctor is an important step in assuming an active role in your health care. Be sure to tell the physician everything that happened leading to the injury: what you felt, signs and symptoms, and any additional information to aid in diagnosing the injury. Do not feel rushed or intimidated by confusing terminology and tests. You are the consumer and are paying for the doctor's time and services. Do not rely on the nurse, receptionist, or friends to explain your injury and treatment. Make sure you completely understand everything you must do to speed your recovery.

Getting Back into Action

To resume activity, you will need to regain normal range of motion and strength in the injured body part. Move the part as early as possible to regain flexibility. When moving, avoid creating excessive discomfort. This rehabilitation motion will increase circulation and reduce the amount of swelling. Work all the motions of a joint to gain freedom of movement. For example, in an ankle injury, move the ankle up and down, in and out, 10 to 20 times, three to four times a day. Gradually increase the repetitions. If after moving the part, you feel pain, apply ice and reduce the amount of repetitions in the next session. You may be doing too much too soon.

After obtaining full range of motion, begin to build strength. Gradually increase the strength of a part to equal that of the uninjured side. You can use partner resistance, free weights, rubber tubing, and universal or nautilus equipment. If possible, work under the supervision of a qualified physical therapist or other rehabilitation professional, especially in the early stages of rehabilitation, since this is when you are most susceptible to reinjury.

Gradually work your way back to your former activity level. You will not be able to start where you stopped. Frequently, exercisers will try to begin working out at their previous level after merely reducing swelling and pain. Healing may not yet be complete. The result is often reinjury since the weakened area is unable to withstand the stress. Overload should be very gradual with the realization that *more* is not always *better*.

Exercise and Disease Resistance

During exercise, 75 percent to 85 percent of the energy produced is released in the form of heat, producing an increase in body temperature.[17] Much of this heat is dissipated at the skin, but body temperature still is elevated during exercise. This regular increase in body temperature, it is speculated, is inhospitable to some viruses and might decrease incidence of viral infections in exercisers. Moderate exercise also has been found to boost the immune system.[18] However, overtraining leading to exhaustion might weaken the system and increase susceptibility to colds and minor infections. Studies on the relationship between the immune system and physical exercise have produced contradictory results.[19] Nonexercisers who start a new program of intense exercise, exceeding their individual exercise limits or who exercise very sporadically may actually experience weakened immunity for a brief period. Highly trained athletes may weaken their immune systems with acute, exhaustive exercise. Of course, psychological and emotional stress may play important roles here, too—whether it be the anxiety felt by the new, out-of-shape exerciser or by the athlete competing for a championship. Few people exercise so strenuously that they need to worry about any possible adverse effects on immunity. The problem for most Americans is too little exercise rather than too much. For anyone in doubt, a consistent and regular program of moderate exercise is a key component of overall health and well-being, including the immune system. However, the optimal level of exercise for each individual's immune system is unknown.[20]

Should you exercise when you have a cold or feel ill? Many professionals recommend that you decrease the intensity and frequency of workouts or take some days off when you have a cold or feel one coming on.[21] Illness affects lung and heart function as well as skeletal muscles. As a result, performance may be reduced. Some people find that exercising when they have a mild cold makes them feel better. Since illnesses vary in severity and people react differently to them, listen to your body. If you just have a minor head cold and otherwise feel fine, it is probably acceptable to work out. Avoid exercise to the point of exhaustion. Avoid exercise if you have the flu, have a fever, feel achy, feel extremely tired, are heavily congested, or have swollen glands. Exercise does not cure illness. The old adage that "you can sweat out a cold" with exercise is untrue. When you do recover from illness, do not start exercising at the same level as before. Give yourself a few days to build back to normal levels.

Care of the Lower Back

Without question, back pain is one of the most common conditions affecting Americans—second only to the common cold as a reason for seeing a physician.[22] Eighty percent of Americans will experience back pain sometime in their lives.[23] Back pain affects a largely youthful population, with the first back pain episodes afflicting people in their 20s and 30s.[24] One of the main contributors to this epidemic of poor back health is our sedentary lifestyle. Fortunately, most back pain is preventable with exercise, good posture, and good lifting mechanics.

Ways to Avoid Lower Back Pain

Why does back pain occur? How can risk of back injury be reduced? We often take a healthy back for granted until something goes wrong. Back problems are rarely caused by a single, isolated factor. The 32-year-old computer programmer who hurts his back while pulling the lawnmower chain prefers to blame the lawnmower. His condition may actually be a result of several years of abuse and neglect. The pull on the lawnmower chain merely "triggered" the condition. During high school and college years, our bodies are

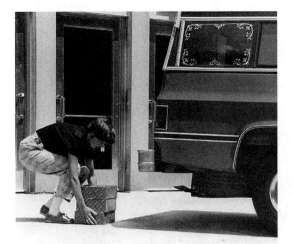

Correct lifting technique.

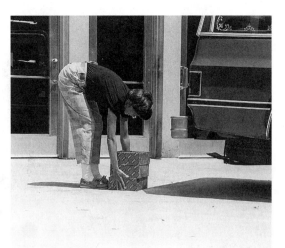

Incorrect lifting technique.

85% of Amer. suffer from low back pain

relatively flexible. As we age, muscles begin to shorten and tighten, decreasing flexibility, especially in the back. Combine this with possible weight gain and declining overall fitness and it becomes evident why back pain afflicts millions. With few exceptions, back problems can be prevented with improved fitness, living and work habits, and posture.

The most important keys to preventing lower back pain are maintaining strong abdominal muscles and back flexibility. Studies show that people who are physically fit have almost ten times less back pain.[25] Many of those who suffer back pain are overweight and have weak, sagging abdominals. This puts the back into an overarched position, placing additional stress on the spinal column. Maintaining normal weight and keeping abdominal muscles strong and tight reduces strain on the spine. Strong abdominals keep the pelvis and spinal column stabilized in a normal position. At the same time, it is important to keep the opposing back muscles flexible. Dr. Paul Hooper[26] believes that the major contributing factors in the alarming incidence of back pain are the shortening and tightening (i.e., decreasing flexibility) of the back muscles and hamstrings. In fact, he feels that stretching the back is even *more* important than strengthening its opposing muscle group—the abdominals.[27]

The one-third of your life you spend sleeping should help, not harm, your back. This makes it very important to select a firm but not extremely hard mattress. Sleeping on a mattress that is too hard will leave the back unsupported. Sleeping on a sagging mattress places the back in an unbalanced position. Water beds, properly adjusted, may provide satisfactory back support as an alternative to a traditional mattress.

The fetal position is the best sleeping position for maintaining a healthy back. Lying on your side, pull your knees up to your chest. This will round the lower back and alleviate back stress. If you must sleep on your back, place a pillow or similar object under your knees to flatten the curve of the lower back. Sleeping on your stomach increases the arch of the back, shortening the back muscles. Placing a small pillow, or even your arm, under your pelvic bone (abdomen) may help straighten your spine enough to sleep without strain.

To decrease back stress when getting out of bed, roll to one side and sit up sideways, using your arms to help. This will eliminate using all of your back and abdominal muscles to get out of bed. This tip is especially helpful if you currently have a back problem.

Good lifting mechanics can reduce the risk of lower back injury. When lifting a heavy weight, bend your knees and use the large muscles of the buttocks and legs. Combining lifting with a twisting force is one of the most common causes of back injury. Instead, lift the object and pivot with your feet rather than your waist.

Common Injuries and Care of the Lower Back

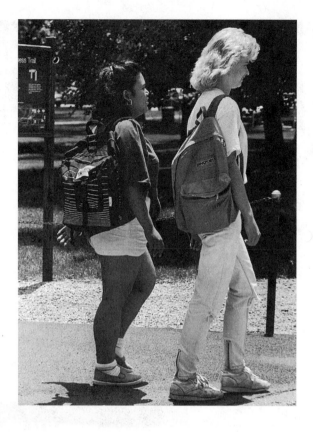

Habitually carrying a heavy backpack on one side may cause back discomfort.

Keep your body close to the object. Standing far away from the object will place undue stress on the lower back. Lift with your back straight rather than bent at the waist. When carrying heavy objects such as books, backpacks, and groceries, try to distribute the load equally and close to the body. Finally, obtain help when lifting heavy objects.

Workplace Considerations

Many Americans will spend the majority of their work time behind desks or in cars. Sedentary jobs and lifestyle make us vulnerable to back pain. How can you maintain a healthy back if your job entails a lot of sitting? Sit close to your work and keep your hips and knees at a 90 degree angle. This will straighten the lower back and prevent slouching. When you sit in a chair, place both feet on the floor. If the chair is too low, it will increase your back curvature excessively. Use a chair that supports your back in its normal slightly arched position. You can place a small pillow or towel against your lower back to maintain that position. Wearing high-heeled shoes is deadly for the lower back. This shortens the Achilles tendon and hamstrings, throws the back into an overarched position, and at the same time overstretches the abdominals. Wear low-heeled shoes to maintain back health.

Maintain good posture while driving, especially when driving long distances. Sitting for extended periods of time in an automobile is a frequent cause of back pain. To maintain normal spinal curvature, place a small pillow between your lower back and the seat. Sit close enough to reach the accelerator and steering wheel without slumping.

If your job requires long periods of standing, you can minimize stress on the back by putting one foot on a low stool. Frequently shift your weight from one leg to another. Some occupations put unusual physical stress on the back. Dentists, chiropractors, nurses, and even musicians may sit, lift, or move in twisted, awkward positions. If you must sit, stand, or work in one position for an extended period of time, get up, stretch, and walk for several minutes. You will feel better, and your back will benefit from the change.

Not to be overlooked is the effect of stress on back health. According to Dr. Paul Hooper, "[T]he accumulating effects of a stress-filled lifestyle produce a 'pro-inflammatory response' that magnifies the impact of otherwise moderate problems. Consequently, an important aspect of injury prevention is the reduction of stress and the use of relaxation therapy."[28]

Lower Back Injuries

The lower back is made up of many tiny ligaments that hold the vertebrae together from the skull to the tailbone. A sudden severe twisting force can injure these ligaments. There are also several groups of muscles, called the *erector spinae muscle group*, that parallel the spinal column. These muscles may be injured by lifting a heavy weight, excessively bending and twisting, or sleeping on a sagging mattress.

If you suffer back pain, what symptoms indicate that you should see a physician? Numbness or tingling in the legs, buttocks, or back may indicate an **intervertebral disc** injury. The intervertebral disc is a cushion that separates the bony vertebrae. Discs are filled with fluid and are flexible through early adulthood but thin and lose their resiliency as we age. A ruptured intervertebral disc will compress nerves, causing pain down the buttocks and legs. Consult a physician who specializes in back pain for these injuries.

Exercises for the Lower Back

Research has shown that 80 percent of patients with back discomfort who visit physicians have no underlying organic disease.[29] Most of these patients are simply deficient in strength and flexibility of key postural muscles. There are several exercises you can do to maintain a healthy back. We recommend the exercise routine in Figure 5.3. These

FIGURE 5.3 ➤
Exercises for the lower back.

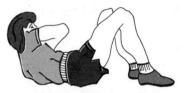

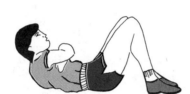

1. Pelvic tilt. Lie on back, knees bent. Press small of back firmly down to floor by tightening the abdominal muscles. Hold for a count of 5.

2. Pelvic tilt with curl. Do a pelvic tilt and, while holding this position, curl head and shoulders up until shoulder blades have been lifted from the floor. Hold briefly. Lower slowly.

3. Pelvic tilt with twist. Do a pelvic tilt and, while holding this position, curl head and shoulders up, twisting right shoulder toward left knee. Hold briefly. Lower slowly. Repeat other side.

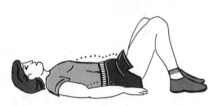

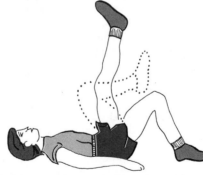

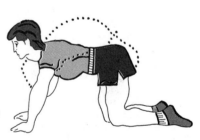

4. Low back stretch. (a) Lie on back. Pull one knee toward chest. Hold for a count of 5. Repeat other leg. (b) Double knee pull. Pull both knees to chest; hold for a count of 5.

5. Lying hamstring stretch. Lie on back. Bring knee toward chest and extend leg toward ceiling. Flex foot. (You may grasp the back of your thigh with your hands.) Hold 20 seconds. Repeat with other leg.

6. Cat stretch. Start on all fours. Round the back upward like a cat. Tighten abdominals. Hold for 5 seconds. Relax and return to starting position. Do not let back sag.

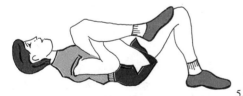

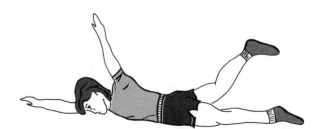

7. Upper back lift. Lie on your stomach with forearms flat on the ground. Tighten abdominals. Lift upper body using back muscles. Do not press with arms. Hold for a count of 5.

8. Alternate arm/leg lift. Lie on your stomach with arms extended in front. Raise one arm overhead toward ceiling while simultaneously lifting the opposite leg. Hold for a count of 5. Repeat with the other arm and leg.

exercises focus on strengthening the abdominals *and* stretching the back. Practice this series daily for best results. The exercises can easily be included as part of your exercise warm-up or cool-down routine. These exercises should not cause any pain, numbness, or tingling in the back and legs. If they do, discontinue them and consult your specialist.

SUMMARY

Much soreness and injury can be prevented. Stretching, strengthening, proper warm-up, sensible progressions, and avoiding overuse are the keys. It is better to block injuries at their source than to pay doctors' fees to treat breakdowns. The pursuit of excellence involves learning to balance your own individual strengths and weaknesses and cooperating with your body instead of assaulting it.

You can prevent lower back problems with proper care and treatment. Maintain leg and back flexibility, strengthen abdominals, utilize correct lifting mechanics, and reduce sources of lower back stress. This is all within your control.

REFERENCES

1. "Exercise Without Injury." *University of California, Berkeley Wellness Letter* 6 (March 1990): 4–5.
2. Peterson, Lars, M.D., and Per Renström. *Sports Injuries: Their Prevention and Treatment.* Chicago: YearBook Medical Publishers, Inc., 1986.
3. Macera, Caroline A. "Lower Extremity Injuries in Runners: Advances in Prediction." *Sports Medicine* 13 (January 1992): 50–57.
4. Macera. "Lower Extremity Injuries in Runners."
5. "Exercise Without Injury."
6. Cook, Stephen D., Mark R. Brinker, and Mahlon Poche. "Running Shoes: Their Relationship to Running Injuries." *Sports Medicine* 10 (July 1990): 1–8.
7. "Fascinating Facts." *University of California, Berkeley Wellness Letter* 8 (January 1992): 1.
8. "Relief: Exercise Injuries, Part II." *University of California, Berkeley Wellness Letter* 6 (May 1990): 4–5.
9. "Relief: Exercise Injuries, Part II."
10. O'Connor, Francis G., M.D., Janet R. Sobel, and Robert P. Nirschl, M.D. "Five-Step Treatment for Overuse Injuries." *The Physician and Sportsmedicine* 10 (October 1992): 128–42.
11. Delhagen, Kate. "Health Watch." *Runner's World* 24 (July 1989): 21.
12. Buroker, Katherine C., and James A. Schwane. "Does Postexercise Static Stretching Alleviate Delayed Muscle Soreness?" *The Physician and Sportsmedicine* 17 (June 1989): 65–83.
13. Warren, Barbara L. "Plantar Fasciitis in Runners: Treatment and Prevention." *Sports Medicine* 10 (November 1990): 338–45.
14. Seder, Joseph I. "How I Managed Heel Spur Syndrome." *The Physician and Sportsmedicine* 15 (February 1987): 83–84.
15. Ellis, Joe. "Shin Splints: Too Much, Too Soon." *Runner's World* 21 (March 1986): 50–53, 86.
16. Matin, Philip, G. Lang, and R. Carretta. "Bone Scanning for Detection of Exercise-Induced Musculoskeletal Injury." *The Physician and Sportsmedicine* 17 (September 1989): 124–35.
17. Costill, David L. *Inside Running: Basics of Sports Physiology.* Dubuque, Iowa: Brown and Benchmark Publishers, 1986.
18. "Does Exercise Boost Immunity?" *University of California, Berkeley Wellness Letter* 8 (March 1992): 6.
19. Weidner, Thomas G. "Literature Review: Upper Respiratory Illness and Sport and Exercise." *International Journal of Sports Medicine* 15 (January 1994): 1–9.
20. Weidner. "Literature Review."
21. Weidner. "Literature Review."
22. "Treat Yourself to Back-Pain Relief." *University of California, Berkeley Wellness Letter* 11 (December 1994): 1–2.
23. Brehm, Barbara A. "Back Basics." *Essays on Wellness.* New York: HarperCollins College Publishers, 1993.
24. Hooper, Paul D. *Preventing Low Back Pain.* Baltimore: Williams & Wilkins, 1992.
25. Collins, John, and Barbara Agenbroad. *What You Can Do for Your Back.* Washington, D.C.: Department of Veterans Affairs, 1991.
26. Hooper. *Preventing Low Back Pain.*
27. Hooper. *Preventing Low Back Pain.*
28. Hooper. *Preventing Low Back Pain.*
29. Brehm. "Back Basics."

SUGGESTED READINGS

Anderson, Marcia K., and Susan J. Hall. *Sports Injury Management*. Baltimore: Williams & Wilkins, 1995.

Arnheim, Daniel D., and William E. Prentice. *Principles of Athletic Training*, 8th ed. St. Louis: Mosby-Year Book, Inc., 1993.

Berman, Judy, Blair Carroll, and Pamela Valdes, eds. *The Back Almanac*. Berkeley, Calif.: Ten Speed Press, 1992.

Buschbacher, Ralph M., M.D., and Randall L. Braddom, M.D. *Sports Medicine and Rehabilitation: A Sports-Specific Approach*. Philadelphia: Hanley & Belfus, Inc., 1994.

Clayton, Lawrence, and Betty Sharon Smith. *Coping with Sports Injuries*. New York: Rosen Publishing Group, 1992.

Cook, Stephen D., Mark Brinker, and Mahlon Poche. "Running Shoes: Their Relationship to Running Injuries." *Sports Medicine* 10 (July 1990): 1–8.

Ellis, Joe. "The Match Game: Finding the Right Shoe for Your Biomechanics and Running Gait." *Runner's World* 20 (October 1985): 66–70.

Francis, Peter, and Lorna Francis. *If It Hurts, Don't Do It*. Rocklin, Calif.: Prima Publishing, 1988.

Guten, Gary N., M.D. *Play Healthy, Stay Healthy*. Champaign, Ill.: Human Kinetics Publishers, 1991.

Hooper, Paul D. *Preventing Low Back Pain*. Baltimore: Williams & Wilkins, 1992.

"Improving Your Posture." *University of California, Berkeley Wellness Letter* 8 (March 1992): 4–5.

Macera, Caroline A. "Lower Extremity Injuries in Runners: Advances in Prediction." *Sports Medicine* 13 (January 1992): 50–57.

McIlwain, Harris H., Debra Fulghum Bruce, Joel C. Silverfield, and Michael C. Burnette. *Winning with Back Pain*. Washington D.C.: Serif Press, Inc., 1994.

McKeag, Douglas B., and Cathleen Dolan. "Overuse Symptoms of the Lower Extremity." *The Physician and Sportsmedicine* 17 (July 1989): 108–23.

Oliver, Jean. *Back Care: An Illustrated Guide*. Boston: Butterworth-Heinemann, 1994.

Renström, P.A.F.H., M.D., ed. Sports Injuries: Basic Principles of Prevention and Care. Champaign, Ill.: Human Kinetics Publishers, 1993.

Ritter, Merrill A., M.D., and Marjorie J. Albohm. *Your Injury: A Common Sense Guide to Sports Injuries*. Dubuque, Iowa: Brown & Benchmark Publishers, 1987.

Root, Leon, M.D. *No More Aching Back*. New York: Villard Books, 1990.

Swezey, Robert L., M.D., and Annette M. Swezey. *Good News for Bad Backs*. New York: Knightsbridge Publishing Co., 1990.

White, Augustus A., III, M.D. *Your Aching Back*. New York: Simon and Schuster Inc., 1990.

YMCA of the USA. YMCA *Healthy Back Book*. Champaign, Ill.: Human Kinetics Publishers, 1994.

chapter 6

Heart Health

➤ Objectives

After reading this chapter, you will be able to:

1. Identify the percentage of deaths in the United States attributable to heart disease.
2. Identify the four primary heart disease risk factors.
3. Identify the eight secondary heart disease risk factors.
4. Identify the controllable and uncontrollable risk factors for coronary heart disease (CHD).
5. Define *arteriosclerosis*, *atherosclerosis*, *angina pectoris*, *myocardial infarction*, and *stroke*.
6. Identify the symptoms of a heart attack.
7. Identify the role of cholesterol and saturated fats in the development of atherosclerosis.
8. Explain the roles of HDL and LDL in heart health.
9. Explain why smoking cigarettes increases heart disease risk.
10. Identify normal blood pressure range and the blood pressure reading that indicates hypertension.
11. Identify the cholesterol reading that indicates high blood cholesterol.
12. Recognize the personality traits of Type A behavior that increase heart disease risk.
13. Recognize five of eight heart disease risk factors that are positively affected by exercise.
14. Identify the two trends that will affect cardiovascular disease in the future.

Terms

- Angina pectoris
- Arteriosclerosis
- Atherosclerosis
- Cardiovascular disease
- Cholesterol
- Collateral circulation
- Diabetes mellitus
- Diastolic pressure

- High-density lipoprotein (HDL)
- Hot reactors
- Hypercholesterolemia
- Hypertension
- LDL cholesterol receptors
- Low-density lipoprotein (LDL)
- Myocardial infarction
- Plaque

- Primary risk factors
- Risk factors
- Secondary hypertension
- Secondary risk factors
- Stroke
- Systolic pressure
- Triglycerides
- Type A, B, and C emotional behavior patterns

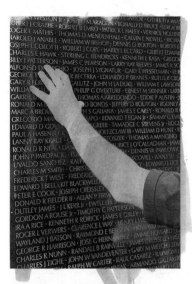

We, not physicians, control our health. One of the most important factors in personal care is behavioral change.

Michael McGinnis, former Deputy Assistant Secretary for Health, U.S. Department of Human Services

the number-one killer in America is not cancer, accidents, or AIDS. It is heart disease (Fig. 6.1). Make no mistake, cancer and other diseases are real threats, but cardiovascular diseases kill almost twice as many victims as all other leading causes of death. The tragedy is compounded because cardiovascular diseases are often inaccurately perceived as diseases of the elderly. On the contrary, based on data from the Framingham Heart Study (Chapter 1), approximately 45 percent of all heart attack victims are under the age of 65, and 5 percent are under the age of 40.[1] These diseases demand attention because they are killing too many Americans who are in the prime of their lives. Don't become complacent! The way you are living your life now determines your future heart health. Many coronary heart disease deaths are preventable. You can reduce your chances of developing coronary heart disease by assessing your current level of risk and by learning ways to reduce those identified risk factors. We now realize that education and behavior change are the keys.

More Americans die each year from heart disease than would have been killed in ten Vietnam wars.

Impact of Cardio-vascular Disease

Cardiovascular disease (CVD) accounts for nearly 43 percent of all deaths in the United States according to the American Heart Association (AHA) statistics.[2] In other words, one out of 2.4 Americans who die each year does so from CVD. How do the death rates from cancer, accidents, and AIDS compare to that from CVD? See Figure 6.1. **Cardiovascular disease** (from *cardio* meaning "heart" and *vascular* meaning "blood vessels") is a condition in which either blood flow through the heart and body is impeded or the electrical impulse of the heart muscle is interrupted. Common forms of CVD include heart attack, stroke, high blood pressure, angina pectoris, irregular heartbeat, congestive heart failure, rheumatic heart disease, and congenital heart disease. More than one in four Americans suffers from these related disorders. Studies show that lower educational levels are directly associated with increased incidence of death from heart disease.[3] Look at Figures 6.2, 6.3, 6.4, and 6.5. What is the leading cause of death for each group?

Heart attack, the most prevalent form of CVD, is still the single largest killer of American men and women (about one of every 4.5 deaths). The cost of CVD in 1995 was estimated by the AHA at $137.7 billion. This figure includes the costs of physician and nursing services, hospital and nursing home services, medications, and lost

FIGURE 6.1 ➤

Leading causes of death in the United States, 1992 estimates.

Reproduced with permission. *Heart and Stroke Facts: 1995 Statistical Supplement,* 1994. Copyright American Heart Association.

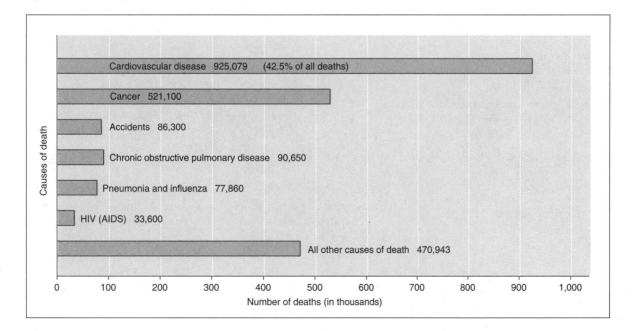

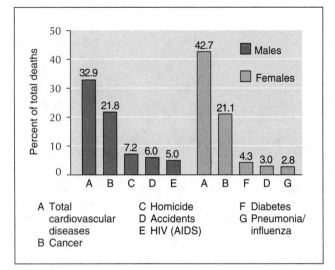

FIGURE 6.2

Leading causes of death for Black males and females. United States: 1991 Final Mortality.

Reproduced with permission. *Heart and Stroke Facts: 1995 Statistical Supplement,* 1994. Copyright American Heart Association.

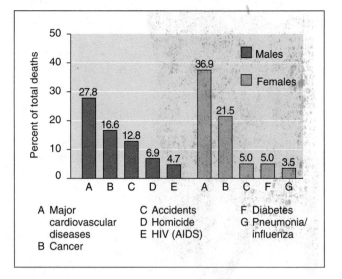

FIGURE 6.3

Leading causes of death for Hispanic males and females. United States: 1990 Final Mortality.

Reproduced with permission. *Heart and Stroke Facts: 1995 Statistical Supplement,* 1994. Copyright American Heart Association.

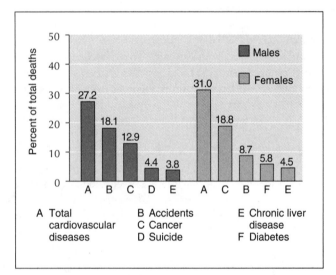

FIGURE 6.4

Leading causes of death for American Indian males and females. United States: 1990 Final Mortality.

Reproduced with permission. *Heart and Stroke Facts: 1995 Statistical Supplement,* 1994. Copyright American Heart Association.

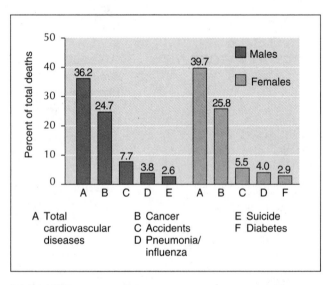

FIGURE 6.5

Leading causes of death for Asian or Pacific Islander males and females. United States: 1990 Final Mortality.

Reproduced with permission. *Heart and Stroke Facts: 1995 Statistical Supplement,* 1994. Copyright American Heart Association.

productivity resulting from disability. While costs for treatment of CVD are spiraling upward, the death rate for these diseases appears to be declining. Advances in medical treatment and education and healthy lifestyle changes can be credited for the declining death rate. However, don't become too complacent about these facts. We still have a long way to go. Cardiovascular disease is the *number-one* health concern in the United States. It is a killer; someone still dies every 34 seconds.[4]

Coronary Heart Disease

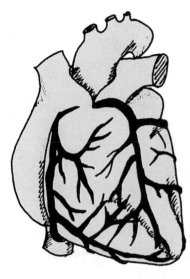

FIGURE 6.6 ➤
Coronary artery system.

The heart is a muscle that works all the time. It never stops beating. Each day, the average heart beats 100,000 times and pumps about 2,000 gallons of blood. Besides providing oxygen and other nutrients to all tissues of the body, the heart must supply itself with oxygen. It has a separate circulatory system, which nourishes only the heart muscle. This system has two coronary arteries, each about the size of a pencil, that subdivide and encircle the entire heart muscle (Fig. 6.6). What is commonly known as "hardening of the arteries" is **arteriosclerosis,** which is a general term for the thickening and hardening of arteries. Some hardening of arteries normally occurs as we age. Coronary heart disease is most commonly the result of atherosclerosis. **Atherosclerosis** (*athero* from the Greek word for "paste" and *sclerosis* for "hardness") is a type of arteriosclerosis. It is a progressive condition in which deposits of cholesterol and other lipids, along with cellular waste products, accumulate on the inner walls of coronary arteries. This buildup is called **plaque.** As the condition progresses, the inner walls of blood vessels become more and more inelastic and clogged and may become totally hardened and blocked. Sometimes, a blood clot forms on the plaque buildup and blocks the entire artery. A heart attack or stroke may result.

There are a variety of causes of atherosclerosis, many of which are related to unhealthy lifestyle choices. One theory attributes atherosclerosis to minor injuries of the inner wall of coronary arteries, which create a roughened region where debris and materials in the blood can attach. Thus begins the atherosclerotic buildup. What injures the lining of our coronary arteries? High blood cholesterol levels, excessive dietary cholesterol and saturated fat, high blood pressure, your reaction to perceived emotional stress, and nicotine are often responsible. All are influenced by lifestyle. Besides causing damage to the smooth lining of our blood vessels, lifestyle factors also contribute to excess plaque in the bloodstream. Atherosclerosis does not suddenly develop at age 65. It is a long, progressive process beginning in childhood.

Angina Pectoris

Atherosclerosis may lead to **angina pectoris,** or chest pain. This pain occurs when a coronary artery becomes partially blocked, causing an oxygen debt in the heart muscle. Often, angina pectoris is brought on by sudden exertion or vigorous exercise when the blood flow to the heart is insufficient to meet its oxygen demands. The Framingham Heart Study estimated that 2.5 million people suffer from angina pectoris with 350,000 new cases occurring each year.[5]

Myocardial Infarction

Myocardial infarction, or heart attack, results when one or more of the coronary arteries is partially blocked by atherosclerosis, and a blood clot (thrombus) plugs the remaining opening. The portion of heart muscle beyond the blockage is deprived of oxygen, resulting in injury or death of that portion of the heart muscle. If a damaged area is large enough or in a vital area of the heart, the individual will die. However, many people do survive a heart attack and are capable of living productive lives (Table 6.1).

table 6.1

WARNING SIGNS OF A HEART ATTACK

- Uncomfortable pressure, fullness, squeezing, or pain in the center of the chest lasting two minutes or longer.
- Pain spreading to shoulders, neck, jaw, arms, or back.
- Severe pain, lightheadedness, fainting, sweating, nausea, and/or shortness of breath.

Not all of these warning signs occur in every heart attack. If some of these symptoms do occur, don't wait. Get help immediately!

source: American Heart Association. *1995 Heart Facts.*

A number of studies have shown that, in some damaged hearts, new blood vessels develop to nourish the area that is being starved of oxygen and other nutrients. This is called **collateral circulation.** Everyone has collateral blood vessels, which are microscopic and closed under normal conditions. However, in some people with coronary heart disease, these seem to enlarge and form a detour around the blockage to provide alternate routes for the blood. Exercise appears to be one practical way to increase myocardial oxygen demand, which in turn may stimulate the development of collateral vessels. In some cases, coronary angiography (X ray) has revealed increased collaterization after exercise training.[6]

Stroke

A **stroke** occurs when blood flow to the brain is blocked. The brain needs a continuous supply of oxygen-rich blood to function. When a blood clot interrupts the flow of oxygen, the brain does not receive the nourishment it needs, and brain cells die. Stroke, primarily caused by atherosclerosis, is the *third* leading killer of Americans (behind heart attack and cancer). On the average, someone suffers a stroke in the United States every minute; every 3.5 minutes, someone dies of one.[7] It is the chief cause of serious disability and a major contributor to later-life dementia. A stroke can result in paralysis of one side of the body, loss of ability to speak or to understand the speech of others, loss of memory, and behavioral change. Because brain cells can't heal, modification of risk factors is very important in the prevention of this disease that affects 500,000 Americans every year, killing about 144,000.[8] It is not solely a disease of the elderly; more than a fourth of all stroke victims are under age 65. Your risk of stroke increases with these factors:

➤ *Hypertension:* If you have high blood pressure, you are two to four times more likely to have a stroke than is someone with normal blood pressure. It is the single most important risk factor for stroke.

➤ *Heart disease:* Sometimes, blood clots forming in the heart can move up to the brain and block blood flow.

➤ *Gender:* About 19 percent more men than women have strokes.

➤ *Diabetes:* Those with diabetes have almost double the risk of stroke.

➤ *Age:* Seventy-five percent of stroke victims are 65 or older.

➤ *Race:* Black Americans have nearly twice as many fatal strokes as whites and more than twice as many as other minorities. Hypertension and sickle-cell anemia are the suspected causes.

➤ *Lifestyle:* These factors can be controlled: high-fat, high-cholesterol diet; *alcohol or cocaine abuse;* smoking; and sedentary lifestyle.

Risk Factors

Risk factors are the conditions, situations, and behaviors that increase the likelihood that an undesirable outcome (injury, illness, or death) will occur. The risk is generally established by multiple scientific studies. A risk factor does not cause the undesirable outcome 100 percent of the time, but of those people who engage in the behavior (or experience the condition), a certain number of them will experience the undesired outcome. The stronger the risk factors link with a negative outcome, the more likely it is that an individual will experience the undesired result.

The riskiness of various behaviors is determined in part through epidemiological research, which involves studying large populations in order to investigate the causes and control of diseases. The famous Framingham Study is an example of this type of research. Research studies on animals and humans, in which conditions are carefully set up to test hypotheses, are often needed to confirm relationships among behaviors, conditions, illness, and death. Over time, clearer and clearer pictures emerge about the degree of danger or risk in a particular situation until health experts can say, "If

FIGURE 6.7 ➤

Danger of heart attack within eight years by risk factors present. For purposes of illustration, this chart uses an abnormal blood pressure level of 150 systolic and a cholesterol level of 260 in a 55-year-old male and female. Taken from Framingham Heart Study.

Reproduced with permission. *Heart and Stroke Facts: 1995 Statistical Supplement,* 1994. Copyright American Heart Association.

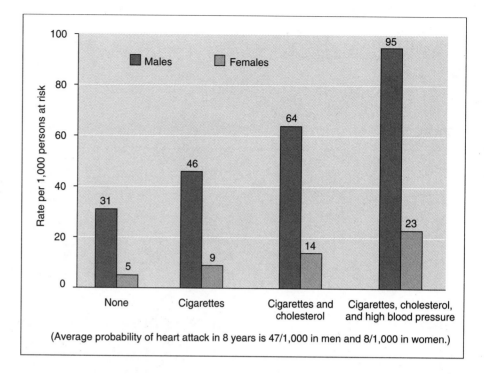

(Average probability of heart attack in 8 years is 47/1,000 in men and 8/1,000 in women.)

you do this, chances are good that this will occur." An example of this is the link between smoking, cholesterol, hypertension, and heart attack seen in Figure 6.7.

CHD researchers have identified several risk factors that may lead to the development of atherosclerosis. The more risk factors you possess, the greater your chances are of developing coronary heart disease. While no one can accurately predict whether you will have a heart attack, you can estimate your odds by evaluating your risk factors. Take the *Are You At Risk* test in the Activities Section (p. 385) to determine your risk and how to reduce it.

Primary risk factors are linked directly to the development of CHD; they increase the possibility of having a heart attack. *All primary risk factors are controllable.*

Controllable Factors
1. High blood pressure
2. High blood lipid level
3. Cigarette smoking
4. Inactivity

The **secondary risk factors** for heart disease contribute to the development of coronary heart disease but not as directly as the primary risk factors.

Controllable Factors
1. Obesity
2. Stress
3. Emotional behavior

Uncontrollable Factors
4. Age
5. Gender
6. Race
7. Positive family history
8. Diabetes mellitus

Notice that some of these secondary risk factors are *controllable*. The choices you make or the way you live have a profound impact in reducing these risk factors. If you possess several uncontrollable risk factors, it is imperative that you adopt a healthy lifestyle.

table 6.2

BLOOD PRESSURE STAGES

CATEGORY	SYSTOLIC/DIASTOLIC	RECOMMENDATION
Normal	less than 130/85	Recheck in two years.
High normal	130–139/85–89	Recheck in one year; begin lifestyle modifications.
Hypertension		
Stage 1	140–159/90–99	Confirm in two months; begin lifestyle modifications.
Stage 2	160–179/100–109	Medical evaluation; begin treatment within one month.
Stage 3	180–209/110–119	Medical evaluation; begin treatment within one week.
Stage 4	210/120 and over	Immediate medical evaluation and treatment.

Primary Risk Factors

1. High Blood Pressure (Hypertension)

Blood pressure is the force exerted by the heart while pumping blood through the body. It is also the pressure of blood against the arterial walls.

There are actually two blood pressure levels, recorded as two separate numbers in fraction form (for example, 120/80). When the heart contracts and pumps blood into the arteries, the pressure increases. This is the **systolic,** or pumping, **pressure** which is recorded as the upper number. The **diastolic,** or resting, **pressure** is the force of the blood against the arteries when the heart relaxes between beats. It is recorded as the lower number. Both the systolic and diastolic numbers are important. High levels of either or of both mean greater risk for heart attack and stroke. Average blood pressure is 120/80, and the acceptable range is 90/60 up to 139/89. High blood pressure, **hypertension,** is generally acknowledged as blood pressure equal to or greater than 140/90. Doctors once called this level of blood pressure *borderline* or *mild* hypertension. This language is falsely reassuring—mild weather is pleasant, but mild hypertension is not. The new term *Stage 1 hypertension* describes it better. Even *high normal* now calls for lifestyle changes and monitoring. Look at the four stages of hypertension listed in Table 6.2.

High blood pressure causes the heart to overwork. Over a period of time, the overworked heart weakens, enlarges, and has a difficult time keeping up with the demands of the body. High blood pressure also causes blood vessels to become inelastic, severely reducing the amount of blood flow to the body's vital organs. Decreased levels of oxygen and other nutrients can produce heart, brain, and kidney damage. Remember, high blood pressure also leads to heart attacks and strokes.

One in four American adults has high blood pressure, and in 90 percent of the cases there is no known cause. However, factors that can increase your chances of developing high blood pressure are heredity, cigarette smoking, male gender, age, black race, obesity, sensitivity to sodium, heavy alcohol consumption, use of oral contraceptives, and a sedentary lifestyle. In a small number of cases, hypertension is caused by a specific condition, such as kidney disease, a tumor of the adrenal gland, or a defect of the aorta. This is called **secondary hypertension.** The cause of secondary hypertension can generally be identified and treated successfully.

How do you know if your blood pressure is too high? The only way of knowing is to have it checked. You cannot feel high blood pressure. High blood pressure has no symptoms, which is why it is so dangerous. You can be hypertensive for years and be unaware of the damage occurring. Of those with high blood pressure, over 46 percent do not know they have it.[9] It is imperative that you know your blood pressure, because high blood pressure, while it cannot be cured, can be controlled or prevented by these specific lifestyle changes:

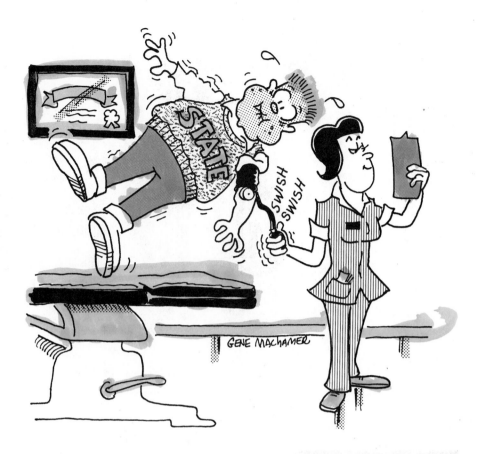

➤ *Maintain a healthy weight.* Losing even 5 or 10 pounds, if you are overweight, can reduce blood pressure.

➤ *Do not smoke.* Smoking does not cause hypertension but does promote heart disease. A hypertensive who smokes is at serious risk.

➤ *Exercise regularly.* For one thing, exercise helps you lose weight and keep it off.

➤ *Eat a well-balanced diet rich in fruits, grains, and vegetables.* This will help you cut back on the consumption of fats and high calorie foods and lose some excess weight.

➤ *Keep your sodium intake low (below 2,400 milligrams daily).* Many people are salt-sensitive, meaning that salt (sodium chloride) elevates their blood pressure.

➤ *If you drink alcohol, do so in moderation.* Drink no more than one drink daily if you are a woman or two if you are a man.

➤ *Take your blood pressure medication, if prescribed.*

➤ *Practice a stress management technique such as meditation,* or one of those discussed in Chapter 7. Harvard Medical School studies have confirmed the value of stress management in the reduction of high blood pressure.[10]

2. High Blood Lipid Profile (Cholesterol and Triglycerides)

Research has firmly linked high levels of cholesterol and other blood fats to the development of arterial plaque, a major cause of atherosclerosis and coronary heart disease. **Cholesterol** is not a true fat but a waxy substance found in the bloodstream. It is manufactured in the liver and is also consumed in foods of animal origin.

Cholesterol is not all bad. It is needed by the body for cell structure and for the manufacture of hormones. The problem with cholesterol is that your body makes most of what it needs, and the normal American diet adds much more. As a result, one-half of all adult Americans have cholesterol levels high enough to require treatment[11] (Fig. 6.8). **Hypercholesterolemia** is the term for high cholesterol levels in the blood.

Ninety-five percent of the fats in the body are in the form of triglycerides, a true fat stored in the fat cells and found in the blood. Both high cholesterol and triglycerides increase the risk of developing atherosclerosis.

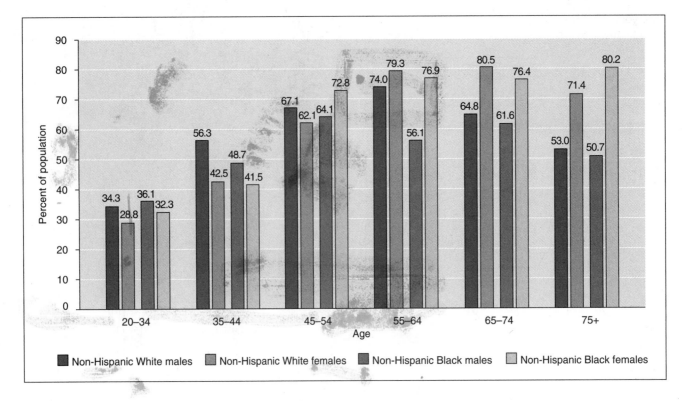

FIGURE 6.8 ➤

Estimated percentage of Americans age 20 and over with serum cholesterol of 200 mg/dl or more by age, sex, and race. United States: 1988–1991.

Reproduced with permission. *Heart and Stroke Facts: 1995 Statistical Supplement,* 1994. Copyright American Heart Association.

When evaluating your blood lipid profile for risk of heart disease, there are two factors to consider: (1) the total amount of cholesterol/triglycerides found in the blood and (2) the way cholesterol/triglycerides are transported in the bloodstream.

Total Amount of Lipids.   Knowing your total cholesterol level provides you with a *rough* estimate of your heart disease risk. Blood cholesterol is measured by analyzing a small blood sample in a laboratory. Total cholesterol level includes the amount of cholesterol carried by high-density lipoprotein, low-density lipoprotein, and very low-density lipoprotein. The National Heart, Lung, and Blood Institute relates cholesterol level to heart disease risk as illustrated in Table 6.3.

Transportation of Lipids.   Like oil and water, cholesterol and blood do not mix. So cholesterol must attach itself to a protein molecule to be carried through the bloodstream. This combination is called a *lipoprotein*. A lipoprotein analysis gives a more accurate picture of your heart disease risk than does total cholesterol alone. A lipoprotein analysis breaks down the total cholesterol into its components, or lipoproteins, of which there are two main types—one that protects and one that damages coronary arteries:

1. **Low-density lipoprotein (LDL).** LDLs are considered "bad" because they carry a large amount of cholesterol. The lower density of the lipoprotein allows it to easily attach to the inner wall of the blood vessel, thus accelerating the atherosclerotics process. A *high* LDL cholesterol level increases your risk for heart disease (Table 6.3). Cigarette smoking, emotional stressors, and diets high in saturated fat have been shown to increase the LDL level. Very low-density lipoproteins (VLDL) are even more dangerous.
2. **High-density lipoprotein (HDL).** HDL is considered to be a "good" form of cholesterol because of the dense structure of the lipoprotein. It is thought that HDL acts as a garbage collector in clearing away plaque and other debris as it flows through the bloodstream to the liver to be excreted from the body. The higher your HDL cholesterol level, the better and the more protection from heart disease it provides. How can you increase your level of HDL? Exercise regularly, don't smoke, and maintain a normal weight. High-fiber and low-fat diets may also increase the HDL cholesterol level.

table 6.3

CHOLESTEROL

RISK	TOTAL CHOLESTEROL (MG/DL)	LDL (MG/DL)	HDL (MG/DL)
Desirable	<200	<130	>60
Borderline High	200–239	130–159	NA
High	≥240	≥160	<35

source: National Heart, Lung, and Blood Institute, U.S. Department of Health and Human Services.
Note: The levels apply to anyone 20 years of age or older.

HDL cholesterol clearing away plaque in arteries.

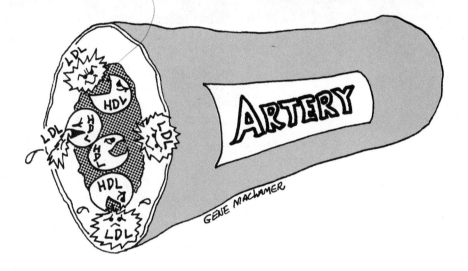

Alcohol consumption has received attention recently as a protective factor against heart attack because it is thought to raise HDL cholesterol in the blood and it might help prevent clotting that leads to plaque buildup inside arteries. Consuming *one* to *three* drinks per week (12 oz. of beer, one glass of wine, or one shot of hard liquor is equal to one drink) is associated with a reduction in the rate of heart attacks. Consuming more than two drinks a day is known to damage the heart. It should be emphasized that a protective effect of alcohol consumption has not been proven, but many adverse effects are well documented. Besides causing automobile accidents and social disruption, excess intake of alcohol can raise blood pressure and triglyceride levels and cause diseases of the liver, pancreas, and nervous system. Even though alcohol consumption above moderate levels adversely affects blood pressure and triglycerides and can damage the heart, alcohol is still *not* considered a primary or secondary heart disease risk factor. To put the benefit of moderate drinking in proper perspective, the reduction in heart disease risk is comparable to what you might achieve by exercising regularly or by cutting blood cholesterol levels through a low-fat diet.

Scientists now believe that the ratio of total cholesterol to HDL cholesterol is a better indicator of risk for cardiovascular disease than the total value alone. To determine your ratio, take a laboratory blood test that will reveal your total cholesterol and HDL cholesterol levels. Next, divide the total cholesterol level by the HDL cholesterol level to find the ratio. For example, if the total cholesterol were measured to be 160 and the HDL cholesterol 40, your ratio would be four (160 ÷ 40 = 4). This would place you

table 6.4

RATIO OF TOTAL CHOLESTEROL AND HDL CHOLESTEROL TO RISK OF CHD

RISK OF HEART DISEASE	RATIO OF TC/HDL-C MEN	RATIO OF TC/HDL-C WOMEN
Very low	under 3.43	under 3.27
Low	4.97	4.44
Moderate	9.55	7.05
High	more than 23.39	more than 11.04

source: *The Wellness Encyclopedia*, University of California, Berkeley.

at lower than average risk, as you can see in Table 6.4. It is generally accepted that a 4.5 or lower ratio (total cholesterol/HDL cholesterol) is excellent for men, and 4.0 or lower is best for women.[12]

Average HDL levels in adult Americans are about 45 to 65 mg/dl, with women averaging higher than men. The female sex hormone, estrogen, tends to raise HDL levels, which may explain why premenopausal women are usually protected from heart disease. Studies suggest that HDL levels above 70 may protect against heart disease, while those below 35 signal coronary risk.[13]

There is genetic variability in how efficiently (or inefficiently) a person metabolizes dietary saturated fat and cholesterol. Some people can eat almost anything and their blood cholesterol levels remain stable. Others find that even a small amount of dietary fat makes their blood cholesterol levels increase. Most of us are somewhere in between on this spectrum.

Drs. Michael Brown and Joseph Goldstein won the Nobel Prize in Medicine in 1985 for their discovery of **LDL cholesterol receptors.** Located primarily in liver cells, these receptors bind and remove cholesterol from the blood. The more cholesterol receptors you have, the more efficiently you can remove cholesterol from the blood. The number of cholesterol receptors is, in part, genetically determined. Lifestyle factors also influence the number. A diet high in saturated fat and cholesterol produces what Brown and Goldstein termed "double trouble." It not only saturates the receptors, it also decreases their number—a bad combination. Only about 5 percent of the population has genetically high cholesterol levels that remain elevated regardless of lifestyle.[14]

Triglycerides are manufactured in the body to store excess fats. They are also known as *free fatty acids*, and in combination with cholesterol, they accelerate the formation of plaque. Triglycerides are carried in the bloodstream by very low density lipoprotein (VLDL). These fatty acids are found in poultry skin, lunch meats, and shellfish. However, they are mainly manufactured in the liver from refined sugars, starches, and alcohol. High intake of alcohol and sugars (honey included) will significantly increase triglyceride levels. Thus, the levels can be lowered by decreasing consumption of the just-mentioned foods, along with reducing weight (if overweight) and exercising aerobically. As a general rule, you should keep your triglyceride level below 250 mg/dl of blood. However, some reports indicate triglyceride levels over 150 should be cause for concern.

You should know your cholesterol level and have it checked annually, especially if you have a positive family history of heart disease. The best way to do this is to have a 12-hour fasting blood test that is analyzed by a reputable laboratory. The over-the-counter tests that don't require fasting are not as reliable. The National Heart Savers Association states that only 8 percent of Americans know their cholesterol level and more than 50 percent have a level that is too high. A diet rich in cholesterol—or worse, one rich in saturated fat (saturated fat is highest in vegetable oils such as tropical and palm and in meat and high fat dairy products)—can increase your blood cholesterol level. Keep fat consumption between 10 percent and 30 percent or less of total calories per day. This small modification in dietary fat can reduce cholesterol levels by 10 percent to 15 percent. (See Chapter 9 for other dietary strategies that affect heart health.) To lower cholesterol, reduce body weight if overweight. Weight reduction alone can lower cholesterol and triglyceride levels. Lowering your stress level also helps offset high cholesterol. Finally, increase daily activity. Try to walk more, use escalators and cars less, be a participant rather than a spectator.

3. Cigarette Smoking

Cigarette smoking is a primary risk factor. Every cigarette package is required by law to carry a consumer warning. One such warning is "Quitting Smoking Now Greatly Reduces Serious Risks to Your Health." Even Ann Landers, the nationally syndicated columnist, gives warning: "Beware, cigarettes are killers that travel in packs." Numerous studies have proven that cigarette smoking causes oral cancer, lung cancer, and emphysema, and in women it is linked to cervical cancer, early menopause, and damage to the fetus during pregnancy. It also leads to the development of wrinkles in both men and women. The number of Americans killed each year from smoking is greater than the number killed during World War II and the Vietnam War combined.[15] No level of smoking is safe!

The American Heart Association reports that smokers have more than twice the risk of heart attack of nonsmokers. Even limited smoking (four to five cigarettes per day) increases CHD risk. Also, smoking increases the risk of developing peripheral vascular disease (narrowing blood vessels in the arms and legs), which may lead to the development of gangrene and eventually amputation.

Passive smoke, synonymous with secondhand smoke, is the cigarette smoke inhaled by nonsmokers from environmental air. Research has shown there are plenty of reasons to worry about secondhand smoke:

1. Nonsmokers may be *more* susceptible to heart and vascular damage from secondhand smoke than smokers are, even though they absorb much smaller doses of the smoke's toxins. That is because smokers develop compensatory responses to some of the adverse cardiovascular effects of cigarette smoke—but nonsmokers do not get the "benefit" of these adaptive responses.[16]
2. Repeated exposure to secondhand smoke causes permanent damage to the heart and arteries.[17]
3. The cardiovascular system is extremely sensitive to the chemicals in secondhand smoke (i.e., carbon monoxide, nicotine, and hydrocarbons).
4. Carbon monoxide, a substance in secondhand smoke (and in inhaled cigarette smoke), damages the smooth inner lining of blood vessel walls. This accelerates the atherosclerotic buildup. Carbon monoxide, higher in the blood of smokers but also found in nonsmokers, decreases the amount of oxygen carried in the blood. It also reduces the heart's ability to use the oxygen it does receive.
5. Even low levels of secondhand smoke increase the stickiness of blood platelets in nonsmokers, making it more likely that a clot will form in the narrowed arteries, which can ultimately lead to a heart attack.
6. Cigarette smoking (as well as secondhand smoke) *decreases* the HDL levels in the bloodstream (the "good" type of cholesterol). Both cause heart rate and blood pressure to rise.
7. Secondhand smoke (and smoking) worsens the damage done by free radicals (i.e., destructive oxygen compounds) to heart muscle cells.
8. When a heart attack occurs, prior exposure to secondhand smoke worsens the damage and makes the outcome more serious.

FIGURE 6.9 ➤

Estimated percentage of U.S. population having selected risk factors for coronary heart disease. More Americans are at risk for heart disease because of physical inactivity than because of any other manageable risk factor.

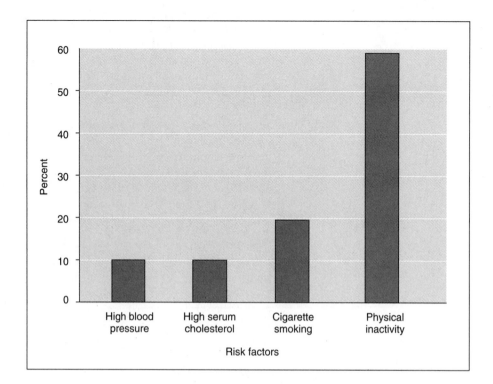

9. Nonsmokers who live with smokers or work where environmental smoke is present have a 30 percent higher risk of dying from heart disease than do other nonsmokers. Secondhand smoke is linked to 40,000 heart disease deaths annually.

10. Heavy smoking in the same workplace or study area gives the nonsmoker the equivalent of mainstream smoking two to three cigarettes a day.

11. Secondhand smoke is a human carcinogen, killing about 3,000 nonsmokers a year through lung cancer. Smoking is everyone's business!

12. The population burden associated with passive smoking and heart disease is estimated to be 30,000 to 60,000 deaths annually in the United States.[18] The simplest and most cost-effective control measure to reduce cost is to *mandate* smoke-free workplaces, schools, and public places.

While studies show that smoking has declined by more than 37 percent since 1965, this downward trend appears to be leveling off, and smoking may be on the upswing again. Smoking promotes heart disease. A nonsmoker should not begin to smoke. Smokers should stop *now*. Ninety percent of smokers who quit do so on their own!

4. Inactivity

Countless studies have linked inactivity to coronary heart disease. The Centers for Disease Control (CDC) in Atlanta has named physical inactivity as our nation's most common cardiac threat.[19] Why? Because only 22 percent of Americans engage in physical activity at intensity levels recommended for health benefits. This leaves close to 80 percent of our population either entirely sedentary or not active enough to reap health benefits.[20] Consequently, it is not surprising to learn that approximately 250,000 deaths (12 percent of all deaths) every year in the United States can be attributed to lack of exercise.[21] Many experts believe today's best buy in the prevention of heart disease is *exercise*[22] (Fig. 6.9).

In yet another ongoing inquiry into the relationship between physical activity and mortality, the Harvard Alumni Study continues to produce results that have led its director Dr. Ralph S. Paffenbarger to conclude that "There's no doubt whatever that insufficient activity will shorten your life." Even exercise of moderate intensity (brisk walking or gardening) is beneficial in improving health and well-being.[23] It is vigorous

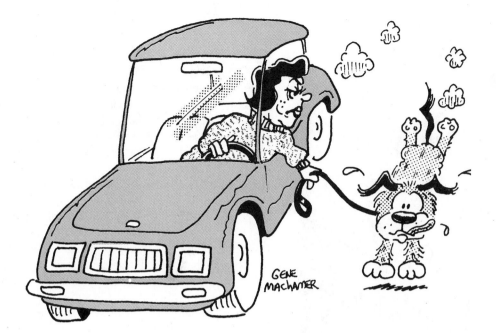

exercise (using the FITT prescription), however, that produces the greatest health benefits and is linked to increased longevity.[24]

The American lifestyle is very sedentary. We no longer have to hunt and grow our own food, build our own homes, or walk to school and work. Our ancestors did not have to build physical activity into their daily lives; it was a part of their lifestyle. Modern conveniences and technology have virtually eliminated physical activity from our lives. The culprits are the automobile, television (now with remote control), elevators, escalators, riding lawn mowers, portable telephones, as well as computers and computer games. You can probably add more to this list.

Vigorous physical exercise is essential to a healthy cardiovascular system. Equally important, however, is overall lifestyle and how long you have been exercising. News from the University of Auckland School of Medicine in New Zealand indicates that the longer you have been exercising, the lower your risk of developing heart disease. The type of regular exercise they found to be protective included light activities as well as those of the intense variety. For example, they noted that the protection given by jogging was similar to that for light activities such as brisk walking, dancing, and calisthenics. It was reported that after five years of regular exercise, the risk of heart disease decreased sharply, indicating that the longer you adhere to an exercise program, the healthier your heart will be.[25] The old saying, "Use it or lose it!" is true. You don't have to run marathons to be physically active. Small increases in daily activity can significantly burn up excess calories, make the heart muscle a stronger and more efficient pump, lower blood pressure, alleviate stress, increase HDL levels, and build self-confidence.

The American Heart Association reports that regular vigorous exercise protects against coronary heart disease and even improves the survival rate after a heart attack.[26] That is life insurance that money cannot buy. The single most important thing you can do to improve your health and well-being is to *exercise*. What is the least amount of exercise you have to do to protect your heart? Significant benefit from exercise comes from expending an extra (beyond daily living requirements) 2,000 calories per week. Expending more calories in exercise than this is not going to change your risk appreciably. Thus, exercise burning approximately 300 calories a day, seven days a week is sufficient—this is about 30 to 45 minutes per day of exercise. Ride your bike, walk to school, play tennis instead of watching others doing these activities. Park at the back of the parking lot instead of right next to the building. There are many ways to add activity to your daily life.

Secondary Risk Factors

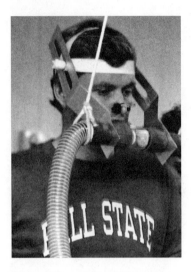

If over 35, you should have a tolerance test before starting an exercise program.

These are factors associated with increased risk of heart disease, though not as directly as the primary risk factors.

1. Obesity

Obesity is uncomfortable, increases the burden on the vital organs, especially the heart, and is directly linked to coronary heart disease. Over a third of the U.S. population is obese or overweight. Childhood obesity rates have increased substantially since 1980 with 21 percent of all 12 to 19 year olds (one in five teens)—now significantly overweight.[27] Hypertension is nearly six times higher in overweight people aged 20 to 44, and high cholesterol levels are twice as frequent in the obese.[28] Eighty-five percent of people with Type II diabetes are at least 20 percent overweight.[29]

In addition, obesity puts women in particular at increased risk of heart disease. A study conducted by the Harvard Medical School of 115,000 women ages 30 to 55 found that of all the women in the eight-year study who developed heart disease, 40 percent had no other risk factors except being 20 percent or more over their ideal weight.[30] Women who had been slim at age 18 and gained weight in adulthood seemed to be at increased risk. The first step in medical treatment for these conditions is usually weight reduction. Obesity is controllable and can be reversed. You can eliminate the obesity risk factor by maintaining reasonable weight (see Chapter 10).

Physical inactivity is a major factor in the development of obesity in men, women, and children. Watching too much television is one of the main culprits. The number of television hours watched per person in this country averages about four per day. Americans should limit TV viewing to about one hour a day to prevent physical and mental inactivity.

2. Stress

Stress is unavoidable. It includes happy, wonderful, and positive events as well as sad, destructive, and negative ones. The birth of a child produces stress as does the death of a family member. Job stress may be particularly unhealthy. High blood pressure is three times more common among people who have jobs with high demands but little control (assembly line worker, waitress).[31] Stress has been found to cause a rise in heart rate, blood pressure, and blood cholesterol, and it can lead to excessive smoking or eating—all linked to coronary heart disease. The type of stress is not that important. Indianapolis 500 race car drivers have higher cholesterol levels after they race than before. Tax accountants have increased cholesterol around April 15. Students have higher cholesterol levels during exams. Stress causes chemical wear and tear on the body by releasing stress hormones into the blood stream (adrenaline). Large amounts of stress hormones are found in the blood streams of people who react to stressful situations with hostile and angry behavior. However, low levels of stress hormones are found in the blood streams of people who react normally to stressful events. How you react to stress seems to be the critical factor. You should recognize stress in your life (both the positive and the negative) and learn to handle the stressful situations in a healthful manner. Coping with stress successfully is vital in today's hectic, in-the-fast-lane lifestyle. Exercise, relaxation techniques, and behavioral modification have been found to be excellent methods for reducing stress. We need to change the way we look at stressful situations. Problems are to be solved, not worried about. Read more about ways to reduce stress in Chapter 7.

3. Emotional Behavior

Several studies have linked emotional behavior to increased risk of heart disease. There are basically three **emotional behavior patterns—Type A, B, and C.** The Type A individual exhibits aggressiveness, competitiveness, and impatience and is easily annoyed. Type As demonstrate a high degree of time urgency—a tendency to do two or three things at the same time. These behaviors may lead to angry, cynical, and hostile behavior. The Type B individual is more relaxed, noncompetitive, patient, and slow to anger. A third emotional behavior pattern, Type C, has been identified recently. Type Cs are actually classified as Type As but they learn to cope with emotional stress by using the five Cs: control, commitment, challenge, choices in lifestyle, and connectedness. Such people welcome change, considering it a challenge. They are committed to goals, gaining confidence as a result (see Chapter 7). Type Cs are called *"hardy"* stress resisters.

Early studies identified Type A people as the ones at greater risk of having heart attacks. However, more recent research indicates it is only when the Type A exhibits the behaviors of *hostility* and *anger* that a serious risk is apparent. These behaviors significantly elevate blood pressure and overstimulate the production of stress hormones. The other Type A behaviors do not seem to be as significant but may be factors in overall poor health and may eventually lead to hostile, angry reactions to stress. Type Bs with these negative behaviors will also suffer adverse health consequences. Twenty percent of apparently healthy people suffer extreme surges in blood pressure when confronted with the challenges of everyday life.[32] They are called **hot reactors** because their systolic blood pressure can rise from 120 to a deadly 300 when stressed. They often go untreated until felled by a stress-induced heart attack or stroke. Hot reactors can be found in all emotional behavior types.

We are not born with hot reacting, angry, and hostile behaviors. These behaviors are learned and, for the sake of our health, we can unlearn them. Learning to modify Type A personality behaviors, especially hostility, anger, and hot reacting, is not difficult, and doing so may add years to your life. How does a "hostile heart" become less angry and cynical—and become a "trusting heart"?

Carry a notebook and record every time you feel angry and/or hostile. Once you have done this for a while, you will start to recognize the situations that provoke these reactions and be able to head off the troublesome behavior. Other suggestions follow:

1. *Stop angry, cynical thoughts*. Every time you have a cynical thought, think to yourself, "STOP!" This is called *thought stopping* and is an effective behavior modification technique when practiced regularly.
2. *Practice laughing at yourself*. Once you realize how silly your anger is in many situations, laughing at yourself will quickly replace fuming.
3. *Be empathetic*. Put yourself in the other person's shoes. Often the other individual is a victim of circumstances, too.
4. *Reason and understand your anger*. There will be times when anyone would be angry in that same situation, but you must say, "I have this trait, and it is bad for my health." Decide if the situation warrants your attention and if you have an effective response. If not, take a "time out" from the situation.
5. *Learn to relax*. Practice the excellent "stress busters" in Chapter 7.
6. *Practice patience and trust*. Instead of getting irritated while standing in a line, concentrate on a relaxing word (such as "quiet") until your anger subsides. Trust that others are not out to cheat you.
7. *Become a good listener*. Pay attention to what others are saying and do not interrupt. This may help you understand the situation better *before* you jump to an angry response.
8. *Live as if you have a serious disease*. You will soon see that the little problems that once riled you up aren't really so important.
9. *Learn to forgive*. Compassion is the strongest medicine for anger. Blame leads to anger; forgiveness heals.

4. Age

Being older has some advantages (wisdom and experience), but protection from CHD is not one of them. As you age, your risk for developing heart disease increases. This does not mean that coronary heart disease is *only* a disease of the old. You don't just suddenly drop dead one day at age 45 from a "heart attack." At any age and certainly at age 18, you have atherosclerotic plaque in your arteries. It accumulates over time, and by the time you've gained "age," you've also increased the private stash of cholesterol in your arteries. There is little that can be done to stop the calendar. Adopting a healthy lifestyle early in life may add years to your life and life to your years.

5. Male Gender

Males have a higher risk of coronary heart disease and stroke throughout their lives than do females. Even after menopause, when women's death rate from heart disease increases, it is less than men's. The increased male risk is not clearly understood. Some credit the

FIGURE 6.10 ➤

Estimated percentage of population with hypertension by race and sex in U.S. adults. Hypertensives are defined as persons with a systolic level ≥140 and/or a diastolic level ≥90 or who reported using antihypertensive medication.

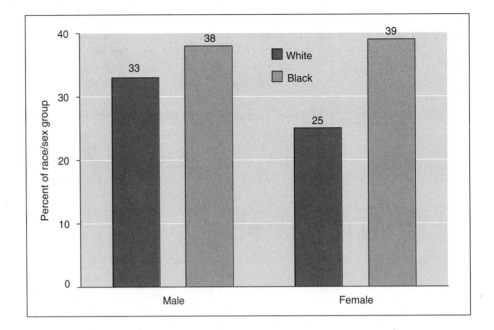

increased risk to the male sex hormone testosterone, which triggers production of low-density lipoproteins, thereby clogging blood vessels. Others say a male's lifestyle may be the culprit. We do know that a female's hormonal makeup is protective until menopause. Female hormones signal the liver to produce more "good" cholesterol (HDL) and make blood vessels more elastic than male's blood vessels, especially during childbearing years.[33]

It is imperative that males modify other risk factors to protect their cardiovascular systems.

6. Race

According to the American Heart Association, African Americans have the greatest risk of all races for heart attack and stroke. It is estimated that due to high blood pressure African Americans have more than 60 percent greater chance of death and disability from strokes than do whites (Fig. 6.10).[34] One explanation for this higher incidence is that many blacks share a mutation in a gene that helps control blood pressure. A hereditary intolerance to sodium may also account for the danger. African Americans have a higher prevalence of diabetes than do whites, and black women have very high obesity rates (Fig. 6.11). Social and economic stresses may also contribute to increased cardiovascular disease risk. It is paramount that early heart health intervention and education programs be supported for African-American populations. Also, being aware of these risks, African Americans should adopt a healthy lifestyle early. See Table 6.5 on page 132 for additional population information.

7. Positive Family History

A family history of heart disease in brothers, sisters, parents, or grandparents increases your risk of developing coronary artery disease. Tendencies toward high blood pressure, stroke, peripheral blood vessel disease, rheumatic fever, high blood lipid levels, obesity, and early heart attack appear to be hereditary. This is why your physician is so interested in your family history. You should find out as much as possible about your family's medical history. You can be alerted early to a possible risk and take preventative measures.

8. Diabetes Mellitus

Diabetes mellitus (which includes both Types I and II) is a condition characterized by the body's inability to produce enough of the hormone insulin or to use it properly. In the normal digestive process, sugars, starches, and other foods are changed to a form of sugar called *glucose*. The blood stream carries glucose to the body cells. There, with the help of insulin, a hormone produced in the pancreas, it is converted to quick energy for immediate use or stored for future needs. In diabetes, this normal process is interrupted. Glucose

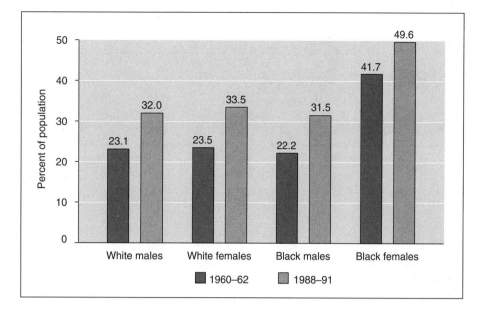

FIGURE 6.11 ➤
Overweight trends by sex and race, adults age 20 and over. United States: 1960–1962 and 1988–1991. Overweight is defined as approximately 20 percent or more above desirable weight.

Reproduced with permission. *Heart and Stroke Facts: 1995 Statistical Supplement,* 1994. Copyright American Heart Association.

accumulates in the blood until some of the surplus is eliminated by the kidneys, passing it off in the urine. Too much sugar in the urine and in the blood are classic signs of diabetes.

Diabetes is found in two forms. In insulin-dependent diabetes (IDDM), also known as Type I or juvenile onset, the pancreas makes little or no insulin. The diabetic must receive insulin injections every day to stay alive and must carefully watch his or her diet and exercise regularly. It occurs most often in children or young adults. Symptoms develop rapidly, usually within a period of months or even weeks.

More common (85 percent to 90 percent of diabetics) is non-insulin-dependent diabetes (NIDDM), also known as Type II or adult onset, in which the pancreas makes insulin but either the amount is insufficiently released or the body cannot properly utilize what is available. This type of diabetes can often be controlled without insulin injections through other medications, diet, and weight management. This form of the disease frequently occurs in people over 40 years old and is usually associated with aging and obesity. Because the onset of Type II is gradual, the disease may go undetected for years. Diabetes seriously increases the risk of developing cardiovascular disease. In fact, more than 80 percent of people with diabetes die of some form of heart or blood vessel disease. Part of the reason is that diabetes affects cholesterol and triglyceride levels by producing a different kind of LDL that is even worse for the arteries than is ordinary LDL. This accelerates atherosclerosis.[35] Even so, Type II diabetes can be delayed or averted by weight management. One condition shared almost universally by Type II diabetics is obesity. The risk of diabetes is two times greater in people who are mildly overweight (20 percent above ideal weight), five times greater in the moderately overweight (20 percent to 30 percent above ideal weight) and *ten* times greater in the obese (30 percent above ideal weight).

Current theories suggest a genetic predisposition to both Type I and Type II diabetes. Several groups of people are at greater risk and should be checking for diabetes at least once a year (with a simple blood glucose test performed in a doctor's office). Women are more prone to Type II than men, especially if they are 40 years of age and have relatives with the disease. African Americans, Hispanics, and especially Native Americans are at higher risk than European Americans.

Symptoms of both types can include hazy vision, excessive thirst, frequent urination, frequent hunger, a weight loss or weight gain, dry skin, a tired washed-out feeling, slow healing wounds, and combinations of these symptoms. Unless detected and controlled, diabetes can ultimately lead to stroke, heart disease, kidney failure, blindness, amputation of limbs, and death. According to the American Diabetes Association, the disease is a leading cause of death in this country and diabetics are twice as prone to heart attack and stroke as are nondiabetics.

table 6.5

DIVERSITY ISSUES

WHO SMOKES?

	Men	Women
All	28.2%	24.4%
White	28.0%	25.7%
African American	32.0%	23.9%
Hispanic	25.6%	13.4%
Asian/Pacific Islander	22.1%	10.5%
American Indian/Alaska Native	30.1%	29.6%

Studies show that smoking prevalence is several times higher among those with less than 12 years of education than it is among those with more than 16 years of education.

WHO HAS HIGH BLOOD PRESSURE (HBP)?

- Men have a greater risk of HBP than do women until age 55. From age 55 to 75, the risks for men and women are about equal; after that, women have a greater risk than men.
- African Americans, Puerto Ricans, and Cuban and Mexican Americans are more likely to suffer from HBP than are Anglo Americans.
- Death rates from HBP in 1992 were 6.2% for white males and 4.6% for white females; 29.3% for African-American males and 21.8% for African-American females.
- 22.8% of Cuban-American males and 15.5% of Cuban-American females have HBP.
- 16.8% of Mexican-American males and 14.1% of Mexican-American females have HBP.
- 15% of Puerto Rican males and 11.5% of Puerto Rican females have HBP.
- 13% of Asian Americans and Pacific Islanders have HBP.

WHO IS PHYSICALLY INACTIVE?

- People with lower incomes and less than a 12th-grade education are more likely to be sedentary.
- Regular exercise is more prevalent among men (44%) than women (38%).
- Black women, the less educated, overweight persons, and the elderly are the most inactive groups.
- In general, whites are more likely to exercise or play sports regularly than are blacks. However, among males ages 18 to 29 a higher percentage of black men (62%) are active than are whites (55%).
- Non-Hispanics are more likely to exercise or play sports regularly (41%) than are Hispanics (35%).

WHO IS OVERWEIGHT (20% OR MORE ABOVE THEIR DESIRABLE WEIGHT)?

- 32% of white males, 31.5% of black males, 33.5% of white females, and 49.6% of black females are overweight.
- Among Mexican Americans, 39.5% of males and 47.9% of females are overweight.
- Among Cuban Americans, 29.4% of males and 34.1% of females are overweight.
- Among Puerto Ricans, 25.2% of males and 37.3% of females are overweight.
- Among American Indians, 33.7% of males and 40.3% of females are overweight.
- Among Native Hawaiians, 65.5% of males and 62.6% of females are overweight.

source: American Heart Association. *Heart and Stroke Facts: 1995 Statistical Supplement.* Dallas: 1995 (7272 Greenville Ave., Dallas, TX 75231-4596).

Treatment for Blocked Coronary Arteries

As you have discovered, most of the risk factors linked to coronary heart disease can be controlled. The way you live, the choices you make, can have a profound impact on the health of your cardiorespiratory system. When coronary arteries do become blocked, usually the first treatments prescribed are diet modification (low fat) and exercise therapy. These are two major areas of one's life that, if maximized, can have positive results. When these methods are unsuccessful, the following procedures may be required.

Drug Therapy

This involves drug treatment affecting the supply of oxygen to the heart muscle or the heart's demand for oxygen. Some drugs (coronary vasodilators) cause the blood vessels to relax, enlarging the opening inside them. Blood flow then improves and more oxygen reaches the heart. Nitroglycerine is the most commonly used drug in this category. Another category of drugs slows down the heart rate or reduces blood pressure, thus decreasing the heart's need for oxygen, reducing its workload.

Angioplasty (or Balloon Angioplasty)

The American Heart Association describes this treatment as a nonsurgical procedure that improves the blood supply to the heart by dilating a narrowed coronary artery. The blocked part of the coronary artery must be identified before this technique is performed. During this process (cardiac catheterization), a doctor guides a thin plastic tube (catheter) through an artery from the arm or leg into the coronary arteries. A liquid dye, visible in X rays, is injected into the catheter and X-ray movies are taken as the dye flows through the arteries. Doctors can identify obstructions in the arteries by tracing the flow of the dye. Once obstructions are identified, another catheter having a balloon tip is inserted inside the first; the balloon tip is inflated at the obstruction site. This compresses the plaque and enlarges the opening of the blood vessel. The balloon is deflated and both catheters are removed. The process injures the vessel wall, causing the area to grow new cells. Some people grow too many cells, reclogging the artery. About 25 percent of the people who have this technique have renarrowed arteries within six months.[36]

Coronary Bypass Surgery

This is a surgical technique in which doctors take a blood vessel from another part of the body (usually the leg) and use it to detour around a blockage in the coronary artery. Blood flow to the heart is restored.

New Techniques

What follows are new techniques under research and showing great promise:

1. *Enzyme therapy:* In this nonsurgical process, enzymes are injected into the blockage, dissolving it.
2. *Laser beam treatment:* This is used to break up the plaque, after which the particles of debris are vaporized.
3. *Vaccination:* Because a virus has been identified in the blocked arteries of heart patients during autopsy, a vaccine might be given early in the life (such as the polio vaccine) to treat some forms of coronary artery disease.
4. *Insertion of a cancer gene:* A gene that slows cancer growth may also help prevent heart patient arteries from reclogging after angioplasty. The retenoblastoma gene is inserted into an ordinary cold virus, it is genetically modified so it cannot spread, and then angioplasty is performed with the virus-coated balloon. The gene does its work until the virus dies; both then become inactive. Reclogging has been reduced in early trials.

The Future . . . Focus on Lifestyle

The cost of treating cardiovascular diseases in this country is staggering (Fig. 6.12 on page 134). Many scientists believe we will be more successful if we focus on prevention rather than rely on expensive, high-tech treatments. "An ounce of prevention is worth a pound of cure" will, in all likelihood, be the slogan of the 22d century. Heart disease

FIGURE 6.12 ➤

Estimated cost of major cardiovascular diseases by type of expenditure. United States: 1995.

Reproduced with permission. *Heart
and Stroke Facts: 1995 Statistical
Supplement,* 1994. Copyright
American Heart Association.

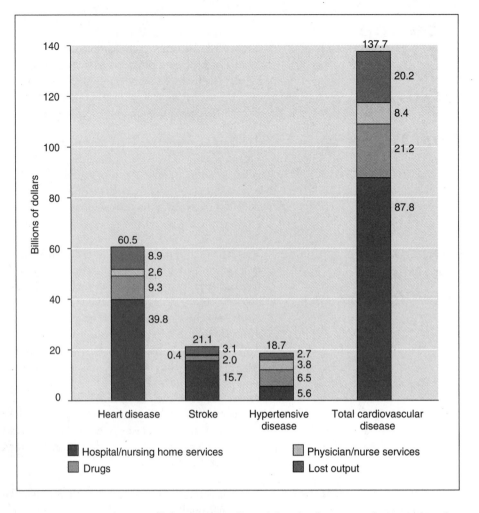

prevention in our future will focus primarily on lifestyle changes and approaches that involve "mind and body" concepts. Many scientists are already substantiating these trends in their research and medical practices.

One example is Dr. Dean Ornish, cardiologist, clinical professor of medicine at the University of California at San Francisco, and pioneer in the treatment of coronary heart disease. He found that after treating his patients with the current, recommended medical procedures—medication, angioplasty (balloon technique), and coronary by-pass surgery, all expensive and dangerous—most did not stay well. Despite the procedures, some died and many returned for further treatment. He began to question the wisdom of such dramatic medical care for coronary heart disease. He found it interesting that lifestyle factors could trigger all mechanisms known to cause CHD. The lifestyle choices we make each day, such as about what we eat, how we respond to stress, how much we exercise, and whether we use tobacco, have a profound impact on our heart's health. With this concept in mind, he developed a plan that focused on lifestyle. His new program, "Reversing Heart Disease," is having significant success in reducing atherosclerosis without medication or surgical procedures. The program involves the following lifestyle changes:[37, 38]

1. A special diet is recommended. The Reversal Diet is 10 percent fat, 70 percent to 75 percent carbohydrate, 15 percent to 20 percent protein, and 5 milligrams of cholesterol per day. In comparison, the typical American diet is 40 percent to 45 percent fat, 25 percent to 35 percent carbohydrate, 25 percent protein, and 400 to 500 milligrams of cholesterol per day. The Reversal Diet

allows but does not encourage moderate alcohol consumption (less than 2 oz. per day). It excludes caffeine, allows moderate use of salt and sugar, and is not restricted in calories.

2. Smoking is prohibited.
3. Thirty minutes a day or one hour every other day of moderate exercise is prescribed.
4. Stress management methods are prescribed every day. These include yoga stretches, progressive relaxation, abdominal breathing, meditation, and imagery.
5. Communication skills should be enhanced and techniques for increasing intimacy are taught.

By adhering to the five steps involved in the "Reversing Heart Disease" plan, Americans can save billions of dollars and thousands of lives every year. Can we afford *not* to stop smoking, dramatically reduce the fat in our diets, make commitment to lifetime exercise and stress management, and become more in tune with each other?

Mind and Body Connection

The traditional risk factors explain only a portion of the known causes of heart disease. Why do some people develop heart disease and others do not? Clearly, all the risk factors are important, but could there be something more? Are there common psychological—and perhaps even spiritual—factors that lead to or prevent coronary heart disease? Is there an unconscious connection between mind, body, and spirit that would explain the unknown causes of heart disease?

Scientists are beginning to examine these questions: Is laughter good for you? Can prayer bring down blood pressure? Does a bad marriage or divorce suppress your immune system? Does listening to others lower blood pressure? Is a cynic more likely to have heart trouble? To each of these questions there is a scientist able to answer "YES!" and provide data to back it up. There is a whole field of mind/body research tapping into the interaction between our immune systems and our bodies, mind, moods, and spirit. Just as we learned the importance of exercise and nutrition to our health, we are now discovering ways to go deeper into inner wellness. Ponder these studies that support the mind/body concept:

➤ Norman Cousins, author, philosopher, and former professor at the Department of Psychiatry and Bio-behavioral Sciences at UCLA Medical School, found that laughter heals because it replaces fear and stress with serenity and homeostasis. He taught others to never underestimate the capacity of the human mind and body to regenerate, even when the prospects seemed most dismal. His research confirmed that positive emotions boost health.[39]

➤ Larry Scherwitz, professor of psychology at the University of California, found that people who overuse the self-centered pronouns "I," "me," or "mine" are twice as likely to have heart attacks. These people are hostile, have a low level of trust in others, and put their own self-centered interests and pleasures ahead of all others.[40]

➤ Redford Williams of Duke University found that cynics, being full of contempt for other people, and angry hostile people have more than their share of heart trouble.[41]

➤ Many scientists have developed psychological tests to measure levels of anger that bring on heart attacks.[42] Studies linking social support (i.e., loving family, happy marriage, one or two close friends, support groups) to vitality, longevity, lowered blood pressure, and healthier immune systems confirm that emotions may very well regulate health. These head and heart factors are powerful medicine.[43,44,45]

➤ Dean Ornish, M.D., is convinced that one cause of blocked coronary arteries stems from three kinds of loneliness (or isolation): (1) we feel isolated from ourselves, (2) we lack "connectedness" and intimate relationships with others, (3) we have a cosmic loneliness of the spirit (or higher part of ourselves). He feels that isolation leads to chronic stress and to illnesses such as heart disease, and that real intimacy and feelings of connectedness with others can be healing. He argues that the ability to be intimate with ourselves, with others, and with a higher spirit—within ourselves—is the key to emotional health and essential to the health of our hearts as well.[46]

➤ Mind/body connection authority, Jon Kabat-Zinn, author of *Full Catastrophe Living*, advocates meditation as a technique to bridge the gap between the mind and the heart to improve health, ease pain, and reduce stress.[47]

➤ Another authority on the mind/body connection, Bill Moyers, author of *Healing and the Mind*, explored the latest research in the field of medicine known as psychoneuroimmunology.[48] He found evidence supporting the ways in which thoughts, feelings, and emotions influence our health. Moyers documents the importance of mind/body interactions in both the prevention and the treatment of illness.

SUMMARY

Heart disease is the number-one killer in the United States today. Extensive studies have identified 12 factors that increase the risk of developing coronary heart disease. These factors lead to the development of atherosclerosis. The most significant factors are high blood pressure, high blood lipid profile, cigarette smoking, and inactivity. These four are labeled *primary* and can be controlled. There are eight additional contributing factors labeled *secondary*. The first three of these are controllable. They are obesity, stress, and emotional behavior—especially negative emotional behaviors such as hostility and anger. The other five secondary risk factors, which cannot be controlled, are age, male gender, race, positive family history, and diabetes. The more risk factors you have and the longer they are present, the greater the chance you have of developing heart disease. By age 20, you already have fatty deposits present in your coronary arteries.

If the coronary arteries become blocked due to advanced atherosclerosis, there are several treatments available. These include exercise and diet modification, drug therapy, angioplasty, and coronary bypass surgery. The cost of treating CVD continues to spiral upward every year. To counter this trend, many scientists are convinced that preventing CVD through lifestyle change is the *key* to heart health.

As was stated earlier, adopting a healthy lifestyle early in life can add years to your life—and life to your years. In addition, great discoveries await us as the field of mind and body research gains wider acceptance in the quest for increased well-being.

REFERENCES

1. *Heart and Stroke Facts: 1995 Statistical Supplement*. Dallas: American Heart Association National Center, 1995: 1 (7272 Greenville Avenue, Dallas, TX 75231–4596).

2. *Heart and Stroke Facts: 1995 Statistical Supplement*, 1.

3. *Heart and Stroke Facts: 1995 Statistical Supplement*, 1.

4. *Heart and Stroke Facts: 1995 Statistical Supplement*, 1.

5. *Heart and Stroke Facts: 1995 Statistical Supplement*, 1.

6. Kavanagh, Terrence, M.D. "Does Exercise Training Improve Coronary Collateralization? A New Look at an Old Belief." *The Physician and Sports Medicine* 17, no. 1 (January 1989): 43, 96–113.

7. *Heart and Stroke Facts: 1995 Statistical Supplement*, 11.

8. *Heart and Stroke Facts: 1995 Statistical Supplement*, 11.

9. *Heart and Stroke Facts: 1995 Statistical Supplement*, 12.

10. Ornish, Dean, M.D. *Dr. Dean Ornish's Program for Reversing Heart Disease*. New York: Random House, 1990, 79.

11. *Heart and Stroke Facts: 1995 Statistical Supplement*, 18.

12. Editors of the University of California, Berkeley Wellness Letter. *The Wellness Encyclopedia*. Boston: Houghton Mifflin Company, 1991, 310.

13. *The Wellness Encyclopedia*, 310.

14. *Heart and Stroke Facts: 1995 Statistical Supplement*, 18.

15. "Fascinating Facts," *University of California, Berkeley, Wellness Newsletter* 6. No. 3 (December 1989): 1.

16. Glantz, S. A., et al. "Passive Smoking and Heart Disease: Mechanisms at Risk." *Journal of American Medical Association* 273, no. 13 (April 5, 1995): 1,047–52.

17. Glantz, S. A., et al. "Passive Smoking and Heart Disease: Mechanisms at Risk."

18. Glantz, S. A., et al. "Passive Smoking and Heart Disease: Mechanisms at Risk."

19. Hurley, Judith, and Richard Schlaadt. *The Wellness Lifestyle*. Guilford, Conn.: The Dushkin Publishing Group, 1992, 91.

20. Pate, Russell, et al. "Physical Activity and Public Health. A Recommendation from The Centers for Disease Control and Prevention and The American College of Sports Medicine." *Journal of American Medical Association* 273, no. 5 (February 1, 1995): 402–7.

21. Russell, Pate, et al. "Physical Activity and Public Health," 402.

22. Morris, Jeremy, N. "Exercise in Prevention of Coronary Heart Disease: Today's Best Buy in Public Health." *Medicine and Science in Sports and Exercise* 26, no. 7 (1994): 807.

23. Kohl, H. W., III, S. N. Blair, R. S. Paffenbarger, et al. "Changes in Physical Fitness and All-Cause Mortality; A Prospective Study of Healthy and Unhealthy Men." *Journal of American Medical Association* 273, no. 14 (April 12, 1995): 1,093–98.

24. Lee, I. M. C., Hsieh, R. S. Paffenbarger. "Exercise Intensity and Longevity in Men: The Harvard Alumni Health Study." *Journal of American Medical Association* 273, no. 15 (April 19, 1995): 1,179–84.

25. Scragg, Robert. "Alcohol and Exercise in Myocardial Infarction and Sudden Coronary Death in Men and Women." *American Journal of Epidemiology* 126, no. 1 (July 1987): 77–85, 531.

26. *Heart and Stroke Facts: 1995 Statistical Supplement*, 21.

27. Koop, Everett C., M.D. *Shape Up American Campaign Report*, 1995.

28. *The Wellness Encyclopedia*, 310.

29. *Heart and Stroke Facts: 1995 Statistical Supplement*, 21.

30. *The Wellness Encyclopedia*, 312.

31. Schmall, Peter, M.D., et al. "The Relationship Between Job Stress, Work Place Diastolic Blood Pressure, and Left Ventricle Max Index." *Journal of American Medical Association* 263 (April 11, 1990): 315, 1929–35.

32. Eliot, Robert S., M.D. *From Stress to Strength*. New York: Bantam Books, 1994, 45.

33. *The Wellness Encyclopedia*, 310.

34. *Heart and Stroke Facts: 1995 Statistical Supplement*, 20.

35. Liebman, Bonnie. "The HDL/Triglyceride Trap." *Nutrition Action* 17, no. 7 (September 1990), 4.

36. *Heart and Stroke Facts: 1995 Statistical Supplement*, 20.

37. Ornish, Dean, M.D. *Dr. Dean Ornish's Program for Reversing Heart Disease*, 60.

38. Ornish, Dean, M.D., et al. "Can Lifestyle Changes Reverse Coronary Heart Disease?" *Lancet* 336 (1990): 61.

39. Cousins, N. *The Healing Heart*. New York: Avon Books, 1983, 45.

40. Scherwitz, L., et al. "Speech Characteristics and Behavior-Type Assessment in the Multiple Risk Factors Intervention Trial (MRFIT) Structured Interviews. *Journal of Behavioral Medicine* (1987): 215.

41. Williams, Redford, M.D., et al. *Anger Kills*. New York: Random House, 1993.

42. Eliot, Robert S., M.D. *From Stress to Strength*, 90.

43. Spiegal, David, et al. "Effect of Psychosocial Treatment on Survival of Patients with Metastatic Breast Cancer." *Lancet* (1989): 209.

44. Syme, Leonard. "Social Determinants of Disease." *Annual of Clinical Research* (1989): 45.

45. Seeman, T., and L. Syme. "Social Networks and Coronary Artery Disease: A Comparison of the Structure and Function of Social Relations as Predictors of Disease." *Psychomatic Medicine* (1987): 75.

46. Ornish, Dean, M.D. *Dr. Dean Ornish's Program for Reversing Heart Disease*, 60.

47. Kabat-Zinn, Jon. *Full Catastrophe Living: Using the Wisdom of Your Body and Mind to Face Pain, Stress, and Illness*. New York: Dell Publishers, 1991, 115.

48. Moyers, Bill D. *Healing and the Mind*. New York: Doubleday, 1993, 71.

SUGGESTED READINGS

Cooper, G. R., G. L. Myers, S. J. Smith, R. C. Schlant. "Blood Lipid Measurements: Variations and Practical Utility." *Journal of American Medical Association* 267, no. 12 (March 25, 1992).

Cooper, Kenneth H., M.D., M.P.H. *Dr. Kenneth Cooper's Preventive Medicine Program Controlling Cholesterol*. New York: Bantam Books, 1987.

Dooley, Denton, M.D., and Carolyn Moore, Ph.D. R.D. *Eat Smart for a Healthy Heart Cookbook*. Woodbury N.Y.: Barron's Educational Series, Inc., 1987 (113 Crossways Park Drive, Woodbury, NY 11797).

Eliot, Robert S., M.D. *From Stress to Strength*. New York: Bantam Books, 1994.

Friedman, M., and R. H. Rosenman. *Type A Behavior and Your Heart*. New York: Knopf, 1994.

Fuchs, C. S. "Alcohol Consumption and Mortality Among Women." *The New England Journal of Women* 332, no. 19 (May 11, 1995).

Healthy People 2000. Washington, D.C. Department of Health and Human Services, No. (PHS) 91-502B, 1990.

Hoeger, Werner W. K. *Principles and Labs for Physical Fitness and Wellness*. Englewood, Colo.: Morton Publishing Company 1988 (925 W. Kenyon Ave., Unit 4, Englewood, CO 80110).

Kabat-Zinn, Jon. *Wherever You Go There You Are, Mindfulness Meditation in Everyday Life*. New York: Hyperion, 1994.

Melby, Christopher, Roseann Lyle, and Gerald Hyner. "Beyond Blood Pressure Screening: A Rationale for Promoting the Primary Prevention of Hypertension." *American Journal of Health Promotion* 3, no. 2 (Fall 1988): 5–11.

Ornish, Dean, M.D. *Dr. Dean Ornish's Program for Reversing Heart Disease*. New York: Random House, 1990.

U.S. Department of Health and Human Services. *Report of the Expert Panel on Population Strategies for Blood Cholesterol Reduction*. PHS & National Institutes of Health, November 1990.

Williams, Redford. *Anger Kills*. New York: Times Books, 1993.

For more information, contact the following organizations:

American Heart Association
7272 Greenville Avenue
Dallas, TX 75231–4596
(214) 750–5300

National Heart, Lung, and Blood
Institute Information Center
4733 Bethesda Avenue, Suite 530
Bethesda, MD 20814–4820
(301) 951–3260

National Stroke Association
1565 Clarkson Street
Denver, CO 80218
(303) 839–1992

American Diabetes Association, Inc.
Two Park Avenue
New York, NY 10016
(212) 683–7444

The Juvenile Diabetes Foundation
International
23 East 26th Street
New York, NY 10010
(212) 889–7575

National Diabetes Information
Clearinghouse
Box NDIC
Bethesda, MD 20205
(301) 496–7433

chapter 7

Coping with Stress

4g's

148's

➤ Objectives

After reading this chapter, you will be able to:

1. Define the terms *stress*, *stressor*, and *stress response*.
2. Explain the three stages of the stress response.
3. Define and give examples of eustress, distress, and optimal stress.
4. Explain how perception and control are involved in stress.
5. Measure the amount of life changes on the Holmes and Rahe Life Event Scale you have encountered this year and be able to predict your susceptibility to a stress-related illness.
6. Explain the difference between daily hassles and daily uplifts and how each affects overall health.
7. Describe six harmful effects of too much stress.
8. Contrast Type A, Type B, and Type C behavior patterns.
9. Describe a hot reactor's behavior and the health consequences of this behavior.
10. Identify your behavior when reacting to stress.
11. List five Type A behavior modification techniques.
12. List five strategies for managing stress.
13. Describe two methods of relaxation that produce the relaxation response.
14. Define and list three benefits of the relaxation response.
15. Describe mindfulness meditation.

father of stress research

Terms

- Autogenic training and imagery
- Biofeedback training
- Catecholamines
- Daily hassles
- Daily uplifts
- Distress
- Eustress
- Fight-or-flight response (Alarm Stage)
- General Adaptation Syndrome (GAS)
- Hatha yoga
- Hot reactors
- Meditation
- Mindfulness meditation
- Optimal stress
- Progressive relaxation
- Psychoneuroimmunology
- Psychosomatic disease
- Reframing
- Relaxation response
- Stage of exhaustion
- Stage of resistance
- Stress
- Stressors
- Stress response
- Transcendental meditation (TM)
- Type A personality
- Type B personality
- Type C personality

Happiness is an inside job.

H. Jackson Brown, Jr., ed. *Dad, a Father's Book of Wisdom*

Lisa was the oldest child of three and the first in her family to go to college. Living on campus was wonderful—it meant new friends, open visitation in the residence hall, and no curfew hours. But, by the end of the school year, her life had changed for the worse.

Her G.P.A. was barely above a "C" average, which was far below her high school performance. There just never seemed to be enough hours in the day to keep up with all the reading. Plus, she felt exhausted most of the time and had trouble waking up for early classes. It was no wonder: The "action" never settled down on her hall before 12:30 or 1:00 A.M. Then, just before final exams, her parents announced that they were getting a divorce. Had her college expenses created a financial burden on the family budget and contributed to the divorce? She felt guilty and partially responsible for her parent's problems. Now she would have to move back home and work full-time at the local discount store to help pay for college. Would it be possible to finish the nursing degree by taking night classes? Antonio, her boyfriend was pressuring her to drop out of school so they could get married. He complained that she devoted too much time to school work and not enough to him. Her mother would now have to go back to work and would expect her to help take care of her younger brothers and assist with the household chores. Feeling fatigued and really stressed out, she wondered, with work and family obligations, when would she study? Would she ever have any time for herself? Was she the only one in college with such problems? How complicated her life had become.

The scene just described is not all that uncommon on the typical college campus. The many challenges faced by college students can be stressful and can cause feelings of anxiety. Stiff competition for grades, career choices, selection of classes, test anxiety, sense of loss of family and home, balancing work and school, peer pressure, inadequate

College students face many stresses.

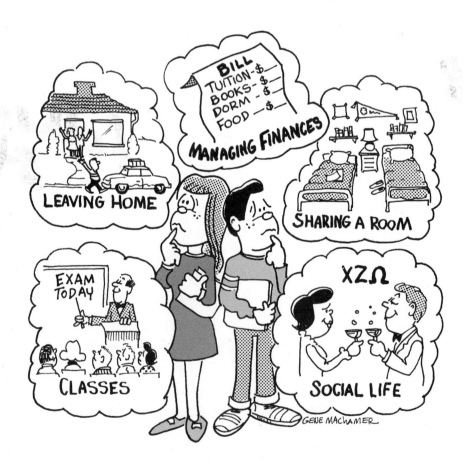

FIGURE 7.1 >

Optimal stress and the relationship to health and performance. Everyone has a point at which the "right" amount of stress improves performance, health, and efficiency.

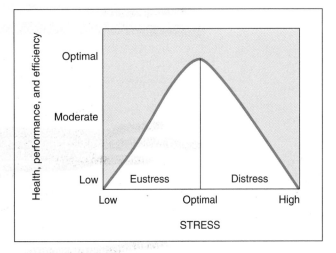

sleep, poor nutritional habits, low physical fitness levels, and increased social involvements all contribute to high levels of stress. Clearly, college is a stressful environment, one that makes demands on you physically, socially, intellectually, and emotionally. It's no wonder that you sometimes feel anxious, irritable, and stressed out. Contrary to what many college students believe, stress does not "evaporate" after graduation. The pace of life has in the past 10 years seemed to be accelerating. Federal Express overnight service is no longer quick enough—the letter needs to be faxed immediately. Receiving one telephone call at a time is not enough; now, with call waiting, two or more can be received at once. Even the traditional places of refuge in the 20th century—the car and the home—are transformed into offices away from offices, with fax machines and computers in the home and telephones and even fax machines in the car. With portable telephones and laptop computers, work stress never ends. We often do not have time to recover from one stressful situation before we face another one.

No one is exempt from stress. This is good since a certain amount is beneficial for an optimal level of health and achievement, plus it helps us cope with emergency situations. Figure 7.1 illustrates how the "right" amount of stress improves health and performance, but how our health and well-being can be adversely affected by excessive stress. Too much stress ultimately exhausts the body's ability to adapt; vital organs wear out, and various illnesses may appear. This is especially true when stress is perceived to be negative or harmful. Since stress is a normal part of life, why do so few people understand it or how to manage it? Improvement in the quality of life is dependent on *balancing* the demands made upon you and developing effective ways to *manage* stress.

What Is Stress?

Dr. Hans Selye, one of the foremost authorities on stress, defined **stress** as the "nonspecific response of the human organism to any demand made upon it."[1] It is the response of the body to any type of change and to any new, threatening, or exciting situation. *Nonspecific* means that the body reacts the same regardless of the cause. **Stressors,** factors causing stress, can be pleasant or unpleasant, either real or imagined, and can be of different types. All cause the body to adapt. For example, *physical* stressors include illness, accidents, injury, heat, cold, and noise. *Psychological* or *emotional* stressors involve parenting, deadlines, poverty, final exams, work overloads (school or job), rejection, depression, holidays, divorce, and marriage.

Dr. Selye described the ways in which we react to stress as either *eustress* (good) or *distress* (bad). In both cases, the physiological response is the same. In the case of **eustress,** which refers to happy, pleasant events (holidays, getting married, etc.), health and performance improve even as stress increases. On the other hand, **distress** refers to unpleasant or harmful stress (flunking an exam, breakup of a relationship, etc.) under which health and performance begin to decline. **Optimal stress** is a point at which the stress is intense enough to motivate and physically prepare us to perform optimally yet not intense enough to cause the body to overreact or to sustain harmful effects.[2] Figure 7.1 illustrates this concept. Optimal stress gives the athlete the competitive edge and the public speaker the enthusiasm to project with charisma. Overstress results in poor performance and produces overreaction, poor concentration, test anxiety, and health problems.[3] When experiencing positive stress, individuals generally feel in control. Negative stress causes out-of-control feelings.

Regardless of the cause, the adaptation (reaction) to stress is both psychological and physiological and leads to what Dr. Selye called the **General Adaptation Syndrome (GAS).** Today, the GAS is simply called the **Stress Response.**

The Stress Response—a Three-Stage Process

Hans Selye summarized the Stress Response in a three-stage process:[4]

1. **Fight-or-flight response (or Alarm Stage):** The body prepares itself to cope with a stressor. The response is a warning signal that a stressor is present. Physiological and psychological responses appear. This is really a primitive survival mechanism that today is rarely needed. See Figure 7.2.
2. **Stage of resistance:** The body actively resists and attempts to cope with the stressor. In this stage, the stress response is channeled into the specific organ system most capable of suppressing it. It is this adaptation process that contributes to stress-related illness. The specific organ system becomes aroused and, if prolonged, it may fatigue and begin to malfunction. Headache, forgetfulness, colon spasms (constipation or diarrhea), asthma, anxiety attacks, and high blood pressure are examples of prolonged arousal.
3. **Stage of exhaustion:** Adaptation energy is exhausted and signs of fight-or-flight reappear. During the exhaustion phase, the organ system involved in the repeated stress response breaks down. Disease or malfunction of the organ system or even death may occur. For example, high blood pressure (caused by excessive stress) promotes kidney and heart damage, which can kill the individual if allowed to continue.

Fight-or-Flight (Alarm)

The body responds to stress, whether emotional or physical (real or perceived), by activating a series of mechanisms collectively known as the fight-or-flight response.[5] This response, which has been a part of our physiological makeup since the beginning of time, prepares us to either fight or to flee to safety by pumping powerful stress hormones and steroids into the blood stream (Figure 7.2). Early humans, faced with daily life-and-death situations, relied heavily on this response for survival. The caveman or -woman could escape the jaws of a hungry lion (stressor) by swiftly running (the fight-or-flight response in action). These mechanisms work best where the danger is clear, well-defined, and short-term (acute not chronic). Many examples of the fight-or-flight response can be found even in today's world. Imagine this scenario: You are crossing the street on your way home when suddenly you see a car fast approaching you. Instinctively, your muscles tense, and you jump back on the curb with such force that you fall back into a newspaper stand and cut your head, which quickly stops bleeding. The fight-or-flight response saved your life (the quick backward jump and the cut that stops bleeding). Other examples of the response, normally described as "superhuman" acts, are in reality the fight-or-flight response in action. Perhaps you can add others to this list:

➤ A person lifts an automobile off an injured individual at an accident scene.
➤ A small child rescues an older child who is drowning in a backyard swimming pool.
➤ After having both arms ripped off by a farm machine, a young farmer manages to telephone for help by dialing 911 with a pencil clenched in his teeth.
➤ A mother knocks down a locked bedroom door to rescue her children from a burning house.
➤ A student outruns a mugger on a dark corner of campus.

FIGURE 7.2 ➤
Physical reactions to stressors.

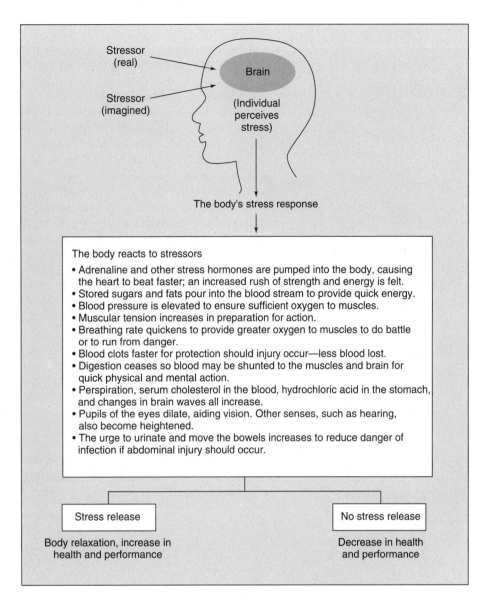

These are only a few examples that have required action to prevent or minimize physical harm. A few minutes after the frightening event (acute stressor), the individuals return to their normal physiological state. Other stressors, the kind you encounter every day, such as noise, arguments, keys locked inside the car, missed deadlines, traffic tickets, or any new situation that causes us to adapt, have the same potential for eliciting the fight-or-flight response.

Physical and emotional stress (too much to do, breakup of a relationship, public speaking, etc.) may be either acute or chronic. We are designed to cope with acute stress much better than with chronic stress.[6] Unfortunately, physical and emotional stress in modern times tends to be chronic rather than acute. The pace of life accelerates every year. We often do not have time to recover from one stressful situation before we face another one.

Innate physiological stress responses (Figure 7.2) have evolved over the centuries to help us survive danger and prepare us for swift action whether or not it is needed. However, the buildup of unused stress products produces excessive wear and tear on the body and may even increase the rate of aging. When stressors inappropriately provoke the fight-or-flight reactions many times a day, the body repeatedly responds as if experiencing real emergencies. The fight-or-flight response is often appropriate and should not be thought of as always harmful. It is a necessary part of our physiological makeup, a useful reaction to many situations in our current world. However, we need to learn how to avoid triggering the stress response except in real emergencies.

Stage of Resistance

The longer our bodies stay in a chronic "on guard" resistance stage, the more likely we are to experience ill effects. Today, we don't have much opportunity to physically play out the fight-or-flight response in acute stress situations because today's stress is mostly chronic. Though we chronically evoke the fight-or-flight response, modern society does not accept the fight naturally associated with it. For example, you obviously do not run away from or hit your boss when he or she reprimands you. Our innate reactions have not changed, but society has. The response is turned on, but we do not use it appropriately. As a result, the body remains in the resistance stage for longer periods. Our sedentary lifestyles decrease the outlets for fight-or-flight hormones that are pumped into the body. The length of time that a stressor is with you is an important factor. Stress becomes harmful when it is prolonged and perceived as negative to the recipient.

Learning stress management skills is important in coping with the stresses of life. People who have learned these skills may still overreact to a stressor but will relax more quickly to their resting physiological state than will people who have not learned these skills.

Stage of Exhaustion

The exhaustion stage of the stress response can ultimately result in death if not countered. Thankfully, it is not often reached. If our bodies are successful in resisting stress, exhaustion does not follow. We usually adapt to the stress and make whatever adjustments are necessary to cope, whether the stress is physical or psychological. Learn and practice regularly one or more of the stress management skills described in this chapter to reduce the unhealthy stress in your life.

Perception and Control

Individuals may respond differently to the same stressor. Whether a particular stressor causes a negative reaction depends on whether the person perceives that stressor as being negative.[7] This concept was confirmed by the research of Dr. Richard Lazarus who asserted that we are, after all, thinking, cognitive creatures. We are able to assess the positive and negative consequences of any situation or threat. One person may *perceive* a stressor as threatening, and as a result, experience a full-blown fight-or-flight response. Another may encounter the same event and not perceive it as a threat. We are all different, and each of us perceives stressors in a different light. How do you perceive snakes, announcement of an exam, competition, being cut off in traffic, being called in to see the boss, a doctor's appointment, being called on to contribute to class discussion, a professor requesting to speak with you after class? These situations do not bother some individuals but are agonizing to others.

In reality, most people's problems have to do with *faulty perception*—that is, unnecessarily seeing a situation as hopeless, harmful, or negative. Fortunately, we each have the power to develop cognitive skills to cope with faulty perception. As Duke Ellington put it, "A problem is a chance to do your best." Before gearing up to fret, fight, or flee, ask yourself, "Does a threat really exist? Is the issue really important to me? Can I make a difference?" If the answer to any of these questions is "no," do not waste your energy. It is not worth it. Some situations are truly threatening and deserve high energy stress responses. When the threat you perceive in a situation is quite real, go ahead and gear up. You can then benefit from the energy generated by your natural stress response by applying it to the situation at hand.

Control is another important factor in the total stress picture. You are in much greater control over your stress than you ever realized. Managing stress means empowering yourself to take control rather than relinquishing the control to events, to other people, to your environment, or to the calendar. People who handle stress best tend to

We all perceive stressors differently.

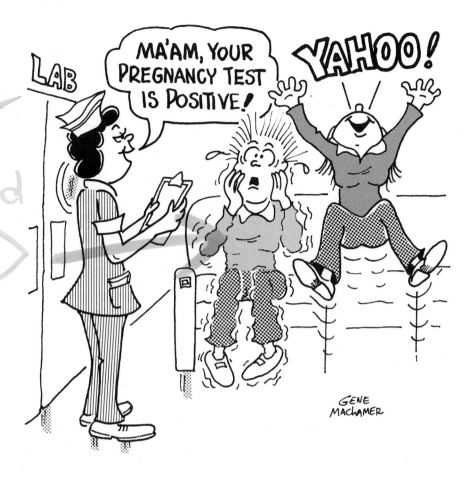

control their lives and look for active solutions to the problems and circumstances of their lives. You are responsible for allowing stressful situations to raise your blood pressure and heart rate. We can all recall events that made us angry one time but did not even faze us the next. Why is this? It is because we *allowed* ourselves to become upset. Perhaps the situation was complicated by nasty weather, lack of sleep, or a buildup of particular events. The bottom line is this particular time we *allowed* the event to provoke an angry response. This does not need to be the case. You cannot control what other people say or do, but you can change how you react to what others say or do. Whether to allow stressful events to provoke physiological reactions, such as increased muscle tension and nervous stomach, is your decision. By taking charge, you can decide whether to be an overstressed, nervous wreck or a calm, collected person.

Other ways to gain control over your life are making healthy lifestyle decisions and getting prepared (organized) at work, school, and home. Control is diminished when you don't. It is your decision to smoke or not smoke, to learn and implement time management skills or not, to exercise or not exercise, to eat nutritionally or to gobble up beer, colas, and greasy junk food. You must decide when to take on added duties and assignments or when to say, "No, sorry, not at this time. I have too many irons in the fire right now." It is, likewise, your decision to regularly practice relaxation techniques or to find excuses for not incorporating these relaxing skills into your daily life. Often, people say they would like to meditate but can't find the time. Nonsense! Why not make a *commitment* to taking control of your life and controlling your stress? Begin now to employ one or more of the stress-coping strategies described in this chapter, restore a sense of control, and reduce symptoms of stress. Remember, only you can decide if you want to manage your stress. It is your responsibility to learn these skills, practice them, and incorporate them into your daily life. You will be a healthier person for it. The key to surviving and even thriving on stress is self control. Take charge of *you*—for *you*.

Measuring Your Stress

In 1967, two psychiatrists at the University of Washington School of Medicine, Thomas H. Holmes, M.D., and Richard H. Rahe, M.D., observed that certain life events coincided with illness.[8] According to the doctors, change, whether for "good" or "bad," causes stress, leaving humans more susceptible to disease. Even simple changes, such as in eating habits, job routine, and housekeeping duties, can increase one's susceptibility to stress-related diseases. After studying medical histories and personal biographies of patients, the doctors found a curious link between life changing events and illnesses such as heart disease, ulcers, and psychiatric problems (depression, anxiety, etc.); they developed a list of life changes that range from minor to severe and assigned points to each one based on the amount of stress evoked (Table 7.1). An adaptation of the *Holmes and Rahe Life Event Scale* has been developed for college students and can be found in the Activities Section (p. 391). Take a few moments to complete the *Life Event Scale*, identifying those events that have occurred in your life during the past year. Add up your score and evaluate your potential for developing a serious illness due to the amount of stress you have had to adapt to this year.

Perhaps you can adapt this list to include factors that concern you personally and then substitute them into this scale. Whether you use the original Holmes and Rahe Scale or the college student adaptation of it, this is an excellent method of measuring the number of stressful events in your life. It can also be an effective tool when used to *anticipate* major life events so that you can control the stress they produce. No one would suggest we get rid of holidays, vacations, weddings, and family reunions. But we should take all life changes, including these positive ones, into account when planning our lives. Scheduling predictable life events such as marriage or recreation provides you with some control over them and is helpful in reducing stress. Realizing there are certain life events you cannot control is equally important in stress reduction. Remember, change is inevitable; that's what living is all about. But keep in mind that you can plan ahead for change and regulate the timing of many events (stressors) to prevent them from draining much of your adaptation energy. Spread change out over a period of time. When you feel in control, you perceive stressful situations as much less stressful; thus, there is less chance of provoking a stress-related illness. Change in life situations alone may not be enough to cause illness. When these changes are perceived as distressing, and result in chronic and prolonged emotional and physiological wear and tear, your risk of illness increases. Some people are more vulnerable to certain types of stress than others. If you would like to find out what type of stress you are most susceptible to and how well you cope with stress take the *Measuring Your Stress and Coping Skills* test in the Activities Section. This test also measures coping skills for dealing with stress.

Establishing coping techniques is a positive way to block the development of a stress illness. Well-timed social support is probably the best coping mechanism we have. When you are experiencing many life changes but have family and friends with whom you can discuss your problems, you probably will avoid a stress illness. Another individual experiencing fewer life changes but with less support may become ill. Ponder the wisdom of Alvin Toffler, author of *Future Shock:* "To survive (today), the individual must become infinitely more adaptable and capable than ever before. He must search out totally new ways to anchor himself. . . ."

Daily Hassles and Uplifts

Studies by Richard Lazarus and colleagues suggest that it is not just the major "life events" that have a negative impact on health, but other factors called *daily hassles*, and these may be even more harmful.[9] **Daily hassles** are the events or interactions in your daily life that you find bothersome, annoying, or negative in some way. These irritating demands include practical problems such as losing things, traffic jams, arguments, inclement weather, and family concerns. Lazarus and colleagues found that the greatest

table 7.1

HOLMES AND RAHE LIFE EVENT SCALE

Determine which of the following events you have experienced within the past year.

MEAN VALUE	LIFE EVENT	MEAN VALUE	LIFE EVENT
(100)	Death of spouse	(30)	Foreclosure of mortgage or loan
(73)	Divorce	(29)	Change in responsibilities at work
(65)	Marital separation	(29)	Son or daughter leaving home
(63)	Jail term	(29)	Trouble with in-laws
(63)	Death of close family member	(28)	Outstanding personal achievement
(53)	Personal injury or illness	(26)	Spouse begins or stops work
(50)	Marriage	(25)	Change in living conditions
(47)	Fired at work	(24)	Revision of personal habits
(45)	Marital reconciliation	(23)	Trouble with boss
(45)	Retirement	(20)	Change in work hours or conditions
(44)	Change in health of family member	(20)	Change in residence
(40)	Pregnancy	(19)	Change in recreation
(39)	Sex difficulties	(19)	Change in church activities
(39)	Gain of new family member	(18)	Change in social activities
(39)	Business readjustment	(17)	Mortgage or loan for lesser purchase (car, TV, etc.)
(38)	Change in financial state		
(37)	Death of a close friend	(16)	Change in sleeping habits
(36)	Change to different line of work	(15)	Change in number of family get-togethers
(35)	Change in number of arguments with spouse	(13)	Vacation
		(12)	Christmas
(31)	Mortgage or loan for major purchase (home, etc.)	(11)	Minor violations of the law

DIRECTIONS FOR LIFE EVENT SCALES

To obtain your score, multiply the number of times an event occurred by its mean value. Then total all of the scores. Your score is termed your **life change units (LCU).** This is a measure of the amount of significant changes in your life to which you have had to adjust. In other words, your LCU is a measure of the stressors you have encountered this past year.

Rating	Score	Implications for Illness
Low stress	≤150	37 percent chance of getting a stress-related illness in the next year or two
Moderate stress	151–300	51 percent chance of getting a stress-related illness in the next year
High stress	≥301	80 percent chance of getting a stress-related illness in the next year

source: Holmes, Thomas H., and Richard H. Rahe. "The Social Readjustment Rating Scale." *Journal of Psychosomatic Research* 11 (1967): 213–18 (Pergamon Press, Inc.).

table 7.2

NATIONAL LIST OF TOP HASSLES AND UPLIFTS

HASSLES	UPLIFTS
1. Misplacing or losing things	1. Being visited, phoned, or sent a letter
2. Troubling thoughts about your future	2. Visiting, phoning, or writing someone
3. Not getting enough sleep	3. Having fun (socializing, partying, being with friends)
4. Filling out forms	4. Completing a task
5. Money problems	5. Recreation (sports, games, etc.)
6. Social obligations	6. Making a friend
7. Concerns about weight and physical appearance	7. Hugging and/or kissing (relating well with spouse or lover)
8. Too many things to do	8. Getting enough sleep
9. Concerns about meeting high standards (not living up to expectations)	9. Being complimented
10. Being lonely	10. Having someone to listen to you
11. Child care problems	11. Eating out

source: Miles, G. T. "Daily Hassles and Uplifts—Short Form: Item Selection and Cross Validation." Masters Thesis, Pennsylvania State University, University Park, 1986.

toll from stress may not come from a divorce, loss of a job, or other traumatic changes, but from an accumulation of the minor, frequent annoyances we experience daily. Having too many things to do, roommate problems, not enough sleep, parking problems on campus, and money difficulties were the most frequently reported hassles of our students at Ball State University. Examine the top 10 hassles that most of the people interviewed (by researchers) seemed to mention (Table 7.2).

Everyday hassles can be the "straw that broke the camel's back" when they are added to your life at a time when it is already overloaded with stressful events. In fact, the average person is as likely to be "nibbled to death" by everyday hassles as to be overwhelmed by tragedies. The way you handle daily hassles to a large degree depends on your score on the Life Event Scales.[10] When scores are high (i.e., you are overstressed), you are more likely to react to daily hassles with less tolerance and a shorter fuse. For example, after Akiko's mother died of cancer, she had to leave college in her first year and enroll at the local community college in her hometown because she was needed at home to care for her younger brothers. On top of all this, she lost her billfold (with driver's license and credit cards) on the very first day of classes at the new school. Now, the hassles of too many things to do, losing the billfold, caring for the home and her brothers, and keeping up at school were overwhelming. She became ill. As with any stressor, the way you perceive it is critical. What constitutes a hassle or an uplift varies greatly from person to person. Concern about weight may not be a hassle to you but may be a real problem to another for whom physical appearance is a top priority.

The counterpart to daily hassles are **daily uplifts.** These are positive events that make us feel good. Fridays, payday, going shopping, and having a date were the uplifts most often listed by our students at Ball State (see Table 7.2). Research has shown that these little daily uplifts can actually reverse the negative effects of daily hassles. An appropriate balance between hassles and uplifts may be the important ingredient in your overall health and well-being. These daily uplifts may actually protect you from stress-related illnesses.

Everyday hassles won't end with college.

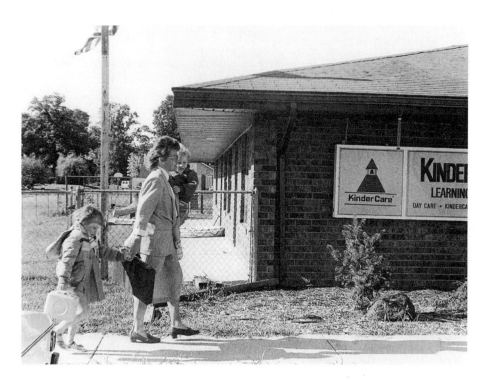

List the events in your everyday life that you find bothersome. How many of them can you eliminate? How many will you simply have to deal with in some manner? List the daily uplifts you find enjoyable. Can you find ways to add to this list?

Type A Behavior and Stress

We all know people who have the "hurry-up-itis" syndrome. They always are rushed, never have enough time, usually need more than eight hours a day to complete a day's work, could not survive without their car phone or laptop computer, and appear to be doing four or five things at one time. The woman who impatiently pushes ahead of you in line at the grocery, the young man who honks the horn of his automobile indicating for you to hurry up, or the friend who constantly looks at his or her watch all exhibit Type A behavior.

The **Type A personality** is described as competitive, ambitious, driven, impatient, workaholic, and always rushed. Type As put big demands on themselves to accomplish more and more in less and less time. They have little time for or interest in hobbies or leisure pursuits and have few intimate friends. The key problem with Type A behavior is stress. Type As put themselves under constant pressure and their bodies react by producing extra amounts of stress hormones.

Type B personality is the opposite—relaxed, casual, unaggressive, and patient. Most Type Bs build time in the day for absorbing activities such as exercise, hobbies, and friendship. They speak more softly, are less obsessed with success, and tend to deal more effectively with stressful situations.

Type A behavior was identified and named in the late 1950s by two cardiologists, Drs. Meyer Freidman and Ray Rosenman.[11] Their research led many to believe that the individual who exhibits Type A behavior is prone to developing coronary heart disease, with increased risk of suffering a heart attack. However, recent research suggests that it may be the personality behaviors of hostility, cynicism, and anger that are the major culprits that increase the risk of heart disease. People exhibiting hostility, cynicism, and anger in response to stress produce greater amounts of hormones that damage the cardiorespiratory system. These traits are also related to atherosclerosis and higher diastolic blood pressure. The problem is that the components of Type A behavior can be harmful because they often lead to the development of hostile, angry behavior. Type Bs exhibiting angry, cynical, and hostile behaviors suffer the same negative effects as Type As.

Do you become enraged when a car in front of you cuts you off? Do you find it intolerable to wait in lines? Do you lash out with gestures, raised voice, and increased heart rate when someone does something that seems incompetent, messy, selfish, or inconsiderate to you? These are examples of angry, hostile behavior. While the debate connecting Type A and illness continues, the evidence is stacking up in favor of a positive connection—even without the hostility, cynicism, and anger. This means that just being a Type A person may have some health risks attached.

The Hot Reactor

Another example of how the combination of angry behavior and stress can be lethal has been discovered by Robert S. Eliot. He has found that 20 percent of apparently healthy individuals are prime candidates for stress-related heart attacks or strokes because of the extreme reactions they demonstrate in response to daily stress. He labeled these people **hot reactors** because, when stressed, they produce astronomical amounts of powerful adrenalinelike chemicals called **catecholamines** that damage the cardiovascular system.[12] Abnormally high blood pressure and dangerous heart muscle lesions are the results of the massive doses of these stress hormones being released into the blood stream. (Systolic readings can raise from 120 to a deadly 300.) Hot reactors are guilty of faulty perception. They perceive nearly every stressor as a life-and-death issue and constantly perceive a loss of control in their daily lives. Daily challenges at work or school (deadlines, friendly competition, dealing with the kids, disagreement with a neighbor) trigger an overblown fight-or-flight reaction. The fight-or-flight reaction is a human response meant to be used only in real life-or-death situations. Squandering doses of these powerful hormones on mundane situations (i.e., missing a green light, standing in a checkout line, and running out of dental floss) is a characteristic of a hot reactor. Hot reactors may be either hard-driving Type As or more placid Type Bs.

Constant stress causes many people to bristle with aggressiveness, hostility, cynicism, and anger. Our increasingly complex world fosters the development of the Type A personality. We reward the student who excels in the classroom, the winning athlete, the "superwoman" (with career and family), the youngest-ever CEO, the secretary who never takes a break, the executives who talk business over lunch, and the college student who is president of a sorority or fraternity, homecoming king or queen, A student, and a member of the tennis team. Our society provides a rich environment for Type A personality development. You should recognize your own behavior pattern. Are you a Type A person or a Type B? Are you hostile and angry or a hot reactor?

Life threatening overreaction to stress is neither innate nor inevitable. People are not born with this trait. They learn it, and they can unlearn it. Reframing is an excellent way to calm hot, angry reactions to stress. Read more about reframing later in this chapter. You can take charge and be in control of your life. Ask yourself, "Is this situation worth dying for?" Stop sweating the small stuff and, remember, it is all small stuff! Assess your reaction to stress by taking the behavior quiz in Table 7.3.

Type A Behavior Modification

Okay, so you are a Type A. What can you do about it? We now know that many Type A behaviors are learned and that even the most severe Type As can learn to modify their behavior and successfully control hot, angry, and hostile reactions to stress in a more healthful way. Try these behavior modification suggestions:

1. Every day find time to be alone. Remind yourself that you are not the general manager of the universe. Everyone can spare 15 minutes or so a day to calm down and reflect on happy memories.
2. Daily practice relaxation techniques, especially meditation.
3. Develop a sense of humor about life. *He or she who laughs lasts.*
4. Laugh more.

table 7.3

QUIZ TO IDENTIFY YOUR TYPE A, ANGRY/HOSTILE, HOT REACTOR BEHAVIOR

Answer yes or no to the following statements:

1. I hate to wait for anyone or anything.
2. I often interrupt others when they are speaking.
3. I am usually rushed. There's never enough time in the day.
4. I feel guilty when I have nothing to do or when I play.
5. I get impatient when others perform tasks that I can do faster.
6. I eat faster than most of my friends.
7. I feel stretched to my limits at the end of the day.
8. I think about other things during conversations.
9. When driving, I get irritated at drivers who cut me off or drive too slowly. I frequently blow my horn and try to pass them.
10. I react with gestures, raised voice, and increased heart rate when someone does something incompetent, messy, inconsiderate, or unfair or after an irritating encounter.
11. I think cashiers will shortchange me if they can.
12. I feel my anger is justified. I feel an urge to punish people—plot to get back at them.
13. I frequently feel irritated when I stand in line or drive.
14. I like to have the last word in an argument.
15. In a checkout express line, if the person in front of me has more items than the limit, I get frustrated.
16. If I see a nonhandicapped person park in a handicapped driver's space, I feel anger inside.
17. When I am angry, I keep things bottled-up inside, pout, and sulk.

Scoring:
Statements 1 through 8 demonstrate Type A behavior. If you said yes to three or more of these statements, you probably fall into the Type A behavior category. Statements 9 through 17 demonstrate angry/hostile/cynical/hot reactor behavior. Even one yes response to any of these statements is too many. Have a friend or loved one who knows you also check the statements for you. Was there a change in any of the responses?

5. Spend more time with friends and make these friendships more intimate.
6. Anticipate stresses and regulate their number and timing when possible.
7. Maintain a flexible schedule. Don't schedule appointments and activities unnecessarily.
8. Learn to say no and to protect your precious time.
9. Delegate more.
10. Talk less, listen more. Listen to others without interrupting.
11. Avoid irritating, competitive people.
12. Allow extra time to do things and to get places.
13. Carry a paperback with you to read while waiting in lines or for appointments.
14. Develop a caring attitude (most people are doing the best they can).
15. Learn to savor food instead of grabbing fast food and eating "on the run."
16. Purposely choose the longest line in which to do your business (at the bank, at the checkout in the grocery store, in a fast-food restaurant, or in a discount department store).
17. Discontinue polyphasic behavior (doing two or more things at once).
18. Practice smiling for a whole day.
19. Build a time each day for exercise or another absorbing activity.
20. Read a good book.
21. Spend an entire afternoon in a museum or art gallery.

Harmful Effects of Stress

All events, emotions, or situations, good or bad, cause you to react and force you to adapt. We are all constantly adapting to new things, things we like and things we don't like. This adaptation to the stresses of life isn't harmful unless you are overloaded with too much in a short period of time—too many life change events and hassles, especially the ones perceived as undesirable or uncontrollable. Stress is part of being alive. In today's society, stress has increased dramatically. Having more stress than one can cope with can lead to dysfunctional behavior (i.e., worry, neurosis, aggressive behavior, depression, domestic violence—even homicide or suicide) or to a psychosomatic disease.

A **psychosomatic disease** (*psycho* refers to the mind; *somatic* refers to the body) is a physical ailment that is mentally induced. These "stress" diseases, as they are frequently called, are not "all in the mind" as some people believe. They are real and can be diagnosed. When stress is prolonged, it can depress the immune system and lower the body's resistance to disease. The mind and the body are an interrelated whole—what affects one ultimately affects the other. **Psychoneuroimmunology** is a specialized branch of medicine that studies the mind/body connection. The stressful consequences of living in modern society—constant job insecurity, inability to make deadlines because of family and school obligations, running a single-parent family, living in poverty—can weaken the immune system and lead to some devastating mind/body diseases. Examples of psychosomatic conditions are hypertension, stroke, coronary heart disease, ulcers, life-threatening gastrointestinal problems, migraine headaches, tension headaches, cancer, allergies, asthma, hay fever, rheumatoid arthritis, and backache. Stress is responsible for two-thirds of all doctor's visits and plays a role in two major killers—heart disease and cancer.[13] How is stress related to cancer? In addition to depressing the immune system, according to some studies, stress increases the incidence of smoking, alcohol consumption, and promiscuous sexual behavior, all of which have been associated with increased risk for developing certain kinds of cancer.

Controlling stress means adapting and changing as circumstances demand. There are a number of common signs of stress (Table 7.4). If you are experiencing five or more of these symptoms, you may be headed toward developing a psychosomatic disease and need to practice the antistress measures in this chapter.

The Stress-Resistant Hardy Person

Have you ever imagined what George Washington or any of our other founding fathers would think about our modern, high-tech, fast-paced world? They might be surprised by computers, fax machines, television with global news, heart transplants, as well as overcrowded calendars, never-ending deadlines, and chronic shortages of time. Certainly, they would agree that we have just cause to feel overwhelmed by our daily schedules and would be glad not to be participating in the 20th century with us. Yet we all know some people who, in spite of it all, seem relatively insulated from the potential negative effects of their hectic pace. Their lives are as full as ours, but they seem to carry on, taking "everything in stride"—often with a sense of enjoyment and fun. Who are these effective copers? Are they born this way or are they bred—learning strategies for coping with stress that protect them from being overwhelmed and feeling stressed-out?

Two psychologists, Dr. R. Flannery of Harvard University Medical School and Dr. S. Kabasa, independently researching these questions discovered that, even when highly stressed, many individuals manage lower incidence of physical illness, lower amounts of anxiety and depression, and increased longevity.[14,15] These stress-resistant individuals were labeled "hardy." The same study found that people lacking "hardiness" were more prone to illness in the face of stress. A hardy soul is a Type A who has been relabeled a **Type C personality** because of the five unique personality traits he or she possesses for adapting to life stress. We call the Type C traits *The Five Cs*:

> *Control:* Control is the opposite of helplessness. The hardy person has a sense of internal control (influence) over life events and their outcomes. They take daily hassles in stride. They think ahead, plan, and make lists of what needs to be

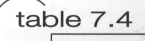

table 7.4

COMMON SIGNS OF STRESS

Check the signs of stress that you have experienced lately.

PHYSICAL

- Headaches
- Asthma attack
- Constipation and/or diarrhea
- Abdominal pains
- Acne flare-up
- Excessive dryness of hair or skin
- Frequent colds, flu, low-grade infections
- Chest pain
- Upset stomach, nausea, or vomiting
- Neck, back, or shoulder pain
- Excess perspiration
- Allergy flare-up, rashes, hives
- Muscle twitches or eye twitches
- Heart pounding, racing, or beating erratically

EMOTIONAL

- Feeling depressed
- Feeling nervous, anxious, fearful
- Feeling burned out
- Feeling that life is out of control
- Feeling that you are being rushed
- Questioning your personal worth
- Feeling very sensitive to criticism
- Often feeling suspicious

BEHAVIORAL

- Disorganization (losing things, making dumb mistakes)
- Trouble getting along with others
- Daydreaming about escaping
- Difficulty making small decisions
- Increased irritability
- Frequent fatigue
- Overeating/overdrinking
- Increased craving (tobacco, sweets, caffeine, drugs)
- Sleep disorders (sleeping too much, sleeping too little)
- Trembling hands
- Focus on unimportant details while not completing more important jobs
- Loss of sex drive
- Restlessness, poor concentration

done. They seek active solutions to problems. Do you feel "in control" of your life? If not, what plan can you implement that will help you gain more control?

➤ *Commitment:* Commitment is the opposite of alienation and is typified by meaningful involvement in one's family, job, and community. The hardy person has a sense of purpose in life and sets short- and long-term goals. Rearing one's children, having friends, participating in community projects, having religious values, reaching career goals, and working to complete "your degree" are examples of personal commitments that help us unstress. List one or two goals to which you have made a commitment.

➤ *Challenge:* The hardy person perceives life change as a potential opportunity and a challenge rather than a threat. Hardy people are highly confident in their ability to do their work. They accept setbacks as a part of life and as an opportunity for growth.

➤ *Choices in lifestyle:* Hardy individuals make lifestyle choices that enhance health and reduce stress. They reduce use of caffeine, nicotine, alcohol, and sugar and incorporate aerobic exercise and relaxation activities into their lives. How much caffeine do you consume every day? Do you practice any of the relaxation techniques found in this chapter? Sydney J. Harris said it best: "The time to relax is when you don't have time for it."

➤ *Connectedness:* Hardy people develop a social network that includes helping and being helped by others. They have developed a sense of "connectedness" to others. They are actively involved with others. Studies show that social interaction is important. It may lower pulse rate and blood pressure, enhance the immune system, and boost the production of endorphins. When you're in a caring relationship with another person, all these health benefits accrue. Do you have one or more close friends to whom you feel "connected" (i.e., sharing troubles, ambitions, and desires) or whom you can count on for emotional support?

Research on the hardy, stress-resistant Type C personality has made it clear that the five interrelated traits of control, commitment, challenge, lifestyle choices (personal health practices), and connectedness (social support) are important factors that buffer us from the ravages of our modern lifestyles and help us to adapt and even flourish in the face of them.[16,17] How many of these hardiness traits do you possess? The *Becoming Stress Resistant and Hardy* exercise in the Activities Section will help you strengthen these traits in your own life. Can you think of two ways you can apply the knowledge of these five traits to your life, bolstering your "hardiness" rating?

Building Skills for Stress Management

Relaxation training is now being recommended, in combination with medication, nutrition, and exercise, not only to reduce stress but to treat chronic pain and illness, such as heart disease, high blood pressure, diabetes, infertility, and even cancer. Relaxation is also being used in easing depression, painful AIDS symptoms, headaches, and back pain. The concept of relaxation as "good medicine," once totally dismissed by scientists, is accepted now, thanks to the work of several pioneers in the mind/body field.

As you have learned, when an individual is stressed, the body responds with an outpouring of hormones to prepare him or her to either fight or to take flight (the stress response). Performance and work decline when you feel stressed out. When relaxed and feeling in control, the mind and body function efficiently and effectively. Dr. Herbert Benson of the Harvard Medical School and founder of the Mind/Body Medical Institute at New England Deaconnes Hospital in Boston, discovered that, with effort and training in the use of meditation, we can learn to quiet down and summon at will the healing changes in body chemistry called the **relaxation response.** Benson found that the relaxation response was the body's built-in defense mechanism against the harmful effects of the inappropriate elicitation of the fight-or-flight response caused by everyday living.[18]

The innate physiological changes produced by the relaxation response, which we can elicit to counteract stress, include the following:

➤ Decreased oxygen consumption and metabolic rate, lessening strain on the body's energy resources
➤ Increased intensity and frequency of alpha brain waves associated with deep relaxation
➤ Reduced blood lactates (substances in the blood associated with anxiety)
➤ Decreased anxiety, fears, and phobias and increased positive mental health (i.e., less anxiety and greater feeling of control)
➤ Significant decreases in blood pressure in hypertensive individuals (which remained lowered throughout the day)
➤ Reduced heart rate and slower respiration
➤ Decreased muscle tension
➤ Increased blood flow to arms and legs
➤ Improved quality of sleep

Dr. Redford Williams, Director of the Behavioral Medical Research Center at Duke University, found that angry, hostile people suffered more heart disease than calm ones.[19] Dr. Williams, like Benson, believes relaxation and other stress-management techniques are critical ways to reduce negative emotions.

Dr. Jon Kabat-Zinn, another stress pioneer, is known for using stress-reduction programs, especially mind/body interactions and mindfulness meditation, to help patients suffering from chronic pain and stress-related disorders at the University of Massachusetts Medical Center. While traditional meditation involves training the mind on a single point of focus, such as a word or phrase, **mindfulness meditation** involves focusing on whatever a person happens to be experiencing at the time—and learning to experience it calmly, whether it is pleasant or unpleasant. Kabat-Zinn describes *mindfulness* as waking up and living in harmony with oneself and the world. He encourages his patients to cultivate some appreciation for the fullness of each moment they are alive. He asserts that it is important to be "in touch" with each moment so that we may live our lives with greater satisfaction, harmony, and wisdom. What he's talking about is conscious attention to behavior. Mindfulness meditation is not an attempt to escape from problems or difficulties. On the contrary, it is a willingness to go nose-to-nose with pain, confusion, and loss. For example, people using mindfulness meditation to cope with chronic pain would not try to distract themselves from the pain but would simply experience the pain without fear or anxiety (emotions that generally make the pain more intense). Like Benson, Kabat-Zinn has found that meditation is a way of slowing down enough so that we can get in touch with who we are, a true mind/body approach to managing the stresses in our lives.[20,21]

You can't change the complexities of life, but you can develop strategies that enable you to cope more effectively. You can learn to relax, to quiet down the mind and body (so you can get "in touch" or "connected to" your inner thoughts, feelings, goals, and values), and successfully manage the stress in your life.

Practice the relaxation techniques in this chapter to find the ones that you feel most comfortable using and that work best for you. For best results, set aside some time every day for relaxation. By following the five simple stress management strategies in this chapter, you will be well on your way to becoming a stress hardy person. Enjoy!

Strategy #1
Exercise

Get physical. Regular exercise is an excellent method for reducing stress, mental and physical tension, anxiety, and aggressive feelings. Exercise allows us to play out the instinctive fight-or-flight response, to use the muscles that are tensed for action, and to reduce the adrenaline being pumped into the bloodstream. A number of studies suggest that exercise reduces the intensity of the stress response, shortens the time it takes to recover from stress, and even helps ward off illness in people who are experiencing stress.[22]

Exercise is a natural way to relax and renew energy. When hassles and problems begin to pile up in the office or at school, change into your workout clothes and take a vigorous run, a swim, or a brisk walk. The effect is amazing. Headaches, tension, anxiety, aggressiveness, and irritability are all diminished. Because research supports the value of exercise in reducing stress, many physicians now recommend exercise to their patients instead of medications such as tranquilizers. Vigorous exercise increases the release of endorphins, brain chemicals that may alleviate harmful effects of stressors by producing a more relaxed state.[23] Besides better stress management, other psychological benefits of exercise, documented by research, are increased self-esteem, increased alertness, and decreased depression and anxiety.[24] Although aerobic vigorous exercise is best, even a relaxing walk can do wonders to relieve tension. Play tennis or racquetball, golf, dance, bowl, swim, rake leaves, garden, bike, or do whatever. Enjoy physical activity. It is the healthiest thing you can do for yourself, and it's inexpensive.

Strategy #2 Relaxation Techniques

2.1 Meditation

Meditation is a mental exercise that affects body processes, producing physical benefits. The purpose of meditation is to gain control over your attention—to internally quiet down, allowing *you* to choose what to focus upon and to block out distracting thoughts.

Meditation originated in the Eastern cultures of India and Tibet and was exported to the Western world by the Maharishi Mahesh Yogi. The Maharishi popularized the **transcendental meditation (TM)** method. In recent years, TM, as well as other forms of meditation, have been subjected to a battery of scientific studies. Especially revealing and conclusive were the findings conducted at the Harvard School of Medicine by Dr. Herbert Benson and at the School of Medicine, University of California, San Francisco, by Dr. Dean Ornish.[25,26] They found that meditation was a simple yet powerful, easy-to-learn, nonchemical stress reducer that produced the relaxation response. They call meditation the "universal stress antidote" and assert that it is totally compatible with modern medicine. Other experts agree that meditation is now mainstream. They feel that the proficient meditator develops a sense of wholeness and is able to face stress, pain, and illness with equanimity and even triumph over his or her problems.[27] Meditation is merely a discipline for training the mind to focus, for developing greater calm, relief, and understanding. This, in turn, leads to a greater sense of control and happiness.

To bring the relaxation response benefits into your everyday life, learn to meditate. Meditation, now recognized as one of the most powerful antidotes for stress, should be practiced for 20 minutes, twice a day. Soon you will be enjoying the relaxing periods of stillness and quietness of the mind that meditation produces. (Use the Activities Section, page 393, for additional practice.) Meditation involves the following four essential elements:

1. *A quiet, comfortable environment.* A place where you will not be disturbed is essential. However, once you become experienced, you will be able to meditate almost anywhere.
2. *A comfortable position.* A position that will allow you to remain in the same position for approximately 20 minutes is necessary to avoid any undue muscular tension. Lying down or sitting in an overstuffed chair may cause you to break your focus and fall asleep.
3. *A mantra, a mental device, or the breath on which to focus your attention.* For starters, you can keep it simple by focusing on your breathing, feeling it as it moves in and out. Use your breath as an anchor to bring you back when your attention is disrupted. A mantra is a silently repeated word, phrase, sound or thought such as *one, love, peace* or *omh.* The mantra should be easy to pronounce and short enough to repeat silently as you exhale. A mental device is an unchanging object such as an

object in the room where you meditate. Gaze at the object fixedly. Select any one of the three methods to help you maintain your focus, to shut out outside stimuli, and to keep you calm. The method may vary but the relaxation benefits do not.

4. *A calm, relaxed attitude.* Relax. Try not to try. Let it happen. The harder you try, the more tense you get. Disregard outside noise thoughts. When distracting thoughts and noise intrude—it is normal that they will occasionally—calmly return focus to the slow, steady repetition of the mantra or the mental device.

2.2 Autogenic Training and Imagery

Autogenic means "self-generating" or "self-induced." The **autogenic training and imagery** technique uses mental concentration exercises to bring about sensations of warmth and heaviness in the limbs and torso and then uses relaxing images to expand the relaxed state. Both meditation and autogenic training lead to the relaxation response. Many who find meditation too easy and boring enjoy autogenic training because of the switches of focus from one part of the body to another and the use of imagery. Autogenic training has been found to be very successful in the treatment of chronic and lower back pain. Otherwise, the physiological and psychological benefits are similar to meditation.

Autogenic training should be done with eyes closed while you are either lying down or in a seated position. Whatever position you choose, be sure that you are relaxed and comfortable. Eliminate muscle tension in any part of the body by changing position slightly. Practice 10 to 30 minutes, one or two times a day, to become skillful at this technique.

The six steps to autogenic training follow:

1. Concentrate on heaviness of arms and legs, beginning with dominant side.
2. Concentrate on warmth of arms and legs, beginning with dominant side.
3. Concentrate on warmth and heaviness of heart and chest.
4. Concentrate on breathing rhythm.
5. Concentrate on warmth of abdominal area.
6. Concentrate on coolness of forehead.

After the six stages of autogenic training have been mastered, transfer body relaxation to mind relaxation by using images of relaxing scenes, such as the following:

➤ Sinking into a mattress
➤ A sack of sugar melting away in the rain
➤ Floating out to sea
➤ A feather floating in the sky
➤ A soaring bird
➤ Clouds drifting by
➤ Ocean surf splashing on the sand
➤ A warm, relaxing fire burning in the fireplace
➤ A sailboat drifting on a calm lake

You should use images you find relaxing. They may be quite different than those of your friends.

2.3 Jacobson's Progressive Relaxation

Edmund Jacobson, a physician, designed for his tense patients a series of exercises that emphasize the relaxation of voluntary skeletal muscles—that is, all the muscles over which you have control. He taught his patients to contract a muscle group and then relax it, progressing from one muscle group to another until the total body was relaxed. The idea was to learn to recognize tenseness and be able to consciously relax whenever it was needed. This method of relaxation, named after its developer, does not produce the relaxation response. However, if practiced regularly, it is very beneficial in helping people relax. It has been used in the treatment of insomnia and psychological conditions such as poor self-concept, depression, and anxiety.

There are many routines of contract-relax exercises for progressive relaxation. Try the progressive relaxation routine in this chapter (Table 7.5) that begins at the head and ends at the feet or develop your own routine. With practice, you will be able to eliminate the contraction phase and focus totally on relaxation.

table 7.5

PROGRESSIVE RELAXATION ROUTINE

1. Lie on your back on the floor in a quiet place with the lights dimmed. Remove shoes. Let feet relax and rotate outward. Arms should be beside body, palms turned upward.
2. Proceed slowly over the body, tensing a muscle group and then relaxing it. Stop if cramping or pain develops.
3. Face: Squint eyes, wrinkle nose, make a face, and then relax. Open mouth very wide, stick out tongue. Close mouth and clench teeth. Now relax.
4. Neck: Nod head downward to touch chin to chest. Relax.
5. Head: Try to touch right ear to right shoulder and left ear to left shoulder. Relax and center head over torso.
6. Shoulders: Shrug shoulders up toward ears: pull shoulders down from ears; press hard against floor. One at a time. Relax.
7. Hands and arms: Squeeze fingers together, making a fist. Relax. Raise right arm, bending at elbow, and "make a muscle" with biceps. Relax. Repeat with left arm. Relax. With arms on floor, stiffen both arms, making a fist. Relax.
8. Back: Try to squeeze shoulder blades together. Relax. Press lower back area into floor. Relax.
9. Abdomen: Suck in abdominal muscles. Relax.
10. Buttocks: Contract buttock muscles. Relax.
11. Thighs: Contract thigh muscles, one at a time and then both at the same time. Relax.
12. Calves: Flex toes back toward head and then extend or point toes away from head, using right leg and then left leg. Relax.
13. Toes: Curl toes under, first right foot and then left foot. Relax.
14. Be aware of relaxed state of body.

table 7.6

ABDOMINAL BREATHING

1. Inhale and exhale fully through mouth.
2. Inhale very slowly and push out your abdomen (stomach) as though it was a balloon inflating. Move your chest as little as possible.
3. Exhale *slowly* and allow stomach to flatten.
4. Repeat the pattern. On each "in" breath, let belly inflate, and on each "out" breath, let it flatten.
5. Each "out" breath is an opportunity to rid body of tension.

2.4 Abdominal Breathing

Most of us breathe in short shallow breaths, expanding only the chest, especially when we're under stress. This is called *thoracic breathing* and is really not the proper way to breathe. It does not allow the lungs to fill and empty completely, and it can increase muscle tension.

During stressful situations, it is even more important to breathe from the abdomen. This method allows more oxygen to enter the body and relaxes the muscles. You can practice the simple steps described in this chapter almost at anytime or in any place, even on the telephone, in class, or at a meeting. Practice at least once a day so that it becomes natural when you use it in stressful or fatiguing situations. This simple procedure has produced excellent results for many (Table 7.6).

Yoga is a relaxing form of exercise.

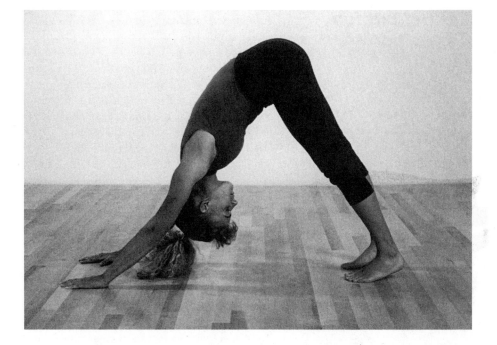

2.5 Hatha Yoga

The most familiar form of yoga is **Hatha yoga,** or physical yoga. It is a discipline that involves the use of various exercises or postures (called *asanas*) in combination with proper breathing rhythm to remove tension and inflexibility in the body. It also improves muscular strength, muscular endurance, and body alignment. Hatha yoga should not be associated with religious or spiritual groups. The physiological and psychological benefits of Hatha yoga have been thoroughly researched, confirming it to be an excellent form of exercise and an aid to improving the health and well-being of those who practice it.

2.6 Massage

When you are bombarded with too much stress, the muscles in the neck, shoulders, and back can become tight and stiff to the point of pain. Without relaxation, these muscles can become chronically tight and can cause much distress. One of the most enjoyable ways to relieve this condition is to have a massage.

These are two popular forms of massage:

1. *Swedish massage*, the most familiar form, involves kneading and rubbing the muscles to increase relaxation and circulation.
2. *Shiatsu*, originating in Japan and China, is a technique that is actually a form of acupressure. Pressure is applied with the thumbs or fingers along acupuncture meridians. The idea is to restore balance so that the "chi" energy (an energy believed to be linked to the life force) flows freely and in a balanced manner.

Massage given by a spouse or friend can be just as pleasant. You can even massage yourself when tight neck and shoulder muscles are tense. Put on your favorite music and enjoy.

2.7 Biofeedback Training

Biofeedback training is a technique in which machines measure certain physiological processes of the body. The machines then convert this information to an understandable form and feed it back to the individual. This process allows a person access to biological information not usually available to one's consciousness. Proponents of biofeedback believe that by mentally recognizing involuntary biological responses such as heart rates, you can control them. With feedback training, stressors themselves are not removed, but the response to them is controlled. Control of physiological arousal is an important step in stress management. A major drawback of biofeedback is the cost and availability of the machines and the lack of trained professionals to operate them.

2.8 Relaxation (Floatation) Tanks

A floatation tank is one of the newest stress-management devices. It is merely an oversized bathtub (or shell) (Fig. 7.3) filled with body-temperature water and placed in a small room. The shell is lightproof and sound insulated. The idea is to reduce sensory stimuli, thereby providing complete relaxation. Epsom salts are dissolved in the water to help you float. The warm water, the quiet, and the darkness combine to create a pleasant sensation of floating in space. You just lie there, body and water becoming one, and relax. The distractions of the everyday world are left behind. Research supports the use of floatation tanks in the management of stress. They are now found in many health clubs in larger cities in the United States.

Strategy #3 Lifestyle Change

3.1 The Impact of Diet

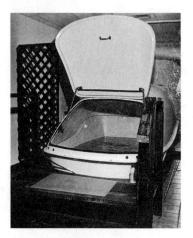

FIGURE 7.3 ➤
Floatation tank.

3.2 Time Management

Proper diet is an important part of your stress-management program and an area in which *you* can definitely exert *control*. A nutritious diet will help you look and feel good, plus it will strengthen your immune system. Many feel that poor diet can increase your susceptibility to stress by causing fatigue and irritability. This is especially true for individuals who are eating too many meals away from home, missing meals, or eating on the run. Unfortunately, there are no miracle foods to boost energy and reduce stress. The best advice for surviving the stress of modern life is to eat three nutritious meals a day and follow these guidelines to help keep you from feeling irritable and uptight:

1. Reduce (below 250 milligrams per day) or eliminate the caffeine in your diet. Caffeine is a stimulant and magnifies the effects of stress (see *caffeine* in Chapter 10). Also, avoid or minimize the use of stimulating drugs (i.e., diet pills and oral decongestants) that may cause added agitation.
2. Limit foods containing sugar, especially if you have been skipping meals. It robs the body of B-complex vitamins and may induce anxiety and failure to cope with stressful situations.
3. Limit your intake of sodium because excessive fluid buildup leads to discomfort and increased stress. Too much sodium (salt) can also increase blood pressure due to the fluid buildup.
4. Limit alcoholic beverage consumption. Alcohol makes people feel relaxed and less stressed while drinking it, but it leaves them feeling more tired the next day.

Insufficient time appears to be the plague of the 20th century. How well you manage your time plays a large role in how much pressure you feel. You should manage your time as if your life depended on it, because it does. The goal of time management should not be the elimination of leisure time (relaxation, etc.); rather, it should be the elimination of life's real time wasters. Use the Time Management Activity on page 401 to practice this important stress-management lifestyle strategy. Time management experts suggest these time-saving tips:

1. Analyze how you spend time and then evaluate that use of time. Keep a diary. You may find you are wasting too much time.
2. Learn to set short- and long-range goals. Write them down. This helps you plan for today and for the future.
3. Learn how to set priorities. Not everything you do is number one on your list of importance. With goals in mind, you will know how to prioritize your activities. Items on the "Do" list must get done; items on the "Maybe" list are those you would like to take care of today, if possible; and those on the "If Possible" list are those you would like to do if all the activities of the first and second lists are completed.
4. Use a planner calendar to schedule your priorities into your day, week, and year. This will help you organize and simplify your life by keeping track of important dates, appointments, and meetings. A planner calendar is very productive. By systematically planning your day, you can more clearly see what needs to be done. Minor tasks need no longer overshadow major ones. A few minutes of planning can control hours of chaos. A planned day allows you to schedule

160

College students have many demands on their time and must plan wisely.

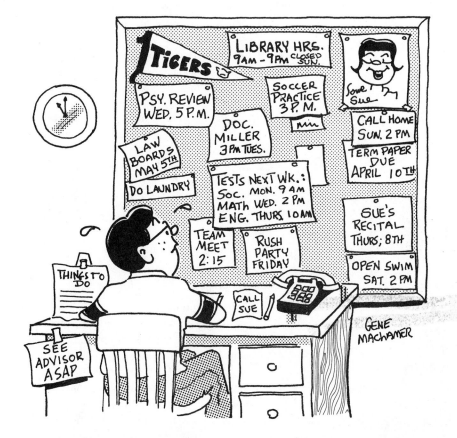

stress-reducing breaks and rest periods and to have time for family, friends, personal development, and hobbies. Gaining control over your life reduces stress.

5. Take 5 to 10 minutes at the end of the day to evaluate how well you managed your time. How many of your goals did you check off today? Good time managers use this technique daily to assess time wasted, reprioritize goals (even dumping some), and maintain progress for achieving all their short- and long-range goals.

6. Adopt the following time-saving strategies:
   - Learn how to stop being inefficient. This is an art that anyone can learn. Go through mail one time only. Start a task with the intention of completing it now. Don't look it over and put it aside for later. You have wasted time looking it over the first time.
   - Know your limits. Don't allow too many demands to be made "on your time." You can say, "No!" Learn to delegate certain activities to others when possible.
   - Practice quick relaxation tricks frequently throughout the day. Get up and go for a drink of water. Give yourself a massage to the neck, shoulders, and forehead. This energizes you to complete tasks more efficiently.

3.3 Alcohol, Drugs, and Cigarettes

Alcohol is a powerful depressant drug that temporarily masks but doesn't solve your problems. In fact, it can increase stress by creating new problems—hangovers, arrests, traffic violations, fights, and accidents. Taking illegal drugs can only increase your stress. Why risk ruining your physical and mental health and the stress of being arrested? Do not smoke cigarettes or use other tobacco products (snuff, chewing tobacco). Nicotine is a stimulant that increases stress.

3.4 Get Plenty of Restful Sleep

Take care of yourself. Most people need seven to eight hours of restful sleep each night. Getting enough sleep can make you more alert, less irritable, and better able to cope with stressful situations. Don't lose sleep over things that you can't control.

3.5 Develop Satisfying Relationships

Having close friends with whom to share the joys and sorrows of living is a huge asset in protecting your health. It has been shown that unhappiness, depression, and feelings of isolation can be caused by lack of close emotional bonds with friends, a spouse, or family members. Intimate relationships and social support can become a powerful life-support system when internal resources have fallen short. Social support can both directly provide reinforcement for healthy behaviors and indirectly buffer disappointments that would otherwise lead to excessive stress.[28] Friends are not just nice, they are a necessity. You have to *be a friend to have a friend*. Make the effort. It's good health and happiness insurance.

3.6 Learn When to Seek the Help and Support of Others

There will be stressful situations you will not be able to deal with alone. Don't be embarrassed to seek professional help. Developing a variety of support groups such as family, friends, coaches, counselors, or physicians can be very helpful. Talking to someone gives a different perspective on worries and concerns.

3.7 Balance Work and Play

Plan for regular recreation (or a time for yourself) and make that time inviolate. It is your special time. Let nothing else interfere. This can include learning to do nothing (loafing) at times and feeling okay about it.

Strategy #4 Reframing

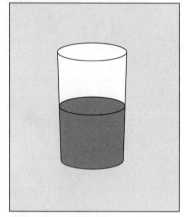

Reframing: Is the glass half empty or half full?

Reframing means consciously reinterpreting a situation in a more positive light. It is a way of looking at life in a positive manner. This makes you better able to deal with problems when they come. Is the glass half empty or half full? Viewing yourself as a sick person because you have asthma is very different, for example, than perceiving yourself as a healthy person who also happens to have asthma. In the case of the driver who cuts you off in traffic, you might tell yourself, "Maybe she had some emergency." This is an excellent way to diffuse anger and negativism. See if you can learn to "reframe" life's stumbling blocks into challenges. Look at the bright side of each situation. Learn to be an optimist. Good things happen to people who expect them. Remember, you are in control of you. Positive emotions and laughter play an important role in keeping well and fit. Optimists have higher hardiness scores, whereas pessimists are more likely to resort to anger and hostility. Laughing is like "internal jogging"—it causes endorphins (pain-relieving chemicals) to be released in the brain. Laughter is like a tranquilizer with no negative side effects. Scientific evidence is beginning to support the biblical axiom that "a merry heart doeth good like a medicine."

Strategy #5 Create a Memory Bank

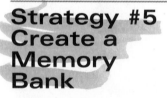

Appreciate and take advantage of opportunities to savor a special experience each day. Do this every day. Store these in your memory bank. When you look back over your life, what special memories do you fondly recall: Roasting marshmallows over a campfire, watching the sunset, smelling a rose, the glow after a satisfying workout, a hug that said "I care"? What can you do today to increase your store of pleasant memories?

SUMMARY

Stress is unavoidable. Optimal levels of stress improve health and performance, but excess levels, especially when chronic and perceived as negative, can be hazardous to your health. Major life events—death of a spouse, marriage, and divorce, for example—are significant stressors. Other more frequent stressors are daily hassles (i.e., missed sleep, rush-hour traffic, losing things). We learn to cope with major life events and daily hassles in a variety of ways. Some are healthy; some are not. Healthy stress-management strategies include exercise, relaxation techniques, lifestyle changes, reframing, and creating a memory bank. Hassles can be countered with the giving and receiving of daily uplifts (i.e., compliments, hugs, and getting enough sleep).

Three stress-coping behavior types—Types A, B, and C—have been identified. Type As are described as rushed, competitive, and impatient. These behaviors often lead to angry, hostile, and cynical reactions when the individual is stressed, which are, in turn, the lethal risk factors for coronary heart disease. Type Bs are more relaxed than Type As but if they demonstrate anger and hostility, they also will develop negative health consequences. Hot reactors perceive every stressor as a life-or-death situation and may be either Type A or Type B. Type Cs are often referred to as "hardy." Type Cs possess The Five Cs: They accept challenges, feel they are in control of their lives, have a strong commitment or purpose in life, make healthy lifestyle choices, and have a strong sense of connectedness to others.

Your wellness is dependent on how well you balance the stress in your life, how well you can modify your angry and hostile behavior, and how successfully you take charge of your life. As one wise person said, "If you can't fight and you can't flee, flow."

REFERENCES

1. Selye, Hans. *Stress Without Distress.* New York: J. B. Lippincott, 1984.
2. Girdano, D. A., G. S. Everly, and Dorothy Dusek. *Controlling Stress and Tension: A Holistic Approach,* 3d ed. Englewood Cliffs, N.J.: Prentice-Hall, 1990.
3. Girdano, D. A., et al. *Controlling Stress and Tension: A Holistic Approach.*
4. Selye, Hans. *The Stress of Life.* New York: McGraw-Hill, 1956.
5. Ornish, Dean. *Dr. Dean Ornish's Program for Reversing Heart Disease.* New York: Random House, 1990.
6. Ornish, Dean. *Dr. Dean Ornish's Program for Reversing Heart Disease.*
7. Lazarus, R. *Psychological Stress and the Coping Process.* New York: McGraw-Hill, 1966.
8. Holmes, T. H., and R. H. Rahe. "The Social Readjustment Rating Scale." *Journal of Psychosomatic Research,* 11 (November 1967): 213–18.
9. Delongis, A., et al. "Relationship of Daily Hassles, Uplifts and Major Life Events to Health Status." *Health Psychology,* 1 (January 1982): 210–14.
10. Kanner, Allen, James Coyne, Catherine Schafer, and Richard Lazarus. "Comparison of Two Modes of Stress Measurement: Daily Hassles and Uplifts Versus Major Life Events." *Journal of Behavior Medicine* 4 (January 1981): 197–201.
11. Friedman, M., and R. H. Rosenman. *Type A Behavior and Your Heart.* New York: Knopf, 1994.
12. Eliot, Robert S., M.D. *From Stress to Strength.* New York: Bantam Books, 1994.
13. Sweeting, Roger L. *A Values Approach to Health Behavior.* Champaign, Ill.: Human Kinetics Books, 1990.
14. Flannery, R., Jr. "Towards Stress Resistant Persons: A Stress Management Approach to the Treatment of Anxiety." *American Journal of Preventive Medicine* 3 (January 1987): 157–60.
15. Kobasa, S. C. "The Hardy Personality: Toward a Social Psychology of Stress and Health." *Social Psychology of Health and Illness,* Sanders, R. S., and Suls, J. (Eds.) Hillsdale, N.J.: Erlbaum, 1982.
16. Flannery, R., Jr. "Towards Stress Resistant Persons: A Stress/Management Approach to the Treatment of Anxiety."
17. Kobasa, S. C. "The Hardy Personality: Toward a Social Psychology of Stress and Health."
18. Benson, Herbert. *The Relaxation Response.* New York: Avon Books, 1976.
19. Williams, Redford. *Anger Kills.* New York: Times Books, 1993.
20. Kabat-Zinn, Jon. *Full Catastrophe Living: Using the Wisdom of Your Body and Mind to Face Stress, Pain and Illness.* New York: Dell Publishers, 1991.
21. Kabat-Zinn, Jon. *Wherever You Go You Are There.* New York: Hyperion Publishers, 1994.
22. "Does Stress Kill?" *Consumer Reports on Health* 7, no. 7 (July 1995): 4.
23. "Does Stress Kill?"
24. Shephard, Roy J. "Physical Activity, Fitness, and Health: The Current Concensus" (American Academy of Kinesiology and Physical Education Papers). *Quest* 47, no. 3 (August, 1995): 288–303.
25. Benson, Herbert, M.D., and Eileen M. Stuart, R.N., M.S., et al. *The Wellness Book.* Boston: Mind and Body Medical Institute, Carol Publishing Group, A Birch Lane Press Book, 1992.
26. Ornish, Dean, M.D. "Can Lifestyle Changes Reverse Coronary Heart Disease?" *Lancet* 336 (July 1990): 129–33.
27. Kabat-Zinn, Jon. *Wherever You Go You Are There.*
28. Moyers, Bill D. *Healing and the Mind.* New York: Doubleday, 1993.

SUGGESTED READINGS

Birkel, Dee Ann. *Hatha Yoga: Developing the Body, Mind and Inner Self.* Dubuque, Iowa: Eddie Bowers Publishing, Inc., 1996.

Cohen, Sheldon, et al. *Measuring Stress: A Guide for Health and Social Scientists.* New York: Oxford University Press, 1995.

Cousins, Norman. "Anatomy of an Illness." *New England Journal of Medicine* 295, no. 26 (December 23, 1976): 1,458–63.

Cousins, Norman. *The Healing Heart.* New York: W. W. Norton and Company, 1983.

Davis, Martha, et al. *The Relaxation and Stress Reduction Workbook,* 3d ed. Oakland, Calif.: Harbinger Publications, Inc., 1994.

Delongis, A., S. Folkman, and R. Lazarus. "The Impact of Daily Stress on Health and Mood: Psychological and Social Resources as Mediators." *Journal of Personality and Social Psychology* 54 (1988): 486–95.

Delongis, A., et al. "Relationship of Daily Hassles, Uplifts, and Major Life Events to Health Status." *Health Psychology* 1 (1982): 119–36.

Donatelle, Rebecca, and Michele Hawkins. "Stress Management, Employee Stress Claims: Increasing Implications for Health Promotion." *American Journal of Health Promotion* 3, no. 3 (winter 1989): 19–25.

Eckenrode, John, and Susan Gore, eds. *Stress Between Work and Family*. New York: Plenum Press, 1990.

Garfeinkel, Perry. "Meditation Goes Mainstream." *Yoga Journal* (March/April 1995): 62–68.

Ginter, Gary, John West, and John Zarski. "Learned Resourcefulness and Situation-Specific Coping with Stress." *The Journal of Psychology* 123, no. 3 (May 1989): 295–304.

Girdano, Daniel, George Every, and Dorothy Dusek. *Controlling Stress and Tension: A Holistic Approach*. 3d ed. Englewood Cliffs, N.J.: Prentice-Hall, 1990.

Greenberg, Jerrold. *Comprehensive Stress Management*. Dubuque, Iowa: Brown & Benchmark Publishers, 1992.

Greenberg, Jerrold. *Your Personal Profile and Activity Workbook*. Dubuque, Iowa: Brown & Benchmark Publishers, 1992.

Jacobson, Edmund. *Progressive Relaxation*, 2d ed. Chicago, Ill.: Chicago Press, 1938.

Jones, Graham, Lew Hardy, eds. *Stress and Performance in Sport*. New York: John Wiley & Sons, 1990.

Kanner, A. D., J. C. Coyne, C. Schaefer, and R. S. Lazarus. "Comparison of Two Models of Stress Measurement: Daily Hassles and Uplifts Versus Major Life Events." *Journal of Behavioral Medicine* 4 (1981): 1–39.

Lazarus, Richard, and Susan Folkman. *Stress, Appraisal and Coping*. New York: Springer Publishing Company, Inc., 1984.

Matheny, Kenneth. *Stress and Strategies for Lifestyle Management*. Atlanta: Georgia State University Press, 1992.

Moyers, Bill D. *Healing and the Mind*, New York: Doubleday, 1993.

Pennebaker, James. *Opening Up: The Healing Power of Confiding in Others*. New York: William Morrow and Co., 1990.

Powell, Trevor. *Anxiety and Stress Management*. New York: Routledge, 1990.

Quick, James, ed. *Stress and Well-Being at Work: Assessments and Interventions for Occupational Mental Health*. American Psychological Association, 1992.

Selye, Hans. *The Stress of Life*. New York: McGraw-Hill, 1956.

Smith, Jonathon. *Cognitive-Behavioral Relaxation Training*. New York: Springer Publishing Co., 1990.

Thoren, P. J., J. Florias, P. Hoffman, and D. Seals. "Endorphins and Exercise: Physiological Mechanisms and Clinical Implications." *Medicine and Science in Sports and Exercise* 22 (1990): 991–94.

Tubesing, Donald. *Kicking Your Stress Habits*. Duluth, Minn.: Whole Person Associates, 1989.

Wagner, B., B. Compas, and D. Howell. "Daily and Major Life Events: A Test of an Integrative Model of Psychosocial Stress." *American Journal of Community Psychology* 16 (1988): 189–205.

Williams, Redford. *Anger Kills*. New York: Random House, 1993.

Williams, Redford. *The Trusting Heart, Great News About Type A Behavior*. New York: Random House, 1989.

RESOURCES

The American Association for Therapeutic Humor, 1163 Shermer Road, Northbrook, IL 60062, (708) 291-0211. Can supply bibliographies on various aspects of humor as therapy and newsletter, *Laugh It Up*.

The Humor Project, 110 Spring Street, Saratoga Springs, New York, NY 12866, (518) 587-8770. Supplies workshops, courses, free information packet on positive power of humor, and magazine, *Laughing Matter*.

Stress Reduction Clinic, University of Massachusetts Medical Center, Worcester, MA 01655, (508) 856-1656.

Mind/Body Medicine Clinic, 2440 E. 5th St., Tyler, TX 75701, (903) 592-2202.

Stress Management Clinic, Rehabilitation Institute of Pittsburgh, 6301 Nortumberland St., Pittsburgh, PA 15217, (412) 521-9000.

Department of Psychology, Toronto Hospital, 200 Elizabeth St., Toronto, Ont. M5G2C4, Canada, (416) 340-3950.

chapter 8

Special Exercise Considerations

➤ O b j e c t i v e s

After reading this chapter, you will be able to:

1. Identify the physiological bases for differences in men's and women's exercise performance levels.

2. List the similarities in men's and women's responses to exercise.

3. Define *amenorrhea, oligomenorrhea, Kegel exercise,* and *stress incontinence.*

4. Identify correct recommendations for exercise during pregnancy.

5. Identify recommendations for safe exercise in hot and cold weather.

6. Identify the best replacement fluids to prevent dehydration during exercise in hot weather.

7. Identify the safe exercises from a list of safe and contraindicated exercises.

8. Recognize the effect of aging on exercise performance.

9. Identify the effects of a regular program of exercise on the aging process.

➤ T e r m s

- Amenorrhea
- Contraindicated exercises
- Dysmenorrhea
- Endorphins
- Estrogen
- Female athlete triad
- Hemoglobin
- Hyperthermia
- Hypothermia
- Kegel exercises
- Menarche
- Oligomenorrhea
- Stress incontinence

Don't wait for your ship to come in. Row out to meet it.

H. Jackson Brown Jr., ed. *Dad, a Father's Book of Wisdom*

his chapter brings together several different concerns related to exercise participation. Six major areas are addressed: females and exercise, males and exercise, environmental considerations, fluid replacement, contraindicated exercises, and aging.

Similarities and Differences in Men's and Women's Exercise Performance

While performance levels may differ, both men and women respond to exercise in a similar manner. Although women have approximately 20 percent lower maximal oxygen uptake than men (due to smaller heart size), with exercise they show similar rates of improvement. Performance levels differ for several reasons. Due to hormonal changes during puberty, a woman adds fat because of estrogen, while a man's muscle mass doubles because of testosterone. The average male has 10 percent to 15 percent body fat and 40 percent muscle tissue, while the average female has 20 percent to 25 percent body fat and 23 percent lean tissue.[1] Therefore, women have half as much muscle tissue to move their weight and more inactive fat weight to carry. In addition, men's greater muscle mass gives them 30 percent to 40 percent greater strength. Women commonly have a smaller heart, a smaller thoracic cage, and lower blood volume than men, all of which may limit performance.[2]

Women have fewer red blood cells than men and about 10 percent to 15 percent less **hemoglobin** (the oxygen-carrying component of red blood cells), so their blood has less oxygen-carrying capacity, which may limit endurance. Even though women are at a disadvantage in terms of physical performance, they benefit equally from aerobic exercise in terms of fitness improvement.[3] Training effect benefits, such as loss of fat from deposit areas, increased bone density, and decreased exercise heart rates, are similar for men and women. When differences in body size are taken into account, fitness gains for men and women are *essentially* the same.

Some women fear that exercise will make them develop large or bulky muscles or a masculine appearance. This is not likely unless a woman is using anabolic steroids and spending many hours in extremely strenuous weight training. Potential for muscular development is genetically determined by levels of the sex hormone testosterone, and women generally have only one-tenth as much of this hormone as men. While women, like men, vary in their potential for muscular size development, what most women want from exercise is exactly what they will gain: decreased fat, increased lean body tissue, and firmer, toned muscles.

Females and Exercise

Once, the sight of a female training on the road or competing in a race was sufficiently unusual that people would stop and stare. As late as 1965, women were threatened with banishment from international competition if they ran races longer than 1.5 miles, and it was 1984 before the first women's Olympic marathon took place. As the interest in fitness as a lifestyle has grown, so has the number of women participants in aerobic activities and athletics. Now that large numbers of females have adopted a physically active lifestyle, research has provided us with new information concerning topics of special interest to women.

Menstruation

Is it safe to exercise during menstruation? Yes. Menstruation is just one small part of the ongoing female reproductive cycle. In the past, women sometimes used this as an excuse to avoid exercise, but now women are encouraged to lead a normal routine during

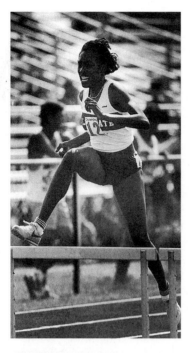

More women are discovering the joys of physical activity.

all parts of the reproductive cycle. Menstrual cycle hormones affect heart rate, ventilation rate, basal body temperature, and blood hematocrit, the red cell portion of the total blood volume.[4] How women experience menstruation varies greatly. Some feel no different than usual; some may experience abdominal and leg cramps, backache, or mood swings, particularly during the first two days of the menstrual flow.

Dysmenorrhea, or painful menstruation, is probably neither caused nor cured by exercise. However, there is some evidence that enhanced fitness generally leads to a reduction in menstrual complaints, although this is still being researched. Some studies indicate that exercise decreases mood swings and relieves depression, anxiety, and irritability.[5] Excess body water lost through perspiration can reduce weight gain due to water retention, relieving premenstrual bloating and edema.[6] While there are no specific exercises that cure severe cramps, participation in a program of regular exercise has been shown to decrease the frequency of minor menstrual cramps. This is perhaps due to increased abdominal tone, increased circulation to the uterus, or increased levels of pain-relieving **endorphins.**[7]

Menstruation should be treated as a normal physiological function, not an illness. As long as she is comfortable, a woman should continue her regular exercise program. For women who want to look and feel their best, exercise is beneficial at any time of the month.

Recent studies indicate that young girls who exercise vigorously may experience a delay in **menarche,** the start of their menstrual cycle, decreasing their risk of cancer later in life.[8] While the average American girl experiences menarche between 11 and 12 years of age, those who train vigorously experience their first menstrual cycle at an average age of 15½, the same as the average age for menarche 100 years ago.[9] This delay may be natural and even desirable, because it reduces the body's lifetime exposure to **estrogen,** a female sex hormone. The more menstrual cycles a woman has over her lifetime, the longer her exposure to estrogen and the greater her risk of cancer of the breast and reproductive organs. In addition, women who exercise tend to be leaner, thus producing less potent estrogen. In one study, women who had been athletic in college and high school as compared to sedentary women had half the incidence of breast and reproductive cancer in later life.[10] The role of exercise in reducing cancer risk is controversial and still under study.

Menstrual abnormalities, such as **oligomenorrhea** (infrequent or irregular menses) and **amenorrhea** (absent menses), occurs in about 3 percent to 5 percent in the general population of women and in up to 10 percent to 25 percent of women athletes.[11] In athletes, the prevalence appears high in sports that require greater intensity, frequency, and duration of training (e.g., distance running and swimming) or sports that emphasize low body weight or involve competition by weight class (e.g., dance, gymnastics, boxing, wrestling). Numerous factors, both physiologic and psychologic, including change in diet or inadequate diet and physical and emotional stress, may affect menstruation abnormally (for example, stressors such as heavy athletic training and competition acting synergistically with other stressors in life). Weight loss and rate of weight loss (with extremely low body fat) have also been identified as probable causes of menstrual abnormalities. Some female athletes who are underweight and nonmenstruating are being diagnosed as victims of the **female athlete triad:** eating disorder, amenorrhea, and osteoporosis.

Exercise-induced oligomenorrhea and amenorrhea are rare in women doing moderate amounts of exercise as part of a fitness program. They are more frequent among those whose menstrual cycles started late, past age 15, or who had a history of irregularity before starting exercise programs. Although no specific body fat percentage has been associated with the development of exercise-induced amenorrhea, the evidence suggests that decreased fat levels may lead to a decreased production of one form of estrogen. Thus, as fat percentages decrease, estrogen levels decline and the evidence of amenorrhea increases. Some scientists have suggested that the critical body fat level may be as low as 13 percent or that there may be no such critical level at all.[12] If such a critical fat percentage does exist, it probably varies widely from individual to individual.

The focus of research is upon how all of the factors mentioned may affect the hypothalamus, thereby influencing the production of important regulatory hormones relative to menstruation and metabolism, including estrogen, epinephrine, and corticoids. Whatever the cause, exercise-induced amenorrhea is generally considered reversible. Normal menstrual cycles resume with as minor a change in lifestyle as a 10 percent decrease in exercise, improved nutrition, or a weight gain of 4 to 5 pounds.[13] Also, exercise-induced amenorrhea does not seem to affect long-term fertility.[14] In fact, while a woman with amenorrhea does not experience a regular menstrual cycle, it is still possible for her to ovulate and become pregnant. She should not rely on this for birth control and should continue her regular birth control method if pregnancy is not desired. Any active woman should be aware of her normal menstrual cycle and should discuss any irregularities with her physician to rule out such conditions as thyroid disorders, ovarian cysts, brain tumors, and pregnancy.

There is concern that low estrogen levels during amenorrhea accelerate bone mineral loss, increasing the risk of osteoporosis. Estrogen, exercise, and calcium must all be present in order for a woman to build or maintain bone mass. An excess of one element will not make up for an absence of another. While people who exercise tend to have greater bone densities than do nonexercisers, loss of estrogen, regardless of age, may cause an irreversible loss of bone strength. A 20-year-old amenorrheic athlete can have the bone density of a 50-year-old.[15] While bone density does increase with a resumption in normal estrogen levels, it does not appear to recover fully. If an amenorrheic athlete has a low estrogen level, lifestyle change and/or low-dose estrogen replacement therapy to prevent bone mineral loss should be discussed with a physician. In addition, a calcium intake of 1,500 mg/day (about 5 cups of milk) is recommended.

Pregnancy

Is exercise advisable during pregnancy? How much? What are the benefits? Are there any limitations or cautions to keep in mind? Are some exercises better than others? Pregnancy is a natural and normal physiological function, not an illness. A pregnant woman is not fragile. She will be healthier and the pregnancy safer if she remains active. Of course, any pregnant woman should obtain medical clearance from her physician before beginning or continuing an exercise program. General advice for a healthy woman having an uncomplicated pregnancy is to continue her regular exercise program, being careful not to get overtired. If she has not been exercising before pregnancy, this is not a time to begin a crash program. A 20-minute to 30-minute walk, three to four days per week, is a program a doctor might approve. Throughout pregnancy, to keep the effort aerobic, a woman should use the "talk test." She should be able to carry on a conversation while exercising without getting out of breath. In early pregnancy, if exercising seems to require more effort, decrease intensity and duration. Particular care should be taken to avoid overheating, which has been linked to increased risk of central nervous system abnormalities (such as spina bifida) in the baby.[16] For this reason, steam rooms and saunas are contraindicated. Pregnant women also should be counseled not to undertake excessive physical activity in a hot climate to which they are not acclimated. A gradual weight gain, which is natural and desirable, is likely to increase stress to joints, ligaments, and muscles. Also, muscles and connective tissues become more lax as they gradually undergo hormonal changes. Increases in the pregnancy hormone relaxin helps to facilitate the baby's birth but makes the pregnant woman more susceptible to strains and sprains. Therefore, during late pregnancy and the early postdelivery period, vigorous increases in flexibility should not be pursued.

In the fifth to sixth months of pregnancy, due to increasing weight and joint flexibility, impact activities may become uncomfortable. At this time, many women switch to low- or no-impact exercises such as walking, swimming, or stationary cycling. While some women continue their normal exercise program right to the day of delivery with no ill effects, don't feel guilty if you feel a need to cut back. Toward the end of pregnancy, if you fatigue easily and exercise seems to require more effort, it is natural to de-

table 8.1

ACOG GUIDELINES FOR EXERCISE DURING PREGNANCY AND POSTPARTUM

PREGNANCY AND POSTPARTUM

1. Regular exercise (at least three times per week) is preferable to intermittent activity. Competitive activities should be discouraged.
2. Vigorous exercise should not be performed in hot, humid weather or when you have a fever.
3. Ballistic movements (jerky, bouncy motions) should be avoided. Exercise should be done on a wooden floor or a tightly carpeted surface to reduce shock and provide a sure footing.
4. Deep flexion or extension of joints should be avoided because of connective tissue laxity. Activities that require jumping, jarring motions, or rapid changes in direction should be avoided because of joint instability.
5. Vigorous exercise should be preceded by a 5-minute period of muscle warm-up. This can be accomplished by slow walking or stationary cycling with low resistance.
6. Vigorous exercise should be followed by a period of gradually declining activity that includes gentle stationary stretching. Because connective tissue laxity increases the risk of joint injury, stretches should not be taken to the point of maximum resistance.
7. Heart rate should be measured at times of peak activity. Target heart rates and limits established in consultation with a physician should not be exceeded.
8. Care should be taken to gradually rise from the floor to avoid a sudden drop in blood pressure. Some form of activity involving the legs should be continued for a brief period.
9. Liquids should be taken liberally before and after exercise to prevent dehydration. If necessary, activity should be interrupted to replenish fluids.
10. Women who have led sedentary lifestyles should begin with physical activity of very low intensity and advance activity levels very gradually.
11. Activity should be stopped and the physician consulted if any unusual symptoms appear.

PREGNANCY ONLY
(1994 Revision of the 1985 Guidelines)

1. There is no maternal heart rate limit. The former recommendation was that the maternal heart rate should not exceed 140 bpm.
2. There is no limit on exercise duration. Formerly, strenuous activities were limited to 15 minutes in duration.
3. No exercise should be performed while lying on the back after the first trimester. This slows blood flow back to the heart and decreases its output. Also, avoid *motionless standing,* which may also decrease heart output.
4. Exercises that employ the Valsalva maneuver should be avoided.
5. Caloric intake should be adequate to meet not only the extra energy needs of pregnancy, but also of the exercise performed.
6. Maternal core temperature should not exceed 38°C (100.4°F).

source: American College of Obstetricians and Gynecologists. *Exercise during Pregnancy and the Postnatal Period (ACOG Home Exercise Programs),* Washington, DC: ACOG, 1994.

crease the activity level. After the fourth month, it is not advised to do exercises that require lying on your back. This position can block the blood supply to the uterus (by compressing the aorta and/or the vena cava), resulting in depression of the fetal heart rate.[17] Throughout pregnancy, a woman needs to listen to her body and adjust exercise to maintain comfort. Note specific pregnancy exercise guidelines from the American College of Obstetricians and Gynecologists in Table 8.1. Also review Table 8.2.

table 8.2

REASONS TO DISCONTINUE EXERCISE AND SEEK MEDICAL ADVICE DURING PREGNANCY

1. Any signs of bloody discharge from the vagina
2. Any "gush" of fluid from the vagina
3. Sudden swelling of the ankles, hands, or face
4. Persistent, severe headaches and/or visual disturbance; unexplained spell of faintness or dizziness
5. Swelling, pain, and redness in the calf of one leg (phlebitis)
6. Elevation of pulse rate or blood pressure that persists after exercise
7. Excessive fatigue, palpitations, chest pain
8. Persistant contractions (more than six to eight per hour) that may suggest onset of premature labor
9. Unexplained abdominal pain
10. Insufficient weight gain during the last two trimesters

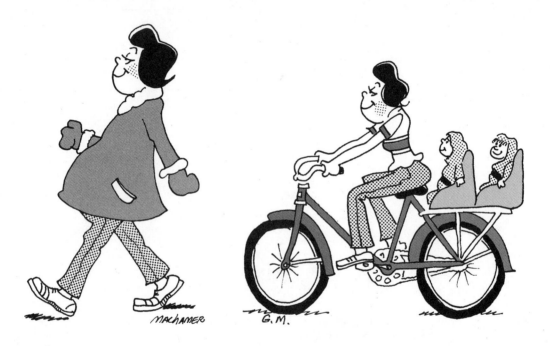

Exercise during and after pregnancy has many advantages.

There are many reasons exercise is important during pregnancy. The physiological changes of pregnancy place a great demand on the body. Labor and delivery are perhaps the most physically demanding events a woman will ever experience. Exercise can maintain optimal fitness, enabling a woman to control weight gain, improve muscle tone, improve posture, decrease backache, and decrease constipation. Exercise can also aid in increasing energy, increasing psychological well-being, managing stress, enhancing sleep at night, and regaining her prepregnancy figure.

While fitness is no guarantee of a quick labor or easy delivery, endurance and increased capacity to deal with the physical stress of childbirth are assets that come from fitness. A fit mother can enjoy a quicker recovery from childbirth and can regain her normal fitness and activity levels in less time than can the unfit.

Stress Incontinence

Stress incontinence, an involuntary leakage of urine when you laugh, cough, sneeze, or exercise, is a common problem, particularly in women over 30 who have given birth. During pregnancy and birth, these muscles become weakened and stretched. One solution is to wear a sanitary pad, but a better approach is to strengthen the perineal muscles that control this function. The pelvic floor is a hammocklike muscle layer attached at the front and back of the pelvis. It supports the pelvic organs, including the bladder, uterus, and rectum. Kegel exercises, named after the Los Angeles physician who developed them, strengthen the pelvic floor muscles and may prevent or cure stress incontinence. As a side benefit, many women report increased pleasure during intercourse.

Kegel Exercise

Kegel exercises are done by contracting perineal muscles, which surround the bladder neck and vagina. To learn the exercise, when urinating stop and start the flow. Hold the contraction for 3 to 4 seconds during the stop phase. The muscle action you take to do this when urinating is the action you must take when doing Kegel exercises. You can do these exercises anytime—contract hard and then release. Do 10 in a row, and work up to five sets of 10 daily. These exercises should be done before, during, and after pregnancy.

Postpartum: Getting Back into Shape

Giving birth and coping with the demands of a new baby are both joyful and stressful for a new mother. The main problem in resuming exercise is not fatigue or shortness of breath, which might be expected, but finding someone to watch the baby while mother takes a well-deserved break. Postpartum recovery times vary greatly. If the delivery has been normal, walking is encouraged in the hospital the day after delivery. This can be continued when the woman returns home. Rest, good nutrition, and a progressive walking program will make recovery faster than will complete inactivity or resuming prepregnancy activity levels too soon. You should not rush into impact activities such as jogging or pursue flexibility increases until you have given loosened joints (due to the hormone relaxin) a chance to recover—6 weeks to 16 weeks.[18] Abdominal curls are important for toning overstretched abdominal muscles and preventing back problems. Also, do Kegel exercises to strengthen pelvic floor muscles.

A nursing mother needs to avoid fatigue and dehydration, which may reduce milk production. Drink eight or more glasses of fluid a day, and nap when the baby does to ensure adequate rest. Wear a good supportive bra, with pads to control leaks, and nurse before exercise for greater comfort. There is no conflict between nursing a baby and moderate exercise. Both help a mother regain her prepregnancy figure.

Breast Support

Does bouncing cause breasts to sag? Some believe that breast movement stretches the skin and ligaments that support the breasts. There is no evidence to support this claim; the main culprits are genetics and pregnancy.[19] Still, a good bra makes exercise more comfortable by reducing breast movement during activity. The best designs flatten breasts to redistribute their mass across the chest wall. This results in less mass for gravity to affect. Racerback and crossback straps prevent slippage off the shoulder. Certain designs are more suited to small-breasted women, while others are more comfortable for large-breasted exercisers. A woman should try different styles to decide what is best for her. A good exercise bra should (1) limit breast movement; (2) have wide straps that do not slip off the shoulders; (3) have a wide band at the bottom to prevent the bra from riding up; (4) have no rough seams or uncovered fasteners to prevent chafing; and (5) be made of nonabrasive materials and be seamless, or at least have seams that do not cross the nipple area.

Males and Exercise

Participation in sports and physical activities no longer ends with graduation from high school or college. Large numbers of men are continuing or beginning lifetime exercise programs.

Exercise appears to lower the hormonal levels of males as it does of females. In one study, testosterone levels of men who ran 40 miles a week averaged 30 percent less than the levels of nonexercisers.[20] The runners' levels were still in a normal range, and the effect was reversible. Sperm count and libido were not affected. While it may lower hormonal levels, overtraining is not associated with decreased fertility in male athletes unless accompanied by anorexic behavior and a high-stress lifestyle.[21,22]

A more common male fertility problem results from constantly wearing tight undershorts. In order for the testicles to maintain normal sperm production, they must be a few degrees cooler than normal body temperature. Their position outside and slightly away from the body accomplishes this. When the testicles are overheated by consistently being held close to the body, sperm production temporarily decreases. A switch to boxer shorts solves the problem.

Environmental Considerations

Exercising in the Cold

All your friends think you're crazy, sharing a narrow roadway with cars that spray you with slush as you exercise on a chilly winter day. Walking, running, and cycling are more complicated in the winter. Still, there is something liberating about a good workout on an icy winter day. Cold weather workouts can be invigorating, comfortable, and safe if you follow these tips:

1. *Layer clothing:* Dress in several thin layers so you can remove or add a layer as needed. Wool and polypropylene clothing wick moisture away from the skin to keep you dry. The outer layer of clothing should be breathable and windproof.

2. *Avoid overheating:* Don't overdress or you'll overheat. You should feel a little cool until you warm up. Do take the windchill factor into account when preparing for your workout (Fig. 8.1).

3. *Avoid overexposure:* While frostbite *is* a possibility if you don't dress properly, there is *no* possibility that you will freeze your lungs or throat. If cold air bothers you, breathe through a bandanna. Frostbite can occur on outer body areas such as the fingers and toes when your skin temperature drops below 32°F. Frostbite can easily be avoided by covering exposed areas and by getting inside and warming up if any body parts feel numb or tingly. **Hypothermia** is a life-threatening condition in which body temperature drops to a dangerously low level. Medical attention should be sought immediately.

4. *Protect exposed parts:* Fingers and toes receive the smallest blood supply and experience winter's chill fastest. Mittens are more effective than gloves which allow cold air to circulate around the fingers. On extremely cold days, it may be advisable to wear two pairs of socks or a thermal insole if the feet get too cold. Up to 40 percent of body heat can be lost through the head. Exposed ears or face can lead to windburn or chapping. To avoid discomfort, wear a hat and spread a thin layer of petroleum jelly on exposed skin areas.

5. *Work with the wind:* Plan out-and-back workouts, heading into the wind on the way out so you can return with the wind to your back. Not only will you appreciate the push when you're tired, but you'll be less likely to be chilled by your own sweat during the return.

6. *Exercise with caution:* Winter weather changes the safety rules for outdoor exercise: Fewer daylight hours, icy roads, and snowy nights lower visibility for drivers. Exercise at midday as often as possible. Avoid high-volume traffic areas, wear bright clothing, and be prepared for potential hazards by remaining alert. Wear waffled or ridged shoe soles to provide extra traction on icy roads.

7. *Stay motivated:* Winter exercising demands greater personal motivation than exercising at any other time of the year. Winter holidays, less daylight, and poor

Wind speed	Temperature (Fahrenheit)																				
Calm	40	35	30	25	20	15	10	5	0	-5	-10	-15	-20	-25	-30	-35	-40	-45	-50	-55	-60
	Equivalent chill temperature																				
5	35	30	25	20	15	10	5	0	-5	-10	-15	-20	-25	-30	-35	-45	-60	-65	-55	-65	-70
10	30	20	15	10	5	0	-10	-15	-20	-25	-35	-40	-45	-50	-60	-55	-70	-75	-80	-90	-95
15	25	15	10	0	-5	-10	-20	-25	-30	-40	-45	-50	-60	-65	-70	-80	-85	-90	-100	-105	-110
20	20	10	5	0	-10	-15	-25	-30	-35	-45	-50	-60	-65	-75	-80	-85	-95	-100	-110	-115	-120
25	15	10	0	-5	-15	-20	-30	-35	-45	-50	-60	-65	-75	-80	-90	-95	-105	-110	-120	-125	-135
30	10	5	0	-10	-20	-25	-30	-40	-50	-56	-65	-70	-80	-85	-95	-100	-105	-115	-120	-130	-140
35	10	5	-5	-10	-20	-25	-35	-40	-55	-60	-65	-75	-80	-90	-100	-105	-115	-120	-130	-135	-145
40*	10	0	-5	-15	-20	-30	-35	-45	-55	-60	-70	-75	-85	-95	-100	-110	-115	-125	-130	-140	-150

Little danger | Increasing danger (Flesh may freeze within one minute.) | Greater danger (Flesh may freeze within 30 seconds.)

FIGURE 8.1 ➤

Windchill readings.

Ball State University Weather Station, Department of Geography.

weather can disrupt a routine. To maintain enthusiasm, set realistic wintertime goals to work toward. Don't worry about your pace. Between the slick footing and the heavy clothing, it's prudent to run relaxed. Just go fast enough to stay warm.

8. *Be safe:* Tell someone your route and when you expect to be back. Better yet, go with a friend.

Don't hesitate to mix your usual exercise with other activities—cross-country skiing or sledding in snow country, aerobics, stair climbing, indoor cycling, or water exercise if you crave a break from the cold. Your heart will benefit as long as you stay in your training zone, and the cross-training will work new muscle groups.

Exercising in the Heat

Given a couple of weeks and plenty of water, the human body can adapt quite well to exercise in the heat. Hot-weather workouts make the body work harder than it does in cool weather. The heart must pump enough blood not only to fuel working muscles but also to carry heat to the skin to be dissipated, reducing work capacity. Drinking plenty of cold fluids is critical in order to maintain sweating, your body's air conditioning system. The body can acclimatize to heat but not to dehydration. Overexertion in hot weather, particularly when coupled with dehydration, can lead to heat cramps, heat exhaustion, heatstroke, or **hyperthermia,** a life-threatening condition in which the body's temperature rises to a dangerous level. Particularly susceptible are people who are over 40, are out of shape, are overweight, have heart disease, or have previously experienced heat injury.

When performing endurance exercise, men and women have similar responses in adaptability to hot weather. Both genders are equally susceptible to heat stress, and both respond by acclimatization. Women seem to sweat less than men in order to maintain body temperature. This may indicate that women have a more efficient means of thermoregulation. However, with endurance training, women's level of sweating equals the level of sweating in men.[23]

To exercise safely in hot weather, follow these guidelines:

1. Respect the heat. Hot, humid, sunny weather poses a potentially life-threatening challenge to your body.
2. Monitor environmental conditions before exercising and adjust your workout accordingly. Exercise in the coolest parts of the day: early morning or after

FIGURE 8.2 ➤

Heat safety index.

Ball State University Weather Station, Department of Geography.

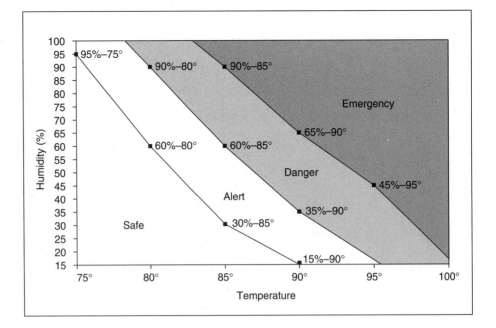

sundown. Avoid the hours between 10:00 A.M. and 4:00 P.M. Postpone the workout when the heat safety index is in the danger zone or above (Fig. 8.2).

3. Avoid dehydration by drinking plenty of fluids before, during, and after a workout. Alcohol and caffeinated drinks are poor choices because they promote water loss through the urine, increasing dehydration.

4. Weigh yourself before and after a workout. This will help you detect water loss. A sudden loss of weight may be a sign you are dehydrated. For every pound you lose, you need to drink 16 ounces of fluids. If you lose as little as 1 percent of your body weight, you may be dehydrating and in serious need of fluids. Drink six to eight glasses of fluids throughout the day whether you are thirsty or not. Studies show that thirst is not a good indicator of your fluid needs. About 15 to 30 minutes before exercise, drink 4 to 8 ounces of fluid. During exercise, drink 4 to 8 ounces of fluid at 15-minute intervals. After exercise, drink at least 8 to 16 ounces of fluid.

5. Wear loose-fitting clothing that allows air to circulate to your body, and expose as much skin to the air as possible to promote sweat evaporation. Light colors are best because they reflect rather than absorb sunlight. *Vinyl or rubber sweat suits worn to lose body weight are definitely contraindicated.* They can lead to dehydration and even death.

6. When becoming acclimated to warmer weather in the spring, decrease exercise intensity and duration. Allow two weeks to gradually increase the workload to normal levels.

7. Ask your doctor about the effects of any medications you take because some can reduce heat tolerance.

8. Stop exercising at the first sign of heat illness (exhaustion, dizziness, nausea, headache, or shortness of breath).

Heavy Sweating During Exercise

One of the hazards of exercising in hot, humid weather is dehydration caused by excessive loss of body water in the form of sweat. Dehydration disturbs cellular fluid and electrolyte balance, thus interfering with muscular contraction. Water losses of as little as 2 percent to 3 percent of body weight have been shown to impair exercise performance, reduce the amount of time a person can exercise, reduce cardiac stroke volume (volume of blood pumped out with each heartbeat), and reduce cardiac output (the amount of blood pumped by the heart over time).[24] Water loss can also interfere with the body's ability to regulate internal temperature, resulting in overheating, which can be deadly.

Sweat is primarily water, but a number of major electrolytes (essential minerals in the form of salts) and other nutrients may be found in varying amounts. Sodium, chloride, and potassium are the predominant electrolytes found in sweat. They help to maintain normal body fluid volume and are involved in nerve impulse transmission and muscle contraction.

Electrolyte Replacement

Is profuse sweating likely to create an electrolyte deficiency? Studies over the years have shown this is not likely to occur, even during prolonged exercise, such as marathon running. This is not to say that electrolyte replacement is not important and that electrolyte deficiency is impossible. After prolonged exercise with heavy sweating, the body's stores of electrolytes are diminished and could eventually become deficient. However, with a normal diet, it is difficult to create an electrolyte deficiency.

Salt tablets are generally not recommended to replace lost sodium and chloride since these electrolytes are abundant in a normal diet. They may be prescribed for those who cannot replace them through normal dietary means. Keep in mind that diets high in sodium have been associated with high blood pressure. Citrus fruits, fruit juices, and bananas are foods recommended for electrolyte replacement.

Fluid Replacement

Rehydration (replacing body fluid volume) is critical to safe, effective exercise involving heavy sweating. For years, we were told that water is the best drink to replace fluids, because that is mainly what you lose when you sweat during a hard workout. But science is dynamic, and conventional wisdom sometimes becomes history in the light of new discoveries. New information, concerning exercise of one hour or more, now gives the slight edge in fluid replacement to electrolyte-containing beverages. This is because fluids are more readily retained in the body's tissues when we consume drinks containing electrolytes.[25] Why? Because plain water tends to slightly increase urination so fewer fluids remain in the body's tissues. Also it has been learned that we will consume more fluids when the beverage tastes good. Since the objective is to replace fluids lost in the tissues, the more you drink, the better. Due to these new findings, many commercial beverages have been produced to help in the process of rehydrating the body. These drinks are commonly known as carbohydrate-electrolyte replacement solutions (CES) or sports drinks. Other than water, the major ingredients in these solutions are carbohydrates in the form of glucose and/or sucrose and some of the major electrolytes. The glucose/sucrose content varies with the different brands, ranging from 1 percent to over 10 percent. Recent studies have shown that sports drinks containing carbohydrates boost endurance and energy as well as help to delay fatigue during exercise.[26] Select a sports drink carefully. Drinks with high carbohydrate concentrations are slow to empty from the stomach, interfering with rehydration, and can cause bloating and nausea. It is best to avoid sports drinks containing carbohydrate concentrations higher than 8 percent (4 percent to 8 percent works best).[27] Experiment during training to find out if you can handle one of these drinks. You should drink early and frequently during your workouts. Don't do anything new for competitive events. So if you are a competitive athlete or marathoner or if you are exercising for several hours at a time in hot humid weather, the fluid of choice for most effective rehydration or prevention of dehydration is a sports drink (not to exceed 8 percent carbohydrate concentration). Water is the next best fluid, followed by fruit juices diluted with 50 percent water. All three are preferable to caffeinated sodas.[28] Caffeine acts as a diuretic, and the carbonation gives you a feeling of being fuller than you are. This new information, which gives sports drinks a slight edge in terms of rehydration, does not mean that drinking water is not a good way to replace lost fluids. Water is still considered to be one of the most effective ways to rehydrate and works just fine for the fitness exerciser and those exercising for less than one hour. Plus, water is convenient and free. Whatever you drink, drink it cold. Cold drinks are better than warm ones because they help cool down the core temperature of the body and empty from the stomach faster.

Contra-indicated Exercises

A few stretching and toning exercises added to an aerobic program can promote balanced fitness by increasing flexibility in tight muscles and by strengthening weak ones. However, not all conditioning exercises commonly done in classes or seen on videotapes are good for everyone. These potentially harmful exercises are labeled **contraindicated exercises.**

By studying people with aches and injuries, fitness experts have learned that some common stretching and toning exercises should be avoided. Others should be modified for safety and effectiveness. Be aware of which commonly done high-risk movements you should avoid and which high-benefit, low-risk exercises to do instead. Here are some examples:

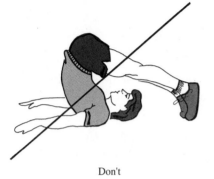

Don't

Yoga plow

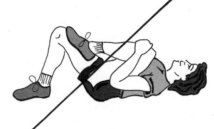

Don't

Single-knee tuck to chest

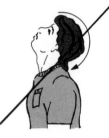

Don't

Head rolls

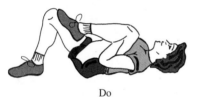

Do

Single-knee tuck to chest

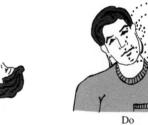

Do

Single-knee tuck to chest

Do

Half-head rolls

1. *Yoga plow:* Sometimes done as a back stretch, this exercise can injure discs, ligaments, and nerves in the neck and back. A better back stretch is a single- or double-knee tuck to the chest.

2. *Knee tuck to chest:* Hyperflexing the knee by pulling it to the body with the arms or hands placed on top of the tibia places undue stress on the knee joint. The hand position should be changed to hug the thigh rather than the shin.

3. *Head roll:* Hyperextension can injure discs in the neck. Safer neck stretches include half-head rolls to the front, turning the head side to side so that the chin touches the right and left shoulders, and touching an ear to each shoulder.

4. *Hurdler stretch:* This stretch can cause groin pull, injure knee cartilage, and overstretch the medial collateral ligament—the one that helps stabilize the knee. It may also cause hip joint discomfort because the femur of the leg that is tucked behind is in a position of extreme rotation in the joint capsule. The alternate hurdler stretch safely stretches hamstrings.

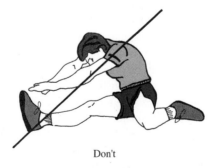

Don't

Hurdler stretch

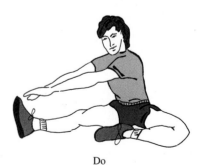

Do

Alternate hurdler stretch

5. *Full squat:* Excessive flexion or extension of the knee is dangerous. To strengthen the quadriceps, substitute half-knee bends for full squats, the duckwalk, deep lunges, and squat thrusts. Deep knee flexion exercises overstress knee ligaments and cartilage.

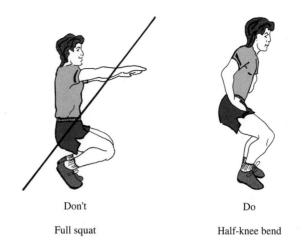

Don't

Full squat

Do

Half-knee bend

6. *Standing toe touch:* This exercise risks the straining of back ligaments. Limit forward flexion in a standing position. As your trunk dips below a 25 degree to 45 degree angle, the lower back muscles cease to work, and the posterior ligaments joining bone to bone must support the load.

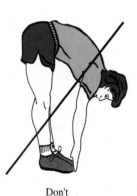

Don't

Standing toe touch

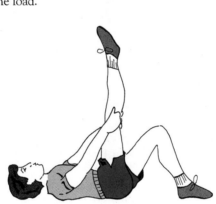

Do

Lying hamstring stretch

Do

Sitting hamstring stretch

7. *Leg stretches at a ballet bar (or other high object):* These may be potentially harmful. When the extended leg is raised 90 degrees or more and the trunk is bent over the leg, it may lead to sciatica problems, especially when the exerciser has limited flexibility. Substitute the back and hamstring stretches suggested in numbers 1, 4, and 6.

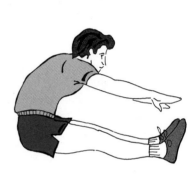

Don't

Ballet bar leg stretch

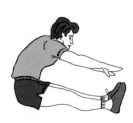

Do

Single-knee tuck to chest

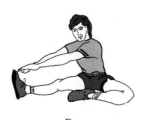

Do

Alternate hurdler stretch

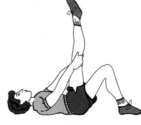

Do

Lying hamstring stretch

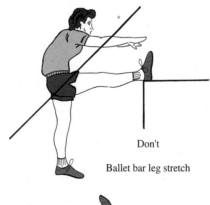

Do

Sitting hamstring stretch

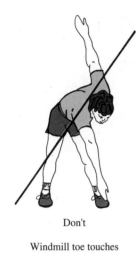

Don't

Windmill toe touches

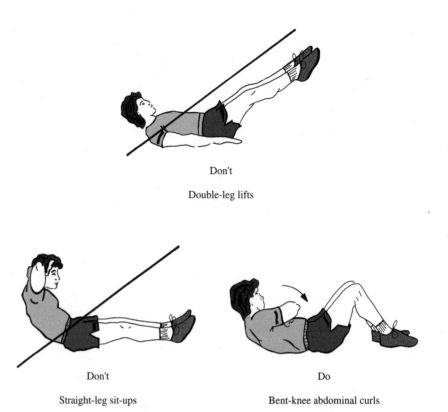

Don't

Double-leg lifts

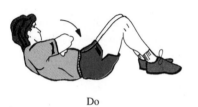

Do

Oblique abdominal curls

Don't

Straight-leg sit-ups

Do

Bent-knee abdominal curls

8. *Leaning forward and twisting the trunk to the side:* These moves are particularly hazardous to the lower back, adding a shearing force to the stress on back ligaments. Avoid swinging hands and the trunk through the knees, windmill toe touches, waist circles, or elbow-knee lunges. There is no exercise you can do standing to tone your waist. The most effective exercise for reducing your waist is aerobic exercise and sensible nutrition. To tone oblique abdominals, the muscles that underlie the waist area, use twisting bent-knee abdominal curls. Lying on your back with heels close to your buttocks and crossing your arms across your chest (or with a hand touching each shoulder), curl the shoulders first toward the right knee and then toward the left knee.

9. *Double-leg lifts, straight-leg sit-ups, and low leg scissors:* These do little or nothing to tone the abdominals. They tighten hip flexors, which in most people are too tight already, causing lordosis (swayback). They may also cause lower back strain. The most effective exercise for toning abdominals is bent-knee abdominal curls in which the lower back stays on the ground while the shoulders curl forward about 3 inches. To avoid jerking on the head or neck, cross your arms across your chest or behind your head with a hand touching each shoulder.

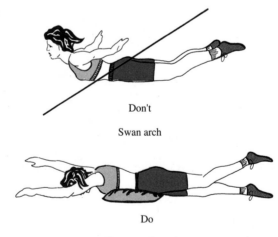

Don't

Swan arch

Do

Single arm/leg raises

10. *The swan arch, prone double-leg raises, and yoga cobra:* These produce excessive back hyperextension and possible back strain. In a prone position, raise your right arm and the opposite leg a few inches off the ground and then switch; this will strengthen the back safely.

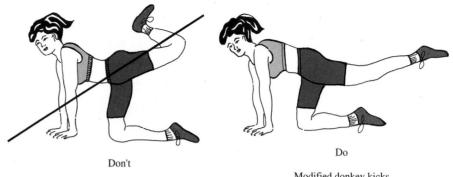

Don't

Donkey kicks

Do

Modified donkey kicks
(can be done with forearms on floor)

11. *Donkey kicks or fire hydrants:* Done on hands and knees with the back hyperextended, these may strain the lower back. To protect the back, hold your abdominals tight, round your back, and raise your leg no higher than 6 inches to 12 inches.

Your body is meant to move in many ways—to bend, twist, and stretch. Some people can do high-risk exercises for years with no ill effects. For others, after only a few repetitions, injury occurs. You may not know into which category you fit until it is too late. The problem is that some movements increase risks to muscles, joints, and connective tissue. While you may need to do deep squats if you are a competitive weightlifter or a yoga plow if you are in a yoga class, these moves don't offer any special benefit for the fitness exerciser. Low-benefit, high-risk exercises should be minimized in programs designed to emphasize personal fitness. Follow these general rules when exercising:[29]

1. Do not hyperflex the knee.
2. Do not hyperextend the knee, neck, or lower back.
3. Do not apply a twisting or lateral force to the knee.
4. Avoid holding your breath during exercise.
5. Avoid stretching long/weak muscles (i.e., abdominals) and avoid shortening already short/strong muscles (i.e., hip flexors). See Chapter 5, Table 5.1.
   a. Most people should avoid aggravating common postural faults: forward head, dorsal kyphosis (rounded upper back), medial rotations of the thigh, and pronation of the foot.
   b. Most people need to stretch the chest muscles, hip flexors, calves, hamstrings, lower back, and medial thigh rotators.
6. Avoid stretching any joint to the point of pain.
7. Be especially careful when using passive stretches with another person (unless the person is a physical therapist).
8. Avoid movements that place acute compressional forces on spinal discs, such as extending and rotating the spine simultaneously (i.e., trunk and neck circling and double-leg lifts).
9. Avoid movements that cause joint impingements or cartilage damage, such as arm circles in the palm-down position.
10. If the nature of your sport regularly requires the violation of good mechanics (baseball catcher assuming a deep squat position or gymnast performing double-leg lifts), make certain that the muscles are as strong as possible to endure the stress.

Aging and Physical Activity

Is your body older than you are? Scientist and well-known physical educator T. K. Cureton estimated that middle age begins for the average person at age 26, because at that age he or she has the physical capacity our ancestors did when they were 40.[30]

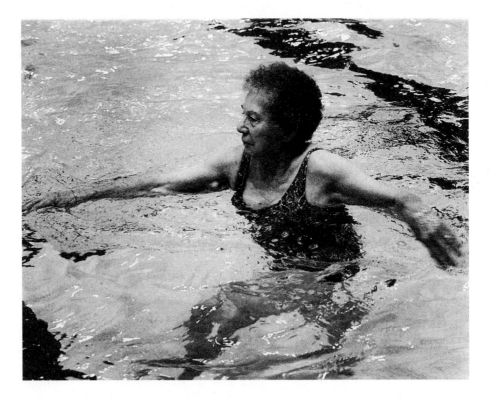

When we retire, we are expected to slow down and take it easy. This often produces disastrous results as atrophy and disuse take their toll. Disorders such as cardiovascular disease, hypertension, and adult onset diabetes don't have to be the natural consequences of aging. We now feel that they are more related to physical inactivity. The body adapts to whatever load is placed on it, and the ability to do work is reduced if the load lessens. However, attitudes are changing. Older adults, encouraged by their doctors and by research revealing the benefits of exercise, are biking, swimming, jogging, lifting weights, and walking in ever-increasing numbers. We know that older adults (even up to age 100) are remarkably responsive to exercise, reaping health benefits. As the health-conscious baby-boom generation matures, they are likely to redefine the concept of aging.

Aging and Performance

Some say, "Growing old isn't so bad, if you consider the alternative." James Dean's "Live fast, die young, and leave a good-looking corpse" does have its proponents, but they are quickly weeded out of the genetic pool. I think a lot more of us would choose to die young, as late as possible. At birth, we each have a 70-plus-year warranty, but the maintenance is up to us. Just like any machine, the human body grows less efficient as it ages. The decline in max VO_2 among the sedentary is about 1 percent for every year after 25.[31] Decreases in strength, flexibility, and endurance and increased body fat proportion with age are often accepted as a natural part of the aging process. These changes may be common, but they are not inevitable. The most significant factor contributing to declines in physiological capacity at any age is *lack of regular exercise*. The "use it or lose it" rule applies here. Unused muscles atrophy, lose elasticity, and grow weak. Ligaments and tendons shorten and tighten, decreasing range of motion and causing aches and pains as they pull across joints. As muscle tissue atrophies, basal metabolism drops, resulting in an increase in body fat even when a person is not eating enough to maintain adequate nutritional levels.

To develop optimal bone strength and mass and to ward off osteoporosis, women need adequate amounts of calcium in the diet, estrogen in the bloodstream, and weight-bearing exercise in their lifestyle. Exercise acts synergistically with estrogen to develop bone strength.[32] Inactivity accelerates bone mineral loss and increases risk of osteoporosis.

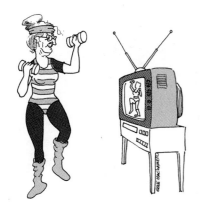

Exercise slows the aging process.

Bone mass begins to decline gradually after the age of 30. The decline is hastened by menopause. While exercise alone cannot prevent osteoporosis, it may help premenopausal women build up their bone densities so they enter menopause ahead of the game. Weight-bearing exercise, such as running and walking, builds up bone mass before this age and slows its decline afterward. Ideally, women should exercise early in life to build bone and later in life to keep it strong. Exercise has been shown to increase mineral content of vertebral and arm bone. Both weight-bearing and other resistance exercise that stresses the bone helps to increase bone content.[33] It is better increased by a combination of aerobic and weight-training exercises than it is by weight training alone. Once osteoporosis has developed, women should still be encouraged to exercise, except, of course, while a fracture is healing. Men also are affected by osteoporosis, but at later ages than women. Recent studies show that men and women 60 and older who train with weights and resistance machines several times a week can quickly double their total body strength.[34] This helps fight osteoporosis by keeping skeletons sturdy. Also, such strength gains have major implications for maintaining independence in later years. Lifelong exercise may also help protect the elderly against falls and the devastating effects of hip fractures. It's never too late to start exercising. Starting late in life is far preferable to not starting at all.

While aging is unavoidable, declines in functional capacity with age are not inevitable. How you age is largely up to you. Cardiologist George Sheehan has said that growing older isn't so bad; it is inactive people who give aging a bad name. Biological aging can be significantly slowed by regular exercise. As much as 50 percent of the functional decline seen in aging is related to disuse and can be prevented with regular aerobic exercise.[35] Older adults who engage in an aerobic exercise program can slow this decline and may even have the same aerobic capacity as that of a sedentary person 25 or more years younger.[36,37]

As one physician observed, "So many things we think are linked to aging . . . actually have to do with lifestyle. Exercise produces a 40-year age offset. A fit person of 70 is the equal of an unfit person of 30 in regard to bones, muscles, heart, brain, sex, and everything else. I see an immense energy in old people who continue [exercise]."[38] Exercise intensity appears to be the key to greatest benefit. A group of master athletes (ages 40 to 75) studied over an 18-year period showed no significant decline in aerobic capacity if they maintained training intensity.[39] *For most elderly fitness exercisers, however, an exercise intensity of 40 percent to 50 percent maximal heart rate reserve is considered adequate.*

The effect of true nonpreventable aging involves a gradual loss of the speed and vigor with which we do activities, but it should not prevent us from doing them. As one older runner observed, "I can do everything I used to. It just takes longer to do it and longer to recover."

Exercise is adult play. At what point was our childhood eagerness to get out and romp replaced by hours of sitting in front of the TV watching others play? Whether aging is an extension of a full and active life or a gradual wasting away is determined by how you choose to live your life.

> We do not stop playing because we are old. We grow old because we stop playing.

Does Exercise Increase Life Span?

While the length of your life may have a strong genetic component, study after study has shown that exercise helps lower the risk of major chronic diseases and premature death. Research recently conducted at the Cooper Institute for Aerobics Research in Dallas found that exercise of *moderate* intensity improved the overall *quality* of life (e.g., enhanced the ability to perform daily tasks, helped with weight control, enhanced psychological well-being) and perhaps increased the *quantity* of life by postponing a heart attack or stroke.[40] A second recent study, which is part of the famous ongoing research of male Harvard alumni, reported that exercise of moderate intensity improved the quality of life but that it took exercise at a *vigorous* intensity level to actually add years to one's life.[41,42] The Harvard men who had expended at least 1,500 calories a

Physical activity is important at every age.

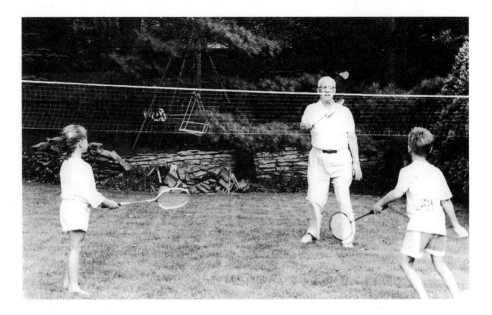

week in vigorous physical activity had a 25 percent lower death rate than did sedentary men. Vigorous activity was defined as fast walking, jogging, playing singles tennis, swimming, and performing heavy, sustained household chores. Studies such as these illustrate that any exercise has health benefits, but more exercise, enough to give your heart and lungs a real workout, is better. While a healthful lifestyle is no guarantee to a longer life, it does stack the odds in your favor.

Are you ever "too old" to begin exercise? No! While the overall impact you can make on the quality of your life is greater if you start exercising young and continue throughout life, there is no age at which the benefits of exercise stop. Frankly, the older you are, the more you need exercise. Table 8.3 shows the benefits of exercise for older adults.

table 8.3

BENEFITS OF EXERCISE FOR OLDER ADULTS

1. Maintenance of a high level of physical and social activity increases the quality of life, enhancing social satisfaction.
2. Increased independence is enjoyed when fitness and health are maintained. Most Americans fear infirmity and dependence more than death.
3. A person who exercises has more energy and can perform daily routines with greater ease.
4. Increased muscle tone and flexibility improve balance, decreasing falls.
5. The more muscle tissue a person maintains, the higher his or her metabolism, making it easier to control weight.
6. Calories burned through exercise allow a person to take in more nutrients.
7. Exercise delays loss of bone mass.
8. With exercise, a person's posture improves, decreasing backache and enhancing appearance.
9. Cardiorespiratory function is enhanced with exercise, improving peripheral circulation and decreasing the risk of atherosclerosis, high blood pressure, and other circulatory problems.
10. Exercise improves the efficiency of elimination.
11. There is decreased depression and stress when a regular exercise program is followed.

SUMMARY

Exercise is meant to be enjoyed throughout life. Regardless of gender or age, the body improves with use and degenerates with disuse. People don't wear out; they rust out. For greatest benefit from an exercise program, it is helpful to be aware of special concerns, such as how to safely exercise in hot and cold weather and how to avoid high-risk exercises. You have learned in this chapter that women respond to exercise the way men do but perhaps a little slower and to a lesser extent. This means training principles are approximately the same, regardless of gender. You have also learned that sports drinks are slightly more strongly recommended than is water for rehydrating the body after prolonged exercise and profuse sweating. Sports drinks contain electrolytes, which enhance fluid retention, contain carbohydrates, delay the onset of fatigue, and boost energy, and they taste good, which increases the likelihood that we will drink more when working out. Water is also a fine rehydrater, especially for the fitness exerciser. As you adjust to a physically active lifestyle, you will find that the benefits far outweigh the effort involved. Exercise will become a habit, and you will begin to look forward to your workout as an important part of your day.

REFERENCES

1. Buschbacker, Ralph M., M.D., and R. L. Braddom, M.D., eds. *Sports Medicine and Rehabilitation: A Sports Specific Approach*. Philadelphia: Hanley and Belfus, Inc. Publishers, 1994.
2. Buschbacker and Braddom. *Sports Medicine and Rehabilitation: A Sports Specific Approach*.
3. Costill, David L. *Inside Running: Basics of Sports Physiology*. Indianapolis: Benchmark Press, Inc., 1986.
4. Seefeldt, Vern, ed. "Menstruation, Pregnancy and Menopause." *Physical Activity and Well Being*. Reston, Va.: AAHPERD, 1986.
5. Cowart, Virginia S. "Can Exercise Help Women with PMS?" *The Physician and Sportsmedicine* 17 (April 1989): 168–78.
6. Seefeldt, Vern, ed. "Mental Health." *Physical Activity and Well Being*. Reston, Va.: AAHPERD, 1986.
7. Buschbacker and Braddom. *Sports Medicine and Rehabilitation: A Sports Specific Approach*.
8. *Cancer Facts and Figures—1995*. Atlanta, Ga.: American Cancer Society, 1995.
9. Zimmerman, David R. "Maturation and Strenuous Training in Young Female Athletes." *The Physician and Sportsmedicine* 15 (June 1987): 219–22.
10. "Sweat Cure: Exercise May Prevent Cancer." *Time* 131 (February 29, 1988): 68.
11. Buschbacker and Braddom. *Sports Medicine and Rehabilitation: A Sports Specific Approach*.
12. Buschbacker and Braddom. *Sports Medicine and Rehabilitation: A Sports Specific Approach*.

13. Munnings, Frances. "Exercise and Estrogen in Women's Health: Getting a Clearer Picture." *The Physician and Sportsmedicine* 16 (May 1988): 152–61.
14. Seefeldt, Vern, ed. "Menstruation, Pregnancy and Menopause."
15. Institute for Aerobics Research. "Young Women and Osteoporosis." *The Aerobics News* 3 (October 1988): 7.
16. McMurray, D., and Vern Katz. "Thermoregulation in Pregnancy. Implication for Exercise." *Physician and Sports Medicine* 10, no. 3 (September 1990): 146–58.
17. University of California, Berkeley. *The Wellness Encyclopedia*. Boston: Houghton Mifflin Co., 1991, 22.
18. Buschbacker and Braddom: *Sports Medicine and Rehabilitation: A Sports Specific Approach*.
19. Buschbacker and Braddom: *Sports Medicine and Rehabilitation: A Sports Specific Approach*.
20. Silberner, Joanne, and Erica E. Goode. "Should Women Stop Jogging?" *U.S. News and World Report* 104 (March 7, 1988): 72.
21. Groves, David. "Study: Hormone Levels in Ultramarathoners." *The Physician and Sportsmedicine* 15 (December 1987): 51.
22. Nash, Heyward L. "Can Exercise Suppress Reproductive Hormones in Men?" *The Physician and Sportsmedicine* 15 (January 1987): 180–86.
23. Buschbacker and Braddom. *Sports Medicine and Rehabilitation: A Sports Specific Approach*.

24. Hamilton, Marc, Jose Gonzalez-Alonso, Scott Montain, and Edward Coyle. "Fluid Replacement and Glucose Infusion During Exercise Prevent Cardiovascular Drift." *Journal of Applied Physiology* 71, no. 3 (1991): 320.
25. Presentation by Ronald Maughan at the Annual Meeting of American College of Sports Medicine in Seattle, Washington, June 1993.
26. Convertino, Victor A., et al. "Exercise and Fluid Replacement. American College of Sports Medicine Position Stand." *Medicine and Science in Sports and Exercise* 28, no. 1 (January 1996): i.
27. Convertino. "Exercise and Fluid Replacement."
28. "Are Sports Drinks Better Than Water?" *The Physician and Sportsmedicine* 20, no. 2 (February 1991): 415.
29. Lindsey, Ruth, and Charles Corbin. "Questionable Exercise—Their Safer Alternatives." *JOPERD* 10 (October 1989): 35.
30. Allen, P., et al. *Fitness for Life*, 4th ed. Dubuque, Iowa: Wm. C. Brown Publishers, 1989.
31. Kasch, Frank, et al. "The Effect of Physical Activity and Inactivity on Aerobic Power in Older Men (A Longitudinal Study)." *The Physician and Sports Medicine* 18, no. 4 (April 1990): 521.
32. Drinkwater, B. "Physical Activity, Fitness and Osteoporosis." In C. Bouchard et al., eds. *Physical Activity, Fitness and Health*. Champaign, Ill.: Human Kinetics, 724–36.

33. Fiatarons, M. A., and E. F. O'Neil, et al. "Exercise Training and Nutritional Supplementation for Physical Frailty in Very Elderly People." *New England Journal of Medicine* 330 (1994): 1769–75.

34. Westcott, Wayne. "Strength Training for the Aging Adult." *Fitness Management* (June 1995): 25.

35. Mullen, Kathleen, et al. "Aging: Adaptations for Wellness." *Connections for Health*. Dubuque, Iowa: Wm. C. Brown Publishers, 1990.

36. Seefeldt, Vern, M.D. "Physical Activity and the Prevention of Premature Aging." *Physical Activity and Well Being*. Reston, Va.: AAHPERD, 1986.

37. Kasch, et al. "The Effects of Physical Activity and Inactivity on Aerobic Power in Older Men (A Longitudinal Study)."

38. Higdon, Hal. "Run for Your Life." *Runner's World* (August 1989): 46–52.

39. Kavanaugh, Terrence, and Roy Sheppard. "Can Regular Sports Participation Slow the Aging Process? Data on Master Athletes." *The Physician and Sports Medicine* 18, no. 6 (June 1990): 562.

40. Kohl, H., III, S. N. Blair, R. S. Paffenbarger, et al. "Changes in Physical Fitness and All Cause Mortality; A Perspective Study of Healthy and Unhealthy Men. *Journal of American Medical Association* 273, no. 14 (April 12, 1995): 1,093.

41. Lee I-M, C. Hsieh, and R. S. Paffenbarger. "Exercise Intensity and Longevity in Men: The Harvard Alumni Health Study." *Journal of American Medical Association* 273, no. 15 (April 19, 1995): 1,179.

42. Paffenbarger, R. S., et al. "Changes in Physical Activity and Other Lifeway Patterns Influencing Longevity." *Medicine and Science in Sports and Exercise* 26, no. 7 (1994): 857–65.

SUGGESTED READINGS

Anderson, Bob, Ed Burke, Bill Pearl. *Getting in Shape: Workout Programs for Men and Women*. Bolinas, Calif.: Shelter Publications, 1995 (P.O. Box 279, Bolinas, CA 94924).

Birkel, Dee Ann, and Susan Freitag. *Forever Fit, a Step-by-step Guide for Older Adults*. New York: Insight Books, Plenum Publishing Corp., 1992.

Costill, David L. *Inside Running: Basics of Sports Physiology*. Indianapolis: Benchmark Press, 1986.

Holstein, Barbara. *Shaping Up for a Healthy Pregnancy*. Champaign, Ill.: Human Kinetics, 1991.

James and Pierre, Richard. *Healthful Aging*. Guilford, Conn.: The Dushkin Publishing Group, Inc., 1992.

Kavanaugh, Terence, and Roy Shephard. "Can Regular Sports Participation Slow the Aging Process? Data on Master Athletes." *The Physician and Sportsmedicine* 18, no. 6 (June 1990): 562.

Kime, Robert. *Pregnancy, Childbirth and Parenting*. Guilford, Conn.: The Dushkin Publishing Group, Inc., 1992.

Lubell, Adele. "Potentially Dangerous Exercises: Are They Harmful to All?" *The Physician and Sportsmedicine* 17, no. 1 (January 1989): 160.

Munnings, Frances. "Exercise and Estrogen in Women's Health: Getting a Clearer Picture." *The Physician and Sportsmedicine* 16 (May 1988): 152–61.

Munnings, Frances. "Osteoporosis: What Is the Role of Exercise?" *The Physician and Sportsmedicine* 20, no. 6 (June 1992): 430.

Myburgh, Kathryn, et al. "Are Risk Factors for Menstrual Dysfunction in Runners Cumulative?" *Physician and Sportsmedicine* 20, no. 4 (April 1992): 312.

Penner, Diane. *Elder Fit: A Health and Fitness Program for Older Adults*. Reston, Va.: American Alliance for Health, Physical Education, Recreation and Dance, 1990.

Roberts, William. "Emergencies in Sports, Managing Heatstroke: On-Site Cooling." *The Physician and Sportsmedicine* 20, no. 5 (May 1992): 351.

Robinson, William. "Emergencies in Sports, Competing with the Cold, Part II Hypothermia." *The Physician and Sportsmedicine* 20, no. 1 (January 1992): 151.

Samuelson, Joan. *Running for Women*. Emmaus, Penn.: Rodale Press, 1995.

Seefeldt, Vern, ed. *Physical Activity and Well Being*. Reston, Va.: AAHPERD, 1986.

Shepard, John, and Lauren Pacelli. "Why Your Patients Shouldn't Take Aging Sitting Down." *The Physician and Sportsmedicine* 18, no. 11 (November 1990): 740.

Sheppard, Roy. *Physical Activity and Aging*. 2d ed. Rockville, Md.: Aspen Publishers, 1987.

Spirduso, Waneen, ed. *Physical Dimensions of Aging*. Champaign, Ill.: Human Kinetics Publishers, 1995.

Stamford, Bryant. "Keeping Cool During Hot Weather Workouts." *The Physician and Sportsmedicine* 20, no. 6 (June 1992): 456.

Stewart, Gordon. *Active Living*. Champaign, Ill.: Human Kinetics Publishers, 1995.

Thornton, James. "How Can You Tell When an Athlete Is Too Thin?" *Physician and Sportsmedicine* 18, no. 12 (December 1990): 879.

Van Norman, Kay A. *Exercise Programming for Older Adults*. Champaign, Ill.: Human Kinetics Publishers, 1994.

White, Jacquline. "Exercising for Two: What's Safe for the Active Pregnant Women?" *Physician and Sportsmedicine* 20, no. 5 (May 1992): 390.

chapter 9

Nutrition

➤ Objectives

After reading this chapter, you will be able to:

1. Describe three ways dietary habits of Americans have changed in the past 75 years, and explain how these changes have affected our nutritional wellness.
2. Identify the percentages of calories recommended in the diet for carbohydrates, proteins, and fats.
3. List the seven dietary guidelines for Americans.
4. List the six major nutrients and describe their main function in the body.
5. Identify the health benefits of soluble and insoluble fiber, and list good food sources of each.
6. Differentiate between complex and simple carbohydrates.
7. Select the correct description of cholesterol, and identify the recommended limit of daily cholesterol consumption.
8. List three foods high in cholesterol.
9. Identify the correct descriptions of saturated, monounsaturated, and polyunsaturated fats, and list three examples of each.
10. Identify three preventive factors relating to osteoporosis.
11. Identify the recommended number of daily servings from the food groups in the Food Guide Pyramid.
12. Give 10 specific examples of small changes that can be incorporated into daily food selections and preparations that could make a significant change in your nutritional wellness.
13. Look at a food label and identify the largest ingredient; calculate the percentage of calories that come from fat, carbohydrate, and protein; identify the sources of fat (including saturated fat); and identify the sources of complex and simple carbohydrates.
14. Identify two ways to eat nutritiously in a fast-food restaurant and as an athlete.

Terms

- Antioxidants
- Carbohydrates
- Cholesterol
- Complex carbohydrates
- Fat
- Fat soluble vitamins
- Fiber
- Glycogen
- Hydrogenation
- Insoluble fiber

- Ketone bodies
- Lacto-ovo-vegetarian
- Lactovegetarian
- Macrominerals
- Minerals
- Monounsaturated fat
- Omega-3
- Osteoporosis
- Polyunsaturated fat
- Protein

- Recommended Dietary Allowances (RDA)
- Saturated fat
- Semivegetarian
- Simple carbohydrates
- Soluble fiber
- Strict vegetarian (or vegan)
- Trace minerals
- Triglycerides
- Vitamins
- Water soluble vitamins

Everything you eat affects you profoundly.

Chinese proverb

fundamental knowledge about nutrition can make a tremendous contribution to your level of wellness. It can help you make food choices that will enhance your health and vitality. This knowledge can also help you to decipher the social influences and messages related to eating. This is just another step toward assuming self-responsibility for your own well-being and health. Learning about nutrition can be exciting. Since eating is a daily activity, you have many opportunities to affect your wellness in a positive way. We are fortunate to live in a country where food is plentiful; we have wide and varied choices.

We tend to see diet as affecting only the physical dimension of wellness. Actually, food can be easily associated with all of the dimensions. Much of our social life revolves around food. Providing food is an important sign of caring. Eating and being fed are intimately connected with our deepest feelings. Table 9.1 gives examples of how food relates to all seven dimensions of wellness. Perhaps you can think of other connections.

After reading this chapter, you should be able to make responsible food choices in your pursuit of high-level wellness. You have heard it before, but it is remarkably true: You are what you eat.

Changing Times

In the agricultural lifestyle of the past, most people grew and prepared their own food. Foods were fresh and simple. Early Americans consumed much greater amounts of fresh fruits, vegetables, and grains and lesser amounts of salt, fats, and refined sugars than Americans do today. In those days, eating out meant eating outdoors—perhaps a picnic or a meal out in the field beside the plow. Today's fast-paced, technological society has contributed to drastic changes in the way we eat. Dual-career and single-parent families are commonplace. As parents juggle careers, child care, social and professional meetings, education, and recreation, meals are often skipped, eaten on the run, or thrown together quickly. As a result, the food preparers are often McDonald's or manufacturers of frozen or processed food. After all, advertisers tell us, "Have it your way!" "Things go better with . . . !" "We do it all for you!" The advertisers' promises are intended to sell products, not necessarily to enhance our nutrition. Supermarket shelves are lined with packaged food products bearing little resemblance to the original farm product. Most are highly processed, often stripped of key nutrients. The result is a new form of malnutrition. Rather than a lack of food, we find ourselves eating too much of the wrong foods. As we have progressed from eating wheat and berries to consuming hot dogs, french fries, and Twinkies, the incidence of heart disease, stroke, hypertension, and cancer has increased. This progression has also cost us our vitality.

To complicate matters, there has been a blitz of nutrition advice in recent years—cut back on eggs, eat more oat bran, eliminate salt, forget red meat, eat organically grown foods, watch the caffeine. Overwhelmed by sometimes conflicting information, many throw up their hands in confusion or disregard nutrition advice entirely.

The 1993 Survey of American Dietary Habits[1] revealed some startling facts regarding nutrition knowledge and behavior in our country. Even though Americans' concerns about nutrition have increased (54 percent of Americans rated nutrition as "highly important," up from 49 percent in 1991), only 37 percent rated themselves as "highly careful" about selecting healthy foods (as compared to 38 percent in 1991). Whereas public awareness of the importance of nutrition continues to grow, action to improve the diet has stalled. A majority of the respondents in the survey felt that changing their dietary habits would mean giving up favorite foods and take too much time. The survey also revealed that most Americans have limited knowledge about dietary guidelines. Only 9 percent of those surveyed could correctly identify the guideline for

table 9.1

FOOD IS ASSOCIATED WITH EVERY DIMENSION OF WELLNESS

DIMENSION	HOW FOOD IS ASSOCIATED
Physical	Food is required for physiological nourishment, genetic growth, and survival.
Emotional	Food is often used as a reward, to soothe feelings, and to ease depression or stress.
Social	Food is often at the heart of social events, celebrations, and family interactions.
Intellectual	Having a healthy relationship with food requires informed consumerism, knowledge about the science of nutrition and sound dietary principles, and the ability to read food labels.
Spiritual	Food is used in rituals and is part of spiritual cleansing. Abstention from eating or eating particular foods often accompanies spiritual growth experiences.
Environmental	The human need for food demands food and crop quality and protection from contamination, protection of the food chain, and strategies for combatting world hunger.
Occupational	Food is often a part of business meetings and social gatherings and breaks at work. Also, the income generated by our occupations determines our food choices. Institutional food preparation is big business.

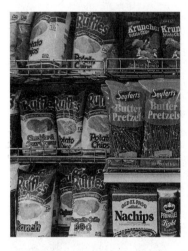

Many of our snacks are heavily processed and stripped of key nutrients.

The Government Takes Action

the percentage of fat in our diet, even though 50 percent of the respondents expressed *concern* about fat in their diet! The percentage who knew about sodium and cholesterol was even lower. Despite the low levels of knowledge, 27 percent of those surveyed rated themselves as "very knowledgeable" about dietary guidelines.

Maintaining healthy dietary habits is crucial to lifelong wellness. In college, you are faced with the perhaps new responsibility of buying and preparing your own meals or making daily cafeteria selections. Data indicate that students are especially unaware of or apathetic about the implications of poor dietary habits on the future development of chronic diseases.[2] Of course, television contributes to the problem by presenting mixed messages about diet and nutrition. We are exposed to hundreds of commercials for sugary, high-fat snacks, often featuring enchanting music, jingles, and appealing characters. In prime-time programming, nutrition is anything but balanced—grabbing a snack is the norm. Yet the models used in commercials are extremely thin, attractive, and seemingly healthy.

Healthful eating *can* be enjoyable and is easier to sustain than most people think. The underlying approach for dietary choices should be to combine basic nutrition *knowledge* with positive and practical *action*. Small, gradual changes can collectively produce substantial and sustainable dietary improvements.

The 1990 government document *Healthy People 2000* lists "improved nutrition" as one of its key objectives, giving attention to diet as a key to health maintenance and preventive medicine.[3] As a service to the American people, the U.S. Department of Health and Human Services distributed a pamphlet entitled *Dietary Guidelines for Americans*. These guidelines (Table 9.2) help answer the question, "What should we eat to stay healthy?" The seven guidelines reflect the newest research on diet and health relationships, with the purpose of giving *practical* suggestions on how to make healthy diet adjustments. It is impossible to specify the perfect diet for every individual. However, these guidelines point out positive directions for everyday food selections that can help you stay healthy.

As you read these guidelines, some questions may be left unanswered. Nutritionists concur that "The main challenge no longer is simply to determine what eating patterns to recommend . . . simply issuing and disseminating recommendations is insufficient to produce change in most people's eating behavior."[4] As in making most lifestyle changes, we need *knowledge* (to identify problem diet behaviors and how to improve

table 9.2

THE 1995 DIETARY GUIDELINES FOR AMERICANS*

1. **Eat a variety of foods.**
   No one food contains all the nutrients in the amounts needed. These nutrients should come from a variety of foods, not from a few highly fortified foods or supplements. Choose the recommended number of servings from each of the five major food groups in the Food Guide Pyramid. Also select a *variety* of foods within each group. The content of your diet over a day or more is what counts!

2. **Balance the food you eat with physical activity—maintain or improve your weight.**
   Many Americans gain weight in adulthood, increasing their risk for high blood pressure, heart disease, diabetes, certain types of cancer, and other illnesses. Therefore, most adults should not gain weight, especially in the abdominal area (where excess fat is most dangerous). Most Americans spend much of their working day in activities that require little energy; try to do 30 minutes or more of moderate physical activity on most days of the week. Healthy low-fat eating and exercise habits can help reduce health risks.

3. **Choose a diet with plenty of grain products, vegetables, and fruits.**
   These foods provide complex carbohydrates, dietary fiber, and other components linked to good health. These foods are also generally low in fat. The antioxidant nutrients in plant foods are potentially beneficial in reducing the risk for cancer.

4. **Choose a diet low in fat, saturated fat, and cholesterol.**
   Diets high in fat and cholesterol have been linked to heart disease, certain types of cancer, and obesity. *Thirty percent* or less of calories should come from fat, with less than 10 percent of calories from saturated fat. All adults are advised to have blood cholesterol levels checked.

5. **Choose a diet moderate in sugars.**
   Sugars and many foods that contain large amounts of them supply calories but are limited in nutrients. They also contribute to tooth decay.

6. **Choose a diet moderate in salt and sodium.**
   Most Americans eat more salt and sodium than they need, and using less will benefit those people whose blood pressure goes up with salt intake. Foods and beverages containing salt provide most of the sodium in our diets, much of it added during processing and manufacturing.

7. **If you drink alcoholic beverages, do so in moderation.**
   Alcoholic beverages supply calories but few or no nutrients. The alcohol in these beverages has effects that are harmful when the beverages are consumed in excess. These effects include altered judgment, potential dependency, and a great many other serious health problems.

source: U.S. Department of Agriculture, U.S. Department of Health and Human Services. "Nutrition and Your Health: Dietary Guidelines for Americans," 4th ed. *Home and Garden Bulletin* no. 232 (1995).
*Recommendations for healthy Americans age two years and over.

them), *motivation* (to make healthy changes), and a *supportive environment* (to maintain changes in restaurants, supermarkets, worksite and school food services, nutrition labeling, and nutrition education in the schools).

So how do you cut salt from your diet? What is a complex carbohydrate? How do you know if your daily diet is under 30 percent fat? What is cholesterol? How do you eat out healthfully? These questions are addressed in the following sections, and we will give practical suggestions as to how to make daily food choices that will enhance your nutritional wellness.

Nutrition Basics

Your body is a priceless machine that needs fuel. This fuel should be composed of six major nutrients: carbohydrates, proteins, fats, vitamins, minerals, and water. These nutrients fulfill three main functions in the body:

1. provide energy,
2. build and repair body tissues, and
3. regulate body processes.

Only the carbohydrates, fats, and proteins contribute energy or calories (kcal) to your diet. To function at optimal efficiency, you need a balance of each of the six essential nutrient groups.

Carbohydrates

Carbohydrates are the major source of energy for the body. In fact, they are the body's preferred form of energy. They provide 4 calories per gram. Carbohydrates are stored in the liver and in muscles in the form of **glycogen.** There is not an RDA for carbohydrate intake. Most dietitians, however, recommend that our daily caloric intake be 55 percent to 60 percent carbohydrate.[5] Carbohydrates have mistakenly earned the reputation of being fattening. If we analyze the two types of carbohydrates, this unearned reputation can be understood. Carbohydrates, with the exception of milk sugar, come from plants. The two types are *sugars*, or **simple carbohydrates,** and *starches*, or **complex carbohydrates.**

Sugars (Simple Carbohydrates)

When you see the suffix *-ose* as an ingredient on a package label (as in sucrose, fructose, dextrose, maltose) or see *corn sweetener, corn syrup, sorghum, sorbitol,* or *honey,* think *sugar.* The presence of these refined and processed sugars in our diet accounts for carbohydrates' "fattening" reputation. Instead of consuming the natural simple sugars found in fruits and vegetables, we consume too much of hidden processed sugars found in sweet desserts, soda, cookies, cereals, candy, jams, and condiments. These refined sugars have been extracted from their natural sources and have little nutritional value other than the calories they contain—hence the name "empty calories." Even if you profess not to eat sweets, you probably consume far more sugar than you realize because it is hidden in so many processed foods. For example, one average 12-ounce cola drink contains 9 teaspoons of sugar. Eight ounces of low-fat fruit yogurt contain 7 teaspoons of sugar. Jell-O is 83 percent sugar. Check your breakfast cereal. Some are nothing more than "candy" fortified with vitamins. Look for cereals with no more than 5 or 6 grams of added sugar per serving.

Starches (Complex Carbohydrates)

The starches are potatoes, rice, whole grains, beans, fruits, and vegetables. These foods are low in calories. They are nutritionally dense, a rich source of vitamins and minerals that provide a steady amount of energy for many hours. What *is* fattening are the calorie-rich additives we often add to these foods (butter, sour cream, jams, gravies, sauces). Complex carbohydrates should comprise 45 percent to 50 percent of our total caloric intake, while simple sugars should be limited to only 10 percent.[6] Carbohydrates supply many vital nutrients such as vitamins, minerals, and water. In addition, they supply an important nonnutrient: dietary fiber. **Fiber** is the part of plant food that is not digested in the small intestine, where most other foods are digested and absorbed into the bloodstream. To many people, *fiber* is synonymous with *oat bran.* Actually, fiber is not a single substance but a large group of widely different compounds with varied effects on the body. Formerly called *roughage* or *bulk,* fiber was once thought of primarily as a filler—it takes up room, leaving less space for high-fat, high-calorie items. That is still one of fiber's potential benefits, plus it is in foods rich in vitamins and minerals. But researchers now recognize that fiber plays a role in reducing the risk of heart disease, cancer, and diabetes.[7] There are two types of fiber: insoluble and soluble. Both play important roles in your nutritional health.

Insoluble fiber is from the cell walls of plants and is not digested by the body. Insoluble fiber absorbs water as it passes through the digestive tract, increasing fecal bulk. It quickens the passage of food through the system, helping to prevent constipation. This type of fiber acts as a deterrent to digestive disorders, including cancer of the colon and rectum, because it decreases the time in which your system is exposed to toxic substances in waste materials. Whole wheat bran is the richest source of insoluble fiber. This valuable bran is lost when whole wheat flour is refined to produce white flour

A fiber profile.

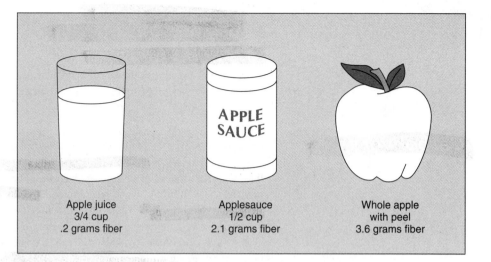

Apple juice
3/4 cup
.2 grams fiber

Applesauce
1/2 cup
2.1 grams fiber

Whole apple
with peel
3.6 grams fiber

(which is used in most breads and cereals). Lentils, skins of fruits and root vegetables, and leafy greens are other good sources of insoluble fiber.

Soluble fiber travels through the digestive tract in a gel-like form, pacing the absorption of carbohydrates. This prevents dramatic shifts in blood sugar levels and can help control diabetes. A diet rich in soluble fiber has also been shown to reduce blood cholesterol levels, especially LDL, thus reducing the risk of cardiovascular diseases. However, this effect primarily occurs when coupled with a diet low in saturated fats.[8] Oat bran, beans, vegetables, and fruits are rich sources of soluble fiber, though most plant foods contain both types of fiber. Animal foods never contain fiber.

According to the National Cancer Institute (NCI), one-third of all cancer deaths may be related to what we eat. Eating between 25 grams and 35 grams of fiber daily is recommended (about double the amount of the current American diet).[9] Since not enough is known about how each kind of fiber (soluble and insoluble) works, the NCI does not recommend any set dietary ratio for either type. Table 9.3 shows the fiber content of some common foods.

Proteins

Hundreds of different kinds of proteins make up the cells of your body. **Protein** is the major substance used to build and repair tissue, maintain chemical balance, and regulate the formation of hormones, antibodies, and enzymes. Protein can also be used as a source of energy, but only if there are not enough carbohydrates or fats available. It is not an efficient source of energy, however. When protein is broken down, the nitrogen part of the protein molecule is left over. The kidneys are overworked trying to excrete this excess nitrogen. Plus, if your body must rely on protein for energy, the protein is not available for building and repairing tissues—its real function.

Each gram of protein provides 4 calories of energy. We need protein daily, and most of us consume more than enough. Protein needs vary throughout the life cycle, due to different growth stages. Growing children need more protein per body weight than adults. Persons age 19 and older can approximate their daily protein need in grams by multiplying their weight (in pounds) by 0.36.[10]

Example: 130 lb. person × 0.36 = 46.8 or 47 grams of protein daily

To give you an idea of how little food this is, 47 grams of protein would be 4 ounces of meat (a piece roughly the size of your palm) plus 2 cups of skim milk. Most Americans consume too much protein.

Good sources of protein are found in both animal and plant sources. Meat, poultry, fish, eggs, and milk products are good sources of animal protein. Since many of these sources also contain high amounts of fat and cholesterol, you are wise to select some plant sources of protein: legumes (beans and peas), whole grains, pastas, rice, and seeds. These plant proteins are also a great source of fiber.

table 9.3

DIETARY FIBER IN FOODS

Almost all fruits, vegetables, and whole-grain products contain some of both types of fiber. You should get your fiber from a variety of the following sources.

GOOD SOURCE OF INSOLUBLE FIBER	GOOD SOURCE OF SOLUBLE FIBER
More Than 5 Grams Total Fiber	
• High-fiber wheat-bran cereal (1 oz) • Lentils (dried, cooked, 1/2 cup)	• Pinto, kidney, navy beans (dried, cooked, 1/2 cup)
2 to 5 Grams Total Fiber	
• Whole-wheat crackers (6) • Banana (medium) • Potato (medium, with skin) • Buckwheat groats (dry, 1 oz) • Shredded-wheat cereal (1 oz) • Brown rice (cooked, 1/2 cup) • Brussels sprouts, broccoli, spinach (cooked, 1/2 cup) • Wheat germ (3 Tbsp) • Whole-wheat flour (1 oz)	• Oat bran, oatmeal (dry, 1 oz) • Barley (dry, 1 oz) • Berries (1/2 cup) • Apple, pear (medium, with skin) • Orange, grapefruit (medium) • Figs, prunes, dried (3) • Okra, cabbage, peas, turnips, sweet potato (cooked, 1/2 cup) • Chickpeas, split peas, lima beans (cooked, 1/2 cup)
1 to 2 Grams Total Fiber	
• Whole-wheat bread (1 slice) • Pasta (cooked, 1 cup) • Rye bread (1 slice) • Corn (1/2 cup) • Low-fiber wheat cereal (1 oz)	• Cauliflower (cooked, 1/2 cup) • Carrots (cooked, 1/2 cup) • Peach, nectarine (medium) • Apricots (2)

Fats

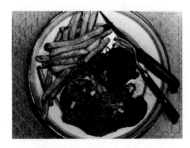

Americans have a tendency to consume a lot of meat. Why is this so?

Fat is the most concentrated form of food energy, providing 9 calories per gram, more than twice the energy provided by carbohydrates and proteins. Fat adds texture and flavor to food. It helps satisfy the appetite because it is digested more slowly. Also known as *lipids*, fats are necessary for growth and healthy skin and for transporting **fat soluble vitamins** in the body. Fats are also linked to hormone regulation. Because of their concentrated form, fats are an efficient way to store energy. Like protein, however, fats are not a good *single* source of energy. Fats burned for energy in the absence of carbohydrates produce a toxic waste product called *ketone bodies*. *Ketosis*, a buildup of poisonous **ketone bodies,** causes fatigue and nausea and overtaxes the kidneys, resulting in nerve and brain damage. Fat is burned more completely in the presence of carbohydrates, another reason to have a diet high in complex carbohydrates (and to avoid weight-loss diets that promote very low carbohydrate and calorie intakes).

An important distinction should be made among the three types of fatty acids. Ninety-five percent of all dietary fat consists of molecules called **triglycerides,** which are made up of fatty acids. The three types of fatty acids are classified according to the number of additional places available for atoms of hydrogen. Table 9.4 on page 192 identifies and compares the three types of fats.

table 9.4

COMPARISON OF THE THREE TYPES OF FATS

	CHARACTERISTICS	EXAMPLES	

Saturated

```
    H   H   H   H
    |   |   |   |
H – C – C – C – C – H
    |   |   |   |
    H   H   H   H
```

- No more room for hydrogen atoms
- In animal products and some vegetable products
- Raises cholesterol levels in the blood
- Solid at room temperature

Coconut oil	Butter
Palm oil	Milk
Cheese	Beef
Hot dogs	Bacon
Chocolate	Lard
Cocoa butter	Pork
Poultry skin	Lamb
Luncheon meats	Veal
Non-dairy cream	Cream
substitutes	Sour cream

Monounsaturated

```
    H   H   H   H   H   H
    |   |   |   |   |   |
H – C – C – C = C – C – C – H
    |   |           |   |
    H   H           H   H
```

- Can accept 2 more hydrogen atoms
- No effect on cholesterol levels in the blood

Peanut oil	Olives
Olive oil	Peanuts
Avocados	Cashews
Canola (rapeseed) oil	

Polyunsaturated

```
    H   H   H   H   H   H   H   H
    |   |   |   |   |   |   |   |
H – C – C = C – C – C = C – C – H
    |       |           |
    H       H           H
```

- Can accept 4 more hydrogen atoms
- Lowers blood cholesterol

Corn oil	Fish
Cottonseed oil	Pecans
Soybean oil	Walnuts
Safflower oil	
Sesame oil	
Sunflower oil	
Mayonnaise	
Almonds	
Most margarines	

C = Carbon Atom

H = Hydrogen Atom

FAT COMPARISON

	Saturated Fat	Monounsaturated Fat	Polyunsaturated Fat	Cholesterol mg/Tbsp
Canola Oil	6%	62%	32%	0
Safflower Oil	10%	13%	77%	0
Sunflower Oil	11%	20%	69%	0
Corn Oil	13%	25%	62%	0
Olive Oil	14%	77%	9%	0
Soybean Oil	15%	24%	61%	0
Cottonseed Oil	27%	19%	54%	0
Chicken Fat	30%	48%	22%	11
Lard	41%	47%	12%	12
Palm Oil	51%	39%	10%	0
Butter	54%	30%	16%	33
Coconut Oil	77%	6%	17%	0

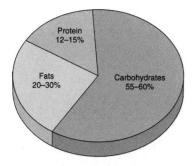

Daily diet recommendations.

An easy observation shows that, with a few exceptions, animal fats are generally more saturated, whereas most vegetable fats are unsaturated. Additionally, all animal fats contain cholesterol, but vegetable foods have no natural presence of cholesterol. Diets high in fat, especially **saturated fat,** have a strong link to heart disease and stroke. They elevate blood cholesterol levels that, in turn, can lead to clogged arteries (atherosclerosis). **Polyunsaturated fat** is the healthier fat to consume.

We eat too much fat. Americans currently consume approximately 37 percent to 40 percent of their daily calories in fats—much of which is saturated.[11] It is recommended that our diet consist of no more than 30 percent fat (10 percent of each type).[12] Some nutritionists emphasize an even more prudent recommendation of only 10 percent to 20 percent of daily calories from fat. The excessive fat in our diet is the main reason America leads the world in heart disease deaths. Thirty to 40 percent of all cancers in men and 60 percent of all cancers in women have been attributed to diet, with excess fat being linked to cancer more frequently than any other dietary factor.[13] Excess dietary fat is linked to cancer of the colon, breast, and prostate. It should be noted that the amount and type of dietary fat eaten—not the amount of cholesterol consumed—have the greatest impact on the blood cholesterol level. Dietary cholesterol also affects the level of blood cholesterol but to a lesser and more variable extent than does the fat content of the diet.[14]

Monounsaturated fat and polyunsaturated oils can be turned into solid saturated fats by a manufacturing process called **hydrogenation.** This technique adds hydrogen atoms to these fats as a way to prolong the shelf life of a product. Avoid completely and partially hydrogenated oils. Like saturated fats, they elevate your blood cholesterol level. Some margarines contain partially hydrogenated oils and may be acceptable if they contain twice as many polyunsaturated as saturated fats. As a rule, if the first ingredient listed on any product is hydrogenated vegetable oil, avoid using it. Table 9.5 shows you how to figure your daily fat allowance in order to adhere to the 30 percent fat-calorie guidelines recommended in the *Dietary Guidelines for Americans.*

With so much emphasis on low-fat eating, some may try to cut their fat grams to almost zero. A little dietary fat is necessary for basic metabolic functions. A minimum of 15 to 25 grams per day should satisfy these requirements.[15]

Cholesterol

Cholesterol is not a true fat. It is a fatlike waxy substance found in animal tissue. It plays a vital role in the body's functioning. Your liver manufactures cholesterol (all that you physically need), and you consume it by eating animal products (meat, egg yolks, cheese, dairy products, liver). Since a diet high in fats and cholesterol has been linked to atherosclerosis, you are prudent to limit animal products in your diet. It is recommended that you reduce cholesterol consumption to 300 milligrams per day.[16] (Remember, vegetable foods contain no cholesterol, unless it is added in processing or

table 9.5

DETERMINING YOUR FAT ALLOWANCE

This example is for a person who consumes 2,000 calories a day:

30% × 2,000 calories = 600 calories

600 calories ÷ 9 (calories per gram) = 66.6 or 67 grams of total fat recommended per day.
(The saturated variety should *only* be 200 calories or 22.2 grams!)

An easy way to *estimate* your fat gram limit per day is to divide your ideal weight in half. Keep your number of fat grams per day under this number. (If your ideal weight is 140 lbs., your fat gram limit should be 70 gms per day.)

food preparation.) Table 9.6 gives you an idea of the amount of fat, cholesterol, *and* sodium in commonly eaten foods. Appendix 8 has a more detailed list.

Fish Oils

Studies of the diets of Eskimos and Asian fishermen have revealed interesting information about fats. Their diets provide 40 percent of daily calories from fats. Yet Eskimos are listed among people with the lowest rates of heart disease in the world. Why? They eat lots of fish, and fish are rich in polyunsaturated fats called **omega-3.** A diet rich in omega-3 fatty acids inhibits atherosclerosis in coronary arteries and can reduce the blood cholesterol level. The best omega-3 sources are salmon, mackerel, herring, tuna, and sardines. Therefore, eating fish once or twice a week is a sound dietary practice.

Vitamins

Vitamins are the organic catalysts necessary to initiate the body's complex metabolic functions. Although these chemical substances are vital to life, they are required in minute amounts. Because of our adequate food supply, symptoms of vitamin deficiencies are rare. However, some factors may alter one's requirements (aging, illness, stress, pregnancy, smoking, dieting). Vitamins fall into two categories: fat soluble and water soluble. Vitamins A, D, E, and K are **fat soluble vitamins** which means they are transported and stored by the body's fat cells and liver. They are stored in the body for relatively long periods (many months). Vitamin C and the B-complexes are **water soluble vitamins.** They remain in various body tissues for a short time (usually only a few weeks). Excesses are excreted out of the body.

Are vitamin supplements necessary? It is important to remember that vitamins do not contain energy or calories. Therefore, extra vitamins will not provide more energy or power. Eating a variety of foods is a preferred way to maintain an adequate intake of vitamins. However, in today's lifestyle, some people may not be consuming a varied and balanced diet. Manufacturer's processing and preserving, food irradiation and chemical pollution, nutrient-depleted soil, and shipping and storage practices have significantly reduced the nutritional value of our foods. Other lifestyle practices, such as smoking, consuming alcohol, and using drugs such as aspirin and oral contraceptives, may increase the need for vitamin or mineral supplementation. Most medical authorities have been reluctant to recommend supplements on a broad scale for healthy people eating healthy diets. However, the accumulation of research in recent years has shown that extra amounts of certain vitamins (especially the antioxidants) may play a significant role in disease prevention.[17] Consult your health professional to assess your personal needs.

RDA

The National Academy of Sciences National Research Council periodically reviews current research on the nutritional needs of healthy Americans in order to establish recommended amounts of nutrients. These recommendations are called **Recommended Dietary Allowances (RDA).** The RDA are the amounts considered to be adequate to meet the nutritional needs of practically all healthy persons. Not all essential nutrients have an RDA. Water, carbohydrates, essential fatty acids, and many trace elements are not included.

In most cases, the RDA are higher than the amount needed to prevent nutritional diseases. For example, the body needs only 10 milligrams daily of vitamin C to prevent scurvy. The adult RDA for vitamin C is 60 milligrams. Since the RDA are established for healthy populations, they do not pertain to individuals who have special nutritional requirements as a result of special physical conditions or use of certain medications.

Minerals

Minerals are inorganic substances critical to many enzyme functions in the body. Two groups of minerals are necessary to the diet: macrominerals and trace minerals. **Macrominerals** are needed in large doses (more than 100 mg daily). Examples are calcium, phosphorus, magnesium, potassium, and sodium. **Trace minerals** are needed in much smaller amounts. Examples are iron, zinc, copper, iodine, and fluoride.

Three minerals deserve special attention: calcium, iron, and sodium.

Calcium

Calcium is the body's most abundant mineral and is critical to many body functions. If the calcium supply in the blood is too low, the body withdraws calcium from the bones.

table 9.6

FAT, CHOLESTEROL, AND SODIUM CHECKLIST

	FAT (GMS)	CHOLES-TEROL (MGS)	SODIUM (MGS)		FAT (GMS)	CHOLES-TEROL (MGS)	SODIUM (MGS)
frozen green beans (1 cup)	0.2	0	17	**McDonald's**			
fish sticks (3 oz, breaded)	10	95	494	Qtr. Pounder with Cheese	29	118	1,150
banana	<1	0	1	Large fries	22	16	200
canned peaches (1 cup)	0.1	0	11	Egg McMuffin	11	226	740
Frosted Flakes (1 cup)	<1	0	247	Chunky chicken salad	3	78	230
toaster pastry	6	0	230	Egg & Sausage Biscuit	35	275	1,250
apple	1	0	1	Hot cakes with syrup	9	21	640
stuffing mix (1 cup prepared)	2	0	1,100	Apple pie	15	0	240
frozen waffle	4	0	256	**Taco Bell**			
hamburger patty (3 oz)	16	74	65				
pork and beans (1 cup)	17	15	1,105	Bean Burrito	12	5	—
cottage cheese (4% fat, 1 cup)	10	34	911	Light Bean Burrito	6	5	—
cottage cheese (2% fat, 1 cup)	4	19	918	Soft Taco	12	30	—
American cheese (1 oz, processed)	9	27	405	Light Soft Taco	5	25	—
				Taco Salad	55	80	—
mozzarella cheese (skim, 1 oz)	5	16	132	Light Taco Salad (without chips)	9	50	—
cr. of chicken soup (1 cup)	12	27	1,046	**Subway**			
canned spaghetti (1 cup)	10	39	1,220				
chicken breast (3 oz, roasted)	7	72	60	Cold cut combo	41	166	2,278
hard boiled egg	5	213	62	Seafood and crab	58	56	2,027
peanut butter (2 Tbsp)	16	0	154	Turkey breast	20	67	2,520
tuna (oil packed, 3 oz)	7	15	301	Roast beef	24	75	2,348
orange juice (1 cup)	0.2	0	3	Ham & cheese	18	73	1,710
bacon (2 slices)	6	11	202	**Other**			
bologna (1 slice)	6	17	335				
glazed yeast donut	11	13	117	Wendy's chili	7	45	750
broccoli (1 cup)	0.3	0	24	Wendy's broccoli & cheese potato	16	0	470
sirloin steak (3 oz)	15	77	54	KFC thigh	30	129	688
fried shrimp (3 oz)	10	150	292	KFC chicken sandwich	27	47	1,060
baked potato	0.2	0	16	Long John Silver's 3 pc. fish	44	100	1,890
potato au gratin (1 cup from mix)	32	0	1,078	Long John Silver's light portion fish with lemon	4	75	900
macaroni and cheese (box mix prepared, 1 cup with 2% milk)	16	15	730	Burger King Whopper	36	104	990
grapes (1 cup)	0.3	0	2	Burger King Bacon Double Cheeseburger	31	105	795
barbeque sauce (2 Tbsp)	<1	0	254	Hardees grilled chicken	9	60	890
pork sausage (2 oz patty)	18	48	732	Hardees biscuit & gravy	24	15	1,250
chocolate coated peanuts (1 oz)	12	0	16	Pizza Hut personal pan pizza (pepperoni)	29	53	—
whole wheat bread (1 slice)	1	0	178				
pepperoni pizza (1 slice) (1/5 of 12″)	17	40	700				

table 9.7

OPTIMAL CALCIUM REQUIREMENTS (RECOMMENDATIONS OF THE NATIONAL INSTITUTES OF HEALTH)

AGE	CALCIUM MG/DAY
6–10	800–1,200
11–24	1,200–1,500
25–65 men and 25–50 women	1,000
pregnant and lactating women	1,200
postmenopausal women on estrogen	1,000
postmenopausal women not on estrogen and adults over 65	1,500

for your information:

1 cup yogurt = 400 mg	1 cup cottage cheese = 150 mg
1 cup milk = 300 mg	1½ oz cheese = 350 mg
1 cup cooked broccoli = 70 mg	3 oz sardines = 370 mg

This inadequate supply of calcium is a major factor contributing to **osteoporosis,** an age-related condition of insufficient bone mass. Healthy bone is living tissue that is continuously being replenished. In fact, an adult body replaces about 20 percent of its bone each year.[18] In osteoporosis, the formation of bone fails to keep pace with lost bone tissue. The result is porous, brittle bones susceptible to fracture. Women are more susceptible to osteoporosis because they have smaller, less dense bones.

In the United States and Canada, osteoporosis affects more than 25 million women over the age of 45.[19] Since some bone loss is normal with aging in both males and females, it is important that you build strong bones now. Consumption of adequate dietary calcium from preadolescence through young adulthood is critical for building bone mass. Current calcium consumption is dangerously low among teenagers, adult women, and the elderly. It's estimated that half of Americans consume less than 600 milligrams of calcium daily.[20]

Your present habits may determine your bone density later in life. In fact, bone continues to be laid down until about age 30, even though adult height is likely to be reached between age 16 and 20.[21] Therefore, the amount of bone mass you have around age 30 influences susceptibility to brittle bones in the future. Mean bone mass remains essentially unchanged between age 30 and the onset of menopause, after which women lose 2 percent to 5 percent each year until approximately five years after menopause. At that time, bone loss becomes more gradual.[22] Osteoporosis cannot be cured—it can only be prevented or its progression delayed. See Table 9.7 for the recommended calcium intake for various age groups.

To keep those bone "banks" filled do the following:

1. Eat calcium-rich foods every day—low-fat dairy products, spinach, broccoli, fish with edible bones (salmon, sardines).
2. Get regular vigorous exercise (exercises that create muscular contraction and gravitational pull on the long bones, such as walking, gentle jogging, and aerobics).
3. Do not smoke. Smoking reduces the production of estrogen, negatively affecting calcium absorption.
4. Avoid excesses of protein, sodium, alcohol, caffeine, and phosphates (in most colas), which accelerate the excretion of calcium in the urine. (Too many young adults are drinking soft drinks rather than milk.)

5. Be sure to consume foods rich in vitamins A and D to enhance absorption of calcium (no need to exceed the RDA, however).
6. If you have a lactose intolerance (have trouble digesting dairy products), lactose-free products are available at some stores. Or experiment with dairy foods lowest in lactose: ricotta, mozzarella, parmesan, American, and cheddar cheeses; tofu; some yogurts; sherbet; 1 percent low-fat cottage cheese.
7. If a high calcium intake through foods is impossible, consider a calcium supplement—ideally in the form of calcium citrate or calcium carbonate, which are more readily absorbed.

Iron

A low intake of iron is a common nutritional problem for women. Due to menstruation, women need to ingest more iron than men (women need 15 milligrams daily; men need 10 milligrams).[23] Iron deficiency may cause chronic fatigue and listlessness. To increase your iron intake take the following steps:

1. Eat foods rich in iron (lean meats, poultry, fish, fortified cereals and grains, green vegetables, beans, and peas).
2. Consume iron-rich foods together with foods high in vitamin C to triple iron absorption (a hamburger and tomato; cereal and orange juice).
3. Keep consumption of tea and coffee under 3 cups per day (caffeine reduces the absorption of iron).
4. Use cast-iron cookware (iron is absorbed into the food in a form that is readily assimilated into the body).

Sodium

Your body needs sodium to survive. The National Research Council recommends 1,100 milligrams to 3,300 milligrams of sodium a day as a safe and adequate range (about one-half teaspoon to 1 and one-half teaspoon of salt).[24] Many Americans consume much, much more than that daily: 5,000 to 10,000 milligrams! We consume sodium most commonly in the form of table salt and in the processed foods we eat. Even if you never salt your food, 90 percent of all processed foods contain sodium—even milk does. In this way, sodium becomes "hidden" in our diet. Sodium is also present in other popular condiments, such as monosodium glutamate (MSG), meat tenderizer, ketchup, salsa, soy sauce, mustard, barbecue sauce, and baking soda. It is even present in many medications—antacids, for instance. Fast-food restaurants often add sodium to their products. Eating a McDonald's Quarter Pounder with Cheese, large fries, and a chocolate shake will give 1,590 milligrams of sodium. This is the total recommended daily allotment of sodium consumed in one meal. Look at Table 9.6 and compare the sodium content in processed and unprocessed foods. Which has more salt, a McDonald's apple pie or french fries? Were you right? "Hidden" salt is a problem in this age of processed foods. Since excess sodium consumption has been one factor linked to hypertension in some sodium sensitive individuals, be conscious of your sodium intake, and try to keep it within the recommended range. (Table 9.8 lists vitamins and minerals, their functions, good food sources of each, and the adult RDA.)

Water

Water is often called the forgotten nutrient. However, it is *the most important* nutrient because it serves as the medium in which the other nutrients are transported. Almost all of the body's metabolic reactions occur in this medium. Water also helps rid the body of wastes, aids in metabolizing stored fat, and helps control body temperature. Water composes approximately two-thirds of your body weight. Your exact percentage of water weight varies depending on your body composition. Lean tissue contains more water than does fat tissue. Lean muscle tissue is about 73 percent water; fat tissue is only 20 percent water. While you could survive for weeks without food, you could only last a few days without water. Some nutritionists claim that the average American is in a constant state of dehydration. Drink plenty of fluids daily. The minimum amount of water a

table 9.8

VITAMINS AND MINERALS

VITAMINS	FUNCTIONS	SOURCES	ADULT RDA*
Fat Soluble			
A	Promotes growth and repair of body tissues; keeps skin cells moist; builds resistance to infection; promotes bone and tooth development; aids in vision	Green leafy vegetables, yellow fruits and vegetables, eggs, butter, margarine, cheese, milk, liver	800–1,000 mcg** RE***
D	Regulates absorption of calcium and phosphorus; promotes normal growth of bone and teeth	Vitamin D fortified dairy products, fish, eggs, fortified margarines, sunlight (absorbed through the skin)	5–10 mcg
E	Essential in preventing oxidation of other vitamins and fatty acids; maintains cell structure	Vegetable oil, green and leafy vegetables, whole grains, egg yolks, nuts, wheat germ	8–10 mg****
K	Aids in blood clotting	Cabbage, cauliflower, spinach, green vegetables, liver, cereals	60–80 mcg
Water Soluble			
C (Ascorbic acid)	Builds resistance to infection; aids in tissue repair and healing; involved in tooth and bone formation	Citrus fruits, strawberries, tomatoes, potatoes, melons, broccoli, peppers, cabbage	60 mg
B_1 (Thiamin)	Needed to convert carbohydrates into energy; promotes normal function of nervous system	Whole grains, fortified grain products, milk, pork, legumes, nuts, meats	1.0–1.5 mg
B_2 (Riboflavin)	Combines with proteins to make enzymes that affect function of eyes, skin, nervous system, and stomach	Meat, dairy products, whole grains, green leafy vegetables	1.2–1.7 mg
B_3 (Niacin)	Aids in energy production from fats and carbohydrates	Meat, poultry, fish, liver, nuts, whole grains, legumes	13–19 mg
B_6	Aids in protein metabolism and red blood cell formation	Whole grains, meat, fish, poultry, legumes, milk, green leafy vegetables	1.6–2.0 mg
Folic acid (Folacin)	Aids in red blood cell formation; aids in synthesizing genetic material	Meat, poultry, fish, eggs, broccoli, asparagus, legumes	180–200 mcg
B_{12}	Aids in function of all body cells and nervous tissue	Animal foods only; meat, poultry, fish, eggs, dairy products	2 mg

healthy person should drink is eight to ten 8-ounce glasses a day. More is recommended if you are overweight, exercise a lot, or live in a hot climate. Water is also a component of many foods (i.e., apples, lettuce, melons, potatoes, green beans, fruit juices). Are you getting enough water? If so, your urine is clear, almost colorless.

Antioxidants

Research is exploding in a new area of dietary study: study examining the power of certain nutrients to ward off chronic diseases. Known as **antioxidants,** vitamin C, vitamin E, beta-carotene, and selenium, when ingested in quantities far beyond the RDA, have

table 9.8—cont.

VITAMINS AND MINERALS

MINERALS	FUNCTIONS	SOURCES	ADULT RDA*
Macrominerals			
Calcium	Aids in bone and tooth formation; aids in utilization of phosphorus; helps muscle contraction and heart function	Dairy products, green leafy vegetables, broccoli, fish	800–1,500 mg
Phosphorus	Aids in all metabolism and energy production	Dairy products, eggs, meat, fish, poultry, legumes, whole grains	800–1,200 mg
Magnesium	Activates important enzyme reactions	Whole grains, nuts, legumes, green vegetables	280–350 mg
Potassium	Regulates body fluids and the transfer of nutrients across cell walls	Citrus fruits, juices, bananas, potatoes	2,000–5,000 mg
Sodium	Regulates body fluids in cells; aids in muscle contraction	Table salt, milk, seafood (abundant in most foods except fruits)	1,100–3,300 mg
Trace			
Iron	Essential for oxygen transport in the blood	Liver, meat, poultry, fish, dried fruit, whole grains, legumes, green vegetables	10–15 mg
Zinc	Aids in metabolism and growth of tissue	Seafood, poultry, eggs, whole grains, vegetables	12–15 mg
Copper	Involved with iron in the formation of red blood cells	Liver, nuts, shellfish, meat, poultry, vegetables	1.5–3.0 mg
Iodine	Forms thyroid hormone, affecting overall metabolism	Iodized salt, seafood	150 mcg
Fluoride	Involved in formation of bones and teeth	Fluoridated water, seafood, green vegetables	1.5–4.0 mg

*Adult RDA values from National Academy of Sciences—National Research Council. *Recommened Dietary Allowances*, 10th ed. Washington, D.C.: National Academy of Sciences, 1989.
**mcg = micrograms.
***RE = retinol equivalents, a measurement of Vitamin A activity
****mg = milligrams

shown promise in warding off cardiovascular disease, certain cancers, hypertension, and even cataracts.[25] Antioxidants are compounds that come to the aid of every cell in the body that faces an ongoing barrage of damage because of the normal oxygenation process (living and breathing), environmental pollution, chemicals and pesticides, additives in our processed foods, stress hormones, and even sun radiation. Studies continue to accumulate about the ability of antioxidants, various carotenoids (the hundreds of phytochemicals in fruits and vegetables that give them their characteristic yellow, green, and orange coloring), and even garlic and green tea to suppress cell deterioration and strengthen the immune system.[26] Many prominent medical investigators (Dr. Kenneth Cooper, Cooper Institute for Aerobics Research; Dr. William Castelli, Director of Framingham Heart Study; and Dr. Jeffrey Blumberg, USDA Human Nutrition Research

Center) advocate supplementing the diet with disease-fighting antioxidants.[27] This exciting new development will continue to command more research and study. The National Cancer Institute alone is now supporting more than 20 research studies on the effects of antioxidants and phytochemicals on cancer.[28] Realizing the power of these substances, Americans need to take action by eating a wide variety of fruits and vegetables—at least five servings per day!

Why not just take a supplement? Millions of Americans do, believing that they cannot get all the antioxidants and phytochemicals into their diets. Remember to consult a knowledgeable health professional before taking dietary supplements, since megadoses of some nutrients can cause side effects and can be toxic.

Antioxidant All-Stars

- broccoli
- green and red peppers
- cantaloupe
- spinach
- carrots
- tomatoes
- strawberries
- kale
- brussels sprouts
- pumpkin
- sweet potatoes
- cabbage

The Well-Balanced Diet

Eating healthy is exciting. Nutritious eating does not doom you to "nutrition martyrdom"—eating flavorless foods, counting grams, measuring portions, or passing up favorite desserts. Eating right means having a wide variety of foods, in moderation, throughout the week. There are no "forbidden" or "bad" foods—only bad eating habits! If you have a high-fat snack one day, make sure you balance it with restraint at other meals. Eating should remain one of life's simple pleasures. Americans are fortunate to have food choices that are varied, plentiful, and safe to eat. Nutritionists often refer to three words when attempting to simplify the principles of good nutrition: *variety, balance*, and *moderation*. Do you eat the same thing for breakfast every day? For lunch? For snacks? Despite our access to diverse foods, we have a tendency to consume relatively few types of foods and often become locked into standard meals that many times are culturally influenced. Why not have spaghetti, rice, chili, or pizza for breakfast rather than eggs, bacon, and donuts? The seven dietary guidelines provide a sound framework for helping us make food choices.

In 1956, the U.S. Department of Agriculture (USDA) introduced the "basic four food groups" to graphically convey healthy nutrition to Americans. For almost four decades, the "basic four" (dairy products, meats, fruits and vegetables, breads and grains) were drawn on school chalkboards and printed in nutrition booklets. As the science of nutrition grew more sophisticated, and the roles of fats and carbohydrates became better understood, the "basic four" design came under fire. Nutritionists argued that giving dairy products and meats equal emphasis with fruits, vegetables, and grains has caused heart disease and some cancers. In 1992, the USDA introduced the Food Guide Pyramid (Fig. 9.1), with grains taking up the largest space on the bottom, as the foundation of our diet. Fruits and vegetables are the next largest component. Meat, dairy, and fats occupy smaller spaces near the top. Eating according to this pyramid, with the greatest emphasis on grains, fruits, and vegetables, is the key to sound nutrition and is in harmony with the *Dietary Guidelines*. Of course, fats and sugars can be added to grains, fruits, and vegetables (with sauces, toppings, and preparation methods), making them less healthy choices. It is up to you to make wise choices.

To further promote healthy eating, the National Cancer Institute initiated a national "Five a Day for Better Health" program to encourage Americans to eat five or more fruits and vegetables every day. When this campaign began in 1991, only 23 percent of the population were consuming this recommended amount.[29] You have probably seen examples of this massive campaign—television and magazine ads, billboards, and even grocery bag notices. Think about your dietary intake during the past three days. Did you consume "five a day"?

FIGURE 9.1 ➤

Food guide pyramid: a guide to daily food choices.

source: U.S. Department of Agriculture, Human Nutrition Information Service; USDA's Food Guide Pyramid, *Home and Garden Bulletin* No. 249 (1992).

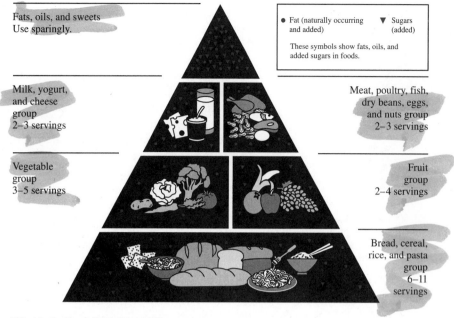

Fats, oils, and sweets
Use sparingly.

● Fat (naturally occurring and added)   ▼ Sugars (added)

These symbols show fats, oils, and added sugars in foods.

Milk, yogurt, and cheese group
2–3 servings

Meat, poultry, fish, dry beans, eggs, and nuts group
2–3 servings

Vegetable group
3–5 servings

Fruit group
2–4 servings

Bread, cereal, rice, and pasta group
6–11 servings

What is the Food Guide Pyramid?

The Pyramid is an outline of what to eat each day. It's not a rigid prescription but a general guide that lets you choose a healthful diet that's right for you.

The Pyramid calls for eating a variety of foods to get the nutrients you need and at the same time the right amount of calories to maintain a healthy weight.

The Pyramid also focuses on fat because most American diets are too high in fat, especially saturated fat.

Fat

● In general, foods that come from animals (milk and meat groups) are naturally higher in fat than foods that come from plants. But there are many low-fat dairy and lean meat choices available, and these foods can be prepared in ways that lower fat.

Fruits, vegetables, and grain products are naturally low in fat. But many popular items are prepared with fat, such as french-fried potatoes or croissants, making them higher-fat choices.

Added sugars

▼ These symbols represent sugars added to foods in processing or at the table, not the sugars found naturally in fruits and milk. It's the added sugars that provide calories with few vitamins and minerals.

Most of the added sugars in the typical American diet come from foods in the Pyramid tip—soft drinks, candy, jams, jellies, syrups, and table sugar we add to foods such as coffee or cereal.

Added sugars in the food groups come from foods such as ice cream, sweetened yogurt, chocolate milk, canned or frozen fruit with heavy syrup, and sweetened bakery products such as cakes and cookies.

What counts as a serving?

Milk, yogurt, and cheese group (2–3 servings)	Meat, poultry, fish, dry beans, eggs, and nuts group (2–3 servings)	Vegetable group (3–5 servings)	Fruit group (2–4 servings)	Bread, cereal, rice, and pasta group (6–11 servings)
1 c. milk or yogurt 1 1/2 oz. natural cheese 2 oz. processed cheese 1 c. frozen yogurt 1 1/2 c. ice cream 2 c. cottage cheese	2–3 oz. cooked, lean meat, poultry, or fish 1/3 c. nuts (Count 1/2 c. cooked dry beans, 1 egg, or 2 Tbls. peanut butter as 1 oz. meat.)	1 c. raw leafy greens 1/2 c. other kinds of vegetables (raw or cooked) 3/4 c. vegetable juice	1 medium apple, banana, orange 1/2 c. chopped, cooked, canned fruit 3/4 c. juice	1 slice bread 1/2 bun or bagel 1 oz. dry cereal 1/2 c. cooked cereal, rice, or pasta 3–4 small, plain crackers

Making Positive Changes

All of this information about nutrition can seem confusing and sometimes appear contradictory; for example, how do you consume enough meat for iron, yet reduce saturated fat? If you make sure you get plenty of calcium, how do you watch out for those high-fat dairy products? Eggs are a good source of protein, but how do you make sure daily cholesterol milligrams don't exceed 300? You certainly hear enough about what *not* to eat. Since we believe in a positive approach to a wellness lifestyle, Table 9.9 gives many tips to help you eat more nutritiously in today's fast-paced world. These suggestions are ways to incorporate the dietary guidelines into sensible and simple practices. In fact, studies have shown that significant changes in your nutritional health can be accomplished with *simple* changes, without excluding commercially prepared foods or drastically reducing the amount of food you eat.[30] For example, using Prochaska's behavior change model (see Chapter 1), clients have been successful in lowering and maintaining their dietary fat intake to below 30 percent of their calories by using five specific action-based techniques:[31]

1. switching to low-fat or nonfat cheeses
2. eating bread, rolls, and muffins without butter or margarine
3. taking the skin off all chicken
4. using low-cal or nonfat salad dressings
5. periodically eating fruit or veggies as snacks

People eat food, not numbers. So rather than focusing on constant measuring, counting, and weighing, dietary change should involve practical changes that can become lifetime habits. It is not advisable or possible to do a complete overhaul of your diet. After reading this chapter, do not go to your refrigerator and throw everything out. It is easier, and usually more lasting, to make small and gradual changes. Realize that no one is perfect or eats perfectly all of the time. Just remember that you do have choices. As you pursue wellness, try to do the best you can with the knowledge that you have about nutrition. Perhaps some of these suggestions could become a central goal for writing a behavior change contract (as discussed in Chapter 1).

A good way to assess your nutritional habits is to record everything you eat for three to seven days in a log. By actually observing types and quantities of food consumed, you can best judge if your diet is nutritionally sound—that is, if it conforms to the *Dietary Guidelines* and mimics the Food Guide Pyramid. Keeping a log can help you set goals for making positive dietary changes. You can write your own food log. (There is a sample Food Log form in the Activities Section at the end of the book.) An appendix with the nutritive value of many foods is also provided at the end of the book. You may prefer to use one of the many computer programs that are available for dietary assessment. It is tedious to keep records for several days, but this experience creates an awareness of food choices and quantities as well as of where improvements can be made.

Nutrition Labeling

Now that you understand the basics of nutrition, how do you find out the actual nutritional content of the foods you are eating? You do this by reading labels. Read about what you are eating. Part of self-responsibility is becoming a nutritionwise consumer. The federal government regulates food labeling. In the past, nutrition labeling was voluntary. Only foods fortified with protein, vitamins, or minerals or making a nutrition claim had to be labeled. As a result, only about half of the processed foods regulated by the Food and Drug Administration were labeled. With a new era of health consciousness, consumers began demanding reliable information on food packages. In 1990, the president signed the Nutrition Labeling and Education Act into law. No longer are food producers and marketers able to mislead, confuse, or make false claims about foods. The goal of the new law is simple: to provide food labeling that the public can understand and count on and that will bring people up-to-date about today's health concerns. The act has three objectives: (1) to clear up confusion; (2) to help consumers make healthy choices; and (3) to encourage food companies to produce healthier foods (to make them work on the "insides" of the package, instead of merely tinkering with the words on the label).[32] The new

table 9.9

THIRTY TIPS FOR NUTRITIONAL WELLNESS

1. Use fresh, unprocessed foods whenever possible.

2. Remove the skin from poultry (the source of most of the fat).

3. Eat low-fat dairy products. There are plenty of reduced fat cheeses available. Switch to skim or 1 percent milk.

4. Try salsa on baked potatoes for a nonfat topping.

5. Trim all excess fat from meats; eat leaner cuts of red meats (i.e., "loin" or "round"). "Select" is lower in fat than "choice" or "prime."

6. Eat fish once or twice a week (baked or broiled, *not* fried or breaded).

7. Instead of focusing a meal around a meat, use a small amount of meat (diced, shaved, chopped, sliced) to mix in with other vegetables and rice or pasta.

8. Steam, bake, broil, or roast foods using a cooking rack to allow fat to drain from the food.

9. Select salad oils, cooking oils, and margarines made with unsaturated fats. Soft, tub margarines with liquid oil listed as the first ingredient are good choices.

10. Try bagels, muffins, or whole wheat toast with jam or apple butter (without butter or margarine), rather than croissants, donuts, sweet rolls, or biscuits.

11. Use a nonstick vegetable oil spray for sautéing.

12. Use deli luncheon meats such as shaved chicken breast and turkey instead of high-fat bologna, salami, beef, or hot dogs.

13. Remove the salt shaker from the table; experiment with recipes by substituting herbs and other seasoning for salt.

14. Use applesauce in place of the oil in brownie, cookie, and cake recipes.

15. Replace snack items such as potato chips, salted nuts, and crackers with fresh fruit, raw vegetables, unsalted, unbuttered popcorn, pretzels, or rice cakes.

16. Use plain, low-fat yogurt as a substitute for sour cream in dips and on baked potatoes. Fat-free sour cream and cream cheese are now available.

17. Eat a meatless dinner several nights a week.

18. Use ground turkey in casseroles, chili, spaghetti sauce, and skillet dinners that normally require ground beef.

19. When making scrambled eggs, separate the eggs, eliminating half of the yolks. If a recipe calls for one egg, substitute two egg whites to reduce the cholesterol.

20. After making soups and broths, chili; scrape off the congealed fat.

21. Substitute fruit juices or plain water for soft drinks.

22. Top off your meals with fresh fruit for a nutritionally "sweet" dessert. Try frozen yogurt, juice bars, vanilla wafers, fig newtons, or angel food cake to satisfy your sweet tooth.

23. Read labels; learn about what you are eating.

24. Take advantage of the new nonfat chips, dips, snacks, cereals, cookies, and crackers that are appearing on grocery shelves almost daily. (Remember, however, that "no fat" doesn't necessarily mean "no calories.")

25. Try canned fruit with natural juices as a tasty topping for pancakes and french toast, rather than use butter and syrup.

26. Top pizzas and baked potatoes with broccoli, mushrooms, zucchini, peppers, and so on rather than meats.

27. Try powdered "nonbutter" sprinkles or "butterlike" sprays as toppings for vegetables.

28. Make burritoes and tacos with beans, peas, and lentils as fillers.

29. Use breads and cereals that list "whole wheat or "whole grain" as the first ingredient.

30. Select cereals with at least 2 grams of fiber but no more than 2 grams of fat per serving.

Serving sizes are standardized to reflect the amounts of foods people actually eat. They are also expressed in both common household and metric measures. (You should note whether you are consuming more than one serving.)

This mandatory list of nutrients includes those most important to today's consumers. In the past, the concern was vitamin and mineral deficiencies. Now the worries pertain to fat, cholesterol, sodium, types of carbohydrates, and protein amounts.

This means that in a 2,000 calorie diet 65 grams is equal to 30 percent fat.

This information can help you calculate what percentage of calories of this food comes from fat, carbohydrates, and protein.
e.g.:
TOTAL FAT = 13g
13g x 9 = 117 calories
117 ÷ 260 = .45
This macaroni and cheese is 45% fat.
TOTAL CARBOHYDRATE = 31g
31g x 4 = 124 calories
124 ÷ 260 = .476
This macaroni and cheese is 48% carbohydrate.
TOTAL PROTEIN = 5g
5g x 4 = 20 calories
20 ÷ 260 = .076
This macaroni and cheese is 7% protein.

MACARONI AND CHEESE

Nutrition Facts

Serving Size 1/2 cup (114g)
Servings Per Container 4

Amount Per Serving

Calories 260   Calories from Fat 120

	% Daily Value*
Total Fat 13g	20%
Saturated Fat 5g	25%
Cholesterol 30mg	10%
Sodium 660 mg	28%
Total Carbohydrate 31g	11%
Sugars 5g	**
Dietary Fiber 0g	0%
Protein 5g	**

Vitamin A 4% • Vitamin C 2% • Calcium 15% • Iron 4%

* Percents (%) of a Daily Value are based on a 2,000 calorie diet. Your Daily Values may vary higher or lower depending on your calorie needs:

Nutrient		2,000 Calories	2,500 Calories
Total Fat	Less than	65g	80g
Sat Fat	Less than	20g	25g
Cholesterol	Less than	300mg	300mg
Sodium	Less than	2,400mg	2,400mg
Total Carbohydrate		300g	375g
Fiber		25g	30g

1g Fat = 9 calories
1g Carbohydrates = 4 calories
1g Protein = 4 calories

** No daily values have been determined for sugars and protein intake.

% Daily Value shows how a food fits into the overall daily diet. For each item, it shows the percentage or recommended daily consumption for a person eating 2,000 calories a day (e.g., 5 grams of saturated fat is 25% of the *recommended* daily value of 20 grams).

Percentage of daily requirements for selected vitamins and minerals

Recommended daily amounts of each item for two average diets. (If you eat less than 2,000 calories, you will have to adjust the Daily Values.)

Based on 10% consumption

Based on 60% consumption

Voluntary components that will be allowed on labels are calories from saturated fat, polyunsaturated fat, monounsaturated fat, potassium, soluble and insoluble fiber, sugar, alcohol, other carbohydrates, and other essential vitamins and minerals.

FIGURE 9.2 ➤
How to read a label.

rules require nutritional labeling on nearly all grocery items. Meat and poultry are exempt. Restaurants, bakeries, delis, and sidewalk vendors are also exempt from nutrition labeling, as are packages smaller than 12 square inches. Figure 9.2 shows a sample label.

Some points to remember when reading labels follow:

1. Check serving size. If not careful, you may actually eat two to three servings if the stated serving size is skimpy.
2. Ingredients are listed in order of concentration in a product, with the ingredient in the largest quantity listed first.
3. Watch for hidden sugars added to a product: syrup, sucrose, molasses, corn sweetener, dextrose, maltose, honey, and so on. They are all sugars.

4. Check fat content. Avoid hydrogenated fats.
5. Some crackers, pastries, cookies, candies, and instant cocoas are made with coconut and palm oil, which are more saturated than beef fat.
6. Select *whole* wheat bread ("wheat flour" means refined *white* flour—the bran and wheat germ have been removed). All whole wheat bread is brown, but not all brown bread is whole wheat.
7. Fortified foods contain added vitamins and minerals that were not originally in the food or were present in lower amounts. Breakfast cereals are commonly fortified. Can you name the vitamin milk is commonly fortified with?
8. Enriched foods have lost nutrients during processing and then had them replaced by the manufacturers. For instance, when wheat is turned into white flour, it loses at least 50 percent to 80 percent of many nutrients. Of these, iron, niacin, thiamin, and riboflavin are replaced; but other nutrients lost in the milling process, such as fiber, zinc, and copper, are not restored.

One of the problems in food labeling has been the confusing descriptors that manufacturers put on food products, for which there have previously been no definitions (for example, *lite* or *light* could have meant light in calories, color, texture, or weight). Under the new labeling law, specific, uniform definitions have been assigned to descriptors used on the label of any product. Table 9.10 defines these label descriptors. Consistency

table 9.10

LABEL DESCRIPTIONS

Free. The product contains no amount of, or only "physiologically inconsequential" amounts of one or more of these components: fat, saturated fat, cholesterol, sodium, sugars, and calories. For instance, "calorie free" means that there are fewer than 5 calories per serving, and "sugar free" and "fat free" indicate that there are less than 0.5 grams per serving.

Low. This food could be eaten frequently without exceeding dietary guidelines for one or more of the following components: fat, saturated fat, cholesterol, sodium, and calories. Thus, the following terms are used:
  Low fat. 3 grams or less per serving.
  Low saturated fat. 1 gram or less per serving
  Low sodium. Less than 140 mgs per serving.
  Very low sodium. Less than 35 mgs per serving.
  Low cholesterol. Less than 20 mgs per serving.
  Low calorie. 40 calories or less per serving.

Lean and extra lean. The following terms can be used to describe the fat content of meat, poultry, seafood, and game meats:
  Lean. Less than 10 grams of fat, less than 4 grams of saturated fat, and less than 95 mgs of cholesterol per serving and per 100 grams.
  Extra lean. Less than 5 grams of fat, less than 2 grams of saturated fat, and less than 95 mgs of cholesterol per serving and per 100 grams.

High. One serving of the food contains 20 percent or more of the Daily Value for a particular nutrient.

Good source. One serving of the food contains 10 percent to 19 percent of the Daily Value for a particular nutrient.

Reduced. A nutritionally altered product contains 25 percent less of a nutrient or of calories than the regular, or reference, product.

Less. A food, whether altered or not, contains 25 percent less of a nutrient or of calories than the reference food.

Light. A nutritionally altered product contains one-third fewer calories or half the fat of the reference food; or the sodium content of a low-calorie, low-fat food has been reduced by 50 percent.

in these terms will help shoppers who do not scrutinize all the numbers on food labels but who want to pick up a "low sodium" or "fat free" version of foods as they walk through the supermarket. Now, shoppers cannot be misled.

Fast Foods

One out of every five Americans eats at a fast-food restaurant daily. Eating out has become routine for many of us. Meal preparation time at home has decreased due to changing lifestyles, and it is evident this trend will not reverse. In fact, adults eat roughly 30 percent of their calories *away* from home, and fast-food restaurants serve four out of ten meals eaten at away-from-home eating establishments.[33] Most fast-food chains now supply nutrient information on their food products. What has this information revealed about the nutrient value of fast food? Are fast foods junk foods? Nutritionists have found that fast-food items do have significant amounts of certain nutrients (especially protein), but many tend to be low in fiber and high in calories, sodium, and fat.[34] How often do you rely on these foods? What other foods are you eating during the day? Occasional visits to fast-food restaurants will have little effect on the nutritive value of your total diet. In response to consumer demand, many chains have become quite diversified and have added many more items to their menus. Many now offer lower-fat items. However, it is difficult to get ample amounts of fruits and vegetables by eating consistently at fast-food establishments. Table 9.11 gives suggestions for healthy eating at fast-food restaurants.

Special Nutritional Concerns

High-level wellness means adjusting to life changes as well as seeking information for special situations. This section discusses dietary considerations for vegetarians, pregnant mothers, the elderly, and those persons engaging in regular, vigorous exercise.

Vegetarian Diet

For a variety of health and moral reasons, many people prefer a vegetarian diet. A vegetarian diet can be very nutritious and healthy. From not eating animal foods, vegetarians normally have lower body fat, blood cholesterol, blood pressure, and rates of coronary heart disease than do meat eaters. Studies show that mortality rates are lower for vegetarians than for nonvegetarians and that they have a lower-than-average risk of various cancers and Type II (adult onset) diabetes.[35] There are different vegetarian diets, however. Careful planning and food selection is important to avoid nutritional deficiencies. All vegetarian diets emphasize the use of vegetables, fruits, and grains as main staples. Some diets exclude all animal products, while some include dairy products and eggs.

Here are the types of vegetarian diets:

1. A **strict vegetarian** (or **vegan**) consumes only plant foods. (Vitamin B_{12} supplementation is recommended since it is not in any plant foods.)
2. A **lactovegetarian** will consume plant foods and dairy products.
3. A **lacto-ovo-vegetarian** will consume plant foods, dairy products, and eggs.
4. A **semivegetarian** only excludes red meat.

Meat is not essential to your diet, but protein is. Therefore, following a vegetarian diet requires careful planning and food selection in order to consume sufficient vitamins and minerals (especially the vitamin Bs, vitamin D, calcium, zinc, and iron). Search for good quality protein sources such as legumes (beans), nuts, grains, and seeds. A thorough knowledge of nutrition is essential. For example, combining a good source of vitamin C with whole grains and legumes will greatly enhance iron absorption from grain and legumes. Drinking fortified soybean milk will help you obtain calcium and vitamin B_{12}.

table 9.11

FAST TIPS FOR FAST FOODS

1. Think about what else you have eaten or will eat in the day. Fit this meal into your total fat, sodium, and calorie intake.
2. Salad bars are a wise choice for vitamins A and C and fiber; go easy on the dressings, high-fat cheeses, bacon, olives, sour cream, and refried beans.
3. Potato bars are another good choice if you avoid the heavy cheese and butter-type sauces, bacon, and sour cream.
4. Chicken and fish sound healthy, but many are coated with fat. Select the baked or grilled without breading or skin.
5. Pizza is a great choice, especially if the toppings are vegetables; avoid the pepperoni, sausage, and olives.
6. Hamburgers—order the small one instead of the "jumbo" burger.
7. Drink low-fat milk or juices instead of a shake or soda.
8. If eating Mexican food, emphasize soft tortillas, beans, chicken, and vegetables (easy on the cheese).
9. For breakfast, avoid croissants, biscuits, sausage, bacon, butter, and the danish. Better choices are pancakes, English muffins, bagels, bran muffins, and whole grain cereals.

Pregnancy

Many women become more nutritionally aware and eat more wisely during pregnancy. This makes sense. After all, it is an enormous responsibility to be in control of the nutritional well-being of another human. Good nutritional habits before conception give the baby an even healthier start. Good nutrition can improve infant birth weight and reduce infant mortality. Pregnancy is not a time to diet. Weight gain and some increased fat deposition is necessary and quite healthy. Be sure to increase calcium, iron, and protein. Your physician may recommend a vitamin supplement, since many vitamin needs are increased. Even though some additional vitamins and minerals are needed, only about 300 extra calories per day are necessary for fetal growth and metabolic expenditure.[36] Even though a woman is "eating for two," normal energy expenditure is not double. Therefore, it is important to eat nutritionally dense foods. Twinkies, chocolate chip cookies, and potato chips offer few nutrients to that growing baby. Alcohol and caffeine should be limited, since they both increase nutrient excretion and adversely affect fetal development.[37]

Aging

Many factors may interfere with good nutrition in older adults: economics, isolation, dentures, chronic health disorders, loss of taste, and medications. Nutrient absorption may decrease, especially for calcium and zinc. The widow or widower whose partner had always prepared the meals might start eating fast foods or frozen dinners. The depressed and lonely surviving partner may eat very little. Proper nutrition throughout life and into later life can minimize degenerative changes and help you maintain productivity and wellness. However, your 65-year-old body will not be the same one you fed at 25. If you decrease activity and your body composition changes (increase in fat, decrease in lean), then caloric intake should be decreased. Maintaining an active lifestyle can keep energy requirements from decreasing drastically. Even though energy needs may drop as you age, nutrient needs do not diminish significantly. You must make your calories count. Be sure to eat adequate fiber and calcium and fewer fats and refined sugars. Most of all, do not fall prey to nutritional quackery (special pills and elixirs of youth).

Nutrition for Sports and Fitness

Do you play competitive basketball? Are you training for a half-marathon? Is lap swimming every morning your fitness routine? Nutrition complements physical activity as you pursue a wellness lifestyle. However, the nutritional needs of an active person vary little from those of the more sedentary. *Everyone* needs a wide variety of healthy foods. If you are physically active, you burn more calories and have less chance of gaining weight (while eating more). Nevertheless, you do not need a special diet. There are many myths surrounding athletic performance and nutrition. An athlete (even a body builder) does not benefit from consuming a lot more protein. The typical American diet contains adequate amounts of protein—even to support an athletic lifestyle. The main fuel for exercising muscles, glycogen, comes from carbohydrates. The best are complex (breads, pastas, cereals, potatoes, rice, fruit), which provide plenty of vitamins and minerals. Persons engaged in fitness activities should consistently follow the 55 percent to 60 percent carbohydrate diet-proportion guidelines. For those engaging in heavy exercise training, a diet with 60 percent to 70 percent of its calories from carbohydrates may be necessary to refuel glycogen stores.[38] High-sugar snacks consumed before exercising can actually decrease performance. Carbohydrate loading (that is, manipulating diet and training in order to increase glycogen stores in the muscles) has not been shown to be effective for athletes participating in events requiring less than one and one-half to two hours of continuous, noninterrupted effort.[39]

The benefits of vitamin and mineral supplementation is a current area of study in regard to nutrition for competitive athletes. Large doses of the antioxidants vitamins C, E, and beta-carotene have shown promise in minimizing muscle damage and soreness in hard-working athletes.[40] Much more research is needed in this area.

Dehydration is a major contributor to poor athletic performance. Athletes, like everyone else, should drink eight to ten glasses of water every day. They should also drink a cup or more of water immediately before exercise and another 1/2 to 1 cup every 15 minutes during exercise. Do not wait until you are thirsty. Thirst is not a reliable indicator of dehydration because it usually does not occur until after 2 to 4 pints of body water are lost. The inclusion of electrolytes in the new sports drinks has been shown to be beneficial for rehydrating athletes. Sports drinks with 4 percent to 8 percent carbohydrate concentrations work best. (See Chapter 8 for more information on sports drinks.) In regard to nutrition, the key to sports and fitness performance is the same key to general wellness and vitality: a balanced diet.

SUMMARY

Even though diet is not singled out as a specific risk factor for coronary heart disease, dietary factors are often interrelated with patterns of physical activity as major contributors to heart disease, stroke, obesity, atherosclerosis, osteoporosis, and some types of cancer. While many dietary components are involved in diet and health relationships, a primary factor is our high consumption of fats (especially saturated fats). These are often consumed at the expense of fruits, vegetables, and complex carbohydrates that may be more conducive to health.

Like many, you may admit to having some poor nutritional habits. You may rationalize this with some of the following:

➤ I'll do better after I get out of school and have more time. (Frankly, you will probably be busier after graduation.)
➤ But I feel fine! (Like smoking, poor eating habits may not noticeably affect your health for years.)
➤ I don't have any control over what the cafeteria serves. (However, you do have *choices* in the cafeteria and between meals.)
➤ I don't have enough money to buy the right foods. (On the contrary, milk is cheaper than soft drinks; a bunch of bananas costs less than a bag of potato chips.)
➤ I'm going to die anyway, so I might as well eat what I like. (Yes, we are all going to die. However, lifetime dietary habits significantly affect the *quality* of the last 10 to 20 years of your life.)

Wellness involves making informed choices rather than rationalizing. Improved eating habits can positively affect your health—both now and later in life. Therefore, learn about the foods you are eating. Read food labels. The heart of good nutrition is *seven dietary principles*, a *pyramid of choices*, and *three simple words*. A diet that emphasizes *variety, moderation,* and *balance* is a big step toward achieving high-level wellness. A variety of foods is available to you, and it is up to you to make responsible choices: complex carbohydrates high in fiber and foods low in fat, cholesterol, sodium, and refined sugars.

REFERENCES

1. *Survey of American Dietary Habits: 1993 Executive Summary.* Chicago: The American Dietetic Association, 1993.
2. Farthing, Maryann C. "Current Eating Patterns of Adolescents in the United States." *Nutrition Today* 26 (March/April 1991): 35–39.
3. Department of Health and Human Services, Public Health Service. *Healthy People 2000: National Health Promotion and Disease Prevention Objectives.* Washington, D.C.: Department of Health and Human Services, 1990.
4. "Improving America's Diet and Health: From Recommendations to Action." *Nutrition Today* 27 (January/February 1992): 34–36.
5. Williams, Melvin H. *Nutrition for Fitness and Sport.* Dubuque, Iowa: Wm. C. Brown Publishers, 1992.
6. Williams, Melvin H. *Nutrition for Fitness and Sport.*
7. "The Importance of Fiber." *University of California, Berkeley Wellness Letter* 8 (April 1992): 4–5.
8. Kantor, Mark A. "Nutrition, Cholesterol, and Heart Disease, Part IV: The Role of Dietary Fiber." *Nutrition Forum* 6 (July/August 1989): 25–29.
9. Nicklas, Theresa, Rosanne P. Farris, Leann Myers, and Gerald S. Berenson. "Dietary Fiber Intake of Children and Young Adults: The Bogalusa Heart Study." *Journal of the American Dietetic Association* 95 (February 1995): 209–14.
10. Williams, Melvin H. *Nutrition for Fitness and Sport.*
11. "Eat Right America." *Journal of the American Dietetic Association* 92 (March 1992): supplement.
12. U.S. Department of Agriculture, U.S. Department of Health and Human Services. "Nutrition and Your Health: Dietary Guidelines for Americans." 4th ed. *Home and Garden Bulletin,* no. 232 (1995).
13. Davis, Judi, and Kim Sherer. *Applied Nutrition and Diet Therapy for Nurses,* 2d ed. Philadelphia: W. B. Saunders Co., 1994.
14. Kantor, Mark A. "Nutrition, Cholesterol, and Heart Disease, Part III: How Diet Affects Blood Cholesterol Levels." *Nutrition Forum* 6 (May/June 1989): 17–20.
15. Davis and Sherer. *Applied Nutrition and Diet Therapy for Nurses.*
16. "Nutrition and Your Health: Dietary Guidelines for Americans."
17. Margen, Sheldon, Joyce C. Lashof, and Patricia A. Buffler, eds. *Nutrition for Optimal Health and Weight Control.* Berkeley, Calif.: The University of California at Berkeley, 1995.
18. Clark, Nancy. "Dairy Tales." *Runner's World* 24 (June 1989): 44–50.
19. Beatty, Denise, and Susan Calvert Finn. "Position of the American Dietetic Association and The Canadian Dietetic Association: Women's Health and Nutrition." *Journal of the American Dietetic Association* 95 (March 1995): 362–66.
20. Margen, Lashof, and Buffler, eds. *Nutrition for Optimal Health and Weight Control.*
21. Beatty and Finn. "Position of The American Dietetic Association."
22. Beatty and Finn. "Position of The American Dietetic Association."
23. National Academy of Science—National Research Council. *Recommended Dietary Allowances.* 10th ed. Washington, D.C.: National Academy of Sciences, 1989.
24. *The Surgeon General's Report on Nutrition and Health,* DHSS publication 88–50210. Washington, D.C.: U.S. Department of Health and Human Services, 1988.
25. Margen, Lashof, and Buffler, eds. *Nutrition for Optimal Health and Weight Control.*
26. Block, Abby, and Cynthia A. Thomson. "Position of The American Dietetic Association: Phytochemicals and Functional Foods." *Journal of the American Dietetic Association* 95 (April 1995): 493–96.
27. Carper, Jean. *Stop Aging Now!* New York: HarperCollins Publishers, 1995.
28. Dickinson, Annette, ed. *Benefits of Nutritional Supplements.* Washington D.C.: Council for Responsible Nutrition, 1993.
29. National Cancer Institute. *5 A Day for Better Health: A Baseline Study of Americans' Fruit and Vegetable Consumption.* Rockville, Md.: National Cancer Institute, 1992.
30. Smith-Schneider, Lisa M., Madeleine J. Sigman-Grant, and P. M. Kris-Etherton. "Dietary Fat Reduction Strategies." *Journal of the American Dietetic Association* 92 (January 1992): 34–38.
31. Greene, Geoffrey W., Susan R. Rossi, Gabrielle Richards Reed, Cynthia Willey, and James O. Prochaska. "Stages of Change for Reducing Dietary Fat to 30% of Energy or Less." *Journal of the American Dietetic Association* 94 (October 1994): 1105–10.
32. "The New Food Label." *Nutrition Today* 27 (January/February 1992): 37–38.
33. U.S. Department of Agriculture, Human Nutrition Information Service. "Eating Better When Eating Out." *Home and Garden Bulletin,* nos. 232–11 (1991).
34. "Eating Better When Eating Out."
35. Margen, Lashof, and Buffler, eds. *Nutrition for Optimal Health and Weight Control.*
36. Davis and Sherer. *Applied Nutrition and Diet Therapy for Nurses.*
37. Davis and Sherer. *Applied Nutrition and Diet Therapy for Nurses.*
38. Adams, Judi. *Carbohydrates: The Athlete's Choice.* Englewood, Colo.: Wheat Foods Council, 1993.
39. Williams, Melvin H. *Nutrition for Fitness and Sport.*
40. Williams, Melvin H. *Nutrition for Fitness and Sport.*

SUGGESTED READINGS

Achterberg, Cheryl, Elaine McDonnell, and Robin Bagby. "How to Put the Food Guide Pyramid into Practice." *Journal of the American Dietetic Association* 94 (September 1994): 1030–35.

Amato, Paul R., and Sonia A. Partridge. *The New Vegetarians*. New York: Plenum Press, 1989.

"Are You Eating Right?" *Consumer Report* 57 (October 1992): 644–51.

Berning, Jacqueline, and Suzanne Nelson Steen, eds. *Sports Nutrition for the 90s*. Gaithersburg, Md.: Aspen Publishers, Inc., 1991.

Carper, Jean. *Stop Aging Now!* New York: HarperCollins Publishers, 1995.

Clark, Nancy. *Nancy Clark's Sports Nutrition Guidebook*. Champaign, Ill.: Human Kinetics Publishers, 1990.

Cooper, Kenneth. *Antioxidant Revolution*. Nashville, Tenn.: Thomas Nelson, Inc., 1994.

Davis, Judi, and Kim Sherer. *Applied Nutrition and Diet Therapy for Nurses*, 2d ed. Philadelphia: W. B. Saunders Co., 1994.

Dickinson, Annette, ed. *Benefits of Nutritional Supplements*. Washington D.C.: Council for Responsible Nutrition, 1993.

Diet and Health: Implications for Reducing Chronic Disease Risk. Washington D.C.: National Academy of Sciences, 1989.

Jones, Jeanne. *Eating Smart*. New York: Macmillan Publishing Co., 1992.

Kurzwell, Raymond. *The 10% Solution for a Healthy Life*. New York: Crown Publishers, Inc., 1993.

Li, Virginia C. "On Diet and Dieting: Reaching High Level Wellness." *Wellness Perspectives* 7 (winter 1990): 61–75.

Margen, Sheldon, Joyce C. Lashof, and Patricia A. Buffler, eds. *Nutrition for Optimal Health and Weight Control*. Berkeley, Calif.: The University of California at Berkeley, 1995.

McBean, Lois D., Tab Forgac, and Susan Calvert Finn. "Osteoporosis: Visions for Care and Prevention—A Conference Report." *Journal of the American Dietetic Association* 94 (June 1994): 668–71.

Meyer, Jean, and Jeanne P. Goldberg. *Dr. Jean Meyer's Diet and Nutrition Guide*. New York: Pharos Books, 1990.

Morreale, Sandra, and Nancy E. Schwartz. "Helping Americans Eat Right: Developing Practical and Actionable Public Nutrition Education Messages Based on the ADA Survey of American Dietary Habits." *Journal of the American Dietetic Association* 95 (March 1995): 305–8.

Munnings, Frances. "Osteoporosis: What Is the Role of Exercise?" *The Physician and Sportsmedicine* 20 (June 1992): 127–38.

National Research Council. *Improving America's Diet and Health: From Recommendations to Action*. Washington D.C.: National Academy Press, 1991.

Peterkin, Betty B. "Dietary Guidelines for Americans, 1990 Edition." *Journal of the American Dietetic Association* 90 (December 1990): 1725–27.

Piscatella, Joseph C. *Controlling Your Fat Tooth*. New York: Workman Publishing Co., 1991.

Piscatella, Joseph C. *Don't Eat Your Heart Out Cookbook*. New York: Workman Publishing Co., 1994.

Rolfes, Sharon Rady, and Linda Kelly DeBruyne. *Lifespan Nutrition: Conception Through Life*. St. Paul, Minn.: West Publishing Co., 1990.

"The New Food Label." *Nutrition Today* 27 (January/February 1992): 37–38.

The Surgeon General's Report on Nutrition and Health. Washington D.C.: U.S. Department of Health and Human Services, DHHS (PHS) publication 88–50210, 1988.

Tribole, Evelyn. *Eating on the Run*. Champaign, Ill.: Human Kinetics Publishers, 1992.

Weisburger, John H. "Nutritional Approach to Cancer Prevention with Emphasis on Vitamins, Antioxidants, and Carotenoids." *American Journal of Clinical Nutrition* 53 (January 1991): 2263–375.

Werbach, Melvyn R. *Nutritional Influences on Illness*, 2d ed. Tarzana, Calif.: Third Line Press, 1993.

Williams, Melvin H. *Nutrition for Fitness and Sport*, 3d ed. Dubuque, Iowa: Wm. C. Brown Publishers, 1992.

RESOURCES

Human Nutrition Information Service, U.S. Department of Agriculture, 6505 Belcrest Road, Hyattsville, MD 20782, (301) 436-7725.

National Center for Nutrition and Dietetics, 216 West Jackson Blvd., Suite 800, Chicago, IL 60606-6995.

National Dairy Council 1(800) 426-8271.

Nutrition Hotline, 1(800)843-8114 or 1(800)366-1655. A registered dietitian will answer your questions Monday–Friday, 10:00 A.M.–5:00 P.M. (EST). Prerecorded messages play 24 hours a day.

chapter 10

Weight Management

➤ Objectives

After reading this chapter, you will be able to:

1. Differentiate between overweight and obesity.

2. Explain the purpose of the Body Mass Index (BMI), and identify a BMI associated with health problems.

3. List seven health conditions associated with obesity.

4. Identify how the location of fat on the body is linked to health risks.

5. Describe how each of the following factors contribute to obesity: energy balance, fat cells, set point, heredity, metabolism, and nutrient composition of food.

6. Define basal metabolic rate (BMR), and identify five factors that affect it.

7. List four reasons crash/fad dieting does not work for permanent weight loss.

8. Define and explain the *yo-yo syndrome* (weight cycling).

9. List six guidelines to follow in evaluating any weight loss plan.

10. Identify and explain the three major components of effective lifetime weight management.

11. Give five examples of behavior modification techniques.

12. List five ways exercise helps in weight management.

13. Identify weight loss myths, fads, and gimmicks.

14. Compare and contrast the eating disorders: bulimia and anorexia nervosa.

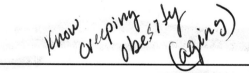

Terms

- Anorexia nervosa
- Basal metabolic rate (BMR)
- Behavior modification
- Body fat
- Body image
- Body mass index (BMI)
- Bulimia

- Calorie (kcal)
- Cellulite
- Eating disorder
- Essential fat
- Fat cells (adipose cells)
- Fat-free mass
- Glycogen

- Lean-body mass (muscle mass)
- Liposuction
- Obesity
- Overweight
- Set point
- Storage fat
- Yo-yo syndrome (weight cycling)

The best way to lose weight is to watch your food—just watch it, don't eat it!

Ed Koch, Former Mayor of New York

americans are obsessed with weight. It is likely that you know your weight within 5 pounds. Every birth announcement gives the baby's weight to the exact ounce. Weight scales are commonplace in American bathrooms and even on street corners. This preoccupation has made weight control a multibillion-dollar business. Americans spend approximately $33 billion yearly on weight-reduction products (including diet foods and drinks) and services.[1]

The craze to lose weight (whether needed or not) is reflected by the millions of Americans who report that they are dieting. Approximately 40 percent of all women and 25 percent of men in the United States are on a diet at any given moment.[2] Bookstore shelves and magazine racks are crammed with diet plans guaranteed to help you lose those extra inches. Television, radio, and newspapers further advertise a multitude of weight-loss options. With all of this attention and effort, one would predict that the American population would be very lean. Actually, obesity is a major health problem in our country. According to data released in 1994 from the Third National Health and Nutrition Examination Survey (NHANES III), approximately 35 percent of women and 31 percent of men age 20 and older are overweight, as are about one-fourth of children and adolescents.[3] While government health goals for the year 2000 call for no more than 20 percent of adults and 15 percent of adolescents to be overweight, the facts indicate we are getting fatter—not thinner.[4] Even with a decline in the consumption of dietary fat and more interest in "healthy" eating and fitness, American adults are gaining weight at an average of nearly 8 pounds a decade.[5] Few dieters attain their weight-loss goals, and most are unable to keep weight off over a period of time. Many health professionals feel that obesity is THE most common and serious health problem facing America today. In fact, if current trends continue, some predict that obesity will replace tobacco as the number-one cause of preventable death in the United States.[6] On the other extreme, the incidence of anorexia nervosa and bulimia nervosa is at an epidemic level. The paradoxes of these facts reveal how complex America's weight problem is.

Maintaining a reasonable body weight is a definite wellness issue. Your body is the vehicle by which you function in society. Being overfat can affect you physically, emotionally, socially, and even occupationally. Since the purpose of wellness is to strive toward full potential, maintaining a reasonable body composition is one step toward achieving wellness. Knowledge gives you the tools to plan your lifetime weight-management scheme. It is important that you understand body composition facts, effective weight-loss principles, weight-management guidelines, and the influence of heredity and environment on weight control.

The Impact of Culture

Why people diet and how they go about dieting is heavily bound in culture. In the 1880s, full-figured actress Lillian Russell was the epitome of beauty. During these times, a surplus of fat was equated with wealth and success. The 20th century brought about a decline in fatness as a social asset. Insurance companies began observing the increased death rate among those extremely overweight. The socially elite began diminishing the enormity of banquet menus. President William Howard Taft, weighing in at 355 pounds in 1909, began facing ridicule for his size. Corsets gave way to exercise, massage, raised hemlines, and penny scales. Hollywood stars, such as Jean Harlow and Gloria Swanson, gave diet and beauty advice that focused on reducing food intake. Thinness became equated with glamour, success, and desirability. After the Depression, the knowledge that excessive fat was linked to heart disease became a publicized issue. Weight reduction became a national pastime—a craze. Mail-order companies began making large profits with their weight-loss gimmicks. The market eventually gave way to new low-calorie foods and drugs designed to fool the body's hunger sensations. At the same time, labor-saving machines reduced the energy output necessary in daily life. The message

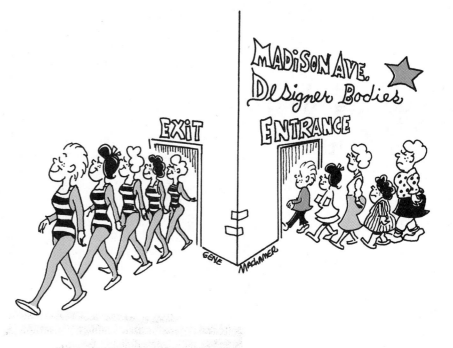

Many feel pressured to pursue the development of a model-like body.

that emerged by the 1960s was, "Thin is in." The desire for an unrealistic slimness, particularly among women, has caused many to be preoccupied with their bodies and with dieting. Diet books become instant best-sellers.

This standard is perpetuated in all channels of social influence: families, peers, and the media. The message is pounded home over and over: "You can never be thin enough." This notion was documented in a 1980 study by David Garner and colleagues.[7] His study of data from *Playboy* centerfolds and Miss America Pageant contestants from 1959 to 1978 indicated a shift toward a thinner ideal shape for women in our culture. The same study showed a significant increase in diet articles in popular women's magazines over the same period. It further demonstrated that American women during this time period were actually *increasing* in weight based on actuarial tables. A recent follow-up study[8] shows that the cultural ideal for women's body size has remained thin and perhaps even thinner. The body size of recent Miss America contestants has decreased even more, and *Playboy* centerfolds' measurements have plateaued at a very low level. This cultural index of the ideal woman's body is now 13 percent to 19 percent below the expected weight for age and height, as determined by actuarial tables. Since a body weight below 15 percent of expected weight is one of the criteria for diagnosing anorexia nervosa, what does this say about our cultural ideals?

With extreme slimness as a cultural norm, it becomes clear why fear of fat, fad dieting, surgical fat removal, and eating disorders abound. At one university, 35 percent of the women and 19 percent of the men reported to have tried to control their weight with fad diets, laxatives, fasting, or self-induced vomiting during the previous month.[9] The overweight, obese, and even normal-weight individuals evaluate themselves in society's mirror, defining themselves as unattractive and as failures. Such harsh evaluations are a result of an acceptance of society's distorted concept of the ideal body. Every day, advertisements suggest that we invest money, time, and hope into trying to reach this ideal. Unfortunately, the results are often feelings of guilt, despair, and inferiority.

Weight management begins with an acceptance of your personal body type and a healthy perception of your body image. Your basic body build and frame size are genetically determined. That is why 140 pounds may look different on you than on someone else. Women, starting at birth, normally have a higher proportion of fat than do men. The much-desired flat tummy is simply unnatural for most women. Once you accept this, you can proceed with being the best you can be. Making wishful statements such as, "If only I looked like that, life would be better," takes away the energy that could be used to take charge of your life and improve *all* dimensions of wellness. The media and fashion industry need to take responsibility for using models who depict fitness and health rather than emaciation. Some already have. With the popularity of fitness and wellness programs in our country, we hope the image is changing. The "one size fits all" standard *must* change.

Understanding Body Composition

Your body is composed of body fat and fat-free mass. **Fat-free mass** includes muscle, bone, body fluids, and organs. Muscles, which are part of your fat-free mass, are often specifically referred to as **lean-body mass** or **muscle mass.** Body fat is classified as either essential fat or storage fat. **Essential fat,** required for normal body functioning, is stored in major body organs and tissues such as the heart, muscles, intestines, bones, lungs, liver, spleen, and kidneys and throughout the central nervous system. Females have additional essential fat in the breasts and pelvic region for child bearing and other hormone-related functions. **Storage fat** is the extra fat that accumulates in adipose cells (or fat cells) around internal organs and beneath the skin surface to insulate, pad, and protect the body from trauma and extreme cold. As you learned in Chapter 4, there are different ways of assessing body composition. Knowing your body composition (especially your percentage of body fat) can help you set realistic weight goals.

Overweight Versus Obesity

Too often, the terms *overweight* and *obesity* are used interchangeably. **Overweight** refers to body weight greater than that which is normal.[10] "Normal" is most often thought of as an average weight for a specific height. The Metropolitan Life Insurance Company began publishing height-weight charts in the 1940s, listing desirable weight ranges for specific heights based on three classes of frame size. These charts, based on mortality rates of persons who purchased life insurance policies, have been widely distributed. Metropolitan regularly updates these charts. You have probably seen one of these charts in a physician's office or magazine and looked to see where you rank. There has been considerable controversy and criticism over the appropriateness of these height-weight charts, since they do not take into account different shapes, skeletal sizes, or variances in muscle development. The frame sizes give too much latitude of choice, and non-Caucasians are underreported in these tables. Also, the mortality data for life insurance purposes does not necessarily correlate to a desirable weight for wellness, vitality, and quality of life.

A more suitable measure for assessing the relationship between weight and health risk is the **body mass index (BMI),** as illustrated in Figure 10.1. This nomogram helps you calculate your BMI, which is a ratio between weight and height. BMI is computed from the following equation:

$$BMI = \frac{\text{weight in kilograms}}{(\text{height in meters})^2}$$

Take a few seconds and determine your BMI. A BMI of 20 to 25 is associated with the lowest risk of health problems for most people. Your health risk increases as your BMI increases. A BMI of 25 to 27 may be associated with health problems for some people. This is the caution zone. A BMI of over 27 is associated with increased risk of health problems such as heart disease, high blood pressure, and diabetes. A disadvantage of using the BMI is that it remains a measure of weight and height, not fatness (it doesn't distinguish between body fat and muscle). The BMI should be used with caution as an *absolute* indicator of obesity. Nevertheless, it is regarded by the scientific community as a means to correlate health risks and body size, especially when more scientific measures are unavailable (see Chapter 4).[11]

Understanding the difference between being overweight and obese is important. A weight scale can only measure how much you weigh, not how much fat you have. Standard height-weight tables do not assess your "fatness." An athlete may be considered overweight according to a height-weight chart but actually be very low in fat, due to muscular development. Overweight can also be a result of increased bone density or fluid. On the other extreme, a normal-weight, sedentary person may actually have too much fat. **Obesity** means an excessive accumulation of body fat.[12] We consider a woman to be obese if she is over 30 percent body fat. A man over 25 percent body fat is obese. A BMI above 27 is nor-

FIGURE 10.1 ➤

Nomogram for Body Mass Index (BMI). BMI (the ratio weight/height² in metric units) is read from the central scale after a straight edge is placed between height and body weight.

source: 1983 Metropolitan Life Insurance Company Tables Courtesy Statistical Bulletin, Metropolitan Life Insurance Company.

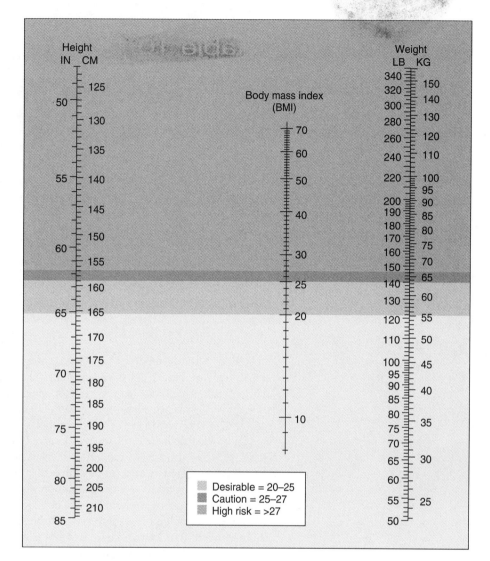

Risks Associated with Obesity

mally classified as obesity. At this level, the excess body fat becomes a severe health threat. Since several medical problems are associated with obesity, it is important that you have an idea of your body fat percentage and your BMI rather than just your weight.

Although women generally face more cultural pressure to be thin than do men, obesity poses significant health threats for both men and women. In *Healthy People 2000*, obesity is identified as a risk factor in five of the 10 leading causes of death.[13] These major killers associated with obesity are heart disease, some types of cancer, stroke, diabetes, and atherosclerosis. Obesity can aggravate high blood pressure, cardiovascular problems, liver disorders, and arthritis. Obesity is often found in conjunction with diabetes and gallbladder disease. Obesity complicates surgery and pregnancy. Pulmonary problems, heat intolerance, and reduced fertility are more prevalent in the obese. Among obese women there is an increased risk of endometrial and breast cancers. Obese men face an increased chance of colon, rectum, and prostate cancer. Obesity restricts mobility, increases fatigue, and decreases overall body efficiency.

The high prevalence of obesity in the United States is not only linked to numerous chronic diseases, but is responsible for a substantial portion of total health-care costs. Obesity health-care costs exceed $70 billion per year.[14] This figure does not include the psychosocial costs of obesity—from lowered self-esteem to eating disorders to severe clinical depression.

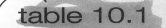

table 10.1

SAMPLE WAIST-TO-HIP RATIOS

$$\text{Waist-to-Hip Ratio} = \frac{\text{Waist circumference}}{\text{Hip circumference}}$$

(see Chapter 4 for specific measuring instructions)

$$\frac{\text{waist}}{\text{hip}} = \frac{26"}{35"} = 0.74 \qquad \frac{\text{waist}}{\text{hip}} = \frac{40"}{42"} = 0.95$$

$$\frac{\text{waist}}{\text{hip}} = \frac{32"}{40"} = 0.80 \qquad \frac{\text{waist}}{\text{hip}} = \frac{40"}{37"} = 1.08$$

$$\frac{\text{waist}}{\text{hip}} = \frac{38"}{42"} = 0.90 \qquad \frac{\text{waist}}{\text{hip}} = \frac{45"}{39"} = 1.15$$

Higher risk is associated with a ratio >0.8 for women and >0.95 for men.

Until recently, modest weight gains throughout adulthood of initially lean individuals were overlooked and even culturally expected as long as the weight and BMI remained within the desirable range. In fact, height-weight guidelines issued by the government in 1990 *increased* the upper limit of desirable weight for persons older than 35 years as compared to the 1985 U.S. guidelines.[15] The newest findings[16] from the ongoing Nurses' Health Study (a 14-year tracking of 115,818 nurses) have revealed that even *modest* (11 to 17 lbs) weight gains after 18 years of age (even while staying in the desirable weight range) increase one's cardiovascular disease risk. The researchers concluded that there is a large fraction of the population who are falsely reassured that their weight is not a health concern because they are not "overweight." The study found that a person's weight at midlife (30 to 55 years) has the greatest influence on heart disease risk. Those with a BMI of 23 to 27 kg/m^2 had a 31 percent increased risk; those with the lowest risk had a BMI below 21 kg/m^2.

Weight-management experts also point to the location of excess fat as a risk factor. Fat distributed primarily in the abdominal area (called *apple-shape obesity*) is characteristic of many men (but also present in some women). This apple-shape obesity is linked to increased risk for coronary heart disease, hypertension, high cholesterol, diabetes, and breast cancer. Fat distributed in the lower extremities, around the hips, buttocks, and thighs (called *pear-shape obesity*) does not present as great a risk.[17] Pear-shape obesity is more common in women. The two types of fat have biochemical differences. Abdominal fat experiences much more enzyme activity, dumping more fatty acids into the bloodstream. Hip-thigh fat activity is more stagnant. Unfortunately, this hip-thigh fat is more difficult to lose than is abdominal fat. Some obesity experts feel that one's waist-to-hip ratio is as important as the BMI in predicting potential weight-related health problems. Waist-to-hip ratio can be calculated by dividing the number of inches around the waistline by the circumference of the hips. See Table 10.1 for examples of waist-to-hip ratios. For example, someone who has a 30-inch waist and 40-inch hips has a ratio of 0.75. A woman whose ratio is 0.80 or higher is at risk, as is a man whose ratio is 0.95 or above. Whereas the distribution of fat has some genetic link, a comprehensive program of a low-fat, reduced-calorie diet and regular exercise can help reduce body fat stores, regardless of where they are located.

While obesity is known to decrease life expectancy, the psychological and social consequences of obesity are often overlooked. Obese people face a tremendous amount of prejudice and discrimination in our society. Their educational and professional opportunities often suffer.

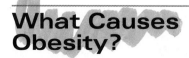

What Causes Obesity?

For years, the popular explanation for obesity was that people became obese simply because they ate too much. Obesity was viewed as a condition resulting from a lack of self-control around food. Today, research points to obesity as a complex puzzle of metabolic, genetic, psychological, behavioral, social, and cultural factors—not solely a result of a lack of individual willpower. It is evident that no single factor results in obesity. In fact, obesity research is in its infancy. In an attempt to explain the causes of obesity, several factors have to be examined. These include energy balance, fat cells, set point, heredity, metabolism, and the nutrient composition of food.

The Energy Balance Equation

The energy balance equation states that energy input (calories consumed) must be equal to energy output (calories expended) for body weight to remain constant. Any imbalance in energy input or energy output will result in a change in body weight. If you eat more calories daily than your body expends in activity, you will store the excesses as fat. If you eat fewer calories than you burn, you will lose weight. It is unrealistic to assume that the equation must be exactly equal every day to maintain your weight. Some days you eat more; some days less. Some days you are more active than you are other days. Obviously, several days of imbalance in one direction will produce a change in body weight.

This explanation assumes that a calorie is a calorie. A **calorie** (actually a **kcal**) is a measure of energy. One pound of body fat equals 3,500 calories of stored energy. Therefore, consuming an extra 3,500 calories will cause you to gain 1 pound of fat. If you burn an extra 3,500 calories with activity, you will lose 1 pound. To cause a reduction in body weight, you simply (1) reduce calorie intake below the energy requirement; (2) increase the calorie output through additional physical activity above energy requirements; or (3) combine the two methods by reducing calorie intake and increasing calorie output. So how do you lose 10 pounds? By creating a calorie deficit of 500 calories daily (by either increasing exercise or decreasing food intake) for seven days, you will lose 1 pound (3,500 calories). By maintaining this deficit, you will be 10 pounds lighter in 10 weeks.

However, weight loss is not necessarily this simple. For some, dieting causes feelings of fatigue, resulting in a decrease of energy expenditure. As body weight is reduced, the energy costs of movement go down proportionately, thus reducing caloric output. Also, individual differences in resting metabolic rates, cellular makeup, and lean tissue need to be considered. That is why knowledge about other factors is necessary to fully understand the complexities of weight loss.

Regardless of the problems that come with relying solely on the energy balance equation as the only way to understand weight loss and weight gain, the equation is the best way of explaining why, in this age of modernization and decreased physical demands, so many Americans are too fat. Most are not active enough to utilize the calories consumed. Food in America is plentiful, available, and relatively inexpensive. It is also high in sugar and fat. Even though many people are consuming lower-fat food items, *low fat* doesn't necessarily mean *low calorie*. While our calorie intake hasn't declined drastically, our caloric expenditure has. Countless labor-saving devices at home and work and our passive leisure-time activities (television, computer games, videos) have contributed to creeping obesity. Sedentariness has become a way of life.

How many calories do you need to maintain a desirable body weight? Table 10.2 on page 218 helps you estimate your daily caloric need based on your activity level. Remember, this is only an approximation and may vary between individuals. To lose or gain weight, the calorie intake must be adjusted upward or downward.

Fat-Cell Theory

The size and number of fat cells in the body determine degrees of fatness. **Fat cells** (also known as **adipose cells**) are storage sites for energy. The body increases fat storage in two ways: by increasing the number of fat cells and by increasing the size of the fat cells. As might be expected, the body increases its number of fat cells during childhood and teenage growth spurts. Fat cells also expand and contract as energy is stored or burned. In fact, they can expand to two to three times their normal size, but they cannot enlarge

table 10.2

DETERMINING YOUR DAILY CALORIC NEEDS

Desirable weight × Activity level = Calories needed daily

ACTIVITY LEVEL	CALORIES NEEDED PER POUND PER DAY
Sedentary (most Americans, office job, light work)	13
Moderately active (weekend recreation)	15
Very active (vigorous exercise 3–4 times per week)	16

Example: 140 lbs (desirable weight) × 15 (moderate activity) = 2,100 calories

Fat cells are with you forever.

endlessly. At some point, new fat cells are created in response to the body's need to store more excess energy. It is now well-accepted that, contrary to earlier theories, increases in fat cell *number* can occur throughout adult life.[18] This capacity to increase cell numbers when a maximum cell size is reached depends on the age and sex of the person as well as on the site of the fat tissue.[19] Unfortunately, once a fat cell has been created, it exists for life. Fat cells do not seem to be destructible.

Therefore, the fat-cell theory proposes that weight reduction in adults is a result of decreasing the size of the fat cells, shrinking them by using the energy stored in them, or not filling them at all. This theory also explains why people who grow a large number of fat cells during childhood have a predisposition to obesity as adults. They can reduce the amount of fat stored in the cells, but the excess number of fat cells is still there, waiting to be filled again.

Knowing that obese children often become obese adults, it is easy to see one way to prevent obesity. Control the development of new fat cells during childhood and teenage years with regular exercise and sensible eating. This makes more sense than letting children become obese in the first place. This fact makes us question why daily physical education is being cut from most school programs. In this day and age, children need more daily exercise, not less.

When going on a low calorie diet, the adult with an excessive number of fat cells gets caught in a trap. A large number of empty fat cells is a biologically abnormal state. The body's natural tendency is to defend its fat cell size. As a result, the appetite control center in the brain is stimulated, causing the dieter to eat more calories. This condition of "starved fat cells" is the reason most dieters (especially in the obese category) eventually regain their lost weight. This is also the reason obese people on treatment programs tend to stop losing weight when their fat cells shrink to normal size.[20] In this way, obesity can become a lifelong condition. *Prevention* is the key.

Set-Point Theory

The set-point theory maintains that every individual is programmed to be a certain weight and that the body regulates itself to maintain that "set" weight. Studies of people in alternating states of semistarvation and gorging have shown that, once intervention ceases, they return to their former weights.[21] What determines your **set point**? The hypothalamus in the brain may act as a body weight thermostat, lowering body metabolism and increasing hunger if fat levels fall below the set point. Here is where the set-point theory and fat-cell theory merge. The set-point mechanism is thought to respond to signals sent out by the fat cells as to the amount of fat in storage. The weight at which this occurs may depend on the number of fat cells. Consider two 200-pound women. Sara has a normal number of fat cells, which are enlarged. Mary has an excessive number of fat cells of normal size. Sara has a greater chance of weight loss, because she can reduce her cell size and still sustain adequate fat volume. Mary faces a harder battle, because her body will work to maintain her cell size. This theory also helps explain why attempts at permanent weight loss by crash dieting are not successful. The body naturally fights against this starvation state.

The set-point theory is based on survival. How else could populations endure famine or our ancestors survive periods of food shortages? Heredity influences the set point, too. Some people have naturally higher set points, causing maintenance of higher levels of body fat. Some individuals have naturally low set points.

Can you change your set point? Some studies show that sustained consumption of a high-fat diet (the typical American diet?) actually raises the set point and that regular, vigorous exercise can lower the set point.[22] Exercise stimulates changes in metabolism, thus causing the body to use fat rather than protect against its losses. Knowing this it is easy to see how our growing sedentary lifestyles and dietary habits are more likely connected to America's obesity problem than are brain thermostat alterations. We've gone from lean to fat because we eat more and exert ourselves less. As one obesity expert states, obesity in "each successive generation may be more easily explained by the availability of gasoline than by the availability of fast food"—or by the set-point theory.[23]

Heredity

"I can't lose weight; it's in my genes!" Many would view this exclamation made by many obese persons as an excuse for their physical state. New research about genetic influences of obesity lends some (but not *total*) credibility to this exclamation. Children with obese parents do have a greater tendency to become obese adults.[24] Is this an inherited tendency or a result of inappropriate behaviors learned and reinforced at home? Studies of families (especially twins) have provided insights to this question. A classic study[25] conducted by Claude Bouchard showed that adult identical twins were similar in *total* fat gain and *distribution* of fat gain when consistently overfed for 100 days. There were huge differences between pairs of twins as to body weight gains, body composition changes, and waist/hip circumference changes. Between twins, however, there were striking similarities. Similar research[26] shows that adult twins tend to be similar in body weight and body mass index regardless of whether they were raised together in the same home or separated in early childhood and raised in different environments.

Obesity rates are higher in certain ethnic groups, especially among women. Data from NHANES III[27] indicate that 50 percent of African-American females and 48 percent of Mexican-American females are overweight (compared to 34 percent of white females). The prevalence of obesity is approximately the same for African-American and white males (32 percent); but 40 percent of Mexican-American men are obese. Obesity rates among Native Americans are also higher than among whites: 34 percent of males; 40 percent of females (Fig. 10.2). Some may explain these differences totally by heredity, when, in fact, cultural differences may be the truer reason. In many ethnic groups, food is more than nutrients. It is the focal point of family gatherings. It eases stress. Limited resources and dependence on commodity foods may also be a contributing factor. Being heavy in some cultures is associated with health, prosperity, and sexuality. Also, African Americans—except for males up to age 25—are very sedentary. Lack of time, single parenting responsibilities, lack of exercise facilities, and the belief that exercise is selfish because it takes time away from family responsibilities could all be reasons.[28]

Even though these facts address a role heredity has in obesity, heredity is only a *tendency* or predisposing factor that can be influenced by environmental components and behaviors. Those people who are predisposed to be overweight or obese will have more difficulty controlling their weight, but it is certainly not impossible for them to attain and maintain a healthy weight.

Metabolism

Every individual expends a certain amount of energy, even at rest, to sustain the vital functions of the body. This energy requirement is called the **basal metabolic rate (BMR)** and accounts for approximately 70 percent of calories burned in one day.[29] A true measure of basal (resting) metabolism is taken when you have been lying quietly but awake and without food for 12 to 15 hours. Most men have a BMR requirement of 1,600 to 1,800

FIGURE 10.2 ➤
Obesity rates of selected ethnic groups in the United States.

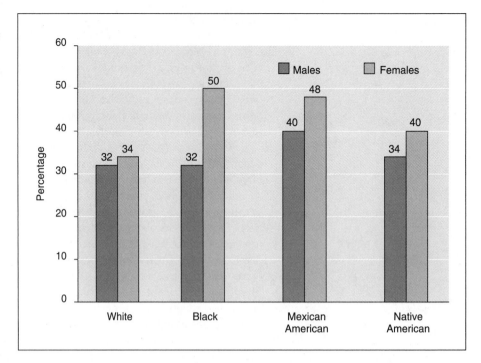

table 10.3

FACTORS THAT AFFECT BASAL METABOLIC RATE

Gender	Women generally have lower BMRs than do men (about 5 percent to 10 percent lower) due to smaller size, greater body fat, and less muscle mass.
Musculature	Increased muscle mass or tone increases BMR. Muscle tissue is more metabolically active than is fat. As muscles atrophy from inactivity, BMR declines.
Age	For both men and women, BMR declines by about 2 percent to 3 percent per decade after age 25. Loss of lean muscle mass typically occurs with aging as well. Maintaining a regular exercise program can help prevent a decline of lean muscle mass and BMR as you age.
Body size	Smaller body surface area results in lower BMR.
Nutritional status	Fasting, very low calorie diets, or long-term undernutrition lower BMR.
Activity level	BMR increases during exercise and may remain elevated somewhat after exercising.
Genetics	We all inherit physiological tendencies, and, as a result, BMR is inherently higher in some people and lower in others.

calories daily; most women need 1,200 to 1,450 calories daily. Since BMR is such a large component of your daily energy expenditure, it can significantly affect body weight over time. It is an important yet highly individual factor in the development of obesity.

Your BMR is a result of several interrelated factors, including age, gender, body size, nutritional status, musculature, activity level, and genetics. Table 10.3 depicts how BMR is affected by each of these factors. Some theorize that the obese have "sluggish" metabolisms. That is, they need fewer calories for normal body functions than the average person, and they turn food into energy very slowly. While some of the obese may have some of the factors that cause a lower-than-normal metabolism, the crucial question remains: Are they fat because their metabolism is low, or is their metabolism low because they are fat? Fat, being storage tissue, is inactive and has a low metabolism, whereas muscle tissue is active and has a high metabolic rate.

Nutrient Composition

The energy balance equation approach to weight loss/gain is based on the premise that all calories are created equal. That is, for weight loss, the *source* of calories is not important as long as the total calorie deficit is greater than the caloric intake. Recent findings report that total caloric intake is not correlated to obesity as much as dietary fat is.[30] The premise is that a calorie is *not* a calorie. Some researchers have even narrowed the association between dietary fat and body fat specifically to saturated fat intake.[31] Saturated fat is converted into body fat with greater ease than are carbohydrates. For every 100 carbohydrate calories consumed, 23 calories are burned up metabolizing it (converting it to a storable form), and about 77 calories are actually stored. In contrast, for every 100 fat calories consumed, only about 3 calories are used to convert it to storable form, leaving a whopping 97 calories available for body fat.[32] (There *is* one predominantly carbohydrate substance that has been found to convert to body fat quite easily—alcohol.[33] This fact confirms the direct correlation between alcohol consumption and weight gain.) Studies show that normal-weight and overweight persons may consume approximately the same number of calories, whereas the overweight persons derive a greater proportion of their calories from fat.[34] When fat intake is reduced and carbohydrate intake is not restricted, people can still lose weight—even when the total daily intake of calories is increased. Knowing this, isn't it absurd that most people's first attempt at losing weight is to go on a radical, restrictive diet?

What About Dieting?

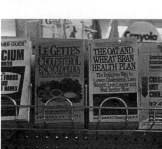

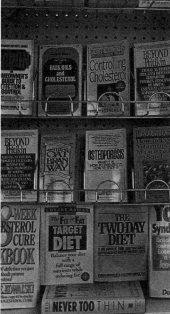

The multitude of diet books, many of which are sources of quackery and misleading information, can be confusing to the consumer.

Most people who want to lose weight think immediately of going on a diet. This notion is reinforced by the number of new fad diets advertised each year. These popular diets are viewed by the user as a temporary inconvenience that will be discontinued as soon as the weight goal has been reached. "Going on" a diet implies "going off" it. Dieters assume that weight will be lost quickly and immediately. Chances are, however, that the excess pounds have accumulated gradually over a period of years. These pounds are maintained by ingrained habits. Most fad diets rely on rigid food choices. Food becomes the enemy and mealtime a battle to be fought. Practicing restraint can result in food cravings, binges, guilt, and self-deprecation. Most popular diets do not emphasize physical exercise. In fact, more than half of the overweight adults trying to lose weight are doing so by eating fewer calories. Less than one-third are increasing physical activity.[35] This is a reflection of our sedentary lifestyle and the emphasis on dieting as a means to control weight. Diets have special appeal and sound so easy. Most of them, however, are nutritionally inadequate, too low in calories, and potentially dangerous.

When you go on a very-low-calorie diet, up to 70 percent of the weight loss during the first three days is water.[36] This is predictable since your body prefers carbohydrates for energy. Being starved of carbohydrates, it uses **glycogen** (stored carbohydrates) for energy. As you use this glycogen, you lose water, since each gram of carbohydrate is stored with 3 grams of water. Your body also uses protein for energy, resulting in a loss of muscle tissue. Crash dieting can cause headaches, ketosis, and loss of bone mineralization. If you go on a very-low-calorie diet (less than 800 calories per day), your body slows its metabolism (BMR) significantly.[37] After all, your body doesn't know that there is a grocery store just a block away. It reacts as if you were dying from starvation. Therefore, your body saves energy by burning fewer calories. This conservation of energy causes the diet to be even less effective. Depression, irritability, fatigue, and feelings of deprivation often follow. The survival urge to eat eventually wins out and weight is regained. When this happens, the crash dieter may become fatter for five reasons:

1. If old eating habits are resumed, the regained weight is fat; some of the weight loss was most likely lean tissue.
2. Metabolism can remain slowed for months.
3. Overeating (especially a preference for dietary fat) may occur in response to the past deprivation.
4. More fat cells can develop as the existing cells fill to capacity and divide.
5. Metabolic alterations can occur (i.e., fat can be stored more efficiently; the body conserves fat stores as a protective phenomenon against future losses).

Yo-Yo Syndrome

Fad dieting does not produce lasting results, and repeated bouts of dieting result in improved efficiency in the body's adaptive response to semistarvation. Since the body interprets drastic dieting as a mortal threat, basal metabolic rate slows in an effort to maintain life. This metabolic response causes greater difficulty in losing weight and greater efficiency in gaining weight.[38] As a result, many obese people have repetitive cycles of weight loss and weight gain. This cycle is known as the **yo-yo syndrome** (or **weight cycling**). In this cycle, fat is often lost slower and regained faster with each repeated dieting bout. Therefore, yo-yo dieting affords the body repeated opportunities to enhance its efficiency at storing energy—a function of fat cells. Yo-yo dieters also tend to regain their weight in the more risky abdominal location. Incessant dieting may actually be one reason many Americans are fatter today than ever.

Much attention has been focused in recent years by both the lay press and professional journals on possible physiological and psychological dangers of weight cycling—even suggesting that staying overweight may actually be safer in terms of heart disease or premature death than riding the diet roller coaster. Experts on a National Institutes of Health task force reviewed 43 human studies on yo-yo dieting, finding that the evidence for the claimed adverse health effects is not convincing or consistent (yo-yo dieting by itself does not increase the risk of dying from heart disease).[39] The scientists admitted, however, that repeatedly regaining hard-lost pounds *may* result in depression and a loss of self-esteem. Millions of overweight people stand to benefit from loss of fat, and worries about weight cycling should not be a deterrent. As with any attempt at changing a habit, you may experience cycles of success and relapse before finally succeeding. This information accentuates even more dramatically the need to learn *skills* for maintaining weight loss and to *prevent* obesity from occurring altogether. Losing weight—and maintaining a healthy weight—is a lifelong commitment.

Reliable Diet Programs

Are there any reliable weight-loss programs? Yes. There are some very good programs available, as long as the dieter understands the purpose and limitations of commercial-based plans. Enrolling in a weight-control program is an investment of time, energy, and money. Ask yourself if you are ready to lose the weight *and* do what it takes to keep it off. Losing the weight is only half the battle. Keeping it off demands lifestyle changes that are lifelong. It is especially important for the morbidly obese to seek professional help in losing weight. These persons would be wise to consult one of the excellent hospital-based programs available in many communities. Since new fad diets appear almost weekly and disappear almost as quickly, it is unrealistic to assess every particular diet for strengths and weaknesses. Instead, use the following guidelines in evaluating any weight-loss plan:

1. It should use real, regular food available in supermarkets.
2. It should provide an energy deficit to allow slow, safe weight loss of 1 to 2 pounds per week.
3. It should encourage the reduction of fat in the diet.
4. It should encourage a safe, personalized exercise program.
5. It should teach lifelong changes that allow freedom and flexibility for individual lifestyles.
6. It should make possible the enjoyment of social situations such as eating out, holidays, and special occasions.
7. It should allow for basic energy needs (never under 1,200 calories daily) and be nutritionally balanced (the Food Guide Pyramid, U.S. dietary guidelines, etc.).
8. It should not be too costly.
9. It should teach techniques for *maintaining* positive behavior change.

A final question to ask yourself when considering a diet plan should be, "Can I live on this diet for the rest of my life?"

The goal of weight loss is fat loss, which takes time and long-term lifestyle change. Many diets are variations on the food restriction theme, are unpleasant, and fail to teach modification of eating behavior. Just about any type of food restriction will result in weight loss. The key is keeping the weight off by learning to live with food.

table 10.4

TOTAL FAT INTAKE PER DAY FOR SPECIFIC CALORIE INTAKE LEVELS

DAILY CALORIE INTAKE	FAT GRAMS/DAY AT 20 PERCENT–25 PERCENT
1,200	27–33
1,600	36–44
2,000	44–56
2,500	56–69

Lifetime Weight Management

The factors that contribute to obesity are so numerous and complex that it is impossible to pinpoint one cause. Having knowledge of the theories of obesity should help you understand some of these complexities. Fat cells, metabolism, set points, genetics, and energy expenditure all play a role. Behaviors that have developed over a period of time are also intricately involved. One unrefuted truth emerges in nearly all weight-control studies: *Permanent weight control involves a lifelong commitment to good eating habits and regular exercise.* There is evidence that young adults in their early 20s gain a disproportionate amount of weight by the time they are 30, making them an important population segment for obesity prevention efforts.[40] If you are in this age group, this fact should help motivate you to commit to a lifetime weight-management plan. Weight management is a lifestyle. Maintaining a reasonable body composition is, rather than isolated bouts of crash dieting or sporadic exercise, a result of lifelong integration of three components: (1) nutritional knowledge; (2) eating management (behavior modification); and (3) exercise.

Nutritional Knowledge

Dieters are notorious for trying faddish diet plans. Thus, it is essential to have a good framework for making sensible, well-balanced food choices. Basic weight-management principles are not different from general good nutritional recommendations (low fat, sugar, and salt and high complex carbohydrates and fiber). Simply cutting the fat from your diet reduces a tremendous number of calories. Studies on the effect of low-fat eating on weight loss have established that (1) weight loss is more closely associated with the percentage of dietary fat than it is with changes in total caloric intake and (2) weight can be lost by reducing dietary fat without any further restrictions of food intake.[41] "I lost weight without eating less!" is often the exclamation of persons who substitute fiber-rich grains, fruits, and vegetables for fat in their diets. It appears that the main causes of obesity are high-fat diets and low levels of physical activity. There is little evidence that excessive caloric intake is the culprit.[42] Of course, carbohydrates and the new nonfat foods have calories, too. Therefore, overall calorie consumption cannot be *completely* ignored. What is considered a low-fat diet? Most dietitians recommend that the diet be composed of a *minimum* of 20 percent fat of total caloric intake.[43] Some fat is necessary, especially for fat-soluble vitamins to be utilized. Therefore, a fat intake of 20 percent to 25 percent of daily calories is a reasonable low-fat diet. (Of course, this is below the American Heart Association's recommended 30 percent.) Table 10.4 translates a fat intake of 20 percent to 25 percent into daily fat grams for various caloric levels. Being aware of caloric values of foods, the food groups, vitamin needs, sources of "hidden" fats, and energy needs can help you make sensible food choices. Learning to read food labels and alter recipes to lower the fat content is where nutritional knowledge plays a major role in lifetime weight management. See Chapter 9 for fat-lowering tips.

Eating is one of life's pleasures. Traditional weight-loss diets often feature a lot of "can" and "cannot have" foods. This "all or nothing" approach to food contributes to binging, overeating, and other abnormal eating behaviors. Sensibility in food choices does not mean that you will never again eat chocolate cake. There should never be guilt or forbidden foods. Instead, lifetime weight management means seeing how much or where chocolate cake fits into your total diet. Reduce, don't eliminate, certain foods. Balance your food choices over time. Control portions. Gradual rather than drastic changes in dietary patterns lead to successful maintenance. Healthful eating does not happen by accident, and it is not always easy. Our culture dishes out food portions adequately described as *mega-* and *super-size*. The 10,000 food advertisements we watch per year on television are not for broccoli and cantaloupe. The commercials say, "Eat, eat, eat" but show a woman who is so thin that she clearly never eats. For lifetime weight management it is essential to learn about the nutritive value of foods and devise strategies for making good choices over the course of each day.

Eating Management

Why do you eat? "Because I am hungry!" you answer. If everyone ate only when they were in the physiological state of hunger, very few would have a weight problem. We are surrounded with opportunities to eat more than we need to. Eating behavior is strongly influenced by psychological, social, and emotional factors. We eat out of emotional needs. We eat when we're happy; we eat when we're sad. Food becomes a substitute for other things.

Controlling eating habits begins with having an understanding of why you eat and what antecedents trigger eating. Do you eat when you are bored? Lonely? Angry? Stressed? Do you eat when you turn on the television? Read? Do you eat when something smells good? When others are eating? When you want to please Aunt Margaret? As discussed in Chapter 1, behavior change is a complex process that involves stages and coping techniques within each stage. You may want to go back to Chapter 1 and review Prochaska's behavior-change theory to see which techniques can be incorporated into eating management. The behavior-change contract can easily be used to manage eating behaviors. You will also find in the Activities Section an *Eating Diary* that can help you understand why you eat.

Behavior modification is based on the premise that all behaviors are learned responses to environmental cues or antecedents. In using these techniques, people make eating a more conscious act, and healthier behavior patterns are integrated into the day-to-day routine. These include slowing the act of eating, altering susceptibility to the cues (separating eating from other activities, such as watching TV), and breaking behavior chains. Table 10.5 gives examples of some behavior modification techniques.

Changing eating behavior demands commitment and perseverance (unlike the magic potion or easy and simple pitches delivered in many popular magazines). Too often, commercial weight-loss programs reward persons simply for the total number of pounds lost, creating undesirable behaviors such as going on crash diets, skipping meals, and using drugs and diuretics. According to some weight-management researchers, "The use of reinforcement for weight loss is inappropriate because weight loss is not a behavior, but the outcome of a complex interaction of many behaviors over time."[44] Appropriate behavior management for weight control includes learning appropriate food choices for a lifetime *and* increasing physical activity. In order to continue with or maintain a weight loss, you must be able to identify your own high-risk situations in which difficulties with feelings or social situations threaten a relapse. Developing and practicing coping strategies for dealing with these situations is an essential part of eating management. Very importantly, behavior change in regard to eating management works best when you are reinforced by social support—family, friends, dietitians, community, and weight-loss groups.

Exercise

Most obese individuals do not consume significantly greater amounts of food than do nonobese individuals.[45] Some even say that we eat less food than Americans did in the 1900s. Are you surprised? Yet we have gotten fatter because calorie output has declined

table 10.5

BEHAVIOR MODIFICATION TECHNIQUES

1. Keep an eating diary to maximize awareness of eating.
2. Eat in one room only; sit at a table—don't stand.
3. Prepackage healthy snacks or meals and take them with you.
4. Keep a weight, fat gram, or calorie graph.
5. Never read or watch TV while eating.
6. Use smaller plates.
7. Always leave some food on your plate.
8. Drink a lot of water throughout the day and during meals.
9. Prepare, serve, and eat one portion at a time.
10. Do not place serving dishes on the table.
11. Grocery shop from a list and never on an empty stomach.
12. Leave the table after eating and clear dishes directly into the compost pile or garbage; brush your teeth immediately or chew gum.
13. Keep problem food out of sight or not in the house at all.
14. Keep healthy food accessible and visible.
15. Eat slowly; chew each bite thoroughly; put utensils down between bites; eat with your nondominant hand; cut food into smaller pieces.
16. Rehearse strategies in advance for eating out, special occasions, and high-risk situations.
17. Substitute alternative activities for eating (write a letter; go for a walk; jog; pay bills; sew; play tennis; etc).
18. Don't do non-food-related activities in the kitchen; stay out of the kitchen as much as possible; close the kitchen down after a meal.

drastically. Our diet hasn't changed as much as our exercise habits have. Television viewing, which substantially decreases activity levels and may influence diet, is a strong factor in obesity.[46] Computers, video games, and VCRs have further decreased overall activity levels. American technology has been ingenious in discovering ways for us to save energy, thus throwing off our energy balance. Electric garage door openers, riding lawn mowers, electric toothbrushes, and drive-in banks are just a few examples of activity-robbing conveniences.

The secret to lifelong weight management is exercise, not dieting. While exercise is an important part of an initial weight-loss program, it is one of the few factors positively correlated with long-term weight *maintenance*.[47] A year-long study[48] of overweight men and women compared body weight losses between two groups: those who dieted only and those who combined diet with exercise (brisk walking/jogging three times per week for 25 to 45 minutes). The diet-plus-exercise group increased loss of body fat, especially in the dangerous abdominal fat area. Regular, aerobic exercise contributes to fat loss in several ways.

It Burns Calories

Table 10.6 shows how many calories you burn per minute in various activities. Note that the larger person burns more energy than does the lighter person engaged in the same activity. Also notice how aerobic activities burn considerably more calories per minute than do light, day-to-day tasks. Most people burn approximately 100 calories per mile whether walking or jogging. If this does not seem like a lot, look at it this way: You only burn about 1 calorie per minute while sitting. Remember that weight gain does not occur overnight; nor does weight loss. A pound of fat is lost by burning 3,500 calories. No one ever said it must all be done at once and only by jogging. Find ways to weave increased energy expenditure into day-to-day living: Walk to work, take stairs instead of elevators, ride a bike on errands.

table 10.6

CALORIC EXPENDITURE PER MINUTE FOR VARIOUS ACTIVITIES

BODY WEIGHT	117	143	170	196
Sitting, quietly reading	0.9	1.1	1.4	1.6
Driving a car	1.8	2.1	2.6	2.9
Household tasks (dusting, sweeping)	2.3	2.9	3.4	3.9
Showering	2.7	3.3	3.9	4.5
Basketball (moderate)	5.5	6.7	7.9	9.2
Bicycling (4.6 min./mile, 13 mph)	8.3	10.2	12.1	14.0
Dance (aerobic, medium)	6.2	7.0	7.8	9.0
Dance (waltz)	4.0	4.9	5.8	6.7
Golf (foursome)	3.2	3.9	4.6	5.3
Racquetball	7.6	9.3	11.0	12.7
Running (8.5 min./mile, 7 mph)	10.8	13.3	15.7	18.2
Swimming (crawl, 50 yds./min.)	8.3	10.1	12.0	13.9
Tennis (recreational)	5.4	6.6	7.8	9.0
Volleyball (moderate)	4.4	5.4	6.4	7.4
Walking (13.3 min./mile, 4.5 mph)	5.1	6.3	7.5	8.6
Weight training	6.2	7.5	8.9	10.3

source: Data from C. Frank Consolazio, Robert E. Johnson, and Louis J. Pecora, *Physiological Measurement of Metabolic Functions in Man* (McGraw-Hill Book Company, 1963), 331–32.

There is some controversy as to whether exercise increases postexercise basal metabolic rate.[49] If there is some slight increase in metabolism after exercise, the total effect on energy balance is minimal. The greatest benefits of exercise in weight control are in the calories burned in the actual exercise and in the positive effects it has on maintaining lean body mass.

It Prevents Loss of Lean Body Mass (Muscle Mass)

Aerobic exercise enhances the burning of body fat. It also tends to build muscle tissue. Since muscle cells are metabolically active, they burn more calories in basal metabolism than do fat cells.

It Is a Natural Appetite Suppressor

Moderate exercise has a tendency to decrease the appetite for a period of time after the workout because blood is diverted from digestive organs to skeletal muscles. You may feel thirsty but not usually hungry. This is why exercising during a lunch break helps you control weight. After exercising, you feel satisfied with a light lunch. Extremely intense exercise tends to lower blood sugar, which stimulates appetite. So to burn fat, keep your exercise at a moderate intensity and work to increase the duration. (Be sure not to view exercise as an excuse for eating more.)

It May Lower Your Set Point

The set-point theorists believe that regular, vigorous exercise is the one sure way to lower your body's fat level. Maintaining an active lifestyle stabilizes the set point at this lower level.

Beware of Fads, Myths, Gimmicks

It Promotes the Maintenance of Weight Loss

Most health professionals agree that losing weight is easy; keeping it off is much more difficult. To avoid the negative consequences of weight cycling, much more attention is being given to *maintenance* of weight loss. Exercise has been shown to be one of the few factors correlated with long-term weight maintenance.[50] A change in lifestyle that includes a consistent exercise regimen across the life span is the fundamental key to successful weight-loss maintenance.

Other Ways Exercise Helps with Weight Management

For overweight, sedentary individuals, exercise may not be a richly reinforcing experience at first. It may be difficult for them to get out and exercise in public. They may feel self-conscious about their bodies. They may have negative feelings about exercise because of past embarrassing experiences. As exercise becomes a satisfying habit, the individual begins to experience a new sense of well-being and power. Anxiety and depression are reduced. As weight comes off, self-image is enhanced. Self-esteem and self-confidence are improved. These psychological benefits received from regular participation in physical activity are often the additional impetus necessary for adhering to a weight-loss/maintenance program. This positive self-concept helps reinforce all other areas of weight management, including food selection, feelings of anxiety, and feelings of control.

Commonly Asked Questions About Weight Control

Q. I have cellulite on my thighs. Is there any special way to remove it?

A. There is no such thing as **cellulite.** It is a slang term used to describe the dimpled fat found primarily on the buttocks and thighs of women. Concentrated areas of fat tend to bulge in some women because, with age, their connective fibers become taut and their skin thin. This fat is like any other fat in that only a comprehensive program of exercise and calorie reduction will remove it. No miracle creams, saunas, diets, or devices specifically break up cellulite. Buying a product that claims to do this only reduces your wallet.

Q. The only place I feel I have too much fat is on my abdomen. Is there any way to just lose fat there?

A. The concept of *spot reduction* (that is, selectively burning off fat from a particular body area) is a myth. No one can dictate where body fat will accumulate or from where it will be removed. Genetics determine your body build and preferred fat storage sites. Exercising a specific body area does not burn fat in just that area. Fat stores from throughout the body are mobilized during exercise. So your abdomen will lose fat only after a combined program of total-body aerobic exercise and calorie management, not solely by doing 100 curl-ups a day. It is possible to "spot tone," however. Those 100 curl-ups create very strong abdominals.

Q. I have read that eating grapefruit with other foods burns excess fat. Is this true?

A. There is no magic food combination that specifically burns fat, just as there is no "negative-calorie" food (that is, food that burns more calories than it contains).

Q. My friend had his stomach stapled and lost a considerable amount of weight. What about this and other surgical treatments of obesity?

A. Surgery for obesity should not be taken lightly and should be considered only as a last resort for the morbidly obese (those at least 100 pounds above ideal weight). Even the nonsurgical means of jaw wiring and inserting balloons in the stomach are drastic measures in tackling obesity. As with any major medical procedure, these methods have inherent risks and medical complications. Also, their long-term effectiveness is questionable, unless a drastic lifestyle change accompanies the procedure. **Liposuction** (suctioning

Weight-loss gimmicks reduce
your wallet not your waist.

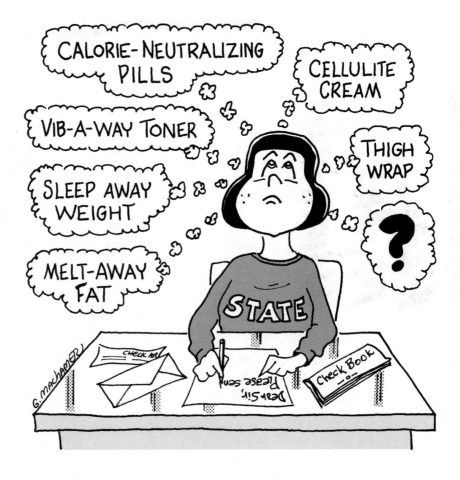

fat from under the skin) has become popular as a method of removing body fat from selected body parts. This surgical procedure, performed by physicians who specialize in cos-
metic surgery, is another questionable approach to weight loss.

Q. I see a lot of weight-loss pills and candies in drugstores and available by mail
order. Are they effective?

A. Over-the-counter products are promoted to do everything from curb the appetite
to magically melt away fat. If you purchase these gimmicks, you are looking for the
"quick fix," not a lifestyle change. Those desperate to lose weight are often easy prey for
drugs and products that promise the metabolically impossible. The side effects (nervousness, sleeplessness, irritability) make such products questionable lifetime weight-
management strategies. Some have caused severe, even fatal, reactions. Ephedrine and
the Chinese herb ma huang are common ingredients in diet/fat burning products that
can cause dangerous reactions.

There is one compound causing a barrage of interest and research because of its
possible link to fat loss and muscle mass retention. This substance, a highly absorbable
form of the trace mineral chromium (i.e., chromium picolinate and niacin-bound
chromium—*not* chromium chloride), is now showing up in supplements on the shelves
of health food and drugstores. Found primarily in brewer's yeast and whole grains,
chromium is involved in carbohydrate and fat metabolism in the body. Chromium deficiency is common in the United States, primarily due to our high consumption of refined and processed foods.[51] For some people, supplementing the diet with absorbable
forms of chromium has helped control blood sugar, lower cholesterol, and utilize body
fat as fuel, while retaining lean body mass.[52] Much more research is needed in this area
before broad-based supplementation is recommended. There is no miracle diet pill, so
any supplementation should be discussed with a physician.

Q. I have seen a lot of advertisements from health salons promoting effortless exercise machines for weight loss. Do they work?

A. Because many people do not understand the basic principles of fat metabolism, they fall prey to the appeal of these ads. After all, they say you don't have to sweat or even change clothes. It takes only minutes. Roller machines, oscillating tables, electrical muscle stimulators, and power-driven vibrators are promoted as equipment that removes fat or breaks up fatty deposits. These devices are worthless gimmicks. They have no value in reducing fat because of the lack of effort on the part of the participant. Remember, fat loss is a result of burning more calories than you consume. Since these machines are doing the work, few calories are burned. Using active machines such as stationary bicycles, rowing machines, stair climbers, and cross-country skiing machines are effective ways to burn calories, because they require *you* to exert energy.

Q. What about body wraps, rubberized suits, and other special weight-reducing apparel? I've worn some of these and they seem to work.

A. Waist belts or body wraps do nothing more than squeeze water out of one tissue area into another. Think about the indentation that occurs on your wrist after wearing a rubber band there for several minutes. This circumference loss is only temporary until rehydration occurs. Rubberized or vinyl suits can be dangerous, especially if worn while exercising. These suits trap the heat and perspiration given off by the body, not allowing the natural process of evaporation—the body's normal cooling process. These suits make you like a turkey basting in its own juices. Water, not fat, is lost by the body, and the danger of life-threatening overheating is possible. Again, as soon as the body is rehydrated, weight is regained.

Q. I am heavily involved in competitive sports. As a result, I am very muscular. When I stop competing, how do I avoid having all of that muscle turn into fat?

A. Your concern is fueled by a common misconception. Muscle can no more turn into fat than a cat can turn into a dog. Neither can fat become muscle. The cellular makeup of each is totally different. If you stop activity altogether, your muscles will atrophy and lose tone. Calories not needed to fuel your body will be stored as fat. To avoid this, continue some regular exercise and modify your calorie consumption, being sure your energy input and output are relatively equal.

Q. I have heard that I will burn more fat if I work out at the lower end of my target heart rate range rather than at a high intensity. Is this true?

A. This low-intensity fat-burning idea is a misunderstanding based on an oversimplification. It is true that the higher the exercise intensity, the more the body prefers to use glycogen rather than fat for fuel. Some have interpreted this to mean that to burn fat, low-intensity exercise is best. However, the type of fuel used during exercise does not make a great deal of difference. The most important exercise variable is *total* caloric expenditure. Because you don't fatigue as quickly when exercising at a low intensity, you may be able to work out for a longer period of time and feel more comfortable while doing it.

Q. Most of my friends talk about wanting to lose weight. But I want to gain some weight. How do I do it?

A. First of all, realize that body build is genetic. Some people are built like greyhounds, some like German shepherds. Once you assess your body type and potential, engage in weight training and a general exercise program to increase your muscle density. You do not want to put on excess fat by indiscriminately eating more food. Protein drinks are not the answer; nor are high fat and sugar snacks. Do make sure you increase your caloric intake some to compensate for the energy burned while exercising, but make healthy food choices. Complex carbohydrates are best. Ways to healthfully increase your caloric intake include the following:

- Replace sodas with fruit juices.
- Replace cookies and doughnuts with nuts, raisins, bran muffins, yogurt, milk, and fruit.
- Replace hamburgers and fries with thick-crust vegetable-topped pizza.
- Prepare hot cereals with milk instead of water; add nuts, peanut butter, fruit, and wheat germ.
- Top cold cereal with bananas or raisins.
- Eat hearty soups.
- Add garbanzo beans, seeds, tuna, croutons, cottage cheese, and lean meat to salads.

Q. I am concerned because my sister is very much overweight. She doesn't act like it bothers her, but I think it does. What can I do to motivate her to lose weight?

A. Often, we have relatives or friends who have health-robbing habits (smoking, being overweight, not exercising). Because we care about them, it is natural to want to help. In the case of your sister, do not nag or criticize her. Instead, set a good example and talk about why you do the things you do (select certain foods, behavior modification tricks, etc.). Try to include her in your practices. Invite her to go on a walk, bike riding, or to an aerobics class. Grocery shop or eat out together. Share recipes and food preparation ideas. Show that you care. Make a pact with her (you will try to stop biting your fingernails, while she tries to lose weight). Be there for her. However, realize that she is ultimately responsible for herself. Nevertheless, be her friend, confidante, and number-one cheerleader.

Eating Disorders

We live in a society obsessed with thinness. In our culture, thin signifies power, success, and control. This indoctrination begins early in life, and the hundreds of hours we spend in front of the television, at the movies, and looking through magazines drives home the message. The famous, the glamorous, and the models are thin. Every day, we see flat stomachs, perfect breasts, flawless teeth, narrow waists, and unblemished complexions. Our culture especially socializes girls to be concerned about their physical appearance. Even though in popular magazines over the last 20 years there has been increasing emphasis on health and fitness, the coverage typically emphasizes body shape and appearance rather than the value of good nutrition and proper exercise. For example, a recent study revealed that *Seventeen* magazine continues to suggest to its young readers that nutrition is "dieting and weight loss" and fitness is "physical attractiveness," thus contributing to the cultural milieu in which thinness is an expectation for women.[53] Women and girls have a tendency to define their worth in relation to what they perceive others think about them. For them, thinness equates with attractiveness and social approval. The message is, "Work hard in school, but be popular and pretty." On the contrary, a male's self-concept is linked to physical dominance and sports competence. Most adolescent boys desire to be bigger and stronger. Studies have shown that females consistently desire to weigh less than their ideal body weight, whereas males do not.[54]

For adolescents, self-esteem is often determined by body image. **Body image** is the mental picture a person has of his or her body, and the associated attitudes and feelings toward it. This image is not necessarily consistent with actual physical appearance. The changes of puberty bring more fat stores to the average girl. As this new physical self meets the mental self, a negative body image may result. More fat is natural and normal to the adolescent female, but it opposes what she thinks everyone prefers. Feeling these pressures, women often compare themselves to a norm of unrealistic thinness. Since few measure up to the fashion industry's ideal, dieting is commonplace. At the same time, obesity is dramatically rising among children in our country: Thin nine year olds are dieting and fretting about their weight. The dilemma of preventing obesity yet avoiding a fostering of thin mania presents a tremendous challenge.

The frequency of dieting among teenage girls is alarming. In some cases, dieting is carried to such an extreme that the behavior becomes obsessive. Fear of fat, fad dieting, and a distorted body image can lead to a psychological eating disorder. An eating disorder is defined as "a disturbance in eating behavior that jeopardizes a person's physical or psychosocial health."[55] You should bear in mind that preoccupation with weight and dieting are not synonymous with an eating disorder. An eating disorder is an extremely serious psychopathological state. Eating disorders are now viewed as multidimensional in cause and nature: psychiatric, physiological, and social. Thus, the treatment must include all components. Certain populations are especially at risk for developing eating disorders. These include gymnasts, dancers (especially ballet), cheerleaders, pom-pom performers, distance runners, and models. Even though more women than men suffer from eating disorders, there is a higher than normal incidence of eating disorders in certain subgroups of males where slenderness is encouraged: models, dancers, wrestlers, and long-distance runners.

High school and college-age students are also vulnerable due to academic and social stresses as well as peer pressure to conform. Most social events take place around eating and drinking: parties, dates, late night snacks. Physical attractiveness is important, and the stresses of growing up and leaving home intensify these pressures. Rather than a strict addiction, eating disorders are a response to our societal influences, dieting culture, fat discrimination, overachieving perfectionism, and media images. Two of the most common eating disorders are bulimia and anorexia nervosa. They may occur separately or together.

Bulimia Nervosa

Bulimia is a Greek word meaning *ox* and *hunger*. The disorder was so named because the sufferer eats like a hungry ox. That is, bulimia is characterized by a compulsive need to eat large quantities of food (binging) to the point of gorging, followed by purging through vomiting, use of laxatives, or fasting. Often, the binge is a response to an intense emotional experience, such as stress, loneliness, or depression, rather than the result of a strong appetite. Nevertheless, most bulimics are not aware of what precipitates these uncontrollable binges, nor are they able to stop them. The diagnostic criteria for bulimia are as follows:[56]

1. Recurrent episodes of binge eating (rapid consumption of a large amount of food in a discrete period of time)
2. A feeling of lack of control over eating behavior during the eating binges
3. Self-induced vomiting, use of laxatives or diuretics, strict dieting or fasting, or excessive exercise in order to prevent a weight gain
4. Persistent overconcern with body shape and weight
5. Two binge episodes a week for at least three months

Bulimia is the most common eating disorder. Some surveys suggest the prevalence of bulimia to be as high as 19 percent in college-age women and 5 percent in college-age men.[57]

Bulimia frequently starts as normal, voluntary dieting behavior but later becomes compulsive, uncontrollable, and pathological. The bulimic's eating binge involves a rapid gulping down of enormous quantities of food. Preferred foods are high in calories and sweet tasting and can be eaten rapidly without preparation: ice cream, cookies, candy, bread, cheese, chips, doughnuts. The consumption of this food is not a pleasurable pastime but a compulsion. Up to 20,000 calories can be consumed in one sitting, followed by abdominal pain and discomfort. The binge generates guilt, depression, and anxiety. Purging follows, reducing the anxiety and fear. Then the cycle begins again.

The bulimic is aware of his or her abnormal behavior and has great fear of not being able to stop. He or she has feelings of guilt and shame about the behavior. Bulimia is a secret habit and can continue for many years undetected. The weight of most bulimics is normal or fluctuates within 10 pounds as a result of the binge-purge cycle.

The physical effects of bulimia include electrolyte imbalance (especially potassium), low blood sugar, esophageal lacerations, dehydration, and nerve and liver damage from low potassium. Tooth enamel is eroded by the stomach acid brought up with vomiting. Severe abdominal pain is common. In rare cases, actual rupture of the stomach has occurred. Bone density is lost if the disorder continues for many years.

People with bulimia need professional help and are often tearful and desperate when they finally seek help. Psychotherapy is necessary to understand the underlying cause of the disorder as well as to help reshape the bulimic's feelings of self-worth and self-confidence. Bulimics tend to be extroverted perfectionists—high achievers—and are often academically or vocationally successful. Yet bulimics have troubled interpersonal relationships, low self-esteem, poor impulse control, and high levels of anxiety and depression and are self-critical and sensitive to rejection. It is not uncommon to see other impulsive behaviors among bulimics, including kleptomania, alcohol and drug use, and sexual promiscuity.[58] The treatment goal is to get the bulimic to cope with her stresses and body image insecurities through less destructive ways and to feel more comfortable with herself in today's world. Bulimia is difficult to cure, and some struggle with this disorder for life.

Anorexia Nervosa

Far less common than bulimia, **anorexia nervosa** is a psychological disorder in which self-inflicted starvation leads to a drastic loss of weight. Whereas the bulimic has a general dissatisfaction with his or her body weight, the anorexic is obsessed with achieving thinness. Individuals with anorexia nervosa have an iron determination to become thin and an intense, irrational fear of becoming fat. They vehemently deny their impulse to eat, their appetite, and their enjoyment of food. The term *anorexia* is actually a misnomer, because loss of appetite is usually rare until late in the illness. While bulimics feel shameful about their abnormal behavior, anorexics justify their weight-loss efforts.

Found primarily in early and middle adolescent females, anorexia may result in physical deterioration to the point of hospitalization or even death. Anorexia carries a 19:1 female-to-male ratio, with a prevalence estimated at 1 percent among adolescent girls.[59] The diagnostic criteria for anorexia are as follows:[60]

1. Refusal to maintain body weight at or above a minimal normal weight for age and height (e.g., weight loss leading to maintenance of body weight less than 85 percent of that expected)
2. Intense fear of weight gain or becoming fat, even though underweight
3. A disturbance in the way in which one's shape and weight are experienced, undue influence of body weight or shape on self-evaluation, or denial of the seriousness of the current low body weight
4. In females, amenorrhea for at least three consecutive menstrual cycles

Anorexia often starts as innocent dieting that turns into irrational behavior characterized by severe caloric restriction, fasting, relentless exercising, diuretic and laxative use, and, in some cases, self-induced vomiting. The anorexic pursues and maintains thinness despite an emaciated appearance that is so apparent to others.

Anorexics display an extraordinary amount of energy for exercise and schoolwork in spite of their starvation state. However, they avoid social relationships, have low self-esteem, and are fearful of change. Despite an aversion for eating, anorexics are preoccupied with food. They may prepare elaborate meals for others, collect recipes, carry or hide snacks, and memorize the caloric content of various foods. Bizarre eating habits are commonplace. Anorexics have been known to cut a raisin in two and chew each half for several minutes. In many situations, they may pretend to be eating while putting food into their napkin or feeding the dog under the table.

Family stress and social pressure contribute to this disorder. Most anorexics come from middle- to upper-class families that place a high premium on achievement, perfection, and physical appearance. Their families are often overcontrolling and overprotective. Anorexics exhibit extreme perfectionism accompanied by a profound sense of ineffectiveness. Only by restricting food intake do they feel a sense of control and capable of coping with life's stresses.

Anorexia causes the physiological complications that accompany any malnutritive state: chronic fatigue, dry and scaly skin, hair falling out, lack of menstruation, drops in blood pressure, and cardiac complications. Constipation is commonplace. Bone growth is retarded, increasing the risk of fractures and osteoporosis. Anorexics have an unusual sensitivity to cold due to their low body-fat percentage.

Treatment for anorexia nervosa involves medical, psychological, and nutritional help. The major obstacle to treatment is the patient's denial that any problem exists. The entire family must be involved, since the anorexic's behavior has deep psychological origin: low self-esteem, struggle for control and independence, and fear of physical sexual development.

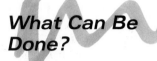

What Can Be Done?

The risk factors for bulimia and anorexia nervosa are similar in many ways—that is, female gender, ambiguity in sex roles for women, and sociocultural emphasis on thinness. Since both eating disorders appear to be increasing in incidence, implementation of prevention programs is desperately needed. The most obvious and effective site for prevention is the schools. However, all segments of society need to absorb some of the responsibility, including parents, coaches, advertising executives, the media, and the entertainment business. Society needs to send the message of healthy acceptance of self and body. Not everyone is meant to be a size 6.

If you suspect a friend, roommate, or relative of having an eating disorder, you probably wonder what you can do to help. Eating disorders are not solely about food and eating but are manifestations of emotional distress. Therefore, just begging someone to start eating or put on some weight is futile. Nor will ignoring the situation or waiting to see what happens solve the problem.

The first step to recovery is indisputable: Locate professional help as soon as possible. Congress has mandated that every state establish a system of community mental health centers to assist people with a variety of psychological problems. These centers are a good source for providing treatment or helping you locate professionals who specialize in treating eating disorders. Even though psychotherapy has become more prevalent and accepted in the last 25 years, some still avoid it. For whatever reason, psychotherapy still carries a stigma with some people.

Since your anorexic or bulimic acquaintance may deny the condition or balk at your suggestion to seek help, it may be very difficult to persuade her or him to seek help. However, both physical and psychological evaluation are crucial at the onset of treatment. You cannot force someone to get help. It is important, however, to be direct and honest while showing sincere concern and support. You may have to be tough, even make the appointment, and insist on accompanying the anorexic or bulimic to see the specialist.

Other Sources of Help

American Anorexia/Bulimia Association, 418 East 76th Street, New York, NY 10021, (212) 734-1114.

Anorexia Nervosa and Related Eating Disorders, P.O. Box 5102, Eugene, OR 97405, (503) 344-1144.

National Association of Anorexia Nervosa and Associated Disorders, P.O. Box 2771, Highland Park, IL 60035, (708) 831-3438.

The National Anorectic Aid Society, 1925 East Dublin-Granville Road, Columbus, OH 43229, (614) 436-1112.

SUMMARY

Obesity should be acknowledged as this country's most important nutrition-related disease. It is a complex disorder, no longer considered just a problem of overeating or lack of willpower. It is caused by multiple factors—some within your control and some beyond. Genetics, environment, and culture combine to complicate the simple act of nourishing our bodies. It is important to understand body composition and be able to differentiate between overweight and obesity. Since many health problems are associated with obesity, concern with weight control should begin sufficiently early in life to reduce the risk of developing obesity. Prevention is the treatment of choice. The factors affecting obesity give insight into the complexities of losing excess body fat.

"Monday I start my diet" is far too often the battle cry for losing weight. This diet mentality has actually contributed to the obesity problem. Dieting and concerns about appearance have also contributed to the increasing incidence of eating disorders. Because successful weight management has been elusive for many obese individuals, the marketplace has provided many legitimate as well as unfounded claims about products and services. Therefore, consumer education is essential. Effective weight management involves nutritional knowledge, behavior management, and exercise. Whereas dieting is temporary, restrictive, and negative, lifestyle weight management is a positive, flexible means of dealing with food for life and health. It is a lifestyle of low-fat eating and regular exercise, amidst established cultural patterns and social and economic forces. No gimmick or gadget can replace this lifestyle approach.

Regular exercise is the key ingredient in maintaining a healthy body composition. Technological advances have increased the quality of our lives in many ways but have eliminated much daily physical exertion. It is a challenge to find ways to fit activity into your life. However, lifelong weight management and total wellness depend on it. Only when we start considering food as fuel and accepting a range of healthy body weights will obesity begin to be eradicated.

REFERENCES

1. National Academy of Sciences. "Summary: Weighing the Options—Criteria for Evaluating Weight-Management Programs." *Journal of the American Dietetic Association* 95 (January 1995): 96–105.
2. "A New Spin on Yo-Yo Diets." *University of California, Berkeley Wellness Letter* 11 (January 1995): 1–2.
3. Kuczmarski, Robert J., Katherine M. Flegal, Stephen M. Campbell, and Clifford L. Johnson. "Increasing Prevalence of Overweight Among U.S. Adults: The National Health and Nutrition Examination Surveys, 1960 to 1991." *Journal of the American Medical Association* 272 (July 20, 1994): 205–11.
4. Department of Health and Human Services, Public Health Service. *Healthy People 2000: National Health Promotion and Disease Prevention Objectives.* Washington, D.C.: Department of Health and Human Services, 1990.
5. Kuczmarski, et al. "Increasing Prevalence of Overweight."
6. Hawks, Steven R., and Paul Richins. "Toward a New Paradigm for the Management of Obesity." *Journal of Health Education* 25 (May/June 1994): 147–73.
7. Garner, David, Paul Garfinkel, Donald Schwartz, and Michael Thompson. "Cultural Expectations of Thinness in Women." *Psychological Reports* 47 (October 1980): 483–91.
8. Wiseman, Claire V., James J. Gray, James E. Mosimann, and Anthony H. Ahrens. "Cultural Expectations of Thinness in Women: An Update." *International Journal of Eating Disorders* 11 (January 1992): 85–89.
9. "The New American Body." *University of California, Berkeley Wellness Letter* 10 (December 1993): 1–2.
10. Williams, Melvin H. *Nutrition for Fitness and Sport,* 3d ed. Dubuque, Iowa: Wm. C. Brown Publishers, 1992.
11. "Body Mass Index Makes Comparisons Easier." *Obesity & Health* 5 (January/February 1991): 8.
12. Williams. *Nutrition for Fitness and Sport.*
13. *Healthy People 2000.*
14. National Academy of Sciences. "Summary: Weighing the Options."
15. U.S. Department of Agriculture, U.S. Department of Health and Human Services. "Nutrition and Your Health: Dietary Guidelines for Americans." 3d ed. *Home and Garden Bulletin,* no. 232 (1990).
16. Willett, Walter C., JoAnn E. Manson, Meir J. Stampfer, Graham A. Colditz, Bernard Rosner, Frank E. Speizer, and Charles H. Hennekens. "Weight, Weight Change, and Coronary Heart Disease in Women." *Journal of the American Medical Association* 273 (February 8, 1995): 461–65.
17. Stamford, Bryant. "Apples and Pears: Where You 'Wear' Your Fat Can Affect Your Health." *The Physician and Sportsmedicine* 19 (January 1991): 123–24.
18. " 'Unhappy' Fat Cell Seeks Balance." *Obesity & Health* 6 (March/April 1992): 25.
19. " 'Unhappy' Fat Cell Seeks Balance."

20. " 'Unhappy' Fat Cell Seeks Balance."
21. Keesey, Richard E. "A Set-Point Theory of Obesity." *Handbook of Eating Disorders*. Kelly D. Brownell and John P. Foreyt, eds. New York: Basic Books, 1986, 63–87.
22. Bennett, William Ira. "Beyond Overeating." *The New England Journal of Medicine* 332 (March 9, 1995): 673–74.
23. Bennett. "Beyond Overeating."
24. "What Causes Obesity." *Reebok Instructor News* 5 (Winter 1992): 4–5.
25. Bouchard, Claude, et al. "The Response to Long-Term Overfeeding in Identical Twins." *The New England Journal of Medicine* 322 (May 24, 1990): 1477–82.
26. Stunkard, Albert J., Jennifer R. Harris, Nancy L. Pedersen, and Gerald E. McClearn. "The Body-Mass Index of Twins Who Have Been Reared Apart." *The New England Journal of Medicine* 322 (May 24, 1990): 1483–87.
27. National Institutes of Health. *Strategy Development Workshop for Public Education on Weight and Obesity: Summary Report*. Washington, D.C.: U.S. Department of Health and Human Services, 1994.
28. National Institutes of Health. *Strategy Development Workshop*.
29. Davis, Judi Ratliff, and Kim Sherer. *Applied Nutrition and Diet Therapy for Nurses*, 2d ed. Philadelphia: W. B. Saunders Co., 1994.
30. Dattilo, Anne M. "Dietary Fat and Its Relationship to Body Weight." *Nutrition Today* 27 (January/February 1992): 13–19.
31. Dattilo. "Dietary Fat and Its Relationship to Body Weight."
32. Hands, Elizabeth S. *Food Finder*, 3d ed. Salem, Ore.: ESHA Research, 1990.
33. Suter, Paolo M., Yves Schutz, and Eric Jequier. "The Effect of Ethanol on Fat Storage in Healthy Subjects." *The New England Journal of Medicine* 326 (April 9, 1992): 983–87.
34. "Issues in Weight Control." *Journal of the American Dietetic Association* (supplement) 92 (January 1992): 17–22.
35. "Weight-Loss Regimens Among Overweight Adults." *The Journal of the American Medical Association* 262 (September 1, 1989): 1163, 1167.

36. Williams. *Nutrition for Fitness and Sport*.
37. Williams. *Nutrition for Fitness and Sport*.
38. Leibel, Rudolph, M.D., Michael Rosenbaum, M.D., and Jules Hirsch, M.D. "Changes in Energy Expenditure Resulting from Altered Body Weight." *The New England Journal of Medicine* 332 (March 9, 1995): 621–28.
39. National Task Force on the Prevention and Treatment of Obesity. "Weight Cycling." *The Journal of the American Medical Association* 272 (October 19, 1994): 1196–1202.
40. King, Abby C., and Diane L. Tribble. "The Role of Exercise in Weight Regulation in Nonathletes." *Sports Medicine* 11 (May 1991): 331–49.
41. Davis and Sherer. *Applied Nutrition and Diet Therapy for Nurses*.
42. Hawks and Richins. "Toward a New Paradigm for the Management of Obesity."
43. Davis and Sherer. *Applied Nutrition and Diet Therapy for Nurses*.
44. Robison, Jonathon, Sharon Hoerr, Karen A. Petersmarck, and Judith V. Anderson. "Redefining Success in Obesity Intervention: The New Paradigm." *Journal of the American Dietetic Association* 95 (April 1995): 422–23.
45. King and Tribble. "The Role of Exercise in Weight Regulation in Nonathletes."
46. Gortmaker, Steven L., William H. Dietz Jr., and Lilian W. Y. Cheung. "Inactivity, Diet, and the Fattening of America." *Journal of the American Dietetic Association* 90 (September 1990): 1247–55.
47. King and Tribble. "The Role of Exercise in Weight Regulation in Nonathletes."
48. Wood, Peter D., Marcia L. Stefanick, Paul T. Williams, and William L. Haskell. "The Effects on Plasma Lipoproteins of a Prudent Weight-Reducing Diet, with or Without Exercise, in Overweight Men and Women." *The New England Journal of Medicine* 325 (August 15, 1991): 461–66.

49. Poehlman, Eric T., Christopher L. Melby, and Michael I. Goran. "The Impact of Exercise and Diet Restriction on Daily Energy Expenditure." *Sports Medicine* 11 (February 1991): 78–101.
50. King and Tribble. "The Role of Exercise in Weight Regulation in Nonathletes."
51. Hendler, Sheldon Saul, M.D. *The Doctors' Vitamin and Mineral Encyclopedia*. New York: Simon and Schuster, 1990.
52. Kamen, Betty. *The Chromium Connection: A Lesson in Nutrition*, 3d ed. Novato, Calif.: Nutrition Encounter, Inc., 1994.
53. Guillen, Eileen O., and Susan I. Barr. "Nutrition, Dieting, and Fitness Messages in a Magazine for Adolescent Women, 1970–1990." *Journal of Adolescent Health* 15 (September 1994): 464–72.
54. "Body-Weight Perceptions and Selected Weight-Management Goals and Practices of High School Students—United States, 1990." *The Journal of the American Medical Association* 266 (November 27, 1991): 2811–12.
55. Harris, Robert T. "Anorexia Nervosa and Bulimia Nervosa in Female Adolescents." *Nutrition Today* 26 (March/April 1991): 30–34.
56. *Diagnostic and Statistical Manual of Mental Disorders*. 4th ed. (revised). Washington, D.C.: American Psychiatric Association, 1994.
57. Harris. "Anorexia Nervosa and Bulimia Nervosa in Female Adolescents."
58. Harris. "Anorexia Nervosa and Bulimia Nervosa in Female Adolescents."
59. Harris. "Anorexia Nervosa and Bulimia Nervosa in Female Adolescents."
60. *Diagnostic and Statistical Manual of Mental Disorders*.

SUGGESTED READINGS

Anderson, Arnold E. *Males with Eating Disorders*. New York: Brunner/Mazel, Publishers, 1990.

Bailey, Covert. *The New Fit or Fat*. Boston: Houghton Mifflin Co., 1991.

Bennion, Lynn J., Edwin L. Bierman, and James M. Ferguson. *Straight Talk About Weight Control*. New York: Consumers Union, 1991.

Berg, Frances M., ed. *Health Risks of Obesity*. Hettinger, N.D.: Healthy Weight Journal, 1993.

Berg, Frances M., ed. *Health Risks of Weight Loss*. Hettinger, N.D.: Healthy Weight Journal, 1993.

Brehm, Barbara A., and Betsy A. Keller. "Diet and Exercise Factors That Influence Weight and Fat Loss." *IDEA Today* (October 1990): 33–46.

Brownell, Kelly D., and John P. Foreyt, eds. *Handbook of Eating Disorders*. New York: Basic Books, Inc., 1986.

Brownell, Kelly D., Judith Rodin, and Jack H. Wilmore. *Eating, Body Weight and Performance in Athletes: Disorders of Modern Society*. Philadelphia: Lea and Febiger, 1992.

Cassell, Jo Anne. "Social Anthropology and Nutrition: A Different Look at Obesity in America." *Journal of the American Dietetic Association* 95 (April 1995): 424–27.

Fallon, April E. "Body Image and the Regulation of Weight." *Psychological Perspectives on Women's Health*. Vincent J. Adesso, Diane M. Reddy, and Raymond Fleming, eds. Washington D.C.: Taylor and Francis, 1994.

Ferguson, James M. *Habits Not Diets: The Secret to Lifetime Weight Control*. Palo Alto, Calif.: Bull Publishing Co., 1988.

Foreyt, John P., and G. Ken Goodrick. *Living Without Dieting*. New York: Warner Books, 1992.

Frankle, Reva T., and Mei-Uih Yang, eds. *Obesity and Weight Control*. Rockville, Md.: Aspen Publishers, 1988.

Gilbert, Sara. *The Psychology of Dieting*. London and New York: Routledge, 1989.

Gortmaker, Steven L., William H. Dietz, and Lilian W. Y. Cheung. "Inactivity, Diet, and the Fattening of America." *Journal of the American Dietetic Association* 90 (September 1990): 1247–55.

Harris, Robert T. "Anorexia Nervosa and Bulimia Nervosa in Female Adolescents." *Nutrition Today* 26 (March/April 1991): 30–34.

Hawks, Steven R., and Paul Richins. "Toward a New Paradigm for the Management of Obesity." *Journal of Health Education* 25 (May/June 1994): 147–53.

Hsu, Lee Keung George. *Eating Disorders*. New York: Guilford Press, 1990.

"Issues in Weight Control." *Journal of the American Dietetic Association* (supplement) 92 (January 1992): 17–22.

Jablow, Martha M. *A Parent's Guide to Eating Disorders and Obesity*. New York: Delta Publishing, 1992.

Jenson, Heather. "Bulimia Nervosa: Predictors of Recovery and Treatment Intervention." *Journal of Health Education* 25 (November/December 1994): 338–40.

Kane, June Kozak. *Coping with Diet Fads*. New York: The Rosen Publishing Group, 1990.

Kano, Susan. *Making Peace with Food: Freeing Yourself from the Diet/Weight Obsession*. New York: Harper & Row, 1989.

Katch, Frank I., and William D. McArdle. *Nutrition, Weight Control and Exercise*. 4th ed. Philadelphia: Lea and Febiger, 1993.

King, Abby C., and Diane L. Tribble. "The Role of Exercise in Weight Regulation in Nonathletes." *Sports Medicine* 11 (May 1991): 331–49.

Li, Virginia C. "On Diet and Dieting: Reaching High Level Wellness." *Wellness Perspectives* 7 (Winter 1990): 61–75.

Logue, Alexandra Woods. *The Psychology of Eating and Drinking*. 2d ed. New York: W. H. Freeman and Co., 1991.

"Losing Weight: What Works, What Doesn't." *Consumer Reports* 58 (June 1993): 347–57.

Miller, Wayne C. *The Non-Diet Diet: A Simple 100-Point Scoring System for Weight Loss Without Counting Calories*. Englewood, Colo.: Morton Publishing Co., 1992.

National Institutes of Health. *Strategy Development Workshop for Public Education on Weight and Obesity: Summary Report*. Washington D.C.: U.S. Department of Health and Human Services, 1994.

Ornish, Dean. *Eat More, Weigh Less*. New York: HarperCollins, 1993.

Papazian, Ruth. "Never Say Diet?" *Healthline* 11 (October 1992): 4–7.

Schlundt, David G., and William G. Johnson. *Eating Disorders: Assessment and Treatment*. Boston: Allyn and Bacon, 1990.

Schwartz, Hillel. *Never Satisfied: A Cultural History of Diets, Fantasies, and Fat*. New York: The Free Press, 1986.

Seid, Roberta Pollack. *Never Too Thin*. New York: Prentice-Hall Press, 1989.

Shisslak, Catherine, Marjorie Crago, and Mary E. Neal. "Prevention of Eating Disorders Among Adolescents." *American Journal of Health Promotion* 5 (November/December 1990): 100–106.

The University of California, Berkely Wellness Reports. *Nutrition for Optimal Health and Weight Control*. New York: Health Letter Associates, 1995.

Tribole, Evelyn, and Elyse Resch. *Intuitive Eating: A Recovery Book for the Chronic Dieter*. New York: St. Martin's Press, 1995.

Williams, Melvin H. *Nutrition for Fitness and Sport*, 3d ed. Dubuque, Iowa: Wm. C. Brown Publishers, 1992.

Wolf, Naomi. *The Beauty Myth: How Images of Beauty Are Used Against Women*. New York, N.Y.: W. Morrow, 1991.

chapter 11

Cancer Prevention

➤ Objectives

After reading this chapter, you will be able to:

1. Identify how cancer deaths rank in overall death statistics.

2. List five primary prevention factors for reducing cancer risk and the three major controllable risk factors included in that list.

3. Give four guidelines for preventing sun overexposure.

4. Give four guidelines for selecting foods that reduce cancer risk, and apply the guidelines to a menu.

5. List three secondary prevention factors for cancer.

6. Recognize the proper procedure and schedule for conducting a breast or testicular self-exam.

7. Identify cancer's seven warning signals.

[handwritten: tobacco usage, sun exposure, diet]

➤ Terms

- Antioxidants
- Benign
- Beta-carotene
- Cancer
- Carcinogens
- Crucifera *[handwritten: veg]*

- Free radicals
- Human papilloma virus (HPV)
- Malignant
- Melanoma
- Metastasis

- Phytochemicals
- Precancerous
- Primary prevention
- Secondary prevention
- Tumor

You may not have been responsible for your heritage, but you are responsible for your future.

Anonymous

 wellness lifestyle implies taking responsibility for your own health and making wise choices. The purpose of this chapter is to discuss how to decrease cancer risk, which is strongly affected by personal lifestyle choices. You will learn which behaviors increase health risks and how to decrease these risks to enhance your own state of wellness.

Cancer Incidence

Cancer is the second leading cause of death overall in the United States.[1] According to present rates, about one in three Americans will eventually have cancer. Even though gains have been made in cancer treatment and survival, the total number of cancer deaths has increased. Today, it is more likely that we will be affected by cancer since we are living longer and there is more time for carcinogens to affect cells. While cancer is most common in people over 55, it can strike at any age. The earlier a cancer is detected, the simpler the treatment and the higher the survival rate. For this reason, it is important to understand cancer risk factors and warning signals and to practice self-exams.

Diversity Issues

Rates of incidence of certain types of cancers differ among countries, races, and socioeconomic groups. Some differences occur because of cultural habits practiced for a lifetime. For example, in Japan, salted and pickled foods are consumed in abundance and rates of stomach cancer are higher than in the United States, where consumption of these products is lower. In the United States, a diet rich in high fat meat and processed and refined food results in high rates of colorectal cancer, which is rare in countries where the diet consists largely of unrefined grains, fruits, and vegetables.

Likewise, cultural influences affect rates of certain types of cancer among socioeconomic groups. Smoking is an example. At one time, smoking symbolized sophistication, affluence, and maturity, and over half the population smoked, but this has changed. Nevertheless, while smoking has declined to about 29 percent of the population, 50 million Americans, mainly the less educated, still smoke.[2] Also, many teenagers are taking up smoking, which foreshadows grim health problems for that group in the future.

Not only cultural influences, but racial background or genetics can affect cancer rates. People with brown, olive, or black skin have a measure of protection against skin cancer provided by melanin, a natural skin pigment. Darkly pigmented blacks can have up to 30 times more melanin than people with pale white skin and are less likely to suffer skin damage due to sun exposure. However, blacks are more prone to a type of melanoma that most often appears on the palms, soles, nail beds, and mucous membranes.

What Is Cancer?

Cancer is not a single disease, but a group of over 100 different diseases, all characterized by abnormal cell growth and replication. Normally, cells grow and are replaced in an orderly manner. Enough new cells grow to replace those that are worn out and injured. Cancer cells lack controls to stop the growth process and continue to grow and multiply without restraint. This loss of control of cell growth may be due to a variety of factors. Ultraviolet radiation from sunlight, tobacco smoke, viral infections, diet, and chemicals in food and in the environment all have been implicated.

It is possible that all of us at some time experience potentially cancerous changes in our cells. These **precancerous** cells usually die or are destroyed by the immune system. Few live long enough to cause harm. If one abnormal cell survives, it can replicate into billions of cells, forming a lump or **tumor**. Tumors may be benign or malignant. **Benign** tumors are usually nonthreatening. Although they can grow large enough to interfere with organs and bodily functions, they seldom cause death. They usually resemble surrounding tissue, remain localized, and spread by expansion, like a wart or mole. They do not spread to other parts of the body. They can be removed completely by surgery and are not likely to recur. **Malignant** tumors are cancerous. They differ from surrounding tissue and tend to spread through **metastasis**. In metastasis, cells break away from the primary tumor and migrate to other tissues through the lymph or blood systems where they continue to grow. They have lethal potential because they invade and destroy normal tissues and spread to other parts of the body.

How to Cut Your Risk of Cancer (Primary Prevention)

People hear so much about cancer, they often get the feeling that everything causes cancer. If everything causes cancer, then there seems to be no use in trying to avoid it. They feel that there is little they can do to make a difference in their cancer risk or that it is not worth the effort. They are wrong. Cancer, like heart disease, is largely preventable. Approximately 85 percent of cancers may be related to lifestyle and environmental factors over which you have control.[3] These cancers occur as a result of cumulative exposure to **carcinogens**, substances that cause cancer, over a period of time. The avoidance of factors that might lead to the development of cancer is termed **primary prevention**. The major primary prevention factors are controllable: tobacco usage, sun overexposure, and diet. Other primary prevention factors include reducing alcohol consumption, avoiding hazards in the workplace, and minimizing exposure to radiation and environmental contamination. Choices you make daily can greatly cut your cancer risk. It is a matter of education and habit change. What follows is discussion of what you can do.

Avoid Tobacco in Any Form

This includes cigarettes, pipes, cigars, snuff, and chewing tobacco. Tobacco contains many carcinogens that increase the risk of developing several types of cancers. (See Chapter 12 for additional information on the effects of tobacco.) In addition, when a smoker is exposed to other carcinogens, there seems to be a synergistic effect that multiplies cancer rates beyond what would be expected from the effect of each alone. For example, smoking combined with the use of alcohol greatly increases the risk of cancer. The number of smokers is decreasing in the United States. However, the use of smokeless tobacco, especially "dipping snuff," has increased.[4] Whereas tobacco use is most often implicated in lung cancer, tobacco products can produce a variety of oral cancers, including cancer of the lip, tongue, mouth, and throat.

The good news is that cancers caused by smoking are 100 percent preventable. If you are a nonsmoker, don't start. If you are a smoker, quit.

Reduce Sun Exposure

Overexposure to the sun is the main cause of skin cancer. It is estimated to strike one of every six Americans, making it the most common cancer.[5] We have been a nation of sun worshipers and are seeing the consequences. How ironic that the price of a "healthy" tan can be premature skin aging and wrinkling and skin cancer. It is never good to lie in the sun to tan, but you can still enjoy outdoor activities and minimize negative effects by following the guidelines in Table 11.1 on page 240.

Eat Healthfully

About one-third of all cancer deaths are related to diet.[6] Certain foods seem to be related to an increase or decrease in some kinds of cancers; for instance, a high-fat diet seems to play a role in the development of breast, colon, and prostate cancers. A multitude of studies show that by eating high-fiber foods, fruits, and vegetables and by avoiding high-fat red meat, bacon, and processed meats, we could significantly reduce our overall cancer risk. The food pyramid in Chapter 9 and the seven dietary guidelines are excellent models to follow. However, many Americans are not making these simple dietary adjustments. A 24-hour diet survey of 12,000 Americans by the National Cancer Institute indicated that 40 percent had eaten no fruit, 20 percent had not consumed a single vegetable, and 80 percent had consumed no whole grain breads or cereals.[7] Eating a variety of fruits, grains, and vegetables is not only more healthful, but actually less expensive than buying a lot of high-fat meat and highly processed foods such as hot dogs, fries, chips, doughnuts, and junk cereals.

table 11.1

handwritten: 1200% increase since 1935

handwritten: 1/6 purple   40% of all Cancers

HOW TO REDUCE SUN EXPOSURE

1. Avoid prolonged exposure to the sun when ultraviolet (UV) radiation is strongest, between 10:00 A.M. and 3:00 P.M., even on overcast days.
2. Plan activities for early morning or late evening.
3. When you will be working or playing outside for even 15 to 20 minutes, *apply a sunscreen rated SPF 15 or higher.* Newer formulations protect from both UVB and UVA radiation. Reapply every two hours or after swimming or perspiring.
4. Avoid tanning, even in tanning parlors or with sunlamps. There is no such thing as a safe tan. Tanned skin is damaged skin. The UVA light emitted by tanning booths still can cause sunburn, premature skin aging, and increased risk of skin cancer.
5. Protect children from too much sun. Skin damage occurs with each unprotected sun exposure and accumulates over a lifetime. Perhaps most of the damage is done in childhood and adolescence. Even one bad burn in childhood can double the risk of skin cancer.
6. Know what skin cancer looks like and examine your skin at least once a month. If you find unusual moles or skin spots, have them examined by your physician.

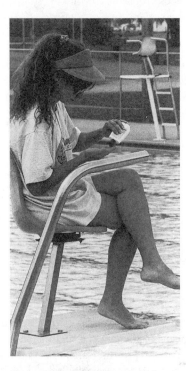

If you have an outdoor job, be aware of sun overexposure.

Concerns have been voiced about pesticide and chemical residues in fruits and vegetables, as well as about irradiation of fresh produce and poultry. There is no doubt that the production, processing, and transportation of food in our mass-market world raises some serious concerns that necessitate further research. Nevertheless, we do know that sun exposure, a fatty diet, and tobacco products are three highly controllable areas where your behavior has a major impact. Taking positive steps in these three areas makes more sense than worrying about food products over which you have little control.

By making positive choices in your daily diet and following the guidelines listed here, you can promote good health now and can reduce your cancer risk in the future. A sample one-day dietary plan incorporating many of these suggestions is given in Table 11.2.

1. *Decrease fat intake:* A high-fat diet appears to be related to several types of cancers, including breast, prostate, lung, uterine, and skin cancer.[8] Information on dietary fat is found in Chapter 9 in Table 9.6. Table 9.11 gives 23 tips for nutritional wellness, and Table 9.13 illustrates healthy choices at fast-food restaurants.
2. *Eat more high-fiber foods:* These include whole grain breads and cereals, beans, fruits, and vegetables (Table 11.3). Fiber, the nondigestible part of plant cells, seems to protect against colon cancer by speeding potentially harmful substances through the digestive tract and reducing contact time between carcinogens and the intestines.[9] More examples of high-fiber food choices are given in Table 9.3.
3. *Eat cruciferous vegetables:* Broccoli, cauliflower, brussels sprouts, cabbage, turnip greens, and other members of the mustard family help prevent certain cancers from developing. **Phytochemicals** (plant chemicals) unique to **crucifera** (cabbage, turnip, and mustard family) stimulate liver enzymes responsible for inactivating toxic chemicals.[10]
4. *Include foods rich in vitamins C and E, folic acid, and beta-carotene in your diet each day:* Citrus fruits, tomatoes, green peppers, baked potatoes, broccoli, and strawberries are high in vitamin C. Dark-green and deep-yellow fresh vegetables and fruits such as carrots, corn, spinach, winter squash, peaches, and apricots contain up to 500 or more natural carotenoids. While much research has focused

table 11.2

ONE-DAY SAMPLE MENU

Breakfast	Whole grain cereal, toast, or lowfat muffin; skim milk; and fruit.
Lunch	Tuna or chicken sandwich made with whole grain bread; lowfat dressing; soup, salad, or vegetables; and skim milk.
Dinner	Pasta or rice dish with small amount of meat; beans; two vegetables; whole grain bread; and skim milk.
Snacks	Lowfat popcorn; fruit; frozen yogurt; pretzels; or raw vegetables with a lowfat dip.

table 11.3

WAYS TO INCREASE FIBER INTAKE

INSTEAD OF	EAT
White bread	Whole grain bread
White rice	Brown rice
Mashed potatoes	Baked potato in the skin
Orange juice	Orange
Applesauce	Unpeeled apple
Processed cereals	Whole grain cereals
Potato chips	Popcorn, plain or lightly seasoned
Always increase fluid intake with increases in dietary fiber.	

on **beta-carotene**, many other carotenoids are stronger **antioxidants**, and it may be that a combination of these and other phytochemicals make them cancer-protective. Green and leafy vegetables, whole grains, egg yolks, nuts, and wheat germ contain folic acid and vitamin E. Folic acid is a B vitamin that guards against cell mutations and chromosome abnormalities that may be involved in initiation of cancer. Folic acid works synergistically with antioxidant vitamins to neutralize **free radicals**, potentially dangerous substances that produce pre-cancerous cellular damage.[11] More information on food sources of these nutrients is given in Chapter 9, in Table 9.7.

5. *Consume charcoal-grilled, salted and nitrite-cured, smoked, and pickled foods in moderation:* Charring and cooking meats at high temperatures for long periods of time produces carcinogens. The preservative nitrate in processed meats such as hot dogs, luncheon meats, bacon, beef sticks, and beef jerky forms cancer-causing substances when broken down by the body.

6. *Drink lowfat milk daily:* Calcium appears to neutralize potentially carcinogenic substances in the digestive tract, reducing the risk of colorectal cancer. Also, processed cheese contains a cancer inhibitor, a form of linoleic acid, which may be incorporated into body cells of people who consume it, locking in a defense against cancer.[12]

Is taking a vitamin pill effective in reducing cancer risk? The debate rages on. While some experts recommend vitamin supplements, others feel that this causes us to get more vitamins than our bodies can use, and the excess are excreted in the form of expensive urine. Both groups agree on this: Pills cannot make up for a bad diet. There is good evidence that a diet rich in certain fruits, vegetables, and whole grain products lowers the risk of some types of cancer, but it is not yet clear whether it is the antioxidants, folic acid, or another of the dozens of phytochemicals in these foods that makes them cancer-protective.[13] A plant may be more than the sum of its nutrients. While taking a pill probably won't hurt, no one compound, or even a small group of compounds, will replace hundreds of nutrients, many of which we are only beginning to learn about. Don't count on a vitamin to replace a diet abundant in fruits and vegetables.

Manage Weight

Cancer is also linked to obesity. Obese individuals increase their risk of cancer of the breast, colon, and reproductive organs. The more overweight a person is, the greater the risk. People who carry extra weight in the abdomen are at higher risk for breast and endometrial cancer.[14,15] The good news is that those who are apple-shaped (as opposed to pear-shaped, having bigger thighs and hips) can reduce their risk by losing weight.[16] It appears to be fairly easy for apple-shaped people to lose weight where it counts since fat leaves the abdomen first. While the explanation for the reduced risk is uncertain, researchers believe that weight loss reduces the amount of sex hormones available to stimulate possible precancerous cell growth in the reproductive organs.

Reduce Alcohol Consumption

Avoid alcohol or limit alcohol intake to two drinks a day or less. Excessive alcohol consumption increases the risk of several cancers. Esophageal and liver cancer occur more frequently among heavy drinkers of alcohol especially when the drinking is accompanied by cigarette smoking or chewing of tobacco. Coupled with poor diet, alcohol increases the risk of developing colon cancer because it interferes with folic acid metabolism.

Other Ways to Reduce Cancer Risk

Make regular exercise a habit. There is evidence that the body's immune system may help in preventing cancer.[17,18] Research has shown that exercise enhances overall health and well-being and strengthens the immune system. Researchers also speculate that exercise decreases the production of some reproductive hormones in both men and women, decreasing the risk of cancers that depend on these hormones to develop.[19]

The results of the Harvard Alumni study should convince sedentary Americans to become more physically active in order to improve health and reduce their cancer risk. Researchers reported that males who burned at least 1,000 calories a week in physical activity had half the risk for colon cancer of inactive men.[20] Researchers speculate this is true for women, as well. (One thousand calories is the approximate equivalent of walking 10 miles.) Other studies show the more you exercise, the more protection you get. Exercise appears to prevent colon cancer by helping to speed food through the digestive system, leaving less time for carcinogens to remain in contact with the colon. As you already know, exercise is the key to weight management.

Avoid excessive exposure to ionizing radiation. Ionizing radiation includes X rays, radon, and UV radiation. While most medical X rays emit low-dose radiation, it is still wise to use protective shields to cover body areas not being X rayed. There is also a potential problem of radioactive radon gas in the home in certain areas of the country. You can buy an inexpensive radon detector to test for radon, which increases the risk for lung cancer, especially in cigarette smokers. If you detect radon, professionals can advise you regarding steps to take to increase ventilation and seal the home against radon infiltration.

Be aware of hazards in the workplace. Exposure to asbestos and other industrial materials increases risk, especially when combined with smoking. Minimize exposure to these products by wearing protective clothing and equipment and by following standard safety procedures.

Limit your exposure to PCBs and the insecticide DDT. PCBs are chemicals that were once used in a wide variety of products including paint, pesticides, plastics, adhe-

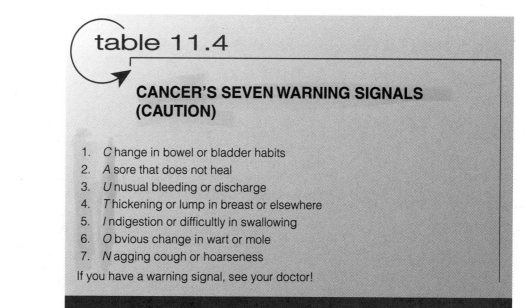

table 11.4

CANCER'S SEVEN WARNING SIGNALS (CAUTION)

1. *C*hange in bowel or bladder habits
2. *A* sore that does not heal
3. *U*nusual bleeding or discharge
4. *T*hickening or lump in breast or elsewhere
5. *I*ndigestion or difficultly in swallowing
6. *O*bvious change in wart or mole
7. *N*agging cough or hoarseness

If you have a warning signal, see your doctor!

source: Courtesy of American Cancer Society.

sives, ink, fire retardants, and electrical insulation. Both PCBs and DDT were banned by the U.S. Environmental Protection Agency in the 1970s, but because contamination of the environment was so widespread, they are still found in the food chain. These chemicals have been found in large amounts in the fat samples of some women who have breast cancer. Not all chemicals are carcinogenic, but a few others that are proven carcinogens include benzene, vinyl chloride, arsenic, aflatoxin, chloroform, formaldehyde. Read and follow label instructions with household and garden chemicals and use natural products when possible (i.e., soap spray to kill aphids).

Early Detection (Secondary Prevention)

Secondary prevention is taking action to diagnose cancer as early as possible. This includes three parts: knowing cancer's warning signals (Table 11.4), practicing self-exams, and getting regular cancer-related checkups by a physician. If cancer is detected in its early localized stages, it is easier to treat. Once metastases spread from the primary site, cancer becomes much more difficult to cure. Although not all cancers can be detected through self-exams, such exams, along with awareness of cancer's seven warning signals, can alert a person to the need to consult a physician.

See your physician for cancer-related checkups. Even if you have no symptoms, it is important for early detection of cancer to have periodic cancer-related checkups (Table 11.5 on page 244). Until all cancers can be prevented, it is important to protect yourself with knowledge about cancer signs, self-exams, early detection, regular checkups, and prompt treatment.

For most people without symptoms, cancer-related checkups are recommended every three years from ages 20 to 39 and annually for those over age 40. People who are at high risk for certain cancers may need tests more often.

Common Cancers

While many types of cancers exist, some are much more common than others. The most common cancers in order of occurrence for men are prostate, lung, and colon/rectum. In the 15- to 34-year-old age group, testicular cancer is the most common. For women, the most common cancers are breast, lung, colon/rectal, and uterine.[21] Although they are the most frequently occurring cancers of all, affecting nearly one in six Americans, skin cancers are not usually included in cancer statistics since almost all nonmelanoma skin cancers are easily cured if detected early.[22] Even so, there are an estimated 8,800 skin cancer deaths yearly.[23]

table 11.5

CANCER CHECKUPS

Breast	Do a monthly self-exam; clinical examination of the breast every three years from ages 20 to 40 and then every year; a screening mammography by age 40, one every one to two years from age 40 to 49, and yearly from age 50.
Colorectal	Have a digital rectal examination by a physician during an office visit yearly after age 40; the stool blood test every year after age 50; the proctosigmoidoscopy examination every three to five years after age 50.
Cervical	Get an annual Pap test and pelvic exam if you are a woman who is or has been sexually active or are age 18 or over. After three or more consecutive satisfactory annual exams, the Pap test may be performed less frequently at the physician's discretion.
Testicular	Do a monthly self-exam.
Skin	Perform a monthly self-exam.
Prostate	Have an annual rectal/prostate examination as part of your regular annual checkup if you are a man over age 40.

table 11.6

WHAT IS YOUR SKIN TYPE?

SKIN TYPE	SUNBURN AND TANNING HISTORY	SPF
I	Always burns, never tans	20–30
II	Burns easily, tans minimally	15–20
III	Burns moderately, tans gradually to light brown	15
IV	Burns minimally, tans well to medium brown	15
V	Rarely burns, tans profusely to dark	10–15
VI	Never burns, deeply pigmented	10–15

Skin Cancer

Skin cancer accounts for 40 percent of all cancers, and sun overexposure during childhood and teen years accounts for much of it. Well-browned skin is a sign of injury to the skin, not a sign of health. While anyone can get skin cancer, people are most susceptible if they work out in the sun, live in sunny climates, or have blonde or red hair, light-colored eyes, or fair skin which doesn't tan easily (Table 11.6).[24]

There are three types of skin cancer that may be caused by UV radiation: basal cell, squamous cell, and malignant melanoma. Basal cell cancers, the most common, are raised pearly nodules that involve the outer layers of skin. Squamous cell cancers are either wart-like growths that ulcerate in the center or pinkish, raised, opaque nodules. These cancers are rarely fatal, do not tend to metastasize, and can be removed by a physician.

Malignant **melanoma**, which usually starts out as a dark wart or mole, has a deadly tendency to metastasize and may be fatal. The problem is particularly severe for men and whites. Men die of melanoma at twice the rate of women.[25] People with naturally dark skin, type VI, have a built-in measure of protection. About 98 percent of malignant melanoma occurs in whites.[26] Contributing to increasing rates of skin cancer is the fact that, in the upper atmosphere, the thinning ozone layer now allows more of the

FIGURE 11.1 ➤
ABCD test for malignant
melanoma.

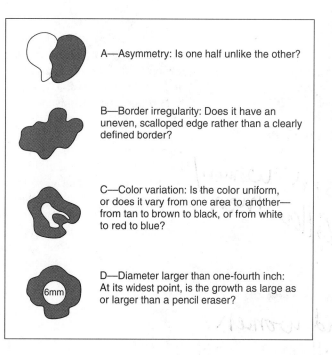

A—Asymmetry: Is one half unlike the other?

B—Border irregularity: Does it have an uneven, scalloped edge rather than a clearly defined border?

C—Color variation: Is the color uniform, or does it vary from one area to another—from tan to brown to black, or from white to red to blue?

D—Diameter larger than one-fourth inch: At its widest point, is the growth as large as or larger than a pencil eraser?

sun's damaging ultraviolet radiation to reach the skin. As a result, skin cancer rates are increasing by about 4 percent per year, faster than any other cancer. Approximately 90 percent of all skin cancers can be prevented by protecting the skin from the sun's rays.[27]

Do tanning beds provide a safe tan? Tanning beds used to emit only UVA ("tanning") rays, but now many approximate natural sunlight, emitting a mix of UVA and UVB ("burning") radiation. UVA rays penetrate deeper into the skin than UVB and can cause serious damage. Both kinds injure the skin, collagen, and immune response and encourage wrinkling and skin cancer. It is a myth that tanning beds will provide a safe "base" tan before a midwinter vacation. The protection is minimal, and you will still burn unless you apply sunscreen. Are the new self-tanning lotions safe? While many previous products turned the skin orange, some newer products contain an FDA-approved dye, dihydroxyacetone (DHA). It stains skin a light brown and is safe to use because it appears to work only on the outermost skin layer. Best results are obtained for people with skin types II and III who have applied the product two to four times within one day. Skin darkened with a dye does not provide UV protection, and you still need to wear sunscreen to guard against burns.

While young people often think of themselves as immune to skin cancer, nearly one-third of all melanomas occur in people under age 45. The most common sites are the upper back and back of the legs, but it can occur anywhere from the scalp to the soles of the feet. You don't have to be a dermatologist to recognize a potential melanoma. It is important to know what skin cancer looks like and to examine your skin at least once a year. Learn where your moles are and what they look like, and then you will notice if there are any changes. If you find unusual moles or skin spots, the American Academy of Dermatology suggests using the ABCD test for early detection of malignant melanoma (Figure 11.1). Besides moles, watch for sores that do not heal, unusual bumps, and chronically scaly, red, or pinkish patches of skin. If detected early, skin cancer has an 85 to 99 percent cure rate.

Lung Cancer

Lung cancer is a rare disease except among smokers. Exposure to sidestream cigarette smoke increases the risk for nonsmokers. Lung tissue damage and cellular changes that precede lung cancer have been observed in 93 percent of active smokers but in only 6 percent of exsmokers and 1 percent of nonsmokers.[28] If a smoker quits, these early precancerous cellular changes are reversible, and the damaged bronchial lining often returns to normal. If the smoker continues, the abnormal cell growth may progress to cancer.

Lung cancer, the leading cancer killer for both men and women, has a low survival rate because it is seldom discovered in its earliest stages. By the time it has grown large enough to produce noticeable symptoms or to be visible on X ray, it is already well advanced. It metastasizes readily through the bloodstream to the brain and other organs and is difficult to treat. The five-year rate for lung cancer survival is 13 percent and has not changed, despite advances in cancer treatment, in 40 years.[29]

Colon and Rectal Cancer

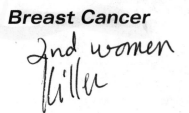

A genetic tendency to develop noncancerous polyps in the colon, combined with a diet high in animal fat and low in fiber, may cause half, perhaps all, colon cancer. One study found that adults whose childhood diets were low in salads and cruciferous vegetables or high in processed meats were more likely to get colon cancer as compared to adults who ate healthier diets. This does not mean that you are doomed by poor childhood eating habits but that eating vegetables and cancer-preventative foods is good insurance at any age. Dietary habits and preferences are formed young and practiced over a lifetime. Chronic exposure to carcinogens in high-fat and highly refined and processed foods can eventually stimulate precancerous changes in cells.

Breast Cancer

Breast cancer is the most common cancer in women, but it is more curable than lung cancer, so it ranks as the second leading cancer killer. It is estimated that the lifetime risk of breast cancer is one out of nine by age 85.[30] Getting older is the most important risk factor for breast cancer. Young women should not feel complacent because breast cancer can occur at any age. Although rare, about 2 percent of breast cancers are in men. Other risk factors for breast cancer include the following:

➤ A sister or mother who has had breast cancer, especially if it occurred before menopause; early onset of menstruation (before age 12)
➤ Experiencing menopause after age 50 (both situations increase the lifelong exposure to high estrogen levels
➤ Obesity
➤ Never having given birth

These factors together account for only 25 percent of all breast cancer. White women have a somewhat higher risk than black or Hispanic women or those of Asian origin.

The incidence of breast cancer is slowly rising, but no one knows why. It could be partly because more women are being diagnosed at earlier ages, thanks to mammography. It might be partly attributed to some as yet unidentified dietary or environmental factor (i.e., PCBs or DDT).[31] High fat intake is currently a suspect. A breast self-exam can detect cancer in its early, curable stage and should be practiced monthly (Figure 11.2).

Prostate Cancer

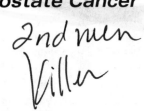

This is the most common cancer (excluding skin cancer) and the second leading cause of cancer deaths in men.[32] The warning signs of prostate cancer are weak or interrupted urine flow; inability to urinate or difficulty starting and stopping urine flow; the need to urinate frequently, especially at night; blood in the urine; pain or burning on urination; and continuing pain in the lower back, pelvis, or upper thighs. Most of these symptoms are nonspecific and may be similar to benign conditions such as infection or prostate enlargement.

Prostate cancer generally occurs in men over 50; risk increases with age. Studies indicate that dietary fat may increase the risk of this cancer.[33]

Testicular Cancer

Most people think that cancer is a disease old people get. Cancer of the testicle is different. It is not one of the most common types of cancer in this country, but it is the most common cancer in young men between the ages of 15 and 34.[34] Warning signs include a swelling or hard lump in the testicle, a dull ache in the lower abdomen and groin, a sensation of heaviness, and pain in the testes. Your risk of getting testicular cancer is 40 times higher if you have a testicle that never descended into the scrotum or descended after age six.

FIGURE 11.2 ➤

Breast self-examination.

Courtesy of American Cancer Society.

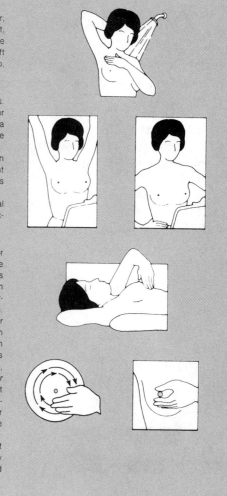

Breast Self-Examination

1. In the shower:
Examine your breasts during bath or shower; hands glide easier over wet skin. Fingers flat, move gently over every part of each breast. Use the right hand to examine the left breast, left hand for the right breast. Check for any lump, hard knot, or thickening.

2. Before a mirror:
Inspect your breasts with arms at your sides. Next, raise your arms high overhead. Look for any changes in the contour of each breast: a swelling, dimpling of skin, or changes in the nipple.

Then rest palms on hips and press down firmly to flex your chest muscles. Left and right breast will not exactly match; few women's breasts do.

Regular inspection shows what is normal for you and will give you confidence in your examination.

3. Lying down:
To examine your right breast, put a pillow or folded towel under your right shoulder. Place right hand behind your head—this distributes breast tissue more evenly on the chest. With left hand, fingers flat, press gently in small circular motions around an imaginary clock face. Begin at outermost top of your right breast for 12 o'clock, then move to 1 o'clock, and so on around the circle back to 12. A ridge of firm tissue in the lower curve of each breast is normal. Then move in an inch, toward the nipple, keep circling to examine *every part of your breast*, including nipple. This requires at least three more circles. Now slowly repeat procedure on your left breast with a pillow under your left shoulder and left hand behind head. Notice how your breast structure feels.

Finally, squeeze the nipple of each breast gently between thumb and index finger. Any discharge, clear or bloody, should be reported to your doctor immediately.

Lives could be saved if more testicular cancers were detected and treated early. The five-year survival rate of testicular cancer is 91 percent.[35] Treatment does not mean losing your "manhood" or your ability to have normal sex, and it doesn't mean you can't have children.

Men themselves discover most testicular cancers by learning how to examine their testicles. In doing this once a month, you can greatly increase the chances of finding a testicular cancer early if it does occur. All young men should learn and practice the monthly testicular self-examination, detailed in Table 11.7 and Figure 11.3 on page 248, from adolescence on. The technique is simple.

Uterine Cancer

With the widespread use of Pap smears for early detection, the death rate from uterine cancer has declined. Cervical cancer, often seen in young women, has been linked to the **human papilloma virus (HPV)** which can be spread through sexual contact. Risk factors for cervical cancer include a history of viral genital infections such as herpes and genital warts, becoming sexually active at an early age, or having had several different sex partners.

A Pap test, in which cells from the cervix and uterine lining are examined under a microscope, is a simple procedure that can be done at intervals by physicians as a part of each pelvic examination. If cervical cancer is detected at an early stage, it can easily be removed.

table 11.7

TESTICULAR SELF-EXAMINATION

1. Perform the examination once a month, after a warm bath or shower, when the scrotal skin is most relaxed.
2. Examine each testicle gently with the fingers of both hands by rolling the testicle between the thumb and fingers.
3. Feel for a small lump, about the size of a pea, generally on the front part of the testicle. There is a natural structure at the back of each testicle called the *epididymis*. Learn what it feels like so you will not confuse it with an abnormal lump.
4. If you do find a lump, tell your physician about it *right away.* Remember, not all lumps are cancerous. Don't let fear keep you from getting the medical attention that could save your life. Cancer will not go away if you ignore it.

FIGURE 11.3 ➤

Testicular self-examination.

Courtesy of American Cancer Society.

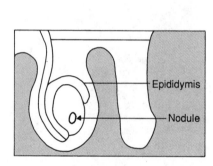
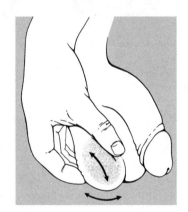

SUMMARY

You can significantly increase your chances of living a healthy, active life, free of disabling disease, by making wise daily personal choices. Your risk of cancer can be greatly decreased with primary prevention awareness. This involves reducing dietary fat; increasing consumption of complex carbohydrates and foods rich in vitamins A, C, and E and folic acid; reducing consumption of alcohol; and avoiding overexposure to sunlight and carcinogens. Secondary prevention is also important. It includes awareness of cancer's seven warning signals, having medical checkups, and performing regular self-exams. Any tobacco product is deadly. Smokers have an increased chance of heart disease, cancer, respiratory disease, and premature death as compared to nonsmokers. Smokeless tobacco causes oral cancer, gum disease, and tooth loss. Smoking is quickly losing its appeal and has fallen to an all-time low as nonsmokers begin to assert their right to breathe clean air. Cancer is not inevitable. Acting to control risks in your immediate environment is a powerful way to enhance your total wellness.

REFERENCES

1. American Cancer Society. *Cancer Facts and Figures—1996.* Atlanta, Ga.: American Cancer Society, 1996 (1599 Clifton Road, N.E., Atlanta, GA 30329-4251).
2. Greenwald, P., and E. J. Sondik, eds. *Cancer Control Objectives for the Nation: 1985–2000.* Bethesda, Md.: National Cancer Institute, 1986.
3. The United Cancer Council. *Cancer Prevention: Fact and Fiction.* Washington, D.C.: U.S. Government Printing Office.
4. *Cancer Facts and Figures—1996.*
5. The Skin Cancer Foundation. New York: 1992.
6. U.S. Department of Health and Human Services. *Nutrition and Health: A Report of the Surgeon General.* Washington, D.C.: U.S. Government Printing Office, 1988.
7. Jennings, Eileen. *Apricots and Oncogenes: On Vegetables and Cancer Prevention.* Cleveland: McGuire & Beckley Books, 1993.
8. "Blocking Skin Cancer Through Diet?" *Tufts University Diet and Nutrition Letter* 12, no. 2 (April 1994): 2.

9. Gray, David S., M.D. "The Clinical Uses of Dietary Fiber." *American Family Physician* 51, no. 2 (Feb. 1, 1995): 419–24.

10. Saltman, Paul, et al. *The University of San Diego Nutrition Book*. Boston, Mass.: Little, Brown, and Co., 1993.

11. Jennings. *Apricots and Oncogenes*.

12. Eichner, E. R. "Exercise, Lymphokines, Calories, and Cancer." *The Physician and Sportsmedicine* 15 (June 1987): 109–16.

13. Jennings. *Apricots and Oncogenes*.

14. Shapira, D. V., N. B. Kumar, G. H. Lyman, et al. "Upper Body Fat Distribution and Endometrial Cancer Risk." *JAMA* 266, no. 13 (1991): 1808–11.

15. Shapira, D. V., N. B. Kumar, G. H. Lyman, et al. "Abdominal Obesity and Breast Cancer Risk." *Annals of Internal Medicine* 112, no. 3 (1990): 182–86.

16. Shapira, D. V., N. B. Kumar, G. H. Lyman. "Estimate of Breast Cancer Risk Reduction with Weight Loss." *Cancer* 67, no. 10 (1991): 2622–25.

17. Woods, Jeffrey A., and J. Mark Davis. "Exercise, Monocyte/macrophage Function, and Cancer." *Medicine and Science in Sports and Exercise* 26, no. 2 (1994): 147–57.

18. Hoffman-Goetz, Laurie. "Exercise, Natural Immunity, and Tumor Metastasis." *Medicine and Science in Sports and Exercise* 26, no. 2 (1994): 157–63.

19. "Fitness and Cancer." *The Physician and Sportsmedicine* 19, no. 12 (December 1991).

20. Lee, I. M., R. S. Paffenbarger, C. Hsieh. "Physical Activity and Risk of Developing Colorectal Cancer Among College Alumni." *Journal of National Cancer Institute* 83, no. 18 (1991): 1324–9.

21. *Cancer Facts and Figures—1995*.

22. *Cancer Facts and Figures—1995*.

23. *Cancer Facts and Figures—1995*.

24. "Even Though You Don't Burn, You Still May Be at Risk." *Healthline* 12, no. 7 (July 1993): 12.

25. *Cancer Facts and Figures—1996*.

26. *Cancer Facts and Figures—1996*.

27. *Cancer Facts and Figures—1996*.

28. U.S. Department of Health and Human Services. *Cancer of the Lung. Research Report*. Washington, D.C.: U.S. Government Printing Office, 1993.

29. *Cancer Facts and Figures—1996*.

30. "One in Nine American Women Will . . ." *University of California, Berkeley Wellness Letter* (July 1992).

31. Watson, Traci. "Breast Cancer's Deadly Masquerade?" *U.S. News & World Report* (February 7, 1994): 59–60.

32. *Cancer Facts and Figures—1996*.

33. *Cancer Facts and Figures—1996*.

34. *Cancer Facts and Figures—1996*.

35. *Cancer Facts and Figures—1996*.

SUGGESTED READINGS

American Cancer Society. *Cancer Facts and Figures—1996*. Atlanta, Ga.: American Cancer Society, 1996 (1599 Clifton Road, N.E., Atlanta, GA 30329-4251).

American Health Research Institute Staff. *Food—Good, Bad, Cancer Potential and the Delaney Clause: Index of New Information and Medical Research Bible*. New York: Random House, Inc., 1994.

Barraclough, Jennifer. *Cancer and Emotion: A Practical Guide to Psych-Oncology*. New York: Wiley Publishers, 1994.

Becker, Gail. *Antioxidant Pocket Counter: A Guide to the Essential Nutrients That Can Help Fight Cancer*. New York: Random House, Inc., 1994.

Coping: Living with Cancer Magazine. Nashville, Tenn. (219 N. Carothers, Nashville, TN 37064).

Dreher, H. *Your Defense Against Cancer*. San Francisco, Calif.: HarperCollins Publishers, 1994.

"The Alcohol/Breast Cancer Connection." *University of California, Berkeley Wellness Letter* 10, no. 6 (March 1994): 1–2.

Holt, Tamara. *Broccoli Power*. New York: Dell Publishers, 1993.

Jennings, Eileen. *Apricots and Oncogenes: On Vegetables and Cancer Prevention*. Cleveland: McGuire & Beckley Books, 1993.

Lerner, Michael. *Choice in Cancer* (videotape). Bolinas, Calif.: *Commonweal* (Box 316, Bolinas, CA 94924): 1993.

Lewis, Claire, et al., eds. *The Psychoimmunology of Human Cancer: Mind and Body in the Fight for Survival*. New York: Oxford University Press, 1994.

Simonton, O. Carl, M.D., and Reid Henson. *The Healing Journey, The Simonton Center Program for Achieving Physical, Mental, and Spiritual Health*. New York: Bantam Books, 1994.

Washington, Harriet. "The Back to the Future Diet." *Harvard Health Letter* 19, no. 8 (June 1994): 6–7.

Whelan, Elizabeth. *The Complete Guide to Preventing Cancer: How You Can Reduce Your Risks*. Buffalo, N.Y.: Prometheus Books, 1994.

RESOURCES

American Cancer Society, Inc., National Headquarters, 3340 Peachtree Road NE, Atlanta, GA 30326, 1 (800) ACS-2345.

Cancer Information Clearinghouse, National Cancer Institute, Building 31, Room 10A18, 9000 Rockville Pike, Bethesda, MD 20225.

Cancer information number, 1 (800) 4-CANCER for all areas except Alaska 1 (800) 638-6070, Hawaii 1 (800) 524-1234.

Living With Cancer, Inc., P.O. Box 3060, Long Island City, NY 11101.

Sexually Transmitted Disease Hot Line, 1 (800) 227-8922.

Y-Me Breast Cancer Support Program, 1 (800) 221-2141.

Internet Addresses

Information on CancerNet from the National Institute of Health. Name: National Institute of Health. Gopher: //gopher.nih.gov.

Database on alternatives to conventional medicine, including acupuncture, homeopathy, chiropractic, osteopathy, diet therapy, herbalism, holistic treatment, traditional Chinese medicine, ayurvedic medicine, yoga, meditation. Name: Allied and Alternative Medicine (AMED). Contact: Data-star through Dialog 1 (800) 334-2564. Telnet: //dialog.com.

Gopher server of the National Institute for Cancer Research and the Advanced Biotechnology Center of Genoa, Italy. Contact: gophman@istge.ist.unige.it. Gopher://istge.ist.unige.it.

Information service for the National Cancer Center in Tokyo, Japan. Contact: ncc-gopher-news@gan.ncc.go.jp. Gopher: //ncc.go.jp.

chapter 12

Substance Abuse

➤ Objectives

After reading this chapter, you will be able to:

1. Give three out of five reasons alcohol/drug dependence is considered a disease.
2. Define the following terms: drug, addiction, alcoholism, tolerance, passive smoking, 'roid rage, and synergy.
3. List five factors that affect alcohol absorption.
4. Describe the effects of alcohol on the central nervous system and personal behavior.
5. Differentiate between alcohol use, abuse, and alcoholism.
6. Identify family behaviors that reduce one's risk of alcohol-related problems.
7. Identify the blood alcohol concentration (BAC) at which a person is regarded legally drunk.
8. Describe the "Zero . . . One . . . Three Rule for Lower-Risk Drinking."
9. Explain why a person may not feel intoxicated but have a BAC of 0.10 percent or more.
10. List the harmful effects of alcohol on the body.
11. Choose a correct guideline to follow if you overindulge in alcohol.
12. Choose a correct guideline to follow if a friend passes out from alcohol overindulgence.
13. List five tips/strategies for drinking less or not at all.
14. Evaluate your personal alcohol use.
15. Differentiate between fetal alcohol syndrome (FAS) and fetal alcohol effect (FAE).
16. Identify the health hazards related to passive smoking.
17. Identify the two most common illegal drugs used in the United States today.
18. Identify the side effects of marijuana, cocaine, anabolic steroids, caffeine abuse, LSD, and heroin.
19. Describe the relationships between cocaine and crack and between crank and ice.
20. List four drugs that affect physical performance and describe how they do so.
21. List three of four common kinds of nonprescription drugs that can lead to physical dependence if overused.
22. Describe how prescribed drugs can be abused.

Terms

- Addiction
- Alcohol (ethyl alcohol, ethanol)
- Alcoholism
- Amotivational syndrome
- Amphetamines
- Anabolic steroids
- Binge drinker
- Blackout
- Blood alcohol concentration (BAC)
- Caffeine
- Cocaine
- Crack
- Crank
- Delta-9-tetrahydrocannabinol (THC)
- Diuretics
- Drug
- Fetal alcohol effect (FAE)
- Fetal alcohol syndrome (FAS)
- Flashbacks
- Heroin
- Ice
- LSD (Lysergic Acid Diethylamide)
- Marijuana
- Narcolepsy
- Nitrosamines
- Passive smoking
- Psychedelic drugs
- 'Roid rage
- Synergistic reaction
- Testosterone
- Tolerance

Everyday, ordinary people accomplish extra-ordinary things.

Unknown

We all live in a drug saturated environment. We have drugs for everything—anxiety, depression, infection, and pain. A **drug** is a chemical that alters a person's physical or mental condition. The question is not whether to use drugs, since most people do, but, rather, when, where, why, and how much to use them. Most of us use over-the-counter drugs, such as aspirin. Others of us use prescribed drugs for a medical condition. Still others misuse and abuse legal and illegal drugs at the cost of our bankbooks, our relationships, and even our lives (Table 12.1). Alcohol is addressed first because it is the most abused legal drug in our society. This chapter includes alcohol use assessments, responsible drinking guidelines, and strategies for drinking less to help you make decisions and take action about your alcohol use. Other drugs addressed are tobacco, illegal recreational drugs, drugs affecting physical performance, and over-the-counter and prescription drugs. Before we discuss specific drugs, let's examine addiction in general.

table 12.1

SUBSTANCE USE IS NOT JUST A COLLEGE PROBLEM— IT BEGINS MUCH EARLIER

Drugs used today are more potent, more dangerous, and more addictive than ever. Initial drug use occurs at an increasingly early age. It erodes the self-discipline and motivation necessary for learning and is closely tied to dropping out of school. Fifty-seven percent of all high school seniors in the United States have used an illicit drug at least once before they finish high school. Thirty-six percent have used an illicit drug other than marijuana. Smoking cigarettes is considered to be a bridge to other drug use, including alcohol. High school seniors who smoke a half a pack of cigarettes a day are *six* times more likely to try cocaine as are nonsmokers, *eight* times more apt to smoke pot, and *three* times more liable to binge drink. Further, teen smoking is linked to other high risk behaviors: fighting, carrying weapons, attempting suicide, and engaging in early, frequent, and unprotected sexual intercourse. Look at substance use in the average class of 30 high school seniors:

- Fifteen or more have tried marijuana at least once.
- At least one uses marijuana daily.
- Twenty-three have reported being around people who were smoking marijuana.
- Twenty-seven have tried alcohol.
- At least one uses alcohol almost daily.
- Seventeen report that they are often around people who are using alcohol to get high.
- Ten say most or all of their friends use enough to get drunk at least once each week.
- Five have tried cocaine.
- Seven have tried nonprescription sedatives and tranquilizers.
- Six have tried inhalants.
- Four have tried hallucinogens.
- Seven have tried amphetamines.
- Six use cigarettes daily.

source: National Institute on Drug Abuse, 1987.

Addiction

Addiction is a pathological or abnormal relationship with an object or event.[1] It is an illness that progresses from a definite, though often unclear, beginning toward an end point. Beginning as a voluntary, pleasurable act, it then becomes a reflective and compulsive behavior. The most insidious of all addictions is alcoholism, which has been recognized as a disease by the American Medical Association since 1956. This recognition eliminates notions that the alcoholic is a weak-willed person, who could quit drinking if he or she wanted. Recognizing alcoholism and other drug dependence as a disease implies five points:

1. *The disease can be described.* The compulsion to drink (or to use other drugs) is manifested in habits that are inappropriate, unpredictable, excessive, and constant.
2. *The course of the disease is predictable and progressive.* It will get worse; it is as simple as that. Sometimes, there will be plateaus when the drinking and/or drug behavior seems to remain constant for months or even years. But over time the course of the disease will move inevitably toward greater and more serious deterioration. This deterioration can be physical, mental, and spiritual.
3. *The disease is primary.* Alcoholism/drug dependency is a primary disease. Other problems the victim may have cannot be treated until the dependency is treated.
4. *The disease is permanent.* Once you have it, you have it. Trying to learn to use drugs/drink moderately will not work. The chances for successful treatment are much better in the earlier stages of the disease.
5. *The disease is terminal.* If you have a chemical addiction and do not successfully arrest it, you will die from it. Whether the chemical complicates a heart condition, high blood pressure, liver problems, or a bleeding ulcer or precipitates a stroke or suicide, it is still the agent that causes the death.

A useful assessment for recognizing any chemical dependency is to ask, "Is the alcohol or other drug causing *any* continuing disruption in my life—or the lives of those close to me?" (i.e., physical, mental, emotional, social, or economic). If the answer is "yes" and you do not stop drug use, despite damage to home life, school performance, or career, then your chemical usage constitutes harmful dependence. This question is useful in assessing any type of compulsive behavior, including gambling, shopping, and having sex.

Addictive Behaviors Other Than Alcohol or Drug Usage

In past years, the focus of the term *addiction* has been centered exclusively around the use of alcohol and other drugs. Recently, a more neutral term, *dependence*, has been substituted for addiction. *Dependencies* or *addictionlike* behaviors may include objects or events such as food, gambling, sex, shoplifting, work, spending, exercise, and television. Even though these addictive objects or events are different, they all produce the desired and pleasurable mood change the addict seeks:

➤ The gambler feels excited when studying a racing form.
➤ The alcoholic feels relaxed and happy when drinking at the neighborhood bar.
➤ The food addict feels rewarded and comforted when eating or shopping for food.
➤ The shoplifter senses a thrill when stealing a magazine from the drugstore.
➤ The sex addict gets aroused when browsing in a pornographic bookstore or when searching for a new sex partner.
➤ The addictive spender feels exhilarated during a shopping spree.
➤ The workaholic feels an extreme sense of accomplishment while working all day on Sunday.

All of these objects and events have a normal, socially acceptable function. Food is to nourish, gambling is for fun and excitement, sex is for intimacy, and drugs are to help overcome illness. Most people have a normal, healthy relationship with these things, but dependent behavior results in an abnormal relationship. Dependent individuals seek a pleasurable mood change to fulfill personal needs. The addict turns to the addiction just as someone else may turn to a spouse or best friend for support,

table 12.2

HOW ADDICTIONS AFFECT THE WELLNESS DIMENSIONS

Physical	Addicts don't take very good care of their bodies. Addictions over time affect various parts of the body—an alcoholic's liver, a bulimic's throat. The added stress of addiction takes its toll on the heart and every other organ of the body; malnourishment is common; the body's immune system breaks down. A body is more accident prone. Suicidal thoughts may become actions.
Social	Addicts become withdrawn and isolated from others, become loners, and interact only with the object or event of addiction. Their responsibility to family, school, job, etc. diminishes.
Emotional	Feelings of guilt and shame increase; depression is common; unresolved issues increase; mood swings increase; anxiety increases; fits of rage for no reason occur; and paranoia develops (the addict starts to question everyone and everything).
Intellectual	Logic breaks down; the addict's behavior doesn't make sense to him/her; schoolwork falters; he/she loses touch with world events; judgment is impaired.
Spiritual	Addicts are not "connected" in a meaningful way to the world around them; they lose feelings of belonging and being an important part of the world; they lose the sense of knowing themselves; the importance of self drifts further and further away; values and priorities shift; addicts begin to rationalize.
Occupational	The quality of job/school performance decreases as the addict becomes more and more preoccupied; absenteeism increases; relationships at work/school deteriorate; promotions and recognition decrease.
Environmental	Addicts show little concern for the health and well-being of the environment. The addiction (compulsive behavior) consumes his/her energies.

nurturing, and intimacy. As the addiction progresses, the addict becomes more and more preoccupied, withdrawn, and isolated. Table 12.2 illustrates how this type of behavior affects all the dimensions of wellness.

We know that chemical addictions produce physiological dependence resulting in withdrawal symptoms when the substance is denied. When the object of other dependencies (i.e., food or gambling) is withdrawn, withdrawal symptoms also result (i.e., anxiety, irritability, or moodiness).

A person can switch an addictive relationship from object to object and event to event. For example, former alcoholics can become chain smokers. Switching from object to object helps create the illusion that the problem has been taken care of, when in reality one dangerous relationship has replaced another.

Many experts predict that compulsive gambling will soon become a serious national problem.[2] There may be good cause for this concern: Consider the millions of dollars spent in the legal and illegal gambling industry every day. Commercial bingo, dog and horse racing, state and interstate lotteries, and video gambling are all on the increase. Gambling casinos are no longer confined to Nevada and New Jersey; they can now be found on Indian reservations and floating up and down our rivers, and they are being built in more and more states every year. Sports gambling is also booming. As gambling becomes legal in more states, the number of problem gamblers rises proportionally. Current figures estimate that between 3 percent and 11 percent of the entire adult U.S. population are compulsive gamblers.[3] Gambling is meant for amusement, recreation, and excitement, but it can turn into a devastating compulsion in some individuals. Take the self-assessment in Table 12.3 to determine if you have or someone you know has a gambling problem.

Individuals with addictions or who exhibit addictivelike behaviors to substances, objects, or events need professional help. A partial listing of organizations, agencies, and resource centers that give information and assistance with addictions can be found at the end of this chapter.

table 12.3

DO YOU HAVE A GAMBLING PROBLEM?

YES	NO	
		1. Do you frequently gamble with more money than you can afford?
		2. Do you bet on something whenever you can or gamble more than you intended?
		3. Have your ever lost time from school or work because of gambling?
		4. Is gambling making your home life unhappy or is it having a negative effect on your relationships with others?
		5. After losing, do you go back as soon as possible to recoup your losses?
		6. Have you ever lied about your gambling or stolen or borrowed money to gamble or to pay a gambling debt?
		7. Have you ever felt guilty about how much you gamble or about what happens when you gamble?
		8. Have you ever been criticized for your gambling or is it affecting your reputation?
		9. Are you reluctant to use gambling money for "normal" expenditures?
		10. Do you ever gamble to escape worry or trouble?
		11. Have you ever considered suicide as a result of your gambling?
		12. Does gambling make you careless about the welfare of your family or friends?

Scoring: One "Yes" answer indicates you *may* have a problem. Two or more "Yes" answers indicate that you could be addicted or heading that way.

Addictive Personality

Is there such a thing as an addictive personality? Do some individuals possess such a personality? This controversial topic continues to produce heated debate among psychologists. Although the addictive personality type has not been confirmed by research, some experts feel that this personality type does exist. They believe the addictive personality may be found in persons who don't know how to have healthy relationships, have been taught not to trust people, and have never learned to "connect" with others, community, their emotions, and spiritual powers greater than themselves.[4]

These experts believe that early life experiences determine whether a person will live in a state of dependency. They argue that the family environment is the most important determinant because the family is where we learn about relationships. For example, in abusive families, the children are often treated as objects, thus developing low self-esteem and mistrust in people. Also, in neglectful families, children may learn to be passive, to feel dead inside, and they will seek out someone or something that makes them feel alive. This theory reflects the idea that people often form addictions because of the positive feelings (mood change) they experience when using a particular substance or repeating a behavior.

Experts claim there is no single characteristic or constellation of traits that is inevitably associated with addiction. So who is vulnerable? Possibly the individual who

➤ has a low sense of self-esteem;
➤ has a sense of alienation;
➤ is unable to turn to others for comfort;
➤ possesses a need for instant gratification;
➤ is impulsive;
➤ displays antisocial behavior (is willing to go outside the boundaries of what is normally accepted);

- ➤ cannot control strong feelings;
- ➤ rebels against authority;
- ➤ likes to try exciting and dangerous things;
- ➤ lies easily;
- ➤ is a perfectionist—a high achiever;
- ➤ seeks approval from others;
- ➤ fears personal criticism;
- ➤ is overly concerned with how others perceive him or her; or
- ➤ tends to be submissive and dependent.

Many people display these characteristics without becoming addicts. This leads some experts to believe that the personality disorders and antisocial behavior that accompany chemical abuse are the result of this abuse, not the cause of it. They claim there is no way to predict who will become an addict.[5]

Alcohol

Alcohol is the most misunderstood drug in America. Some say alcohol is a beverage, and others say that it is a drug. They say it is a mood-altering chemical in liquid form or that it is sinful and dangerous. Others say it is a rite of adulthood and is safe. What a conflicting set of statements. What is alcohol and what does it do? **Alcohol** (technically known as **ethyl alcohol** or **ethanol**) is a central nervous system depressant. The central nervous system (CNS) is composed of the brain and the spinal cord. A CNS depressant is a chemical that slows brain functions. Alcohol slows reaction time, dulls alertness, and impairs body coordination. It intensifies emotions, lowers inhibitions, and increases risk-taking behaviors. It also disrupts judgment and reasoning power. On the positive side, alcohol is a good social lubricant; on the negative, it can be unhealthy and unsafe if abused.

Alcohol Absorption

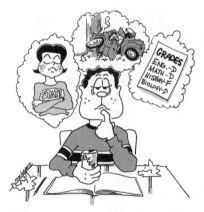

There are many consequences of abusive drinking.

Most healthy bodies process alcohol in the same manner. Alcohol is water soluble and is transported throughout the body by the blood, which is mostly water. The amount of alcohol in the blood is expressed as a percentage; for example, 0.10 percent **blood alcohol concentration (BAC)** or blood alcohol level (BAL). With the first sip, alcohol briefly irritates tissues of the mouth and esophagus. Alcohol rapidly enters the bloodstream through the small intestine and, to a small degree, through the stomach. A fraction exits in breath, sweat, and urine. Alcohol is chiefly metabolized (i.e., chemically broken down) in the liver, through which the entire blood supply circulates every four minutes. Enzymes in the liver metabolize alcohol into acetaldehyde, a highly toxic chemical. This is converted into acetate and, finally, into carbon dioxide and water. The process is slow, taking roughly *three* hours for each ounce of pure alcohol. Despite vigorous folklore, virtually nothing will speed up liver function or sober up the intoxicated. A person who is drunk and drinks coffee does not become sober, only wide awake.

The mind-altering effects of alcohol begin soon after it hits the bloodstream. Within minutes, alcohol enters the brain, numbing nerve cells and slowing their messages to the body. In the heart, cardiac muscles strain to cope with alcohol's depressive action, and the pulse quickens. If drinking continues, alcohol builds in the bloodstream and disrupts the centers in the brain that govern speech, vision, balance, and judgment. As more alcohol is ingested, the drinker may lose consciousness. Alcohol is a hazardous anesthetic, with a narrow range between deadness and dead. At a BAC of 0.4 to 0.6 percent, the drinker is comatose and in danger of dying from respiratory failure.[6]

Speed of Alcohol Absorption

How quickly alcohol is absorbed into your bloodstream depends on five factors: body weight, gender, speed of consumption, food intake, and beverage imbibed. How is alcohol absorption affected by body weight and gender? It is not a myth that a man can drink the same amount of alcohol as a woman of equal weight and have a lower (BAC). This means a woman can get drunk faster than a man does. There are several explanations for this. First, women generally weigh less than men do, so the same amount of alcohol is concentrated in a smaller body mass. Second, even at the same weight, women

FIGURE 12.1 ➤

Percentage of alcohol in beer, wine, and liquor by volume.

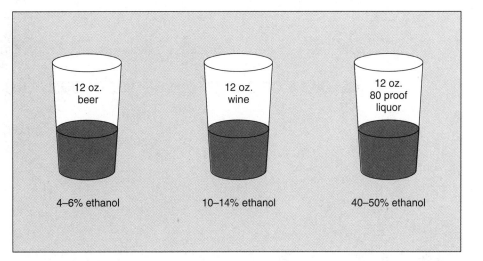

typically have a higher percentage of body fat and less body water than men do. Since alcohol dissolves much more readily in water than in fat, the difference in body composition means that, when alcohol enters a woman's body, it becomes more concentrated and therefore has a more potent effect than the same amount of alcohol would in a man's body. Third, there is an enzyme in the gastric system (small intestine and stomach) that metabolizes alcohol before it is absorbed into the bloodstream. This enzyme is found in greater amounts and is more active in men than in women. So, even if a man and a woman weigh the same, have the same proportion of body fat, and drink the same amounts, more alcohol is likely to reach a woman's blood, brain, and liver than a man's. This phenomenon leaves women more susceptible to liver disease. Alcoholics, especially women, have the added problem of virtually no gastric alcohol metabolism.[7]

Speed of consumption and food intake also affect the rate of alcohol absorption. A 12-ounce can of beer sipped over an hour's time is not absorbed into the bloodstream as fast as a beer that is gulped down quickly. Food in the stomach inhibits alcohol absorption. Without inhibitors in the stomach, alcohol is absorbed extremely fast through the stomach walls and small intestines. Carbonated drinks, such as champagne, rum and coke, and whisky and soda, are absorbed even faster than water-diluted drinks.

There are three major types of alcoholic beverages: beer, wine, and distilled spirits (i.e., hard liquor such as whiskey, vodka, gin, and brandy). All differ as to alcohol content. For example, the alcohol in one 4-ounce glass of wine is 10 percent to 14 percent by volume, in one 12-ounce beer it is 4 percent to 6 percent by volume, and in 1¼ ounces (one shot glass) of distilled spirits it is 40 percent to 50 percent by volume (see Fig. 12.1). However, a standard serving of any one beverage contains approximately the same amount of alcohol. Thus, one 4-ounce glass of wine, one 12-ounce beer, one 12-ounce wine cooler, and one shot glass of liquor all provide approximately the same amount of alcohol.

Often, wine coolers are not perceived as alcoholic beverages because of their fruit juice base and sweet taste. Beware. They contain the same amount of alcohol as beer or any other alcoholic beverage (about 4 percent to 7 percent). These drinks may provide the bridge from soft drinks to other alcoholic beverages for many young people. One person's wine glass is another person's beer mug, so always measure your drinks.

Your alcohol history determines how quickly you feel the effects of this drug. It is based on your lifetime alcohol consumption, the frequency of your drinking, and the tolerance you have acquired. The number of drinks it takes for you to feel a "buzz" increases as your tolerance to alcohol increases. **Tolerance** is the body's physical adjustment to the habitual use of a chemical. Due to alcohol tolerance, an experienced drinker with a BAC of 0.10 percent may not feel drunk. On the other hand, an inexperienced drinker may feel intoxicated at that same BAC because a tolerance has not developed (Table 12.4 on page 258).

table 12.4

PERCENTAGE OF BLOOD ALCOHOL CONCENTRATION (BAC)

NUMBER OF DRINKS*	Body Weight (pounds)				
	120	140	160	180	200
2	0.06	0.05	0.05	0.04	0.04
4	0.12	0.11	0.09	0.08	0.08
6	0.19	0.16	0.14	0.13	0.11
8	0.25	0.21	0.19	0.17	0.15
10	0.31	0.27	0.23	0.21	0.19

EFFECTS RELATED TO BLOOD ALCOHOL CONCENTRATION (BAC)

BAC	Effect
0.04	Reduced visual acuity (as much as wearing dark glasses), slight euphoria, and loss of shyness
0.05	Relaxed state; judgment impaired, caution reduced
0.08	Inhibitions lowered; unexpected behavior
0.10	Movements and speech impaired; legally intoxicated
0.20	Very drunk; loud and difficult to understand; emotions unstable, staggering/muscular coordination reduced; has the appearance of a "sloppy" drunk
0.30	Loss of consciousness
0.40+	Onset of coma; possible death due to respiratory arrest

source: Mothers Against Drunk Driving and PRIDE.
*One drink equals 1½ oz. of 80-proof alcohol, 12 oz. beer, or 4 oz. wine

If you are in a "chugging" contest, many of the previously mentioned factors come into consideration. Chugging is not proof of maturity or a route to social acceptance. Chugging will only make you drunk, incoherent, and accident prone. It is dangerous and may cause convulsions, blackouts (loss of memory during a period of drinking), passing out (unconsciousness), vomiting, nausea, and even death. There are between 200 and 400 alcohol poisoning deaths annually in the United States.[8] Nearly all are due to chugging contests.

Considering all the factors that affect alcohol absorption rate, is your level of alcohol use a low- or high-risk behavior?

Impact of Alcohol

Alcohol is by far the most devastating drug—wrecking families and friendships, impairing health, wrecking careers, and filling jails, hospitals, and morgues. In 1990, it cost U.S. society an estimated $136 billion and more than 100,000 lives.[9] Alcohol accounts for 50 percent of all deaths from motor vehicle crashes, one-third of all drownings, and about half of all deaths caused by fire.[10] Alcohol is linked to half of all homicides, a third of all suicides, and two-thirds of all assaults. Social workers report that alcohol is a factor in nearly 50 percent of their domestic violence cases. Over 36 percent of the male population in prison report that they were under the influence of alcohol at the time of

table 12.5

COLLEGE DRINKING: AND PROBLEMS DRUNKS CAUSE SOBER STUDENTS

- 85% drank alcoholic beverages.
- 44% binged in the two-week period. (Binge drinking is defined as *five* drinks at one setting for men and *four* at one setting for women.)
- 19% were frequent bingers (at least three times in the two-week period).
- 2% thought they were problem drinkers.

Frequent binge drinkers describe their past 30 days:
- 63% did something they regretted.
- 61% missed class because of drinking.
- 60% of men (49% of women) drove after drinking.
- 54% forgot where they were or what they did while drunk.
- 46% fell behind in schoolwork.
- 22% did not use protection during sex.
- 11% got into trouble with campus or local police.

Binge drinking was most common at
- colleges in Northwestern and Northcentral states.
- residential colleges (10% or more of students live on campus).
- co-ed colleges.

Binge drinking was least common at
- colleges in the West and South.
- traditionally black colleges.
- commuter colleges.
- women's colleges.

Sober students are affected in a number of ways: At the big drinking schools, sober students were twice as likely as those at the lowest drinking level schools to be insulted or humiliated; to be pushed, hit, or assaulted; and to experience unwanted sexual advances from drinking students. They were two and one-half times as likely to sustain property damage, to end up taking care of a drunken student, and to have their study or sleep time interrupted by classmates' drinking.

source: The Alcohol Studies Program at Harvard School of Public Health survey of 17,592 students on 140 campuses nationwide during a two-week period in 1994. Wechsler, Henry, et al. "Health and Behavioral Consequences of Binge Drinking in College." *Journal of American Medical Association* 272, no. 21 (December 7, 1994): 1,672–77.

their crimes.[11] The greatest tragedy of all is that the *number-one killer* of teenagers is *drinking and driving*.[12] The majority of these drinkers started early, before they had even turned 13.[13] As you can see in Table 12.5, almost 90 percent of college students report some drinking, ranging from occasional to heavy. Alcohol consumption is one of the major reasons for absenteeism among college students. It is involved in 90 percent of campus rapes, 25 percent of student deaths, and 40 percent of academic problems, and it is the major contributor to campus violence, property damage, and the disruption of sleep and study time.[14] Thousands of college students drop out because of drinking. See Table 12.5 to learn how nondrinking college students are affected by the drinking of their classmates.

Health and Long-Term Effects of Alcohol

Alcohol is a toxin, and its harmful effects on the body are great. A few drinks may make you drowsy and can interrupt patterns of sleep. Over time, heavy drinking can cause brain damage (it speeds the death of brain cells), damage nerve endings, and increase the risk of heart disease and cancer (mouth, throat, stomach, intestines, pancreas, and liver). It can depress the immune system and cause gastritis, pancreatitis, anxiety, delirium tremens (DTs), and malnutrition. Alcohol is a primary cause of liver failure. When alcohol is present in the liver, it preempts the breakdown of fats, which then accumulate within the liver cells. As fatty cells enlarge, they can rupture or grow into cysts that replace normal cells. After years of heavy drinking, fibrous scar tissue, or cirrhosis, impedes the normal flow of arterial and venous blood through the organ, resulting in liver failure and death.

Does drinking alcoholic beverages guard against heart disease? Recent studies of men suggest *light-to-moderate* alcohol intake (*one to three drinks per week*) is the amount associated with a reduction in mortality.[15] This is due to a reduced risk of coronary artery disease because of increased HDL level. However, among women with similar levels of alcohol consumption, an increased risk of breast cancer was noted that complicates the balance of risks and benefits.[16] Light-to-moderate intake of alcohol appears only to reduce mortality risk in some women who are at high risk for coronary heart disease in the first place. Also, while light alcohol consumption may reduce coronary artery disease, it has destructive effects on the heart muscle itself. This is especially true in women who appear to be more susceptible to cardiomyopathy (or heart muscle destruction)—even when they drink less than men.

So this one bit of HDL information about the "protective" relationship of alcohol consumption and heart disease should not be perceived as a "green light" to drink. Keep in mind the cons overwhelmingly outweigh the pros of drinking alcoholic beverages.

Use, Moderate Use, and Abuse

About two-thirds of Americans use alcohol.[17] These individuals enjoy an occasional alcoholic beverage (no more than one to two drinks per week). Others, however, drink in moderation or abuse alcohol. *Moderate* drinking means no more than *two* drinks a day for most men, no more than *one* drink a day for most women, and no more than *five* drinks per week. Who is the alcohol abuser? It is the individual who drinks more than *three per day* or more than *five drinks per week*.[18] The alcohol abuser is also the **binge drinker** (i.e., five or more at one setting for men and four or more at one setting for women). Any time a person consumes this amount of alcohol at one setting it is considered to be binging—regardless of if it is only once per week or even once per year. The alcohol abuser is the drinker who considers alcohol to be something other than a beverage to be consumed with meals or to celebrate special occasions. Alcohol abusers "use" alcohol as a medication to kill pain, to alter emotions (when mad or depressed), to help them sleep, or to cope with life. If you drink when pregnant or drink and drive, you are an alcohol abuser. See Table 12.6.

The morning after a night of abusive drinking, you may experience the following conditions: oversensitivity to light and sound; a hangover; dehydration; nausea; bloodshot eyes; "bags" under the eyes; and **blackout** (cannot remember all or parts of the night before). To avoid abusing alcohol follow the Zero . . . One . . . Three Rule for Lower-Risk Drinking in Table 12.7.

Alcoholism

No one plans on becoming an alcoholic, yet alcoholism is on the rise (Table 12.8 on page 262). Even newborn infants may be addicted if the mother abused alcohol during pregnancy. Most alcoholism is a result of abusive drinking. The difference between the alcoholic and the alcohol abuser is control over drinking. The abusive drinker can stop. The addict cannot. Ask yourself, "Do you *want* it, or do you *need* it?"

Alcoholism is a drug (chemical) dependence. It involves progressive preoccupation with drinking, leading to physical, mental, or social dysfunction. Approximately one of ten Americans is an alcoholic. The point where heavy drinking merges into alcohol dependence is blurry. The behaviors may appear to be the same. For example, both the addict and abuser may suffer from blackouts, passing out, arrests, hangovers, absenteeism, accidents, violence, poor job or school performance, and poor relationships.

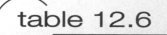

table 12.6

USE, MODERATE USE, AND ABUSE OF ALCOHOL

USE

- No more than one to two drinks per week

MODERATE USE

- Two per day for men; one per day for women; no more than five per week
- Use of alcohol to celebrate special occasions
- Use of alcohol as a beverage with meals

ABUSE

- More than three per day or more than five per week
- Binge drinking (i.e., five or more at one setting for men and four or more for women)
- Use of alcohol
    - —to medicate or kill pain
    - —to alter emotions
    - —to get drunk
    - —to induce sleep
    - —to cope with life's problems
    - —when pregnant

source: Anna Lamb, Alcohol Education Coordinator. Ball State University, Muncie, IN 47306, (317) 285–8437.

table 12.7

THE ZERO . . . ONE . . . THREE RULE FOR LOWER-RISK DRINKING

0 = No level of drinking is recommended. Never drink and drive—even one block.

1 = Drink only one alcoholic beverage per hour if you do drink.

3 = Never drink more than three alcoholic beverages per day (or more than five per week).

source: Concept partially developed by Enjoy Michigan Safety Coalition. Funded by Michigan Office of Highway Safety Planning.

Heredity explains some alcoholism because a history of alcoholism in the family puts you at higher risk. What you inherit is not the disease but a predisposition to the disease. Scientists are looking for biological markers (i.e., variations in neurotransmitters, certain blood enzymes, and brain waves) to eventually identify influential genes. One researcher reports that there are different types of alcoholics, just as there are different types of diabetics and schizophrenics.[19] He claims that a cluster of symptoms is needed in order to lead to dependence. Abusive drinking and craving are pivotal.

table 12.8

PROFILE OF ALCOHOLISM IN THE UNITED STATES

Alcoholism is one of the United States' most serious public health problems. Evidence shows that exposure to alcoholism predisposes people to become alcoholics themselves. Here is a look at percentages of Americans who have been exposed to alcoholism:

- 42.8% of adults have lived with, been married to, or had a blood relative who was an alcoholic or problem drinker.
- 18.1% of adults have lived with an alcoholic or a problem drinker at some time during their first 18 years of life.
- Far more women than men have been married to alcoholics or problem drinkers.
- Half of all traffic deaths can be traced to drunk driving; 54% to 74% of those convicted of drunk driving are alcoholics.
- Health care costs for untreated alcoholics are at least 100% higher than for nonalcoholics.
- 20% to 40% of all U.S. hospital beds are occupied by persons being treated for alcoholism or complications of alcohol abuse.

source: National Center for Health Statistics, 1988.

table 12.9

SOCIAL SELF-ASSESSMENT

You are least likely to have problems with alcohol if

1. you were exposed to alcohol in relatively small quantities early in life by your family or within the context of a religious or cultural group;
2. your family members viewed alcohol as a food and consumed small quantities, primarily at mealtime;
3. your parents set a good example by practicing lower-risk drinking behaviors;
4. your family did not view drinking alcoholic beverages as a means of demonstrating maturity, adulthood, or masculinity/femininity;
5. abstinence with respect to the consumption of alcoholic beverages was accepted as a legitimate choice;
6. drunkenness was not an acceptable form of behavior;
7. alcohol was viewed as a beverage and not as the central focus of a group activity;
8. rules and rituals associated with drinking were known and understood by all group members and they were both reasonable and agreeable to those members.

source: National Institute on Alcohol Abuse and Alcoholism.

The way in which you were introduced to alcohol as a child strongly influences your attitudes and drinking behavior as an adult. Table 12.9 lists factors indicative of those who would experience the fewest problems with alcohol in adulthood. How do you stack up with these factors?

The *alcohol abuser* needs to change his or her drinking behavior by quitting or following the Zero . . . One . . . Three Rule for Lower-Risk Drinking. The *alcoholic* must quit. No alcoholic should ever quit "cold turkey" (abruptly) without proper supervision, however, as the body has become dependent upon alcohol. When you abruptly stop us-

table 12.10

DRINKING HABITS QUIZ

1. Do you think about drinking often?
2. Do you drink more now than you used to?
3. Do you avoid situations in which it would be impossible to get a drink if you wanted one?
4. Do you sometimes gulp your drinks?
5. Do you often take a drink to help you relax?
6. Do you drink often when you are alone?
7. Do you sometimes forget what happened while you were drinking?
8. Has your drinking ever created problems between you and friends, between you and your parents, or with the law?
9. Have you ever injured yourself or another person after drinking?
10. Do you need a drink to have fun?
11. Do you ever just start drinking without really thinking about it?
12. Do you drink in the morning to relieve a hangover?
13. Are you a binger?
14. Do you have more than five drinks a week?

Scoring: If you answered "yes" to four or more questions, you may be a problem drinker.

source: National Institutue on Alcohol Abuse and Alcoholism.

ing alcohol, you will probably experience some withdrawal symptoms, which can be dangerous. Some of these symptoms are profuse sweating, coldness, tremors or shakes, nausea, headaches, and hallucinations (auditory or visual).

It is imperative to identify early the 20 percent of drinkers whose lives can potentially be shattered by addiction to alcohol. Most people have few difficulties with alcohol; many others cross the line into alcoholism, and those who do deny it furiously. That is the paradox of alcohol.

Anyone who drinks should ask the following questions: Does anyone in my family (even one member) have a history of alcoholism or drug abuse? Am I drinking too much? When am I drinking? Where am I drinking? What am I drinking? Why am I drinking? Are most of my friends heavy drinkers? Do I seek out events at which alcohol will be served? Do I have to have a drink? Do I make up excuses to drink? Do I intend to control my alcohol intake but never do?

If you are not satisfied with your answers, consider getting a professional assessment. Take the quiz in Table 12.10 to find out if you have a drinking problem.

For those with an alcohol problem, help is available. There is hope. Many people have gone to treatment centers, hospitals, clinics, and self-help groups for assistance in dealing with drinking problems.

One popular group that offers assistance to alcoholics of all ages is Alcoholics Anonymous (AA). AA was founded in 1935 by two alcoholics: a stockbroker and a surgeon who met in Akron, Ohio. They discovered that leaning on each other for emotional support was crucial to keeping them on the wagon. The group they started had only 100 members during the first four years. It now has a worldwide membership of over two million. AA is a fellowship of mutual and spiritual support that has endured in simplicity. There are no dues and no minutes; the only condition for membership is *a desire to stop drinking.*

Strategies for Dealing with Alcohol

Alcohol is an accepted drug in today's society, but you don't have to go along with the crowd. Who controls and makes decisions about your life—you or others? Take charge. Here are some helpful strategies for you and ways you can help others who have abused alcohol.

Strategies for drinking less or not at all include the following:

1. It is increasingly more acceptable to say, "No thanks" to alcohol.
2. Let your waistline be your incentive. Alcoholic beverages are loaded with "empty" calories (high in calories, low in nutrients). There is some evidence that alcohol not only adds calories to the diet but also keeps the body from burning dietary fat properly. Alcohol in the bloodstream slows down fat metabolism more than 30 percent while speeding up the burning of carbohydrates. This unused fat gets deposited on the thighs, hips, and stomach.[20]
3. If you do drink, follow the Lower-Risk Drinking Guidelines found in Table 12.7. Switch to juice or soft drinks after the three-drink maximum.
4. At restaurants, order food first, not an alcoholic beverage. That way you will have less time to drink.
5. After exercise, or when extra thirsty, avoid carbonated alcoholic drinks. They are absorbed too fast, and you may be tempted to gulp them down. Drink a glass of cold water first.
6. Don't hold the drink in your hand. Put it down somewhere—this will help slow down consumption.
7. Try cocktails without the alcohol (i.e., a Bloody Mary without the vodka) or nonalcoholic beer.
8. Dilute your drinks with water, ice, or extra fruit juice.
9. Make sure your drinks are accurately measured.
10. Volunteer to be the designated driver (you may even get free soft drinks).

If friends pass out from drinking alcohol, do the following:

1. *Put them on their stomach.* If you put them on their side or back, they may vomit, inhale the vomit, and suffocate.
2. *Do not give them anything to eat or drink.* They are unconscious. You could cause them to choke.
3. *Be sure they are breathing normally—not shallow, but deeply.* Shallow breathing means the brain is shutting down and involuntary bodily functions are ceasing. Call for help!
4. *Cover them with a sheet, not a blanket.* If they have overdosed on alcohol, their internal body temperature has fallen. Shivering stimulates them and helps to keep them alive. Too much external warmth will stop that vital stimulation.
5. *If they are shivering, call for medical help!*
6. Gently shake them and call them by first name. They will probably respond in some manner. *If they don't respond at all, call for medical help!*

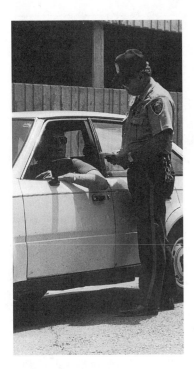

Irresponsible drinking complicates your life.

Alcohol and the Law

Society has responded to the alcohol problem with legislation. All 50 states now have a drinking age of 21 years. You are breaking the law if you are under the age of 21 and are using, possessing, or transporting alcohol. These laws partly discourage some students from drinking, which lowers the potential for accidents. Drinking to *any* extent reduces the ability of *any* driver (see Table 12.4). Fifty percent of all fatal auto accidents in this country are alcohol related.[21]

Most states have defined *driving under the influence of alcohol* as driving with a blood alcohol content (BAC) of 0.10 percent. Whether or not a person feels intoxicated is not the point; the point is whether he or she registers 0.10 on a breathalyzer (see Table 12.4). The rationale for the law is that it may act as a deterrent to drinking and driving. Some states have dropped the figure to 0.08 percent; at least two states are considering 0.05 percent as presumption of intoxication. The point is, there is no safe drinking BAC. Look at Table 12.11 for some sobering statistics.

table 12.11

SOBERING FACTS ON DRINKING AND DRIVING

1. Drunk drivers are 25 times more likely than sober drivers to have accidents.
2. About 23,000 persons are killed each year in alcohol-related accidents. About 450 persons die each week, and every 20 minutes another life is lost in an alcohol-related accident.
3. More than 36 percent of the persons who die in alcohol-related accidents are passengers, drivers of the other vehicle, and pedestrians.
4. About one of every two Americans will be involved in an alcohol-related accident in their lifetime.
5. Social drinkers are a greater menace than commonly believed, as their critical judgment is impaired with a low BAC and they outnumber the obviously intoxicated drivers.
6. More people are arrested for drunken driving—1.8 million a year—than for other crime in the United States. Yet the average drunken driver drives hundreds of times, thousands of miles, before being caught.
7. The average BAC of those arrested is 0.17 percent—equivalent to a 160-pound man drinking nearly 10 beers in two hours.
8. Of repeat offenders within seven years 24 percent are convicted for a second time, 8.6 percent for a third time, and 4.3 percent for four or more times.

source: National Highway Transportation Safety Administration.

Here is the message: You could be one of the persons who dies in the next 20 minutes due to alcohol-related accidents. Or you could be crippled or permanently injured for life. Do not let it be you. Most think it won't happen to them.

Fetal Alcohol Syndrome (FAS) and Fetal Alcohol Effect (FAE)

Fetal alcohol syndrome (FAS) is a condition acquired by the unborn fetus and caused by the mother drinking alcohol during pregnancy. The alcohol passes through the placenta (within minutes) and affects the unborn child. There is no other cause for the FAS. Women need to understand that the placenta does not keep unwanted chemicals away from the fetus. We now know that what a mother eats, drinks, or smokes passes to her unborn child. Humans are supposed to be the wisest of creatures, yet it is not uncommon to see pregnant women drinking alcoholic beverages, smoking, and taking drugs they would never consider giving to their children. Then they expect their babies to come into the world healthy and cuddly.

Alcohol damages the vulnerable, developing brain and may impair placental function as well. This damage is irreversible. We are unsure exactly which brain cells of the fetus are destroyed; the expectant mother who drinks is denying her child development of his or her full potential. The damage can range from severe physical deformity, clumsiness, behavioral problems, and stunted growth to mental retardation. Alcohol is one of the leading causes of mental retardation in the Western world.[22] No one is certain how much alcohol it takes to cause damage to the fetus. Some women drink very little and their babies are still affected.

A far greater number of babies have more subtle symptoms that are rarely attributed to their mothers' alcohol consumption. This less severe manifestation of FAS is called **fetal alcohol effect (FAE)**. The mother of a child diagnosed with FAE did not necessarily drink less during pregnancy than the mother of a child with FAS, but, for some biological reason, the FAE child was not as damaged physically. The FAE child shows traits of impaired memory, poor judgment, and reduced capacity to learn from experience. Many FAE children go through life undetected and misjudged. They often drop out of school or wind up on the margins of society.[23] Recent reports indicate an increasing frequency of both FAS and FAE.[24] Drinking while pregnant is like playing

Russian roulette with your baby's life. Why take chances with your baby's future? The message is this: There is no known safe level of alcohol consumption during pregnancy. FAS and FAE are totally preventable, but abstinence is the only way to guarantee that a baby will suffer no ill effects from alcohol.

Tobacco

If you are a regular smoker, you may be losing about six minutes of life expectancy for every cigarette you smoke. For most smokers that means a life expectancy reduced by five to eight years. The U.S. Surgeon General has described cigarette smoking as "the chief preventable cause of death in our society."[25] To put things in perspective, more people die from smoking-related diseases than from alcohol, cocaine, heroin, suicide, homicide, car accidents, and AIDS combined. Over 400,000 people die each year because they smoked cigarettes. That is more than seven times the total U.S. battle fatalities during the Vietnam War.[26] The Federal Drug Administration and the American Medical Association have declared nicotine to be an addictive drug that should be regulated. Despite all the frightening statistics, the warnings, and the publicity given to the health risks of smoking, each year thousands of young people start smoking.

Smoking Is Becoming Socially Unacceptable

Little was known about the health consequences of smoking until 1964 when the first Surgeon General's report on smoking and health was published. At that time, nearly half of our population smoked.[27] In the years since, millions of people have quit, and now smokers are less than a quarter of the population. The decline in smoking has been influenced by the proliferation of restrictive work site and public smoking policies. Once considered sophisticated, smoking now seems to be most prevalent in the lower socioeconomic and the least-educated groups. Studies reveal that smoking is twice as high among those with less than a high school education than it is among those with a college education.[28]

Before World War II, smoking was considered a masculine activity, and few women smoked. After World War II, with increasing emancipation, women began smoking in ever-increasing numbers. As a result, lung cancer deaths for women tripled. While proportions of adult men and women smokers have dropped since 1964, surveys indicate that men have given up smoking more often than have women.[29]

Smoking may have been considered glamorous once, but, today, attitudes are changing. Smoking commercials have been banned from radio and television since 1971. Cigarette advertisements and packages carry health warnings. Over 70 percent of adult smokers have either tried to quit smoking or would like to try.[30] Nonsmokers are tired of passive smoking—breathing air polluted by tobacco smoke—and are gaining the right to breathe clean air in workplaces and public areas.

Why Do People Smoke?

The most important influences in starting to smoke are family and friends. In families where one or both parents smoke, children are twice as likely to be smokers than are children of parents who are nonsmokers.[31] Many teenagers start smoking because they think everybody else does, and they want to be like their friends or appear more adult. They don't think much about the costs or health risks of smoking. Powerful advertising directed at young people (e.g., Joe Camel) deemphasizes the harmful factors. The tobacco industry spends over $4 billion on advertising to convince young people they should take up smoking. For young people, cigarettes are considered to be a gateway drug—the first drug many use as a stepping stone to illicit drugs and heavy drinking (see Table 12.1).

Nicotine, a drug in cigarette smoke, is addicting, as anyone who has tried to quit smoking has quickly discovered. Nicotine is an alkaloid drug synthesized by the tobacco plant in the same fashion that the opium poppy (the source of heroin) and the coca plant (the source of cocaine) synthesize their addictive substances. Habituation to nicotine may occur after smoking only three packs of cigarettes. Once a person is hooked on nicotine, it can be difficult for the person to quit. Indeed, experts say that addiction to nicotine can be just as strong as addiction to cocaine or heroin. Without a steady supply of nicotine, withdrawal symptoms may occur. A person may become irritable, anxious, and hostile and crave tobacco. Nicotine withdrawal may also produce headaches, nausea, and inability to concentrate. Although 70 percent of smokers want to stop smoking and 34 percent attempt to quit each year, only 2.5 percent successfully stop smoking each year.[32] The high rate of relapse is a consequence of the effect of nicotine dependence. Smokers' families and friends should be more aware that smoking is not just a nasty habit, but a form of drug dependence.

Health Risks of Smoking

Of the 41,000 potentially toxic chemicals in cigarette smoke, the three major toxic substances are nicotine, carbon monoxide, and tar. Nicotine stimulates the cardiovascular system. Increased heart rate and blood pressure place a burden on the heart muscle, which then needs more oxygen. Carbon monoxide, a toxic gas, immediately reduces the blood's ability to carry oxygen and ultimately damages the inner surface of coronary arteries, increasing the rate of atherosclerosis. When combined with vasoconstriction, a narrowing of the arteries, this artherosclerosis can cause ischemia (lack of oxygen) and coronary tissue damage. Smoking also increases arrhythmias, increases stickiness and clotting of blood cells, and decreases levels of HDL.[33] This is why twice as many smokers as nonsmokers die from heart attacks. Also, smoking contributes to peripheral vascular disease, which is the hardening of the arteries in the lower legs. This condition can affect the ability to walk and may eventually lead to amputation of the legs.

Tar contains potent carcinogens. It also contains chemicals that irritate lung tissue and may promote chronic bronchitis and emphysema. These substances can paralyze and destroy the cilia that line the bronchi, allowing tar and other particles to accumulate in the lungs. This causes *smoker's cough*, which is the body's attempt to rid itself of the buildup of particulate matter. Long-term contact between lung tissue and tar can cause cellular changes leading to the development of cancer.

The reduction in a person's life expectancy due to smoking parallels increasing cigarette usage. Mortality is higher the younger a person started smoking, the longer a person has smoked, the deeper a smoker inhales, and the higher the tar and nicotine content of the tobacco used. If a smoker is overweight, has moderately elevated blood pressure, or has a high cholesterol level, the risk of having a heart attack skyrockets.[34]

If you've smoked for many years, does it do any good to quit? Yes. Heart attack risk declines by about half in the first year after quitting. Risk continues to decrease with each year of abstinence until, after 10 to 15 years, an exsmoker has almost the same risk of dying as if he or she had never smoked (see Fig. 12.2). People who quit smoking may gain weight, but the weight gain is less of a health risk than continuing to smoke. The average weight gain is 6 pounds for men and 8 pounds for women, which brings them to average weight levels of persons who have never smoked. Regardless of how long or how much a person has smoked, quitting is beneficial.

Smokeless Tobacco

Cigarette smoking is not the only form of tobacco that presents health risks. Smokeless tobacco—snuff and chewing tobacco—is surging in popularity among young adult males. Advertised by athletes, smokeless tobacco seems to be viewed as a safe alternative to cigarette smoking, which is forbidden by coaches on athletic teams. The tobacco industry wants you to believe that snuff and chewing tobacco provide all the pleasure of cigarettes minus the risks. But the evidence shows otherwise. Highly carcinogenic tobacco **nitrosamines** are released in concentrations 1,000 times higher in smokeless tobacco-saliva mixtures than in cigarette smoke.[35] Snuff and chewing tobacco cause many problems ranging from bad breath to cardiovascular disease and cancer. A decrease in the ability to taste and smell, stained teeth, gum damage, tooth loss, and wear on the chewing surfaces of the teeth caused by grit in the tobacco are commonly experienced. Use of smokeless tobacco also causes leukoplakia, a precancerous condition that produces thick, rough, white patches on the gums, tongue, or inner cheek.[36] Experts predict an oral cancer epidemic beginning in two or three decades if the current trend continues.

In addition, smokeless tobacco is addictive. Nicotine from the smokeless tobacco is absorbed directly into the bloodstream from the mouth (one of the most efficient delivery systems known) and eventually produces dependency. Recently, tobacco companies

FIGURE 12.2 ➤
When smokers quit.

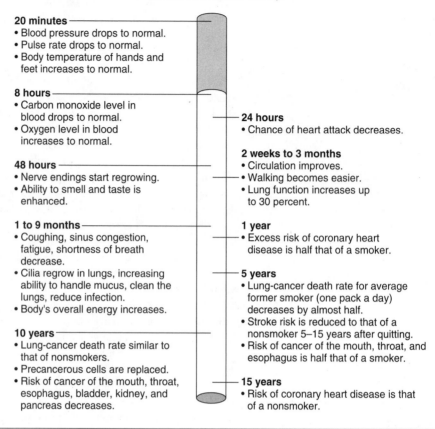

Within 20 minutes of smoking that last cigarette, the body begins a series of changes that continues for years. All benefits are lost by smoking just one cigarette a day, according to the American Cancer Society.

20 minutes
- Blood pressure drops to normal.
- Pulse rate drops to normal.
- Body temperature of hands and feet increases to normal.

8 hours
- Carbon monoxide level in blood drops to normal.
- Oxygen level in blood increases to normal.

48 hours
- Nerve endings start regrowing.
- Ability to smell and taste is enhanced.

1 to 9 months
- Coughing, sinus congestion, fatigue, shortness of breath decrease.
- Cilia regrow in lungs, increasing ability to handle mucus, clean the lungs, reduce infection.
- Body's overall energy increases.

10 years
- Lung-cancer death rate similar to that of nonsmokers.
- Precancerous cells are replaced.
- Risk of cancer of the mouth, throat, esophagus, bladder, kidney, and pancreas decreases.

24 hours
- Chance of heart attack decreases.

2 weeks to 3 months
- Circulation improves.
- Walking becomes easier.
- Lung function increases up to 30 percent.

1 year
- Excess risk of coronary heart disease is half that of a smoker.

5 years
- Lung-cancer death rate for average former smoker (one pack a day) decreases by almost half.
- Stroke risk is reduced to that of a nonsmoker 5–15 years after quitting.
- Risk of cancer of the mouth, throat, and esophagus is half that of a smoker.

15 years
- Risk of coronary heart disease is that of a nonsmoker.

have been accused of manipulating the chemical recipes of their products. This chemical change supposedly allows more nicotine to be absorbed into the bloodstream, thus making the product gradually more addictive. The tobacco industry furiously denies these charges. Many people feel that the dependency produced by smokeless tobacco is harder to break than that produced by smoking.

Are You a Passive Smoker?

Nonsmokers, who outnumber smokers three to one, are growing tired of **passive smoking**—breathing air polluted by tobacco smoke, especially when they read reports from the American Heart Association and the Environmental Protection Agency (EPA). New reports state that passive smoking causes between 30,000 and 60,000 deaths per year.[37] As you learned in Chapter 6 (Heart Health), secondhand smoke harms the cardiovascular systems of nonsmokers more than smokers. This is because the smoker's cardiovascular system has adapted to the ill effects of cigarette smoke.[38] Nonsmokers exposed to secondhand smoke exhibit an increased rise of fatal and nonfatal cardiac events. This is due to the extreme sensitivity of the cardiovascular system to the many chemicals in secondhand smoke. This sensitivity accelerates atherosclerotic heart lesions and increased tissue damage following a heart attack.[39] In 1993, the EPA officially declared secondhand smoke to be a human carcinogen that causes about 3,000 nonsmokers a year to die from lung cancer and about 12,000 a year to die from other cancers. The EPA also reported that children exposed to secondhand smoke are at an increased risk of bronchitis, pneumonia, and asthma.

Nearly all employers in the United States have restricted smoking in the workplace because of the effects of smoke-filled air on the nonsmoker. The problem is that passive smokers involuntarily inhale toxic fumes produced by the cigarette of the mainstream

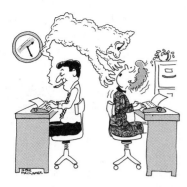

Smoking is everybody's business.

smoker. What nonsmokers may not realize is that these highly toxic substances are found in higher concentrations in sidestream than in mainstream smoke. Even though smoke is mixed with environmental air, it still causes eye and nasal irritations, sore throats, coughing, and headaches in nonsmokers. Families of smokers have more respiratory problems and more days of absence from work or school due to illness than do families of nonsmokers. Children of smokers have more colds, more ear infections, reduced lung function, and a greater chance of being hospitalized for acute respiratory infections than do nonsmokers' children.[40] Studies have indicated that nonsmoking spouses of heavy smokers have double the risk of lung cancer of nonsmokers. The same may be true for their risk of emphysema, bronchitis, and other respiratory diseases.

The decision to smoke can no longer be considered a private matter. Past solutions, such as separating smokers and nonsmokers within the same room, are inadequate. The Surgeon General states that this helps but does not eliminate exposure. The AHA concludes, "the only sure way to protect nonsmokers from environmental tobacco smoke is to eliminate smoking from areas that smokers share with nonsmokers." This once radical step is rapidly gaining acceptance—all indoor smoking may soon be a thing of the past.

It does not make sense to strengthen your heart and lungs with regular exercise only to be at the mercy of smokers when you venture into public. Get involved and start campaigning for eliminating exposure to secondhand smoke.

Why Should You Quit?

The simple act of quitting smoking can add years to a person's life (Figure 12.2). Even more important, it increases the chance that those years will be healthy and active, drastically decreasing the chances of suffering painful, incapacitating, and costly illnesses. Overall quality of life will improve. You will save money, since cigarettes are expensive. A pack-a-day habit sends nearly $700 a year up in smoke. You can say goodbye to tobacco stains on your teeth and fingers. Your breath, hair, clothes, and surroundings will smell fresher. Your smoke will no longer annoy or harm other people, and this will particularly benefit your own family. No longer will cigarette burns or messy ashes ruin furniture, carpet, and countertops. Your risk of setting an accidental fire will be reduced. Your ability to taste and smell will return. As the effects of smoking are reversed, you will eliminate smoker's cough and increase your endurance so that you will have more energy all day long. Besides reducing your health risks, you will overcome a potential drug addiction that may have taken control of your life.

How to Quit Smoking

In the past few years, millions of Americans have quit smoking. Of smokers who quit, most have done it on their own. There are many ways to quit. Some people try to gradually reduce the number of cigarettes they smoke. Others quit cold turkey. A new product is helping many quit by weaning them away from nicotine. The product is a small patch worn on the skin that minimizes the usual withdrawal symptoms. It is available by prescription only. It works by painlessly releasing decreasing doses of nicotine through tiny blood vessels near the surface of the skin. An even more successful cessation program is an approach combining nicotine chewing gum, nicotine patches, and behavior modification counseling.[41] The number-one determinant of success, however, is simply the smoker's own desire to quit, based on some strong motivational goal, like saving money or improving health. If you are a nonsmoker wishing to help a smoker who is trying to quit, you should know that the support of family and friends is the second most important factor in successfully breaking the grip of the nicotine habit.

Giving up smoking can be a long-term process, and some people must try several times before they quit for good. It is not easy. Smokers have about the same success rate as those trying to break alcohol or heroin addiction. This doesn't mean that a person can't quit, because every year thousands of people do. But it takes effort, desire, support, and a firm commitment. If a person quits smoking and then starts again, he or she should not be considered weak. Some former smokers say they still crave cigarettes long after they quit smoking. The smoker who does not succeed in quitting on the first try should try and try again. Mark Twain said it best: "It's easy to *quit* smoking, I should know—I've done it dozens of times."

Substance Abuse   269

If you're ready to toss those cigarettes, *Clearing the Air: A Guide to Quitting Smoking*, available from the American Cancer Society, gives these recommendations:

➤ *Set a target date for quitting*. Then list all the reasons why you want to quit. Review these whenever you crave tobacco.

➤ Before you quit, *change to a brand you find distasteful*, and then taper off a little more each day. Smoke only half of each cigarette. Smoke only during even hours of the day.

➤ *Involve friends and family*. Tell them when and why you are going to quit and ask for their support.

➤ *On the day you quit*, toss out all cigarettes and matches. Go to the dentist to have your teeth cleaned. Keep very busy and concentrate on getting through that one day without tobacco.

➤ After quitting, *change your normal routine*. Spend as much time as possible away from places and situations that you associate with smoking. Go jogging, drink more fluids, get plenty of rest.

➤ When you get the "crazies," *chew on carrots, pickles, sunflower seeds, sugarless gum*. Take a shower. Never allow yourself to think, "One won't hurt." It will.

➤ *Mark progress*. Each month, celebrate the anniversary of your quit date. Put aside the money you've saved by not smoking and treat yourself to something special. You deserve it.

The Clock Strategy

Another strategy for quitting smoking is to let the clock tell you when to smoke. The clock strategy was reported to be twice as successful in the long term as quitting cold turkey.[42] With this method, you assign specific times of day for lighting up and decrease the total number of cigarettes by ⅓ each week. You'll follow a schedule with longer and longer intervals between cigarettes (decreasing cigarettes by ⅓ each week) before finally quitting altogether. By repeatedly putting nicotine urges on hold for manageable periods, smokers gain practice and self-confidence for when they finally quit.

The key to why the clock strategy seems to work so well lies in breaking the link between everyday smoking cues and the habit of lighting up. If you wish to quit smoking, try this new strategy. We wish you success!

Marijuana

A drug that some people consider safe is marijuana. It is the United States' most widely used illegal drug and trails only alcohol and tobacco in popularity as a social or recreational drug.[43] **Marijuana** (sometimes called *pot* or *grass*) is a CNS depressant. It is a psychoactive drug (i.e., mind affecting or mind altering) made from the leaves and flowers of the cannabis sativa plant. The leaves and flowers are dried and crushed, causing the marijuana to have a tobaccolike appearance. When marijuana is rolled in papers, the end product is a cigarette called a *joint*.

Although there are at least 421 ingredients in marijuana, **delta-9-tetrahydrocannabinol (THC)** is the principle psychoactive ingredient. When in smoke, THC is rapidly absorbed by blood in the lungs and transported to the brain in less than 30 seconds. Because the strength of marijuana has increased 15 percent since its strength in the 1980s, the effects of smoking a joint may last several hours with the peak occurring 20 to 30 minutes after inhalation. THC is fat soluble and is stored in fatty tissues of the body, brain, and reproductive organs. Due to this, complete elimination of a single dose is slow and may require one month or more before the body is drug free. During this time, marijuana residuals can be detected in the urine.

The mind-altering effects of marijuana are the basis for its widespread popularity. Low-to-moderate doses may induce a sense of well-being and euphoria and produce feelings of relaxation ("mellowing out"). Marijuana use also causes short-term memory loss, damaged brain cells, increased appetite, reduced comprehension, various respiratory conditions, increased heart rate, lowered sperm count, and abnormal menstruation. Users can experience bad trips or anxiety/panic reactions, such as sudden panic, fears of dying or going insane, and paranoid thoughts. Because marijuana burns hotter than tobacco, it results in more lung and throat damage than do cigarettes. According to Robert Gilkeson, M.D., THC changes the cell membrane, causing it to be less efficient with less energy, particularly in the brain and testicles.[44] Amotivational syndrome is also linked to marijuana use. A person with **amotivational syndrome** experiences low energy, apathy, and little drive to do anything. Students exhibit this syndrome by not going to class, not completing assignments, "vegetating" on a chair, or appearing not to care about anything. Amotivational syndrome is thought to be linked to changes in the cell membranes.

Drinking alcohol while smoking marijuana is dangerous. Marijuana inhibits vomiting, causing the alcohol to remain in your system. This increases the chance of alcohol poisoning. Use of marijuana severely reduces the ability to drive a car. It impairs motor coordination, impairs judgment and perception, and decreases awareness of external stimuli (such as flashing lights).

Even though illegal, marijuana has been used in medicine for over 2,000 years. In 1965, THC was commercially synthesized. However, it was not until 1985 that the U.S. Food and Drug Administration (FDA) approved it for medical purposes. Marijuana and synthesized THC are designated as controlled substances under federal law (Controlled Substance Act of 1970).[45] This law includes all drugs with no medical use and/or high potential for abuse. Marijuana is available only with a physician's prescription in capsule, liquid, or naturally cultivated cigarette form. It is administered orally, intravenously, as drops, or as a cigarette to be smoked. It is sometimes prescribed for relieving the nausea accompanying cancer chemotherapy. More recently, it has been used to stimulate the appetite in AIDS patients to help overcome the debilitating weight loss associated with this disease. When conventional therapies have failed, marijuana has been somewhat effective when used alone or in combination with other drugs to treat the following conditions:[46]

➤ *Glaucoma:* It sometimes helps reduce the vision-threatening intraocular pressure.
➤ *Epilepsy:* It sometimes protects against minimal and maximal seizures.
➤ *Asthma:* It sometimes produces a bronchodilation effect.
➤ *Multiple sclerosis:* It sometimes reduces muscle spasticity.

Marijuana has not been found superior to ordinary medications in the treatment of anxiety, depression, pain relief, or drug/alcohol abuse. In some cases, it hasn't even been helpful. However, the therapeutic potential for medical marijuana merits continued study.

Cocaine and Crack

Cocaine and crack (a cocaine derivative) are controlled substances. They are potent, rapid-acting drugs. Cocaine comes from the coca plant, which is mainly harvested in Central and South America. Cocaine is extracted from the coca leaf during a simple two-step chemical process involving sulfuric and hydrochloric acid. This process separates cocaine from the other chemicals in the coca leaf and results in cocaine hydrochloride (or *street cocaine*). Cocaine hydrochloride is the fine, opalescent, white, fluffy, odorless, and bitter-tasting drug that is sold for illegal, recreational use. It is the second most widely used illegal drug in the United States.[47] Until the early 1980s, cocaine was used mainly by the wealthy. Today, it is truly an equal opportunity drug used by members of all socioeconomic groups.

Cocaine is a euphoriant and a central nervous system stimulant whose effects last from 20 minutes to several hours, depending on the drug's purity. There are several ways to take cocaine, and the speed with which the cocaine user achieves a high varies with each method. It may take 10 to 30 minutes to feel cocaine's effects when the drug is swallowed, three minutes when it is snorted, one-half minute when it is injected, and a few seconds when it is smoked. While it may be swallowed, this is not as effective as other methods because of poor absorption in the gastrointestinal tract. The most common method is to snort the drug (sniff it through the nose). The powder is first chopped fine with a razor blade and arranged into lines on a piece of glass. The user may then inhale the cocaine through a rolled-up dollar bill, straw, or "coke spoon." Injecting cocaine produces an intense and exhilarating rush, but one that is short-lived because of the drug's rapid metabolization by the liver. Cocaine may also be smoked in the form of either freebase cocaine or crack.

Freebase cocaine is separated from ordinary street cocaine (cocaine hydrochloride) in a process that results in a purer and more intense form that can be smoked. (Cocaine hydrochloride—the street, powder form—cannot be smoked.) In this process, the drug is freed from the parent compound by mixing it with water and ammonium hydroxide. The cocaine base is then separated from the water using a fast-drying solvent such as ether, leaving unadulterated cocaine freebase. Small amounts of the base are then placed in the neck of a specially designed water pipe and smoked at high temperature over a torch. All of the freebase components are readily available in the retail marketplace. Smoking freebase cocaine creates a rush that is rapid, powerful, and short-lived, much like the high from injected cocaine. While the euphoria and feelings of energy last only a few minutes, the other effects (such as pupil dilation, increased blood pressure, and heart rate) are prolonged and can be dangerous. Also, the ether used in the process is extremely volatile and may explode.

Crack is crystallized freebase cocaine sold in the form of ready-to-smoke "rocks." The rocks of processed cocaine are smoked in a pipe, or placed in cigarettes or joints of marijuana. As a ready-to-smoke drug, crack spares the user the delay and bother of having to extract the potent freebase form of cocaine from cocaine hydrochloride. The rocks are nicknamed *crack* because of the crackling sound they make as they are smoked. Before crack came on the market, cocaine smokers had to make the freebase themselves, using dangerous, highly flammable chemicals such as ether. The extraction process was complicated and costly as well. Because crack is such a pure drug (about 90 percent pure cocaine) and approximately five times more potent than using cocaine, smoking crack gives the user a far more intense and rapid euphoria than does snorting cocaine. One puff of a pebble-sized rock produces an intense high that lasts about 20 minutes. The user can generally get three or four hits off one rock. The high is always followed immediately by an equally unpleasant crash, characterized by irritability, agitation, and intense cravings for more of the drug.

Crack is usually purchased in small plastic vials containing two or three rocks. Crack, costing $5 to $20 per vial, is more affordable per dose than cocaine. However, most people cannot stop after one vial and may use five or more vials to keep the high. Even though crack is sold in inexpensive units, this has nothing to do with the actual price of the drug. Crack's price per gram is almost double that of cocaine powder. Crack only appears cheaper—much as buying a single cup of coffee for 50 cents seems cheaper but is actually much more expensive than buying a whole pound of coffee for $3.99. The deceptively low initial price of crack makes it possible for just about anyone to start using the drug. Some users go on a three-day crack binge, depleting their body and bank accounts. They quit only because they are out of money or out of crack or because their bodies cannot take it anymore.

Addiction to crack takes less time to develop than addiction to snorting cocaine. Some users can become psychologically addicted after smoking it just a few times. Crack addiction is accelerated by the speed with which it is absorbed through the lungs (it hits the brain within 4 to 6 seconds) and by the intensity of the high.

Some people may start using cocaine to lose weight (it depresses the appetite) or to enhance alertness and relieve fatigue (it stimulates the central nervous system). As a stimulant, this drug also causes blood pressure, heart rate, and body temperature to rise. Because the heart and breathing are accelerated and because cocaine acts as a vasoconstrictor (narrows blood vessels), cocaine can be dangerous to anyone with heart or respiratory problems. The increase in the number of strokes in the early 1990s has been linked to cocaine use.

Cocaine users develop tolerance and eventually need more and purer forms of the drug to get the same effect. If addiction occurs, withdrawal symptoms will develop. Eventually, the addict uses cocaine to avoid the unpleasant depression or crash that always follows the rush. How do you know if you are addicted to cocaine? Put simply, and as stated earlier in this chapter, continuing to use a drug (any drug) despite negative consequences constitutes addiction.

Consequences of using any form of cocaine may be severe. Since cocaine is an illegal drug, users risk arrests, fines, and jail terms. Some states are considering prosecuting women who take drugs during pregnancy and give birth to addicted babies.

Eventually, smoking crack and freebase cocaine may cause paranoia, other psychoses, lung and liver damage, depression, insomnia, impotence, nausea, vomiting, anxiety, and isolation. People who smoke crack (whether for the first or the 50th time) are risking their lives. The intense high can be too much for the body, causing respiratory arrest, heart attack, convulsions, and death. Snorting cocaine can lead to chronic rhinitis (runny nose), nasal congestion, perforation of the nasal septum, and greater vulnerability to upper respiratory infections. Injecting cocaine increases the risk of contracting AIDS, hepatitis, and other infectious diseases if needles are shared.

Heroin

Heroin (sometimes called *smack, junk, H,* and *hard stuff*) is a psychoactive drug that depresses the CNS. Pure heroin is a white powder with a bitter taste. It may vary in color from white to dark brown due to impurities remaining in the manufacturing process or the presence of additives. Heroin is a semisynthetic drug made by treating morphine with acetic anhydride to yield diacetylmorphine. It was first introduced into medical practice in 1898 as a cough suppressant because it had fewer undesirable side effects than morphine. The drug quickly lost favor in the United States due to its great drug-dependency potential. Heroin, a controlled substance, is no longer used medically.

Users are seldom aware of precisely what they are buying on the street from pushers. It may be mixed or cut with substances such as powdered milk, sugar, starch, quinine, and even strychnine and arsenic. By the 1980s, a cheaper and more potent form of heroin, originating in Mexico and known as *black tar* or *tootsie roll,* was being widely used in the United States.[48]

Heroin is illegal and a highly addictive narcotic. It exerts its primary addictive effect by activating both the region of the brain that is responsible for producing the pleasurable sensations of reward and the region that produces the classic physical dependence syndrome. Together, these actions account for the user's loss of control and the drug's habit-forming action.

Heroin is usually mixed into a liquid solution and injected into a vein (*mainlining*). It can also be injected under the skin, sniffed, and taken by mouth. Recent increases in sniffing heroin indicate that purer and cheaper forms are available on the street. Many crack users are switching to snorting heroin because it is cheaper, more plentiful, and carries less of a stigma than crack. Another sign of increased purity is the increasing rate of fatal overdoses. Heroin today is often 65 percent pure, 15 years ago, it was only 6 percent pure.[49] Lately, some pushers, in order to be more competitive, are offering super-pure heroin (90 percent pure) to users. This too potent heroin is known as *Poison, People's Choice, China Cat,* and *Red Sun* and has been linked to a string of overdose deaths. After taking the drug, a euphoric rush occurs. Reddening of the face and constriction of the pupils may also follow. Emotionally, a sense of calm and tranquility develops. Tensions and worries diminish and physical activity is reduced. Eventually, a stuporous period with splendorous daydreams occurs. This high lasts three to six hours. Tolerance to heroin develops quickly. After several weeks of continued use, the user needs to increase the dose in order to achieve the desired rush. Eight to 12 hours after the last dose is taken, withdrawal symptoms appear if another fix is not taken.

Many health problems related to heroin use are caused by uncertain dosage levels (due to fluctuations in purity), use of unsterile equipment, contamination by cutting agents, or use of heroin in combination with other drugs such as alcohol or cocaine. Typical problems include skin abscesses, inflammation of the veins, overdose, allergic reaction, heart valve infection, malnutrition, viral hepatitis B, as well as addiction and withdrawal symptoms. Utilization of unsterile needles by multiple individuals (needle sharing) increases the risk of exposure to HIV. Any drug-abusing lifestyle may depress the strength of the immune system and the body's ability to withstand infection.

The signs and symptoms of heroin use include euphoria, drowsiness, respiratory depression, constricted pupils, and nausea. Withdrawal symptoms include watery eyes, runny nose, yawning, loss of appetite, muscle cramps, and insomnia. Elevations in blood pressure, pulse, respiration rate, and temperature occur as withdrawal progresses. Withdrawal takes approximately one week. Symptoms of heroin overdose include shallow breathing, clammy skin, convulsions, and coma. Death may result. Heroin use during pregnancy is associated with stillbirths, sudden infant death, and below-normal birth weight. The newborn infant is likely to demonstrate the heroin withdrawal process.

LSD

LSD (Lysergic Acid Diethylamide), a controlled substance, is a dangerous and unpredictable hallucinogenic drug. Hallucinogens are grouped under a larger category of drugs called **psychedelic drugs,** which are known for their mind-expanding or mind-affecting capabilities. LSD was discovered in 1938 by Dr. Albert Hofmann, a Swiss chemist, who was seeking to develop a drug to improve blood circulation. This illegal drug is manufactured from lysergic acid which is found in ergot, a fungus that grows on rye or other grains.

LSD, commonly referred to as *acid,* is sold on the street in many forms, including tablets or pellets called *microdots,* gelatin chips known as *windowpanes,* and thin squares of absorbent paper soaked in liquid LSD called *blotter acid.*[50] Several factors account for the recent resurgence in popularity of this drug. First, the potency of today's LSD is less than it was at the height of its popularity in the 1960s and 1970s. Currently, the strength of LSD ranges from 20 to 80 micrograms per dose. During the 1960s and early 1970s, the dosage ranged from 100 to 200 micrograms or higher per unit. This weaker LSD tends to produce more manageable reactions. Second, the packaging of the product is more appealing to young users. Blotter acid is quite enticing and seems almost harmless when packaged on absorbent paper featuring cartoon characters, stars, moons, and dragons. Blotter acid is difficult to detect because it is so small and light; it can be carried in textbooks or pockets and even sent in greeting cards through the mail. Third, LSD is affordable; a hit runs about $3 to $5 in most areas of the country.

The effects of LSD are unpredictable. They depend on the amount taken; the user's personality, mood, and expectations; and the surroundings in which the drug is used. Usually, the user feels the first effects in 30 to 90 minutes after taking the drug. The physical effects include dilated pupils, increased body temperature, increased heart rate and blood pressure, sweating, loss of appetite, sleeplessness, dry mouth, and tremors. Sensations and feelings change much more dramatically than do the physical signs. The user may feel several different emotions at once or swing rapidly from one emotion to another. If taken in a large enough dose, the drug produces delusions and visual hallucinations. The user's sense of self and time changes. Sensations may seem to cross over, giving the user the feeling of hearing colors and seeing sounds. These changes can be frightening and can cause panic attacks.

Users refer to their experience with LSD as a *trip* and to acute adverse reactions as a *bad trip.* Bad trips are long lasting, taking about 12 hours to end. Some LSD users experience severe, terrifying thoughts and feelings, fear of losing control, and fear of insanity. Some fatal accidents and suicides have occurred during states of LSD intoxication because of the user's highly suggestive state and feelings of invulnerability. Examples of this include users walking out in front of fast-moving automobiles and jumping out of high windows.

Many LSD users experience **flashbacks,** a recurrence of certain aspects of a person's drug experience without the user having repeated its use. A flashback occurs suddenly, often without warning, and may occur within a few days or well over a year after LSD use. Flashbacks usually occur in people who have used hallucinogens chronically or who have underlying personality problems. However, people who are apparently normal also have flashbacks.

Bad trips and flashbacks are only part of the risks of LSD use. Relatively long-lasting psychoses, such as schizophrenia, severe depression, mania, and paranoia, may afflict users. Most users of LSD voluntarily decrease or stop its use over time. LSD is not considered to be an addicting drug since it does not produce compulsive drug-seeking behavior as does use of cocaine, amphetamines, heroin, alcohol, and nicotine. LSD does produce tolerance, however, the one characteristic it has in common with many of the other addictive drugs. Thus, the user is required to take progressively higher and higher doses in order to achieve the state of intoxication previously achieved. This is an extremely dangerous practice given the unpredictability of the drug.

Crank and Ice

Crank, a term once used as a street name for cocaine, has emerged on the drug scene as an alias for methamphetamine (a synthetic form of amphetamine). The drug is also called *speed, meth,* and *crystal.* Crank is a powerful CNS stimulant, odorless, yellow or off-white in color, and sold in capsules, chunks, or crystals. *Eightballs,* approximately one-eighth of an ounce, are considered to be a day's supply. Crank is often sniffed, inhaled, or injected to produce a greater high. The rush, an effect greatly desired by the abuser, is a highly pleasurable sensation experienced almost immediately after intravenous injection. It lasts from two to four hours. **Ice,** the street name for crystallized crank, sometimes called *crystal meth,* is smoked, like crack cocaine. It is quickly overtaking crack cocaine as the drug of choice for many addicts. Experts claim that ice is more dangerous than crack cocaine because it is more addictive. The high caused by smoking crack lasts about 20 to 30 minutes, but ice users can feel a high lasting as long as 24 hours, followed by symptoms of depression and acute psychoses, including hallucinations. Ice costs about the same as crack, from $80 to $125 a gram, but is cheaper to use since each dose is smaller and the effects last much longer (between 8 and 24 hours).[51]

Ice, used in Asia for years, was imported to Hawaii in the early 1980s and has since spread to the West Coast. This drug is not new. It has been around since the 19th century (one past user was Hitler). What is new is the source: The drug, once manufactured and aggressively marketed by youth and motorcycle gangs on the West Coast, is now controlled by Mexican crime families who are quickly spreading it eastward across the United States. The main ingredient for the manufacture of the drug, ephedrine, originates in Asia and Europe. It is then shipped to Mexico. Next, it is smuggled across the U.S. border and resold to the operators of stove-top labs located in places as varied as rural shacks and motel bathrooms. Crank can be easily manufactured in the home laboratory by a "cook" with a high-school education in chemistry and $500 worth of equipment by extracting pure methamphetamine from common industrial chemicals. The recipe is on the Internet, available to those who know where to look. Some law enforcement officials fear crank and its smokable form, ice, will be the basis for a national drug crisis during the 1990s. The aftereffects of crank and ice are similar to those of crack and cocaine: lethargy, severe depression, paranoia, and cardiopulmonary damage. Many users develop a tolerance for these drugs quickly and need larger and larger doses to gain the effect they seek.

Drugs Affecting Physical Performance

In the world of competitive athletics, where the margin between winning and losing may be only a fraction of a second, athletes looking for an edge are tempted by illegal drugs. Anabolic steroids are taken to build muscle. Amphetamines may be taken to mask fatigue; caffeine to enhance performance. Diuretics may be used to cause rapid weight loss or to mask anabolic steroid use. All of these drugs can adversely affect your health.

Anabolic Steroids

Anabolic steroids are an artificial form of the male hormone **testosterone.** Testosterone is secreted by the testes of a mature male in quantities of 2.5 mg to 10.0 mg daily. This hormone stimulates the bone, muscle, skin, and hair growth that are characteristically found in the adult male. Steroids were first developed in the 1930s to build body tissues and to prevent the breakdown of tissue that occurs in some diseases. In the 1950s, a few

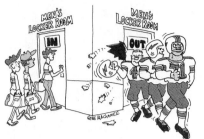

Overly aggressive behavior is a symptom of steroid use in males.

foreign countries experimented with giving testosterone to their male and female athletes. Because these athletes dominated many international competitions, a U.S. doctor developed a form of anabolic steroid that could help build muscle yet minimize masculinizing side effects.[52] Initially steroids were used only by weightlifters in small doses, but athletes assumed that larger doses would build even more muscle. Today, anabolic steroids are widely used and abused by both male and female athletes, from young teens to professionals, at all levels of competition. Many athletes "stack" them—that is, take a combination of brands in quantities of 100 mg or more daily.

While these drugs increase muscle mass and have some legitimate uses (i.e., treatment of hormone disorders, treatment of multiple sclerosis and anemia), they have numerous adverse side effects (Table 12.12). Anabolic steroids can alter mood and behavior. Significant increases in depression, violence, sexual arousal, and distractibility were seen in young male athletes in one study.[53] When taken by men, steroids shut down the body's production of testosterone, causing breast growth, testicular atrophy, prostate enlargement, and premature cessation of bone growth. Large doses of anabolic steroids trigger masculine changes in women. Deepened voice, male pattern baldness, and increased facial and body hair are irreversible. Females experience loss of body fat, enlarged clitoris, decreased breast size, and changes in or absence of menstruation. The

table 12.12

THE BAD NEWS ABOUT STEROIDS

Established side effects and adverse reactions from anabolic steroids follow:

- Acne
- Aggressive, combative behavior ("'roid rage")
- Anaphylactic shock (from injections)
- Breast development (soreness or swelling in men)
- Cancer
- Cholesterol increase
- Clitoris enlargement
- Death
- Depression
- Diarrhea
- Edema (water retention in tissue)
- Fatigue
- Feeling of abdominal or stomach fullness
- Fetal damage
- Frequent or continuing erections (mature males)
- Frequent urge to urinate (in mature males)
- Gallstones
- HDL (which helps reduce cholesterol) decrease
- Heart disease
- High blood pressure
- Hirsutism (hairiness—irreversible)

- Impotence
- Increased chance of injury to muscles, tendons, and ligaments, plus longer recovery period from injuries
- Increased risk of coronary artery disease (heart attack, stroke)
- Insomnia
- Kidney disease
- Liver disease
- Liver tumors
- Male pattern baldness (irreversible)
- Menstrual irregularities
- Priapism (painful, prolonged erections)
- Prostate enlargement (which can result in blockage of the urinary tract)
- Rash
- Sterility (reversible)
- Stunted growth
- Testicular atrophy
- Unnatural hair growth
- Unpleasant breath odor
- Unusual bleeding
- Yellowing of the eyes or skin

Used with permission. Department of Health and Human Services. HHS Publication No. (FDS) 88–3170) "Athletes and Steroids: Playing a Deadly Game" by Roger W. Miller.

athlete who uses steroids faces a variety of other steroid side effects: acne, mood swings, changes in sex drive, and uncontrollable, aggressive behavior, or **'roid rage**.

The popularity of anabolic steroids is attested to by the growth of a large black market and quack steroid products. Many of the black-market brands come from underground labs and foreign countries and are of questionable quality and purity.

Steroids can be deadly dangerous. Unfortunately, to the high school junior trying to make first-string linebacker, the long-term effects of steroids may not seem important. However, steroid use can lead to sterility, kidney disease, liver tumors, bleeding ulcers, cancer, cardiovascular problems (high blood pressure, stroke, lowered high-density lipoprotein), and death. One surprising risk to the user who injects anabolic steroids is the exposure to HIV.

Even though steroids may be easily accessible through health clubs and spas, they are illegal if purchased without a physician's prescription. Some physicians have readily written prescriptions for athletes, but this practice is decreasing as doctors become more aware of the drug's dangerous side effects.

Amphetamines

Amphetamines (*speed, uppers, crank, bennies, meth,* or *crystal*) are powerful central nervous system stimulants. They are controlled drugs, meaning legislation has severely restricted even medical use. Their use without a prescription is illegal. Currently, amphetamines are legitimately used for short-term diet control in obesity and **narcolepsy** (uncontrollable attacks of deep sleep). They increase blood pressure, heart rate, respiratory rate, and metabolic rate; suppress the appetite; and place the body in a state of stress. The ability of amphetamines to relieve sleepiness and fatigue, to decrease appetite, and to increase alertness, confidence, and short-term performance has led to extensive nonmedical use, particularly by people involved in activities that demand stamina and long periods of wakefulness: long-distance truck drivers, pilots, flight attendants, and entertainers. They have also been used by students cramming for exams and by athletes trying to enhance their performance. These drugs do not increase maximal oxygen uptake. While they do enhance endurance by masking fatigue, under the influence of amphetamines, an athlete may go out in a race too hard and burn out midway. Also, a person using amphetamines in competition may be seriously injured and not be aware of it.

Common side effects include headaches, mood swings, rapid heartbeat, restlessness, insomnia, and anxiety. Use of amphetamines over a prolonged time period increases tolerance of the drug and results in a need for larger doses. Large doses can lead to high blood pressure, anorexia, convulsions, and psychosis. Use of amphetamines during exercise in a hot environment may result in an elevated body temperature and death. Amphetamine injections, when needles are shared, may expose the user to needle diseases such as hepatitis and AIDS.

Diuretics

Diuretics cause the body to pass water by increasing urine output. They are useful in treating edema and mild hypertension. Diuretics are useless in producing true weight loss, since they result in loss of water, not fat. Any water lost is quickly regained over the next 24 hours. When used by wrestlers to temporarily decrease weight in order to compete, the resulting dehydration produces weakness and fatigue, along with increased susceptibility to heat illness. Diuretics have also been used, ineffectively, by some athletes attempting to mask anabolic steroid use. Urine tests for steroids are sufficiently sensitive to detect amounts as minute as a drop in a swimming pool of water.

Caffeine

Caffeine is probably the most common drug used by adults and children in our society. It occurs naturally in coffee, tea, colas, cocoa, and chocolate and is added to some prescription and nonprescription drugs. Table 12.13 lists average amounts of caffeine found in commonly used drinks, food, and drugs. Caffeine is a powerful central nervous system stimulant. In healthy, rested people, a dose of 100 milligrams (about 1 cup of coffee) increases alertness, banishes drowsiness, quickens reaction time, enhances intellectual and muscular effort, increases heart and respiratory rates, and stimulates urinary output.

Ingestion of one to two cups of coffee an hour before prolonged exhaustive exercise produces a glycogen-sparing effect by promoting fat use, which may enhance

table 12.13

COMMON SOURCES OF CAFFEINE

	MILLIGRAMS		MILLIGRAMS
Coffee (6-oz. cup)		Tea (5-oz. cup)	
Brewed, drip method	80–175	Brewed	40
Decaffeinated, brewed	3	Instant	30
Instant	60–100	Vivarin	200
Decaffeinated, instant	2	NoDoz (1 Tablet)	100
Espresso (2 oz.)	90–110	Cold-allergy remedies	
Chocolate		Triaminicin	30
Dark chocolate (1 oz.)	5–35	Dristan A F Decongestant	16
Chocolate cake (1 slice)	20–30	Pain Relievers	
Milk chocolate (1 oz.)	1–10	Excedrin	65
Chocolate-flavored syrup (1 oz.)	4	Anacin Maximum Strength	32
Soft drinks (12 oz.)		Midol	32
Mountain Dew	54	Weight Control	
Mellow Yellow	52	Dexatrim Extra Strength	200
Coca-Cola	45	Diuretics	
Diet Coke	45	Permathene H_2 Off	200
Mr. Pibb	40	Aqua-Ban	100
Dr. Pepper	39		
Pepsi-Cola	38		
Diet Pepsi	36		

performance in endurance activities.[54] It also tends to mask fatigue. This effect decreases as fitness increases, however, resulting in little or no benefit for highly trained athletes. If a competitive edge is desired, an athlete is wiser to drink a sports drink or plain water. Caffeine produces dehydration and, in some individuals, abnormalities in heart electrical function, both of which hinder performance.

While moderate use of caffeine is generally harmless, overconsumption can produce a toxic reaction known as *caffeinism*. A 300 mg dose for many people produces sleep disruption, nervousness, irritability, restlessness, muscle twitches, headaches, heart palpitations, and gastric disturbances. In addition, some women report increased incidence of premenstrual syndrome (PMS) or fibrocystic breast disease (noncancerous breast lumps) related to caffeine consumption. How much caffeine is too much? Although tolerance varies from one person to another, intake of less than 200 mg per day is a wise limit.

Caffeine use is habit forming, and those who try to abruptly stop a long-term pattern of heavy consumption often experience withdrawal symptoms. Headaches, lethargy, irritability, and difficulty concentrating are common symptoms that will gradually diminish over a few days to two weeks.

Over-the-Counter and Prescription Drugs

Legal drugs are often subdivided into over-the-counter drugs (OTCs) and prescription drugs. There are over 300,000 OTCs available in the United States. Aspirin is the most common form, but most cold medicines, cough syrups, and laxatives also fall into this category. OTCs are not addictive if used correctly, and they must have clear warnings and instructions printed on labels for consumer use and protection. Still, there is a difference between *safe* and *harmless*. OTCs can do damage if used incorrectly, and some can lead to physical dependence if overused.

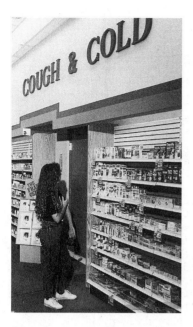
Over-the-counter drugs should be used with caution.

Four common kinds of nonprescription drugs are especially likely to produce adverse side effects or dependence:[55]

1. *Nasal sprays.* After several days' use, these can produce a "rebound" effect, making your nose more congested than ever. The rebound effect is the result of increased swelling of the nasal tissues. If you use a spray, limit use to one or two days.
2. *Laxatives.* The most habit-forming laxatives are the so-called stimulants, which work by stimulating the walls of the intestines. A diet high in fruits, vegetables, and grains, plus 2 quarts of fluids a day will almost always eliminate constipation. Laxatives should not be used to induce weight loss.
3. *Eyedrops.* These blood vessel constrictors will whiten bloodshot eyes, but like nasal sprays, they can produce a rebound effect.
4. *Alcohol/codeine cough syrups.* Codeine, a narcotic, works directly on the part of the brain that controls coughing. In many drugstores, you can obtain codeine-containing cough suppressants simply by signing at the cash register. Some of these medications contain substantial amounts of alcohol, which is dangerous for anyone with an alcohol problem.

Most prescription drugs are put to good use (for example, antibiotics used for treating infection), but many are abused. Prescription drugs that are sometimes abused include amphetamines, barbiturates, narcotics, and tranquilizers. These drugs are used for a wide range of purposes such as to stimulate and/or depress the CNS, overcome fatigue, suppress hunger, induce sleep, deaden the senses, relieve pain, and control anxieties.

There seems to be a pill for every need. Unfortunately, once prescribed, drugs are often taken in amounts and combinations not anticipated by the prescribing physician. Some physicians prescribe drugs more readily than do others, and some fail to stress the importance of reading labels carefully and taking drugs only as directed. Drugs prescribed to diminish physical or mental anguish are sometimes used for social purposes, leading to drug abuse.

Synergistic reaction, a major problem with drug use, is a phenomenon that occurs when various drugs are taken in combination, where the cumulative effect is greater than the effects of the drugs when taken separately. This results in an exaggerated drug effect or a prolonged drug reaction. Used alone, alcohol and tobacco are linked to oral cancer. Used together, the risk escalates. The same is true for alcohol and oral contraceptives in connection to increased risk of stroke and coronary heart disease. Two of the world's most widely prescribed drugs, Zantac and Tagamet (used by millions of people with persistent heartburn and ulcers), act synergistically with alcohol. One study reported[56] that in individuals who drank one and one-half glasses of wine with a meal and were taking Zantac, BAC increased 34 percent. For those taking Tagamet, BAC increased 92 percent. Especially hazardous is the combination of alcohol and barbiturates. This combination can kill a person or leave him or her in a persistent vegetative state.

SUMMARY

The wellness journey does not include substance abuse. Before drinking alcohol, smoking, or using other drugs, consider what these substances do to you. Your mind and body are capable of handling stress and emotional and physical pain without the help of drugs. You can feel happy, sexy, sad, angry, and joyous and experience love without artificial chemicals to enhance your feelings or to help you cope with life's challenges. The fact is, these substances magnify your problems. The single biggest killer of young adults is not heart disease, stroke, or cancer. It is accidents. Over half of all fatal accidents are alcohol or drug related. Use of many substances leads to tolerance or addiction as well as health problems. No other drug, not even alcohol, even comes close to nicotine in terms of deaths, illness, and other economic costs such as fires. Drugs do not make you a better athlete, either. On the contrary, inappropriate substance use can ruin your health, relationships, and future.

Before using any substance, whether over-the-counter, illegal, or prescribed, remember that you have choices. What you do now will affect your future. Be responsible and choose wisely.

REFERENCES

1. Nakken, Craig. *The Addictive Personality: Understanding Compulsion in Our Lives*. Center City, Minn.: Hazelton Foundation. New York: Harper and Row Publishers Inc., 1988.
2. National Council on Problem Gambling, 1(800)522-4700.
3. National Council on Problem Gambling.
4. Nakken Craig. *The Addictive Personality: Roots, Rituals, and Recovery*. Center City, Minn.: Hazelton Foundation, 1988 (5012-0176).
5. *The University of California, Berkeley Wellness Encyclopedia*. Boston: Houghton Mifflin Company, 1991: 67–70.
6. Gibbons, Boyd. "Alcohol the Legal Drug." *National Geographic* 181, no. 2 (February 1992): 291–95.
7. Frezza, Mario, M.D., Carlo DiPadora, M.D., Gabriele Pozzato, M.D., Madalesa Terpin, M.D., Enrique Barano, M.D., and Charles S. Lieher, M.D. "High Blood Alcohol Levels in Women: The Role of Decreased Alcohol Dehydrogenase Activity and First-Pass Metabolism." *The New England Journal of Medicine* 322 (April 11, 1990): 95–99.
8. *PRIDE (Parents' Resource Institute for Drug Education)*. Evanston, Ill.: Signal Press, 1990 (1730 Chicago Avenue, Evanston, IL 60201).
9. "Alcohol the Legal Drug."
10. "The Fact Is . . ." Rockville, Md.: National Clearinghouse for Alcohol and Drug Information, 1990.
11. "The Fact Is . . ."
12. *PRIDE*.
13. *The Wellness Encyclopedia*.
14. "Health and Behavioral Consequences of Binge Drinking in College."
15. Fuchs, C. S. "Alcohol Consumption and Mortality Among Women." *The New England Journal of Medicine* 332, no. 19 (May 11, 1995): 671–80.
16. "Alcohol Consumption and Mortality Among Women."
17. *Healthy People 2000, National Health Promotion and Disease Prevention Objectives*. Washington, D.C.: U.S. Department of Health and Human Services, Public Health Service, 1990.
18. Anna Lamb. Alcohol Education, Coordinator, Ball State Health Center, Ball State University, Muncie, Ind.

19. "Alcohol the Legal Drug."
20. "The Effect of Ethanol on Fat Storage in Healthy Subjects." *The New England Journal of Medicine* 326, no. 15 (April 9, 1992): 671–75.
21. *Healthy People 2000*.
22. Burgess, Donna. "Fetal Alcohol Syndrome and Fetal Alcohol Effect: Principles for Educators." *Phi Delta Kappan* 74, no. 1 (September 1993): 49–51.
23. Gibbons, Boyd. "The Preventable Tragedy—Fetal Alcohol Syndrome." *National Geographic* 181, no. 2 (February 1992).
24. "Trends in Fetal Alcohol Syndrome." *Journal of American Medical Association* 273, no. 18 (May 10, 1995).
25. *Healthy People 2000*.
26. American Heart Association, American Cancer Society, and American Lung Association. "Smoke-Free Class of 2000 FACTS." Dallas: 1995.
27. U.S. Department of Health and Human Services. *The Health Consequences of Smoking: Cardiovascular Disease*. Washington, D.C.: U.S. Government Printing Office, 1983.
28. "Cigarette Smoking Among Adults." *Journal of American Medical Association* 273, no. 5 (February 1, 1995).
29. *Heart and Stroke Facts: 1995 Statistical Supplement*.
30. *Healthy People 2000*.
31. U.S. Department of Health and Human Services. "If Your Kids Think Everybody Smokes, They Don't Know Everybody: A Parents Guide to Smoking and Teenagers." Washington, D.C.: U.S. Government Printing Office, 1995.
32. "Cigarette Smoking Among Adults." *Journal of American Medical Association* 273, no. 5 (February 1, 1995).
33. American Heart Association. *Heart and Stroke Facts: 1995 Statistical Supplement*. Dallas, Tex.: American Heart Association National Center, 1995 (7272 Greenville Avenue, Dallas, TX 75231–4596).
34. *New England Journal of Medicine* 324 (1991): 739–45.
35. American Cancer Society. *Cancer Facts and Figures—1995*. New York: American Cancer Society, 1992.
36. *Cancer Facts and Figures—1995*.
37. *Heart and Stroke Facts: 1995 Statistical Supplement*.

38. Glantz, S. A., et al. "Passive Smoking and Heart Disease: Mechanisms at Risk." *Journal of American Medical Association* 273, no. 13 (April 13, 1995).
39. "Passive Smoking and Heart Disease: Mechanisms at Risk."
40. *Healthy People 2000*.
41. *Cancer Facts and Figures—1995*.
42. Cinciripini, Paul, et al. "The Effects of Smoking Schedules on Cessation Outcome: Can We Improve on Common Methods of Gradual and Abrupt Nicotine Withdrawal?" *Journal of Consulting and Clinical Psychology* 63, no. 3 (June 1995): 388–92.
43. Sweeting, Roger. *A Values Approach to Health Behavior*. Champaign, Ill.: Human Kinetics Books, 1990.
44. Gilkeson, Robert, M.D. "Effects of Drugs on Learning." Sixth Annual Conference of the Indiana Federation of Communities for Drug-Free Youth, Inc. Indianapolis, Ind. (October 30, 1987).
45. National Institute on Drug Abuse (NIDA), U.S. Department of Health and Human Services (5600 Fishers Lane, Rockville, Maryland 20857, 1-301-443-6245).
46. Carroll, Charles R. *Drugs In Modern Society*, 3d ed. Dubuque, Iowa: Brown & Benchmark Publishers, 1993.
47. Schlaat, Richard, and Peter Shannon. *Drugs*, 3d ed. Englewood Cliffs, N.J.: Prentice Hall, 1990.
48. *Drugs in Modern Society*.
49. NIDA.
50. *Drugs in Modern Society*.
51. *Facts About Crank. Prevention Information Series*. Bloomington, Ind.: Indiana Prevention Resource Center for Substance Abuse, Indiana University, 1990.
52. Miller, Roger W. "Athletes and Steroids: Playing a Deadly Game." *FDA Consumer*. Washington, D.C.: Department of Health and Human Services, 1986.
53. Su, T. P., et al. "Neuropsychiatric Effects of Anabolic Steroids in Male Normal Volunteers." *Journal of American Medical Association* 269 (1993).
54. Costill, David L. *Inside Running: Basics of Sports Physiology*. Indianapolis, Ind.: Benchmark Press, Inc., 1986.
55. *The Wellness Encyclopedia*.
56. NIDA.

SUGGESTED READINGS

Alcohol and Women. Rockville, Md.: National Institute on Alcohol Abuse and Alcoholism, 1990.

"Alcohol Related Deaths of American Indians—Stereotypes and Strategies." *JAMA* 267, no. 10 (March 11, 1992).

Barnard, Charles. *Families with an Alcoholic Member*. New York: Human Sciences Press, 1990.

Blum, Kenneth. *Alcohol and the Addictive Brain: New Hope for Alcoholics from Biogenetic Research*. New York: Free Press, 1991.

Blumberg, Leonard. *Beware the First Drink*. Seattle, Wash.: Glen Abbey Books, 1991.

Cahalan, Don. *An Ounce of Prevention: Strategies for Solving Tobacco, Alcohol and Drug Problems*. San Francisco: Jossey-Bass Publishers, 1991.

Cocores, James. The *800-COCAINE Book of Drug and Alcohol Recovery*. New York: Villard Books, 1990.

Cox, Miles, ed. *Why People Drink: Parameters of Alcohol as a Reinforcer*. New York: Gardner Press, 1990.

Flynn, Laura. "Beyond AA: Alternatives for Alcoholics Who Resist the Program's Religious Approach." *Health* 23, no. 6 (July/August 1992).

Fortman, Stephen P., and Joel Killen. "Nicotine Gum and Self-Help Behavioral Treatment for Smoking Relapse Prevention: Results from a Trial Using Population-Based Recruitment." *Journal of Consulting and Clinical Psychology* 63, no. 3 (June 1995).

Frances, Richard, and Sheldon Miller. *Clinical Textbook of Addictive Disorders*. New York: Guilford Press, 1991.

Frankle, Mark, and David Leffers. "Athletes on Anabolic-Androgenic Steroids, New Approach Diminishes Health Problems." *The Physician and Sportsmedicine* 20, no. 6 (June 1992).

Giles, H. G. *Alcohol and the Identification of Alcoholics: A Handbook for Professionals*. Lexington, Mass.: Lexington Books, 1991.

Gold, Mark, M.D. *800-COCAINE*. Summit, N.J.: The Pia Press, Bantam Books, Inc., 1990.

Kelly, P., et al. "Cocaine and Exercise." Med. Sci. Sports & Ex. 27, no. 1 (1995).

O'Brien, Robert, and Morris Chafetz. *The Encyclopedia of Alcoholism*. New York: Facts on File, 1991.

Scaffa, Marjorie, Sandra Crouse-Quinn, and Robert Swift. *Making Choices: A Personal Look at Alcohol and Drug Use*. Dubuque, Iowa: Brown & Benchmark Publishers, 1992.

Schlaadt, Richard. *Alcohol Use & Abuse*. Guilford, Conn.: The Dushkin Publishing Group, Inc., 1992.

Schlaadt, Richard. *Drugs Society and Behavior*. Guilford, Conn.: The Dushkin Publishing Group, Inc., 1992.

St. Clair, Harvey. *Recognizing Alcoholism and Its Effects: A Mini Guide*. New York: Karger, 1991.

RESOURCES

Al-Anon Family Group Headquarters, P.O. Box 862, Midtown Station, New York, NY 10018, (212) 302-7240.

Alcoholics Anonymous, 175 Fifth Avenue, New York, NY 10010, (212) 473-6200.

Alcoholics Anonymous World Services, P.O. Box 459, Grand Central Station, New York, NY 10163, (212) 686-1100.

American Cancer Society, (800) ACS-2345.

American Heart Association, (800) AHA-USA1.

American Lung Association, (800) LUNG-USA.

Boost Alcohol Consciousness Concerning the Health of University Students (BACCHUS of the United States, Inc.), c/o Campus Alcohol Information Center, University of Florida, Gainesville, FL 32611, (800) COCAINE.

Gamblers Anonymous, International Service Office, P.O. Box 1713, Los Angeles, CA 90017, (213) 386-8789.

Mothers Against Drunk Driving (MADD), 669 Airport Freeway, Suite 310, Hurst, TX 76053, (817) 268-6233.

Narcotics Anonymous, P.O. Box 9999, Van Nuys, CA 91409, (818) 780-3951.

National Association of Children of Alcoholics, P.O. Box 421691, San Francisco, CA 94142, (415) 431-1366.

National Clearinghouse for Alcohol and Drug Information, P.O. Box 2345, Rockville, MD 20852, (301) 468-2600.

National Council on Alcoholism, Inc., 12 West 21st Street, New York, NY 10010, (212) 986-4433.

National Council on Compulsive Gambling, 444 West 56th Street, Room 3207S, New York, NY 10019, (212) 765-3833.

National Helpline, run by National Council on Problem Gambling, (800) 522-4700.

National Inhalant Prevention Coalition, (800) 269-4237.

National Institute on Alcohol Abuse and Alcoholism, Parklawn Building, 5600 Fishers Lane, Room 16-105, Rockville, MD 20857, (301) 443-3885.

National Service, run by the New Jersey Council on Compulsive Gambling, (800) GAMBLER.

Remove Intoxicated Drivers (RID), (518) 372-0034.

Shoplifters Anonymous, P.O. Box 24515, Minneapolis, MN 55424.

The National Cocaine Hotline, Fair Oaks Hospital, Summit, NJ 07901.

U.S. Department of Human Services, Public Health Service, Alcohol, Drug Abuse, and Mental Health Administration, Rockville, MD.

chapter 13

Preventing Sexually Transmitted Disease

Study green Sheet.

➤ Objectives

After reading this chapter, you will be able to:

1. Identify symptoms of AIDS and the most common sexually transmitted diseases.

2. Differentiate between curable and incurable sexually transmitted diseases.

3. Identify four ways HIV is transmitted.

4. Recognize the latency period for AIDS.

5. List actions you can take to decrease the risk of acquiring a sexually transmitted disease.

Symptoms & warning signs of STD

Terms

- Acquired Immune Deficiency Syndrome (AIDS)
- Chancre
- Chlamydia
- Genital herpes
- Genital warts
- Gonorrhea
- Hepatitis B
- Herpes simplex virus
- Human immunodeficiency virus (HIV)
- Human papilloma virus (HPV)
- Lymphocytes
- Opportunistic diseases
- Pelvic inflammatory disease (PID)
- Sexually transmitted disease (STD)
- Syphilis
- T-cells

Many receive advice. Only the wise profit from it.

Syrus

diseases that are spread through sexual contact were once called *venereal diseases (VD)*, named for Venus, the Greek goddess of love, mother of Cupid. The terms *VD* and *sexually transmitted disease* have often been used interchangeably. However, VD refers to diseases such as gonorrhea, which are nearly always spread through sexual contact. The term **sexually transmitted disease (STD)** refers to a broader category of diseases that are spread primarily through sexual intercourse but also through other intimate behavior, sex play, and, occasionally, nonsexually.

Sexually Transmitted Disease

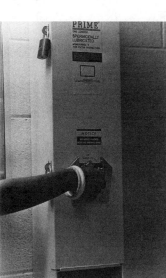

Condom machines are becoming more prevalent.

Today, while **Acquired Immune Deficiency Syndrome (AIDS)** claims the spotlight as the most deadly and feared STD, we are experiencing a silent epidemic of other STDs in the United States. As a group, STDs are the number-one communicable disease problem, but many people are unaware of this because of our cultural reluctance to discuss STDs and fear of public embarrassment. Only colds and flu, which are not officially reported, occur more frequently. It is estimated that one in four Americans will acquire at least one STD in their lifetime.

Changing mores appear to be a major factor in the increasing rate of STDs. Since the 1980s, increasing rates of premarital sexual intercourse among young people have offered more opportunity for the spread of disease.[1] Involvement with alcohol, a concern on many college campuses, is tied to increased sexual activity and lack of commitment to one's sex partner, which increase STD risk.[2] Another factor may be the development of the birth control pill, which resulted in decreasing use of the condom. With concern over AIDS, however, this is changing. Both male and female condoms not only prevent conception but serve as barriers to transmission of STDs.

STDs are most common in people in their late teens to their 20s: 90 percent of reported STDs occur among persons ages 15 to 29[3] (Fig. 13.1). Nevertheless, your risk of acquiring an STD is determined by your behavior, not by your age or sexual orientation. Risk can be reduced or increased by personal choices that you control. If you choose to be sexually active, you are at risk. Your chances of exposure to an STD increase with multiple sexual partners and with increased frequency of sexual activity. Risk of infection is low to zero in a mutually monogamous relationship or if you abstain from sex.

Unfortunately, many people, especially young people, feel that STDs aren't serious or that "STDs only happen to others," and they fail to take precautions. A person may think, "If I get one, I'll just go get it taken care of." While some STDs are curable, some are not. Even some of the traditionally curable STDs are becoming antibiotic

FIGURE 13.1 ➤
STD rates by age.

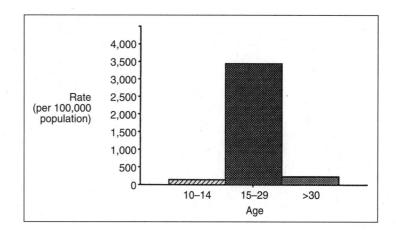

table 13.1

SYMPTOMS OF SEXUALLY TRANSMITTED DISEASE

WOMEN	WOMEN AND MEN
• Pelvic pain	• Abnormal discharge from the penis or vagina
• Bleeding from the vagina between periods	• A burning sensation during urination or bowel movements
• Burning or itching around the vagina	• Sores, bumps, or blisters near the mouth, rectum, or genitals
• Pain deep inside the vagina during sexual intercourse	• Flulike feelings with fever, chills, or aches
	• Redness and swelling in the throat
	• Swelling in the groin

resistant making treatment more difficult. STDs may not seem to be a serious problem because you can't tell by looking at your friends who is infected and who is not. Also, your friends probably are not going to discuss STDs with you as they would discuss their last cold. But silence can be deadly. If you can't see it and don't hear about it, some think, the problem isn't real. They are wrong.

STDs are spread from an infected person to a partner during sexual intercourse, oral sex, or anal sex. Nonsexual infection is possible with some STDs but uncommon. STDs are not spread on toilet seats, in hot tubs, or in swimming pools. The bacteria and viruses that cause STDs need the warmth and moisture of mucous membranes to live. That is why they infect the reproductive organs, rectum, and mouth. After transmission to a new host, the bacteria or virus quickly multiplies and may produce noticeable symptoms in two days to four weeks. Sometimes, an infected person notices no symptoms, however.

Women are particularly vulnerable to STDs, including AIDS, because they have more mucous membranes in their genital tissue than men do. Vaginal and cervical tissue can sustain microscopic tears through which viruses and bacteria, often transmitted by semen, can enter. In addition, women experience early warning signs of STDs much less frequently than men do, resulting in more advanced disease before treatment is sought. STDs are serious and, if left untreated, can cause permanent damage.

Early diagnosis and treatment is important both to prevent serious physical harm and to prevent spread of the disease to other sexual partners. Symptoms of STDs vary with the type of infection and may differ between males and females. Be aware of the warning signs that may indicate the presence of an STD (Table 13.1).

Diagnosis and treatment of STDs is confidential. It is important to contact the STD clinic of your local county health department or see a doctor immediately if you suspect that you may have an STD. Your local family planning clinic can also give information on where to go for help, or you can call one of the hotlines at the end of this chapter. Wherever you are treated, your case will be kept private.

There are over 25 known STDs, some of which are incurable. Most STDs are either bacterial or viral. The most common bacterial STDs, which are treatable, are chlamydia, gonorrhea, and syphilis. Viral STDs, which are incurable, include genital herpes, genital warts, and AIDS (Table 13.2). A person can have more than one STD at a time. Although less prevalent, AIDS is causing much concern because it is not only incurable but fatal.

Chlamydia

Chlamydia is one of the most widespread and damaging of all STDs. It is spread mainly through sexual intercourse but can be spread by the fingers from one body area to another, such as from the genitals to the eyes. Chlamydia, the most common bacterial

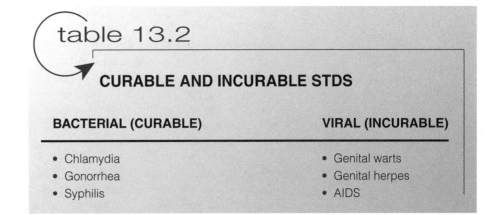

table 13.2

CURABLE AND INCURABLE STDS

BACTERIAL (CURABLE)	VIRAL (INCURABLE)
• Chlamydia	• Genital warts
• Gonorrhea	• Genital herpes
• Syphilis	• AIDS

STD, is estimated to infect 10 percent to 15 percent of college age students.[4] It affects twice as many people as gonorrhea, although it mimics its symptoms, and both diseases often occur together. For this reason, physicians usually treat both infections if one is diagnosed. Early symptoms are usually mild, and if they occur, they appear within one to three weeks of exposure. Chlamydia causes an inflammation of the urethra, which produces a burning sensation during urination. In men, chlamydia can also infect the epididymis, causing painful scrotal swelling. About 80 percent of women and 10 percent of men have no noticeable symptoms and may not even know they are infected. This makes the disease even more difficult to diagnose and cure. As a result, the disease is often not diagnosed until it has done permanent damage.

Untreated chlamydia in women can produce a serious inflammation of the sexual organs called **pelvic inflammatory disease (PID).** PID is extremely damaging and can infect the lining of the uterus, fallopian tubes, and ovaries. This may cause fever and pain in the lower abdomen and scarring and blockage of the fallopian tubes and leave a woman unable to bear children. A new urine screening test for chlamydia makes detection easier than ever. The preferred treatment for chlamydia is tetracycline.

While anyone who is sexually active can get a chlamydial infection, highest rates occur among those who have had more than one sexual partner, have taken a new sexual partner in the past two months, are between 15 and 24 years of age, are of lower socioeconomic status or black race, or are living in an inner city neighborhood.[5]

Gonorrhea

Gonorrhea, the second most common bacterial STD, was named by Galen in 150 B.C. from Greek meaning "flow of seed." At that time, the penile discharge of men infected with gonorrhea was thought to be semen. Actually, the discharge was pus produced from inflammation of the urethra. The gonorrhea bacteria grows and multiplies quickly in mucous membranes such as in the cervix, mouth, rectum, or urinary tract. In women, the most common site of infection is the cervix, but it can spread to the ovaries and fallopian tubes, causing PID. It can be spread directly through sexual intercourse or from the genitals to the mouth with the fingers.

As with chlamydia, gonorrhea often has no symptoms, or the symptoms go undetected as the infected individual continues to spread the disease. Men are much more likely to notice the symptoms than women are. Up to 80 percent of women infected have no symptoms, compared to 20 percent of men. If they occur, symptoms usually appear within two to fourteen days of infection. Gonorrhea often strikes the urethra, causing a burning sensation during urination. Males may notice an unusual penile discharge, as well as swollen lymph glands in the groin. Women may experience an abnormal vaginal discharge, abdominal pain, or vaginal bleeding. A rectal infection may produce anal itching or a discharge. Oral infections usually produce no symptoms, though a few victims may get a sore throat. Early symptoms may clear up on their own, but a person can still be infected and spread the disease to others.

If not treated, gonorrhea may cause permanent damage to the reproductive organs and cause sterility. In men, it may damage the penis, making urination difficult and erection impossible. It can also infect the epididymis, leaving scar tissue that can block the flow of semen from the infected testicle. In women, it can scar the fallopian tubes, making it impossible to bear children. In both sexes, the bacteria can spread to the bloodstream, producing a generalized bacterial infection. It can infect joints with gonococcal arthritis and irreversibly damage heart valves, spinal cord, or the brain. It can be spread from an infected mother via the birth canal to her baby, causing eye infection and blindness if not treated immediately.

Gonorrhea is usually treated with penicillin and antibiotics, although penicillin-resistant strains have developed. In fact, penicillin-resistant cases have doubled since 1988, making treatment more difficult.[6] This increasing occurrence of penicillin-resistant gonorrhea underscores the need for taking protective measures during sexual activity and for being tested once or twice a year even if there are no symptoms.

While overall rates of infection have declined, infection rates for minority adolescents and young adults remain high, especially in inner cities.[7]

Syphilis

For when it has once been received into the body, it does not immediately declare itself; rather it lies dormant for a certain time and gradually gains strength as it feeds.

Fracastoro (1483–1553), *Syphilis, the "French Disease"*

Syphilis was rampant in Europe in the late 1400s, spread during times of war by soldiers who frequented prostitutes and then returned home to their wives and mistresses. It was also reported spread by soldiers who sailed with Columbus to the New World and by many Renaissance explorers who took it beyond the boundaries of Europe. It was first known as the "great pox," in contrast to which "smallpox" was later named, and was at first thought to be a special divine punishment for sexual transgressions. In the 18th century, syphilitics wore wigs and high collars to hide hair loss and throat lesions. Many early treatments used mercury or arsenic but produced side effects that were as bad as the disease. Although syphilis has been a serious health problem during all major wars, it was not until after World War II began that the U.S. Public Health Service started using penicillin to combat it.

Syphilis cases in the United States have increased in the last half of the decade to their highest rate in 40 years and occur mainly in urban heterosexuals in the 20- to 29-year-old age group.[8] Like other bacterial STDs, syphilis is easily spread because its symptoms are often unnoticed or confused with other diseases. In fact, syphilis is known as "the great imitator" because it mimics so many other diseases.

Syphilis occurs in four stages—primary, secondary, latent, and tertiary—depending on how long a person has had it and how far it has progressed. Each stage is described next.

Primary Syphilis

The first sign of syphilis is a **chancre,** or small painless sore, which appears within one to twelve weeks of sexual contact. It may appear on the penis, in the vagina, in the mouth, or in any other area that contacted the bacteria, and it lasts one to five weeks. It is often accompanied by painless swelling of the lymph nodes in the groin. The initial sore may go unnoticed and will disappear if left untreated. The disease then enters a secondary stage two weeks to six months later.

Secondary Syphilis

In the secondary stage, skin rash, fever, headache, sore throat, swollen lymph glands, flulike symptoms, and patchy hair loss may occur. The symptoms are so general that the disease can be misdiagnosed even if medical help is sought. The rash may appear as pink spots or small raised bumps on the palms, soles of the feet, back, chest, arms, legs, face, or abdomen. Small, moist sores may appear in the mouth, and lesions may appear on the genital area. Secondary symptoms, if they occur, may clear up in two to six weeks without treatment but may recur for up to two years. During this time, an infected individual can still spread the disease. If untreated, although the initial symptoms may subside and a person can feel perfectly normal, the disease progresses.

Latent Syphilis

In latent syphilis, the third stage, a person is generally no longer infectious to others unless there is a relapse of moist lesions or unless the disease is passed to a baby during pregnancy. This stage can last for several years with no symptoms, but the infecting bacteria can continue to multiply.

Tertiary Syphilis

While two-thirds of untreated people will have no more symptoms, the one-third who are affected may suffer permanent damage to the cardiovascular or nervous systems. Tertiary syphilis can occur anywhere from three to forty years after initial infection. Complications include heart disease, blindness, brain damage, paralysis, insanity, and death.

Penicillin was discovered to be effective against syphilis in the 1940s. It is still considered the treatment of choice.

Genital Herpes

Genital herpes is another major contributor to human misery. It has no cure. Once you get it, you have it for life. Symptoms usually occur within two to thirty days of having sex. Early signs include itching, tingling, or burning on the genitals. This is followed by small, painful genital sores or blisters that break open and crust over, causing intense itching and extreme pain. In addition, active herpes may be accompanied by fever, swollen glands, and general flulike feelings. Herpes virus is shed from the sores, which are highly contagious. After the blisters appear, they last from one to three weeks and then heal and disappear. Once established, the herpes virus migrates into nerve cells, where it may lie dormant or reactivate to cause recurring outbreaks of sores from time to time. New attacks of the disease appear at intervals, triggered by lowered resistance, fever, sunburn, or even stress.

Genital herpes is caused by the **herpes simplex virus.** A virus invades body cells to live and reproduce. Nearly all herpes infections are caused by Herpes Simplex Type II, which is transmitted from one infected individual to another during intercourse. This is different from the common Herpes Simplex Type I, which causes cold sores to appear on or around the mouth. However, it is possible to spread Type I to the genitals or Type II to the mouth by touching the sores and scratching or rubbing somewhere else. You can also become infected by both types of herpes at the same time. It is important to avoid letting the lesions contact someone else's body through touching, kissing, or sexual contact. Touching an eye after touching a sore can cause a severe eye infection called *ocular herpes*. Simply washing the hands thoroughly after touching a sore can prevent transmission of the virus.

At least two-thirds of the infected individuals are not even aware that they have genital herpes—their symptoms are so mild that they go unnoticed. Because many unreported cases exist, experts estimate that the nationwide infected population may be as large as 30 million Americans.[9] Infections are most common between the ages of 18 and 25 years. Risk factors for genital herpes include having more than one sexual partner, having a greater number of years of being sexually active, exposure to other genital infections, and lower socioeconomic level. While infection is more common in nonwhites, symptomatic infections are more frequent in whites.[10] In women, herpes sores can occur internally and cause no discomfort. However, these infected individuals can still spread the virus to others, and a mother with herpes can give it to her baby. Babies born to infected mothers can become infected with herpes at birth. In infants, the virus can cause blindness, brain damage, and death. For this reason, babies are usually delivered by caesarean section if the mother has genital herpes.

While a person was once thought to be contagious only during herpes outbreaks, current studies indicate that herpes can be spread, particularly from men to women, even if a person does not have symptoms. Women are four times as likely to get herpes from men as men are to get it from women, perhaps because of the greater exposure of vaginal and cervical mucous membranes to the virus during sexual contact.[11]

The severity and duration of symptoms can be decreased with Acyclovir, an antiviral drug. It can also be taken to prevent recurrence of symptoms, although it cannot cure the disease. Thus, the joke "What is the difference between love and herpes?" Answer: "Only herpes is forever."

Genital Warts and Other Human Papilloma Virus Infections

Human papilloma virus (HPV) infections are epidemic among young people of college age. Not all of them cause visible warts.[12] There are over 60 different types of HPV infections, and a person can have more than one type of HPV at a time.[13] Once HPV has invaded cells, depending on its type, it may produce genital warts or genital tract cancers, or there may be no symptoms at all. Both cervical cancer in women and penile cancer in men are associated with HPV, and these all too often occur in sexually active young adults.

HPV is passed through direct skin-to-skin contact through sexual activity. Nonsexual transmission is possible, though rare, since HPV can remain alive for several hours on wet towels or undergarments. HPV infections are more common in women than in men, probably because the warmth and moisture of a woman's vagina provides an ideal place for viral growth.

Genital warts are caused by some types of HPV, are highly contagious, and take one to eight months to appear after exposure. Until the warts appear, there are no symptoms that indicate presence of the HPV virus. Between the time of exposure and the appearance of warts, either partner can have the virus unknowingly and give it to the other. Genital warts may be flat or rounded bumps with a cauliflowerlike appearance. They are often painless but may itch or burn. On men, most genital warts occur on the outside of the penis. In women, they may appear around the vulva and inside the vagina and cervix. They may also appear in the mouth, in the throat, or around the anus, and they do not go away.

Warts can grow and spread, so they should be removed. Warts can be frozen with liquid nitrogen, burned off with an electric needle or laser, or removed surgically or chemically. While these methods can eliminate the external lesions, they do not eradicate the virus, which may become dormant and later reappear or may be destroyed by the body's own immune system.

You can detect some genital warts by self-examination. Men should check the penis regularly. Women should use a mirror to examine the vulva and anus. Warts inside the vagina can be found by a doctor.

A genital wart infection is a major risk factor for cervical cancer, one of the leading cancer killers of women. In some cases, warts turn into precancerous growths called *dysplasia* and later become cancerous. Cervical cancer, thus, is considered a sexually transmitted disease.[14] This cancer infects far too many young women of child-bearing age and is not just a disease of the elderly. Other risk factors for HPV include initiating sexual activity at an early age and having unprotected sex with multiple sexual partners.

An abnormal Pap smear can detect an unseen HPV infection as well as precancerous cellular changes in cervical tissue. There is also a newly developed test that can both detect an HPV infection and indicate the strain of the virus. The Virapap test detects five strains of HPV linked to cancer. Since the Pap smear only detects abnormal changes in cells, it is a good idea to get a Virapap test along with the Pap test to detect latent HPV infections. Benign HPV infections that do not cause warts or cancer do not generally require treatment, but they do signal to the carrier the risk of both and the need for frequent checkups.

Having genital warts doesn't mean you will get cancer, but it does increase your risk. Not having warts doesn't mean you are safe. Since only about 10 percent of human papilloma virus cases have visible warts, it is possible to be infected and unaware of it.

Hepatitis B

Hepatitis B, formerly called *serum hepatitis,* is an inflammatory disease that destroys liver tissue. It is caused by a virus that is spread during vaginal, anal, and oral sex with an infected partner. It spreads through contact with saliva, nasal mucus, sperm, and menstrual blood. It is also spread through sharing contaminated needles (drugs, tattooing, acupuncture) and direct blood contact. Additionally, a mother with hepatitis B can give it to her baby during childbirth. A person infected with the virus can be an asymptomatic carrier and can spread it even though there is no active infection. The incubation period ranges from one to nine months. Many people have no or mild symptoms, which can include lingering flulike feelings: weakness, fatigue, loss of appetite, nausea, vomiting, and fever. This may be accompanied by itching, hives, and joint pain. In a few days, this is followed by brownish urine; loose, light yellow stools; yellowing of the eyes and skin; abdominal discomfort; and liver enlargement; and, in severe cases, liver failure. While many people recover, about 10 percent of people with hepatitis B develop a chronic form of the disease which may produce only mild or no obvious symptoms. Chronic hepatitis may lead to a progressive destruction of liver cells, cirrhosis, or liver cancer. There is an effective vaccine for hepatitis B that is recommended for people at high risk for infection.

Acquired Immune Deficiency Syndrome (AIDS)

AIDS is a threat to all men and women, heterosexual and homosexual alike. In the 10 years after it first appeared, there were 206,000 cases of AIDS reported in the United States, and 133,000 of these people died.[15] Most of these were infected before the virus was discovered in 1981. The toll continues to climb at an alarming rate. It took six years for the first 50,000 cases to be reported, two years for the next 50,000 cases, and two more years for the next 100,000 cases.[16] In 1993, AIDS became the leading cause of death in young people ages 25 to 44.[17] Since then, AIDS cases have increased among women, children, heterosexuals, blacks, and Hispanics and dropped among gay and bisexual men.[18] Teens and young adults are particularly vulnerable to AIDS because they take risks when they may not appreciate the risks—of sex or drug use, for example.

What Is AIDS? What Is HIV?

AIDS is a syndrome, or group of symptoms, caused by the **human immunodeficiency virus (HIV).** The virus itself is not alive but is an infectious agent. It does not kill a person directly but attacks a particular type of **lymphocytes** (white blood cells) called *CD4 +* or **T-cells.** Lymphocytes control cell growth, transport nutrients to cells, and produce antibodies that protect the body against infection. They travel under their own power throughout the body and body fluids. When T-cells sense the presence of a disease, they send messages to other white cells to resist the infection. The virus penetrates T-cells and forces them to make copies of the virus. Then the cells die. Gradually, over a period of years, when enough lymphocytes are destroyed, symptoms of AIDS appear. Victims suffer from an impaired immune system, poor control of cell growth, and poor cell nutrition. A weakened immune system reduces the body's ability to defend itself against **opportunistic diseases** produced by common bacteria, viruses, parasites, and fungi that surround but do not usually have the opportunity to infect people with healthy immune systems. A person suffers infection after miserable infection, is susceptible to unusual cancers, and may become emaciated (slim disease). Another risk is tuberculosis, a contagious lung disease that has increased annually since 1981, mainly because of the AIDS epidemic.[19] Other STD infections, especially those that cause genital lesions, such as herpes and syphilis, may occur concurrently with HIV and may speed the acquisition and transmission of HIV.

What Are Symptoms of an HIV Infection?

Many HIV carriers feel well and have no symptoms for up to 10 to 12 years before the immune system is suppressed enough to cause problems. That is the difference between someone who tests HIV positive and someone who is diagnosed with AIDS. The federal Centers for Disease Control define AIDS as the syndrome of having fewer than 200 T-cells or of testing HIV positive and having one or more specific opportunistic infections. Early warning signs that may indicate a weakened immune system include chronic fatigue, swollen lymph glands, unexplained weight loss, fevers, and night sweats. Poor appetite; persistent diarrhea; an itchy, spreading skin rash; and thrush (a white fungus) in the mouth are also common. (These symptoms are shared by many diseases and do not necessarily mean that you have HIV.) The body's immune system eventually becomes so weak that otherwise rare opportunistic infections may infect the AIDS victim causing life-threatening illness.

For every person with AIDS, 20 to 30 are HIV infected.

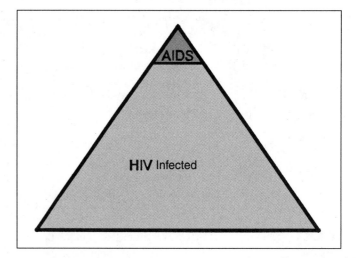

AIDS symptoms include a persistent cough and fever associated with shortness of breath, which may be related to pneumocystis carinii pneumonia; a parasitic lung infection; and tuberculosis. Kaposi's sarcoma, a cancer of the blood vessels, causes pink or purplish lesions on the skin and elsewhere. Women may suffer from persistent vaginal infections, severe pelvic inflammatory disease, and recurrent cervical cancers. In advanced stages of the disease, the virus may also damage the brain and spinal cord, causing memory loss, partial paralysis, or AIDS-related dementia.[20]

Q. Can I tell if someone has HIV?

A. You can't tell by looking. There are many HIV carriers who look and feel fine and don't even know they are infected. A blood test is necessary to detect presence of the HIV virus.

Q. If I get HIV, will I die?

A. It is not known at this time whether 100 percent of HIV-infected individuals will develop AIDS. You can carry the HIV virus in your body for years and experience no symptoms as it gradually destroys your immune system. When enough of the immune system has been destroyed, you may develop AIDS. Some people with AIDS alternate between periods of illness and periods of relatively good health. Generally, however, a person dies within one to two years of diagnosis of full-blown AIDS. It is felt that, given time, probably all HIV-infected individuals will develop AIDS.

table 13.3

HOW HIV IS TRANSMITTED

- Through sexual intercourse with an AIDS carrier
- Through sharing hypodermic needles
- By pregnant women to the fetuses they carry
- Rarely through a transfusion of infected blood

How Does HIV Spread?

HIV is transmitted in body fluids such as blood and semen or vaginal fluid. It is most often spread in one of the four ways shown in Table 13.3.

Some cases of AIDS from tainted blood and blood products occurred before 1985. Today, blood donors are screened, and blood is tested for HIV antibodies to ensure the safety of our blood supply.

HIV: What Is Safe?

AIDS is an infectious disease, but it is not spread through casual social contact with the general public or HIV carriers. You can share a classroom, dining area, or locker room with an HIV-infected individual without risk of transmission. HIV cannot be "caught" like a cold. It is not spread by insects. You cannot get HIV by shaking hands or by touching the clothes of a person infected with HIV. HIV is not spread through eating utensils, dishes, or food handled by a person with HIV. It is not spread through sweat or tears. It is impossible to get HIV by donating blood since clean needles are used for each donor. In studies of households where people with HIV were present, HIV was rarely spread except through sexual contact or from infected mothers to their infants.[21] You cannot get HIV from hugging, body massages, masturbation, or other nonsexual contact. The AIDS virus is fragile. It cannot long survive outside the human body and is easily killed by common household bleach or disinfectant.

Q. Can I get HIV from kissing?

A. There is no risk in a kiss on the cheek, and no case of AIDS has been reported from kissing on the mouth. However, small amounts of the virus are present in saliva and could possibly be transferred to another person during deep kissing, especially if oral sores or cuts exist. To be safe, the Department of Health and Human Services recommends that you avoid deep or prolonged French kissing with someone who may be infected with HIV.

Q. If mosquitoes can spread malaria, can they spread HIV?

A. There has been no recorded case of transmission of HIV from mosquitoes. While a mosquito can pick up and carry HIV in its gut, the virus cannot reproduce there nor travel to its saliva. Flies, lice, ticks, and other insects, likewise, cannot spread the virus.

Should I Be Tested for AIDS?

The Public Health Service recommends you be counseled and tested if you have had any STD, shared drug needles, had sex with a prostitute, or had sex with a man who has had sex with other men. Anyone who has had unprotected sex with three or more partners since 1981 is also at risk. People who have always practiced safe behavior do not need to be tested. For more information, call your local public health agency or the AIDS hotline at the end of this chapter.

Q. Why doesn't a first test always detect HIV?

A. The test doesn't react to the HIV virus itself but to antibodies the body produces to the virus. The time between when a person is exposed to HIV to the time antibodies to the virus appear in the blood is three to six months. A person taking the test shortly after being infected may test negative, but the person can still spread HIV. Several months later, a test will show the infection.

What About an AIDS Vaccine?

There is no vaccine to prevent AIDS, and there is no cure. Drugs such as AZT are being tested to slow the progress of the disease, but results will not be available for many years, due to the long incubation period and slow progress of the disease. Another problem is that the virus rapidly mutates to produce new forms of the virus. A vaccine might be effective for only one viral strain. Scientists feel that an AIDS vaccine may be developed within five to ten years, but it could take another 10 to 12 years to tell if it was effective in preventing AIDS. There is hope that treatments will be found, but the best way to prevent AIDS is to avoid exposure to the virus. We cannot depend on technology for a cure. Behavioral change to prevent infection is the only answer.

Why Should I Be Concerned About AIDS?

Too many young people feel that AIDS can't happen to them. They think that it isn't in their peer group or neighborhood. But when you have sex with someone, you are, in a sense, having sex with all of that person's past partners. There are students on campus who are HIV positive and are having sex. According to Dr. Richard P. Keeling of the American College Health Association Task Force on AIDS, blood samples tested from colleges across the United States revealed that two to three students per 1,000 tested HIV positive.[22] In a university of 20,000 this means 40 to 60 people may carry the virus. Keeling says, "AIDS is a young person's disease. The average age of diagnosis is 32. The incubation period to diagnosis averages 10 to 12 years, so the highest risk time is ages

Is sex under the influence worth it?

16 to 28. The problem doesn't seem real on most college campuses because people silently infected with HIV are not likely to appear ill." Many students who carry HIV look fine and have no symptoms. They may not even know they are infected. However, during intercourse, they can spread the disease to others.

Among gay men, the group with the highest HIV infection rate, significant behavioral change is already dropping the rate of infection and diagnosis. There has been no behavioral change among the next two highest infected groups: IV drug users and their partners and young heterosexuals with multiple partners. Surveys of college students show that while most know how to prevent spread of HIV, over 60 percent report having sexual intercourse with more than one partner and sporadic or no use of condoms.[23] HIV infections among young heterosexuals have increased dramatically in the past five years.[24] Most students know the facts about AIDS, but many do not use condoms or know their sexual partners. Why? Keeling states that there are six reasons:

1. *They feel invincible.* They think, "Things like that don't happen to people like me."
2. *They lack social skills and have low self-esteem.* Many people don't feel comfortable with sexual feelings or behavior and don't feel comfortable talking about these matters or negotiating with a sexual partner to take precautions.
3. *They engage in unwanted sexual behavior.* They become involved in sex without really wanting to—due to peer pressure, role expectations, or alcohol. Alcohol is involved in a tremendous amount of risky sexual behavior on campus. Alcohol increases risk taking and decreases ambivalence and judgment. It is impossible for sex under the influence of alcohol to be safe in terms of prevention of STDs.
4. *They are victims of sexual assault.* Date rape is a common unreported campus problem. If there is no consent, no precautions can be taken.
5. *Society sends mixed messages.* Our society may say, "Just say no," but in advertising and media, it screams, "Just say yes. It will be OK. Just try it."
6. *They share needles.* On campus, this is less a problem of recreational drugs than of anabolic steroids. If needles are shared, it doesn't matter what's in them; they can still spread HIV.

It doesn't matter who you are. It is not who you are that causes AIDS, but what you do. If you do things that can spread HIV, consider the risks. The problem with HIV is that if you make a mistake in judgment, it's irreversible. When you risk AIDS and lose, you lose it all.

How Can I Protect Myself from STDs?

While the facts about AIDS and other STDs are sobering, the good news is that you can reduce your risk of exposure to virtually zero by personal choices. The best prevention for any STD is sexual abstinence or a mutually monogamous sexual relationship with an uninfected partner. There is no safe sex, only less risky sex. No orgasm is worth dying for. Unless you are willing to throw away your future, you must weigh the choices and consequences. If you are sexually active with more than one partner, there are steps that you can take to avoid becoming a victim of AIDS and other sexually transmitted diseases (Table 13.4).

How to Use Condoms

If abstinence or a mutually faithful, single-partner relationship is not your choice, the next best way to protect yourself from sexually transmitted diseases including AIDS is to use a latex condom during sex. While condoms are not 100 percent effective in preventing STDs, if used correctly, it is estimated that they can reduce risk by up to 60 percent.[25] Unfortunately, few people know how to use them correctly, resulting in a failure rate of 40 percent or more. If you are a woman, carry your own condoms, even if you don't plan to have sex (few young adults who have sex plan it). Do not store condoms in a hot place such as a glove compartment or carry them in a wallet for more than one week (they need to be fresh). Use a condom every time, including for oral or anal sex. Avoid skin condoms (i.e., lambskin)—they do not provide protection from all STDs, though they do prevent pregnancy.

table 13.4

HOW TO REDUCE RISK OF STDS

1. Communicate assertively about sexual feelings, activities, partners, and STDs.
2. Choose lower-risk sexual activities that have less likelihood of transmitting STDs.
3. Separate alcohol and drugs from sexual activity. Drunk sex can't be safe sex.
4. Protect yourself. Use latex condoms or dental dams and a spermicide containing nonoxynol-9.
5. Be selective. Limit the number of partners you have sex with. The fewer partners you have, the lower your risk. Do not have sex with someone who has several sex partners or with prostitutes. Prostitutes may also use IV drugs, increasing their chances of exposure to the AIDS virus.
6. Do not use intravenous drugs. If you do, do not share drug needles and syringes. Don't have sex with people who shoot drugs.
7. Observe a partner discreetly for discharge, sores, or rash. While it may not seem romantic, if you see anything that concerns you, don't have sex!

In addition to these guidelines, you should also know the symptoms of STDs, and, if you notice a symptom that concerns you, see a physician. If you are sexually active, have an STD checkup every time you have a health exam. This is especially important for women, who often have no signs of an STD. Have an STD checkup every six months if you have more than one partner. Abstain from sex if you think you have an infection and see a doctor. If you do acquire an infection, make sure that all partners are notified and treated. To prevent infecting others, don't have sex until you have completed treatment and your doctor says you're cured.

FIGURE 13.2 ➤

How to use a condom.

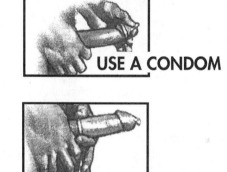
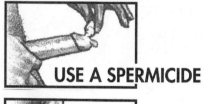
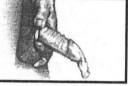

To maximize condom effectiveness, follow these steps (Fig. 13.2):

1. Be careful when opening the package. Be especially careful not to tear the condom with a fingernail or teeth.
2. Put the condom on before penetration, even if ejaculation is not planned. Withdrawal is not effective in preventing STDs. Unroll the condom on the erect penis. Squeeze the air from the top of the condom, leaving about ½-inch space for semen at the tip. Hold the tip as you unroll the condom, making sure there is no air inside. If there is no space at the tip, the force of semen coming out of the penis can break the condom.
3. Apply a water-based lubricant or spermicide such as nonoxynol-9 onto the tip of the condom. Do not use an oil-based lubricant. Vaseline or baby oil quickly deteriorate latex. A few people have allergic reactions to certain spermicides. Do not use a spermicide that causes a rash or irritation, as this could increase chance of infection.
4. Withdraw while the penis is still erect. Hold the rim of the condom to avoid spilling semen. Throw the used condom away. Do not reuse it.

If you or your partner don't like male condoms, you can try a female condom, which works like an extra-large male condom inserted into a woman's vagina. It consists of a 6½-inch long plastic tube with a large ring on each end. One ring holds it in the vagina, and the other ring fits outside the vaginal lips. It is as effective in preventing conception and STDs as the male condom, and it gives a woman the ability to protect herself and her partner, but it is more expensive, is somewhat unwieldy, and has not proved very popular.

Planning Ahead for Safer Sex

When you are in the midst of a passionate embrace, it may not seem convenient to discuss safer sex or how to use a condom, and using either type of condom takes practice. Before beginning a sexual relationship, plan ahead. Think about what you'll say to your partner about using condoms. It may help to use a news story about AIDS to bring up the subject of safer sex. Make your feelings about condom use clear. Tell your partner you want to take precautions because you care about both of you. If your partner won't agree to use condoms, don't have sex.

Choosing Lower-Risk Sexual Activities

There are many ways to show someone you care besides having sex: respect, sharing, trust, commitment. Lasting relationships are built on alternative ways of expressing love and affection. Even if you have decided to have sex, there are lower-risk sex techniques you can use to protect yourself from STDs. Keep in mind that your skin is your largest sexual organ, and your imagination is your most important sexual asset. Consider these options:

No Risk
➤ Kissing with the mouth closed
➤ Hugging
➤ Touching

➤ Massage
➤ Fantasy
➤ Masturbation

Low Risk
➤ Vaginal or oral sex using a condom and spermicide

➤ Masturbating a partner using a latex barrier

Risky
➤ Wet kissing with your mouth open
➤ Anal sex with or without a condom

➤ Vaginal or oral sex without a condom

Coping with Unwanted Sexual Pressure and Avoiding Sexual Assault

Carlos is invited to a party at an off-campus apartment by Maria, whom he met at a football game. He doesn't know anyone at the party but doesn't want to miss the fun. The music is lively and the drinks are free so he has a few drinks and starts feeling relaxed. Maria shows up and invites him to go to her room so they can talk. He agrees. They take their drinks and head toward the bedroom.

Is a woman "asking for it" if she has been drinking? Is consent implied if Maria invites Carlos into her room? If she closes the bedroom door and sits on the bed? Unfortunately, the double standard is alive and well in the United States. Many people come to campus with little experience in sexual matters. What can a person do to prevent unwanted sexual behavior? Dr. Richard Keeling states, "We need to build skills in assertiveness, self-esteem, decision making, running a relationship, and dealing with intimacy. We need a personal commitment that says my life, my future, my potential are more valuable than what's going to happen in this relationship or on this date or in the next 10 minutes."[26] What do you do when he or she wants to have sex and you don't?

It has been estimated that 80 percent of all rape victims are attacked by someone they know, either a date, a former partner, or a casual acquaintance.[27] Many people with active social lives involve themselves in parties and activities with the expectation of meeting new friends and dating partners. There is a tendency to assume this is a safe way to meet people, but placing trust in someone you know only casually can put you in an unsafe situation, particularly if alcohol is involved. Some people have trouble understanding how a person can be raped by someone known. Date rape has been characterized as a four-stage process, and while these stages do not always occur, they show how sexual assault can happen even to someone who exercises caution[28]:

1. *Intrusion.* The offender begins by violating the victim's space in one way or another. He (men can also be raped, but most rapes involve men assaulting women, so we'll use that scenario for our discussion) may start by interrupting while she is talking, talking about personal topics she feels uncomfortable with, or touching her unnecessarily or inappropriately.
2. *Desensitization.* The victim lets down her guard. While the intrusion makes her uncomfortable, she ignores the feelings and thinks, "That's just the way he is" or "He doesn't mean anything by it."
3. *Isolation.* The offender tries to get the victim alone, such as in a car or her home, where she might think she is safe, and uses tactics that put her at greater risk, such as encouraging her to drink alcohol.
4. *Offender denial.* The offender justifies his actions to himself and others by insisting that the victim gave consent and encouraged his behavior. This also increases the victim's feelings of confusion and guilt.

Here is how it might happen: Marcus and Kari were introduced by mutual friends. Marcus has invited Kari to go out to a movie with him. He seems to be a nice guy, so she accepts. They go to the movie and have a couple of beers afterward. Then Marcus takes Kari home. Parked by her home, Marcus engages Kari in a conversation that grows increasingly personal, and he begins making advances that make Kari uncomfortable (intrusion). Assuming that this is typical behavior for him (desensitization), she puts up with it for a while and gently tries to discourage him. She had intended to go to her apartment alone, but Marcus has a long drive home and he asks for a cup of coffee. This seems reasonable, so Kari accepts and Marcus accompanies her to her apartment (isolation). Her belief that she can control the situation and her desire to spare his feelings actually put her at risk. As soon as they are inside the door, Marcus pins her to the wall with a kiss and becomes increasingly aggressive. When she finally tells him to stop, he becomes verbally abusive, calling her a "tease" and a "bitch." Then he forces himself on her. Afterward, he asks her why she invited him to her apartment if she didn't want sex and he insists that it was consensual sex (offender denial).

Unfortunately, these scenes are all too common, and the victim is left feeling somehow responsible for the rape and wondering what she did to cause it or why she didn't head it off. Men can be raped, too—about 10 percent of reported rapes are of men.[29] Many go unreported because of homophobia (in men-on-men rape) and the myth that rape is a crime of desire rather than of violence.

If you are sexually assaulted, follow these steps:

➤ Once out of immediate danger, call the police.
➤ Do not change clothes, shower, urinate, defecate, gargle, take medication, drink alcohol, or do anything else that might destroy evidence.
➤ Go with a trusted friend to a hospital emergency room, where a doctor will ask for information about the assault, conduct a rape exam, and collect physical evidence to be used in court.

If a friend of yours is a victim of date rape, remember the following:

➤ Rape is not a result of uncontrolled passion. It is a violent assault using sex as a weapon.
➤ No one wants to be forced to have sex. No matter what happened, no one wants to be a victim of a crime. A person has handled the situation right if he or she is alive.
➤ You can't control what others think or say about it. Do not isolate yourself or the victim from friends who know about the rape. Neither you nor the victim have any reason to feel shame, embarrassment, or guilt. Your understanding and support are very important.

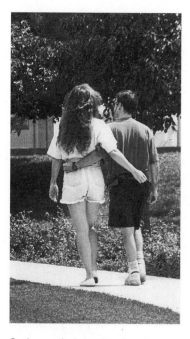

Serious relationships require serious decisions.

➤ If the assault is reported to the police, the victim is not responsible for what happens to the rapist, regardless of what pressure is brought by family or friends of the assailant. The courts are responsible for the outcome and the rapist is responsible for the rape.

To avoid coercive sexual pressure or sexual assault, you must break the chain of circumstances that lead to these outcomes. Here are some tips from the Santa Monica Rape Treatment Center:[30]

Women

➤ *Attend parties with friends you can trust.* Look out for each other. Leave together, rather than alone or with a new acquaintance. If you are attracted to someone you'd like to get to know better, agree to meet for lunch the next day.

➤ *Be selective.* Even if a person you just met seems very nice, find out about him or her from friends and family.

➤ *Avoid isolation.* Don't go to a secluded place or to a wild party with a new acquaintance. Go to concerts, movies, lectures, or restaurants; double date; and stay around people. When you get to know the person well, then you can relax the rules.

➤ *Communicate.* Don't lead someone on. Don't expect a person to know how you feel unless you speak up. Make your feelings, limits, and intentions clear. You have a right to say no to any unwanted sexual contact. If you are being pressured and feel uncertain, ask the person to respect your feelings.

➤ *Listen closely to what a person is saying.* If you think she or he is giving you a mixed message, ask for clarification. On a date when neither person stops to check out what the other person is feeling, the situation can get out of hand.

➤ *Make sure how you say something agrees with* what *you say.* Your body language, how you say something, may come across louder than your words. If you say no with downcast eyes and a smile to soften the refusal, you may end up giving the other person a mixed message. You are more likely to get your message across if you look a person directly in the eyes and say no assertively.

➤ *Be aware.* Pay attention to what is happening. Rely on your gut instinct. If a situation doesn't feel right, exit as quickly as you can and go to a safe place.

➤ *Speak up if you believe someone is at risk.* If you see a woman in trouble at a party or if a friend is using force and pressuring a woman, don't be afraid to intervene. You may save the woman from the trauma of sexual assault and your friend from criminal prosecution.

➤ *Stay sober.* You'll be more likely to make wise decisions if you are sober.

Men

➤ *Don't fall for the stereotype* that when a woman says no she means yes. If she says no to sexual contact, believe her and stop.

➤ *Don't make assumptions about a person's behavior.* Just because a woman drinks heavily, dresses provocatively, or goes with you to your room, don't assume she wants sex. Just because she had sex with you once, don't assume she is willing now. Also, don't assume that because she willingly engages in kissing or other intimate behavior that she wants sexual intercourse.

➤ *Don't assume that silence is consent.* Having sex with someone who is intoxicated, passed out, drugged, or otherwise incapable of giving consent is rape.

Both men and women must be especially careful in situations involving drinking or drugs. These decrease reasoning ability and your ability to make a decision and to communicate effectively. They increase willingness to take risks you wouldn't normally take. Alcohol, a social lubricant par excellence, sets you up for unwanted sexual behavior and STDs. It is involved in approximately half of the incidents of coercive sexual behavior.[31] It decreases the ability to recognize an unsafe situation and to react appropriately. It also decreases the likelihood that you will use a condom. Even if you have one, you may be too drunk to put it on.

SUMMARY

Sexually transmitted diseases have reached epidemic levels in the 1990s. Young adults are at greatest risk. Chlamydia, gonorrhea, syphilis, genital herpes, and human papilloma virus are the most common STDs. AIDS, a new and deadly STD, makes preventative measures more important than ever for those who are sexually active. To reduce risk of STDs, people must take responsibility for their sexual behavior and take protective measures, for themselves and their partners. It is also important to learn skills in communication, assertiveness, negotiation, and relating to others. Awareness of the risk of sexual assault and guidelines for recognizing and preventing it can make dating relationships safer for all.

REFERENCES

1. Centers for Disease Control and Prevention. "Trends in Sexual Risk Behaviors Among High School Students—United States, 1990, 1991, and 1993." *Morbidity and Mortality Weekly Report* 44 (February 24, 1995): 124–32.

2. Murstein, B. I., et al. "Sexual Behavior, Drugs, and Relationship Patterns on a College Campus over Thirteen Years." *Adolescence* 24 (Spring 1989): 125–39.

3. Centers for Disease Control and Prevention. "CDC Surveillance Summaries, Special Focus: Surveillance for Sexually Transmitted Diseases." *Morbidity and Mortality Weekly Reports* 42, no. SS-3 (August 13, 1993): 1–11.

4. Skolnik, Neil S., M.D. "Screening for Chlamydia Trachomatis Infection." *American Family Physician* 51, no. 4 (March 1995): 821–26.

5. Skolnik. "Screening for Chlamydia Trachomatis Infection."

6. Centers for Disease Control and Prevention. "Special Focus: Surveillance for Sexually Transmitted Diseases." *Morbidity and Mortality Weekly Report* 42 (August 13, 1993): 29–39.

7. Bowie, William R., M.D., et al. "STDs in '94: The New CDC Guidelines." *Patient Care* 28, no. 7 (April 15, 1994): 29–53.

8. Centers for Disease Control and Prevention. "CDC Survelliance Summaries, Special Focus: Surveillance for Sexually Transmitted Diseases."

9. Centers for Disease Control. "1993 STD Treatment Guidelines." *Morbidity and Mortality Weekly Report* 42 (1993): 1–102.

10. Clark, Jacquelyn L., M.D., et al. "Management of Genital Herpes." *American Family Physician* 51, no. 1 (January 1995): 175–85.

11. Mertz, G. J., et al. "Risk Factors for the Sexual Transmission of Genital Herpes." *Annals of Internal Medicine* 116 (February 1992): 197–202.

12. Collison, Michele. "Dramatic Increase in Genital Warts Disease Among Students Worries College Health Officers." *Chronicle of Higher Education* 35 (May 31, 1989): A23.

13. Ojanlatva, Ansa. "Human Papillomavirus Infections: The Next Epidemic?" *Health Education* 21, no. 5 (September/October 1990): 18–19.

14. Munoz, N., and F. X. Bosh. "Cervical Cancer—Second Most Common Cause of Cancer Death for Women." In Munoz, N., F. X. Bosh, and O. M. Jensen, eds. *Human Papilloma Virus and Cervical Cancer* (IARC Scientific Publication no. 94). Oxford, England: International Agency for Research on Cancer, 1989.

15. Centers for Disease Control. "The Second 100,000 Cases of Acquired Immunodeficiency Syndrome—United States, June 1981–December 1991." *Morbidity and Mortality Weekly Report 1992* 41, no. 2 (January 17, 1992): 28–29.

16. Centers for Disease Control. "The Second 100,000 Cases of Acquired Immunodeficiency Syndrome—United States, June 1981–December 1991."

17. Centers for Disease Control. "Update: Acquired Immunodeficiency Syndrome—United States, 1994." *Morbidity and Mortality Weekly Report* 44, no. 4 (February 3, 1995): 64–67.

18. Centers for Disease Control. "Update: Acquired Immunodeficiency Syndrome—United States, 1994."

19. Associate Editors of American Family Physician. "Characteristics Associated with Increased Risk of Tuberculosis." *American Family Physician* 51, no. 3 (February 15, 1995): 661.

20. Newton, Herbert B., M.D. "Common Neurologic Complications of HIV-1 Infection and AIDS." *American Family Physician* 51, no. 2 (February 1, 1995): 387–90.

21. Forster, Jeff. "AIDS Comes Home." *Patient Care* 28, no. 12 (July 15, 1994): 19.

22. Keeling, Richard P. Personal communication (September 15, 1992).

23. Ryan, Marilyn, and Lorraine Jones. "Survey of Sexual Attitudes and Practices on Campus." Muncie, Ind.: Ball State University, 1991.

24. Centers for Disease Control and Prevention. "Update: Acquired Immunodeficiency Syndrome—United States, 1994."

25. Gollub, E. L., and M. J. Rosenberg. "Commentary: Methods Women Can Use May Prevent STDs Including HIV." *American Journal of Public Health* (November 1992): 1473.

26. Keeling, Richard P. "Medical Issues." *AIDS in the College Community: From Crisis to Management*. Teleconference. Columbus: Ohio State University (November 16, 1989).

27. Ricker, R. Scott. "Reduction of Date Rape on a University Campus." *Public Health Reports* 107, no. 2 (March–April 1992): 226.

28. McEvoy, A. W., and Jeff B. Brookings. *If She Is Raped*. Holmes Beach, Fla.: Learning Publications, Inc., 1994.

29. Botash, Ann S., et al. "Acute Care for Sexual Assault Victims." *Patient Care* 28, no. 13 (August 15, 1994): 112–14.

30. Roden, M., and G. Abarbanel. *How It Happens*. Santa Monica, Calif.: Rape Treatment Center, Santa Monica Hospital Medical Center, 1987 (Santa Monica, CA).

31. Ricker, R. Scott. "Reduction of Date Rape on a University Campus." *Public Health Reports* 107, no. 2 (April 1992): 226–27.

SUGGESTED READINGS

Cox, Frank D. *The AIDS Booklet*, 3d ed. Dubuque, Iowa: William C. Brown Publishers, 1995.

ETR Associates. *101 Ways to Make Love Without Doin' It*. Santa Cruz, Calif.: ETR Associates, 1995.

ETR Associates. *Safer Sex: Talking with Your Partner*. Santa Cruz, Calif.: ETR Associates, 1995.

ETR Associates. *STD Facts*. Santa Cruz, Calif.: ETR Associates, 1995.

Hiatt, Jane. *Abstinence & HIV*. Santa Cruz, Calif.: ETR Associates, 1995.

Holmes, King K. *Sexually Transmitted Diseases*. Winchester, Mass.: Faber & Faber, 1991.

Jackson, James K. *AIDS, STD, & Other Communicable Diseases*. Guilford, Conn.: Dushkin Publishing Group, 1992.

McCormack, William M. "Pelvic Inflammatory Disease." *The New England Journal of Medicine* 330, no. 2 (January 13, 1994): 115–20.

McIlhaney, Joe S., Jr. *Sexuality and Sexually Transmitted Diseases: A Doctor Confronts the Myth of "Safe" Sex*. Grand Rapids, Mich.: Baker Books, 1990.

Servilio, John. "Just the Facts." *Positively Aware* (July/August 1995): 16–24.

RESOURCES

AIDS Task Force for the American College Health Association, c/o Dr. Richard P. Keeling, Dept. of Student Health, Box 378, University of Virginia, Charlottesville, VA 22908, (804) 924-2670.

CDC AIDS Hotline (U.S. Public Health Service), English, 24 hours daily, (800) 342-AIDS; Spanish, 8 A.M. to 2 A.M. daily, (800) 344-SIDA; deaf and hearing impaired, Mon.–Fri., 10 A.M. to 10 P.M., (800) AIDS-TTY.

CDC National AIDS Information Clearinghouse, (800) 458-5231.

CDC National STD Hotline, (800) 227-8922.

ETR Associates, pamphlets on STDS, (800) 321-4407.

National Gay Task Force AIDS Crisis Line, (800) 227-8922.

National Herpes Hotline, (919) 361-8488.

National Herpes Resource Center, Mon.–Fri., 9 A.M. to 7 P.M., (800) 230-6309.

Teens Teaching AIDS Prevention, (800) 234-TEEN.

INTERNET ADDRESSES

News about AIDS, research, treatments, and issues. Usenet: Newsgroup: clari.tw.health.aids.

Sexual health topics, including STDs, AIDS, contraception. Gopher: Name: Healthline Gopher Server. Address: selway.umt.edu 700. Choose: sexuality. Telnet: Address: selway.umt.edu. Login: health.

Morbidity and Mortality Weekly Report: data on health concerns, including AIDS. Gopher: Name: National Institute of Health. Address: odie.niaid.nih.gov. Choose: AIDS Related Information.

National Institute of Health (NIH): information about health and clinical issues, including CancerNet and AIDS information. Gopher: Name: National Institute of Health. Address: gopher: //gopher.nih.gov.

AIDSLINE: scientific literature from the US National Library of Medicine concerning AIDS, 1980 to the present, updated monthly. Telnet: Address: telnet://dialog.com. Login: AIDS, Medicine.

chapter 14

Planning Wellness for a Lifetime

➤ Objectives

After reading this chapter, you will be able to:

1. Define *quackery* and list six of its nine common characteristics.

2. Discriminate between a credible health product/discovery and a bogus or flimsy finding/promotion.

3. List the four premises on which corporate wellness programs are based.

4. Give 10 examples of wellness programs that corporations might offer their employees.

5. Describe three ways parents can foster wellness habits in their children.

6. Give two examples of behaviors within each dimension of wellness that parents can develop in a young child.

7. List five guidelines for wearing a seat belt properly.

8. List two responsible precautions that you can take to minimize your risk of injury/trouble in each of the following situations:
    a. Airplane travel
    b. Apartment or home fire
    c. In the home
    d. In a hotel

9. List seven responsible precautions you can take to minimize your risk of being attacked, assaulted, or robbed.

10. List three trends and describe how they will affect wellness in the future.

11. List and describe two future challenges we face in regard to wellness.

12. List six environmental concerns that may affect our wellness.

Terms

- Altruism
- Psychoneuroimmunology (PNI)
- Quackery

"The best thing about the future is that it comes only one day at a time."

Abraham Lincoln

t he purpose of this book is to present wellness as a lifestyle where positive choices result in optimal functioning and enhanced living. You have gained knowledge that will help you make informed decisions and you have learned skills for making behavioral change. You are now "wellness educated." With knowledge comes responsibility, so you no longer have the luxury of saying, "I didn't know!" You know what choices contribute to wellness and which ones do not. You can choose to eat right, exercise, and manage stress or you can choose not to. You know the possible consequences of such choices. The challenge of wellness is ongoing, whereas college coursework eventually comes to an end. A new career, different living environments, and family responsibilities will bring many changes to your life. During these changes, the wellness lifestyle can prevail. We hope it will grow for you. Wellness is a process, not a solution. It is a journey, not a destination. A major part of wellness is adapting to change and maximizing your potential amidst change.

Remember that wellness involves a balance among and integration of all seven dimensions of wellness. Too often, *physical fitness* is thought of synonymously with *wellness*. Admittedly, being physically fit has a positive effect on the other dimensions. However, your job satisfaction, family relationships, social ties, emotional health, and spiritual health are equally linked to wellness. This final chapter focuses on some important issues for you to consider as you plan for the future.

Taking Charge

Following a great musician's performance, an admirer said to him, "I'd give my life to play like that." The brilliant performer replied, "I did." We often view a performance of an athlete or artist with envy. Accomplishment is often deceptive, because we don't see the perseverance that produces it. Pursuing wellness also involves a certain amount of perseverance and discipline. Many desire the benefits of wellness living but fail to commit to its precepts. As you take charge of your lifestyle, focus on the positive outcomes of changing a health-robbing behavior, rather than the effort involved. Remember, you do not pay the price for having wellness; you pay the price for *not* having it.

Knowledge and good intentions are a good start. Then focus on self-management techniques and behavior-changing skills (Chapter 1) that put your knowledge into practice through maintainable habits. Be aware of the power of cultural norms, the media, advertising, and sources of social support.

Partners in Prevention

The *Healthy People 2000* document sets high goals for the health and well-being of the American people. It emphasizes personal responsibility and self-empowerment as the means for increasing the quality and quantity of life. Some people need to know the facts in order to make informed decisions. Others need positive influences to motivate them toward appropriate choices. "Still others must have assistance in escaping the bonds of victimization and need support as they move toward self-empowerment. . . . *Healthy People 2000* will become a reality by the year 2000 only through a change of culture in America."[1]

For the wellness lifestyle to permeate our culture, support systems within communities must be available. While emphasizing personal responsibility, we cannot overlook the importance of the collective burden of responsibility of governmental policies, wellness curriculum in the schools, corporate action, and the American family. Even though personal behaviors contribute to the leading causes of death, behaviors occur in and are influenced by the environment. Advertisements, television programs, and popular songs that glamorize drinking, violence, sex, and immoral behavior undermine our nation's health and well-being. For example, cigarette ads show likable young people in upscale settings enjoying smoking. The subliminal message is that cigarettes must not be so bad if such bright, attractive people are not afraid to smoke. Of course, in these

table 14.1

HOW TO RECOGNIZE QUACKERY

Some products use scientific jargon and carry professional-looking logos and endorsements (many of which are bogus). Watch for the following characteristics common in quackery:

1. It sounds too good to be true.
2. It is quick and painless.
3. It has a "secret," "special," "foreign," "magical," "exclusive," or "ancient" formula.
4. It is available only through the mail (most often through a P.O. box number) or telephone and only from one supplier.
5. It is a scientific "breakthrough" or "miracle cure" that has been overlooked by the medical community.
6. It uses testimonials or case histories from "satisfied customers" as the only proof of its effectiveness.
7. It is a single product effective for a wide variety of ailments.
8. It uses pseudoscientific languages: "detoxifies," "revitalizes immunities," "offers enzymatic protection" etc.
9. It displays degrees, credentials, or titles that are from unaccredited or unknown schools.

ads there never are a dirty ashtray, nicotine-stained teeth, or anyone coughing or getting chemotherapy. There is no dangerously underweight baby lying in intensive care. There is no one dying. An important part of wellness education is deciphering these messages and knowing what really does promote well-being.

Individuals, families, communities, corporations, and the government together share the task of enhancing the well-being of all Americans. Since you are wellness educated, part of this challenge of culture change rests with you. Can you think of ways you can affect this change?

Understanding Quackery

The concept of wellness has widespread appeal. Most everyone is attracted to the thought of enhancing the quality of their lives. The expanse of the wellness concept invites a considerable amount of quackery and shortcut schemes. **Quackery** is the promotion of a misleading and fraudulent health claim that is unproven. Most quackery products are foods, drugs, gadgets, or cosmetics that promote physical change—baldness cures, bust enhancers, wrinkle removers, miracle cancer treatments, instant weight loss schemes, bogus AIDS cures, youth elixirs, arthritis cures. These products and schemes are usually developed for the purpose of financial gain. Health fraud is big business in the United States. It is estimated that Americans spend $27 billion per year on quack products or treatments.[2]

Many people erroneously believe that product advertisements are screened by government agencies and that claims on television or in print must be true. This is not so. It is hard to resist the "promise" of effortless, quick shortcuts to health and wellness. Many promoters are wealthy as a result of our willingness to spend money for miracle solutions. Unfortunately, the results are often shattered hopes and wasted money and sometimes endangered health. Misconceptions and half-truths fuel these promotional fires. As an educated wellness consumer, you should be able to evaluate products and plans with intelligence and realism. See Table 14.1 for common characteristics of quackery.

Remember, if it sounds too good to be true, it probably is. Sometimes, television personalities or well-known celebrities write books, represent products in advertisements, or are portrayed as experts in the field of health and fitness. Be wary of the credibility of this type of product/information marketing.

Many hospitals, schools, corporations, community wellness centers, and health organizations offer legitimate programs that can assist you in pursuing a wellness lifestyle. Investigate references and sources before falling for any fly-by-night scheme.

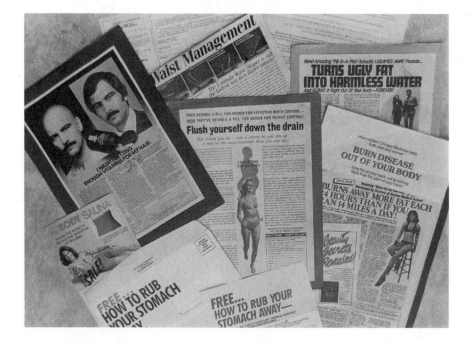

Your physician, the Better Business Bureau, local consumer office, or nearest office of the Food and Drug Administration (FDA) can offer professional advice if you suspect a product makes untrue claims.

Also part of well-informed wellness is distinguishing good quality health research from flimsy or biased data. It seems that every day we hear contradictory information on health, fitness, or nutrition. Is coffee good or bad for you? Is the mega-trim diet safe or not safe? Will an aspirin a day prevent a heart attack? There are no easy answers to these and other questions. However, the more you know about the economics, politics, and methodology of research, the better able you are to form a sound opinion. Ask yourself the following questions as you weigh the evidence:

➤ Where is the work published? In a supermarket tabloid? In a homemaker's magazine? In a scientific journal that uses a board of experts to review the article?
➤ Who paid for the research? (Some companies and foundations might profit from certain outcomes.)
➤ Do my personal biases lead me to want to believe this information?
➤ Are advertisers using this information to sell a product?
➤ Is this only a preliminary finding that has not been fully tested?
➤ Are the researchers from respectable institutions?
➤ Was good scientific methodology used? What was the number of subjects involved in the study? Was there a control group?

Realize that newspaper headlines often report the results of a recent, single study, overgeneralizing its findings. Remember, it takes more than headlines to draw a sound conclusion. Only after weighing *all* of the scientific evidence can sound public health policy be recommended. Unfortunately, you cannot believe everything you read and hear.

Campus Wellness

Many colleges and universities have voiced a commitment to wellness and, as a result, offer a variety of wellness programs to students. Many programs are also available to faculty and staff. Realizing that the collegiate experience involves more than intellectual growth, universities are providing services and activities to promote self-discovery, psychological well-being, career planning, spiritual discovery, health-risk assessment, and lifetime fitness. It is not uncommon for colleges to offer programs for stress management, alcohol education, weight management, smoking cessation, eating disorders, and even investment counseling. Some universities have wellness residence halls, nutrition-controlled food services, academic wellness courses, and even fitness standards for all students. Day-care services, family counseling, and flexible class scheduling are now common on campuses since many students have child-care responsibilities and other jobs. Attending college is a part-time pursuance for many full-time parents and workers. The college campus is no longer viewed as an isolated haven for learning, void of the challenges and realities of life. In response to the diverse needs of students, faculty, and staff, the college environment can enhance your pursuit of wellness with wellness services, information, and programs. Investigate your campus for wellness resources. The variety of expertise and resources found at most universities can prepare you not only for a lifetime career but also for lifetime wellness. Attending a wellness-oriented university is an example of how choosing a supportive environment can enhance your quest for wellness.

Career Wellness

Your job will be a prominent facet of your adult life. You will spend at least 50 percent of your waking hours at work, if you maintain a full-time job or career. Portable telephones, computers, and fax machines have altered the complexion of American work. Twenty-four hour manufacturing and retail shopping, home-based businesses, voice mail, and telemarketing have revolutionized the business place. In fact, in her book *The Overworked American*, Juliet Schor states that working hours are longer than they were 40 years ago: "If present trends continue, by the end of the century Americans will be spending as much time at their jobs as they did back in the 1920s."[3] These realities make the workplace a likely place to receive information and support regarding personal health improvement and wellness living. Leaders in business and industry are beginning to see employee wellness as an asset to be maintained and enhanced. When employees are happy and healthy, productivity increases. The promotion of wellness programs in business and industry is based on four related premises:

1. Prevention is preferable to curing.
2. Teaching people to stay healthy is generally less expensive than treating them when they are ill.
3. Healthful lifestyles offer a better quality of life, higher morale, increased productivity, and possibly increased longevity.
4. Health promotion programs promote a favorable corporate image and help attract healthy, capable employees who see these programs as a valuable employee benefit.

Rising medical insurance costs, employee absenteeism, and sick leaves cut deeply into profits and lead to increases in the costs of doing business. As a result, corporate officials are experimenting with ways of incorporating wellness into the workplace. This exciting avenue for health promotion can bring about changes in behavior for an improved lifestyle as well as enhance personal relationships. Wellness in the workplace can be promoted in a variety of ways. Programs can involve diagnosis (assess current health and habits), education (give information about health enhancement), and/or behavior modification (give help and support in making a specific behavior change). These programs include, among others, smoking cessation, health risk appraisals, back care, stress management, fitness classes, nutrition education, weight management, and cholesterol screening.

Employers realize that the work and nonwork parts of our lives are interactive. That is, job satisfaction is also dependent on family happiness, leisure pursuits, and feelings of worth. Knowing this, employers are actively pursuing a multidimensional approach to supporting employee wellness. Examples are flexible work hours, child care, on-the-job retraining, sports team participation, job sharing, smoke-free work sites, parental leaves, family hikes and picnics, and even children's fitness classes. Several forward-thinking companies are even responding to the needs of employees with elderly parents by providing elder care, as well as providing substance abuse and marital counseling. Since spouses and children of employees account for 40 percent to 60 percent of a company's health-care expenditures, such multidimensional programs can be cost-effective.[4]

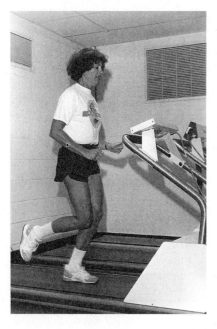

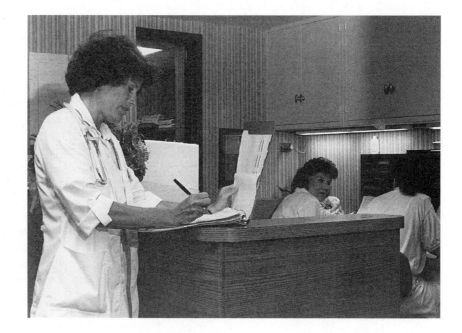

Many companies support employee wellness.

Due to the growing interest in and emphasis on wellness in business and industry, many employers prefer hiring personnel who have already adopted a wellness lifestyle—not smoking, being physically fit, maintaining a reasonable weight. This knowledge is added incentive for you to continue a wellness lifestyle. As a potential employee, your confirmed dedication to wellness may also influence your final selection of a job and your chances of getting hired. You may favor a company that is highly supportive of wellness and provides wellness programs for employees and that company may favor you. Remember how important a supportive environment is in the maintenance of positive lifestyle choices.

Many college students, pressured by school demands, feel they will have more time to exercise and eat right once they graduate. Your life will most likely be just as busy, if not more so, once you begin your career. Time restraints and demands will always be with you. Making wellness living an important part of your current lifestyle will help you to maintain it after graduation, as a habit.

Family Wellness

In all cultures, the family unit is the primary transmitter of values and attitudes in the society. Each partner in a relationship comes with values, norms, and expectations derived from his or her own family. Couples continue to grow, interact, and develop a value framework. If and when children come along, the parental role of maintaining the culture from generation to generation is created. The interacting dynamics of a family unit promote the spiritual, physical, psychological, and social growth of each member.

The family units in today's society are not all identical. Single parents, divorce, combined families, and joint custodies are realities that have changed the American family structure. Dual careers have altered the role of women within the family. Such changes affect the balance between work life and family life, often creating role conflicts, stress, and changing values.[5] Regardless of the makeup of the family unit, nurturance remains essential for all members to strive toward full potential.

The Well Relationship

Many romantic fairy tales conclude with "and they lived happily ever after." Whereas these words *end* these fantasies, marriage is most often the *beginning* of the story of a relationship in real life. Who you marry or choose to spend your life with is one of your most important life decisions. Much of your happiness and life satisfaction will be based on the success of this relationship. Like the wellness lifestyle, a relationship demands

It is important to find time to play together as a family.

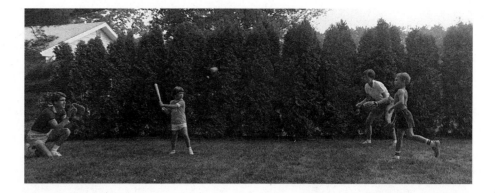

conscious effort, commitment, and even personal sacrifice. It is a partnership that involves change and growth. Many factors influence the success of a marriage relationship. Consider the following key elements that help build a strong and lasting relationship:

1. *Communication:* Partners must be able to share their true feelings.
2. *Compromise:* Each partner must be willing to give a little. Sometimes it's 50:50, sometimes 100:0.
3. *Common values:* Common values and shared goals help maintain focus during tension-filled times.
4. *Likability and respect:* Enjoying each other's company and respecting each other's needs is essential.
5. *Shared responsibilities:* In a world where the two-parent career is the norm, each partner must be willing to share in the responsibilities of home and child care.
6. *Space:* Each partner needs to have his or her own identity and be allowed to grow individually.
7. *Sense of humor:* Laughing and having fun are ways to keep daily problems in proper perspective.

Just as in wellness growth, partner growth is a process. It doesn't happen all at once. Enjoy each step along the path.

The Well Child

It will be your challenge as a parent to initiate wellness living within your child. All dimensions (emotional, social, physical, intellectual, spiritual, environmental, and occupational) demand your attention. If you favor behaviors that promote wellness, your children will follow your example. Family wellness patterns can set the stage for a lifelong pattern of self-responsibility. Since self-responsibility relies on learning and practicing skills, you can be the master teacher of wellness and help your child grow as a decision maker. Children do not learn just in school. They learn by watching you, too. If you exercise, eat nutritiously, read instead of watch television, handle stress, communicate your feelings, and display attitudes of cooperation and respect, your child will, too. In fact, studies show that the strongest predictors of lifetime exercise activity in children are enjoyment of physical activity, family support of physical activity, and direct parental modeling of physical activity.[6]

Recent statistics[7] reveal that more than a third of youths ages 10 to 18 do not engage in enough physical activity to derive any aerobic or endurance benefit. Forty percent of children ages five to eight have at least one major heart disease risk factor. Twenty-one percent of teenagers are overweight (up from 15 percent in the 1970s). Since children with unhealthy habits grow up to be unhealthy adults, part of every parent's responsibility should be to create an environment for children that is conducive to optimum health and wellness. This includes being a positive role model. Aristotle expressed it best when he wrote, "good habits formed at youth make all the difference."

Since the self-concept of most children is formed by the time they start kindergarten, you as parents will be prime molders of this self-concept. A positive self-esteem

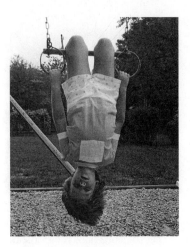

Exercise habits start young.

is an important foundation as the child moves into larger social spheres beyond the family. The child with a high degree of self-worth is able to confront life's situations with confidence. According to psychologists, "A most fundamental ingredient of enduring happiness is confidence in our own ability. . . . Self-confidence gives rise to optimism and hope."[8] Optimism and self-confidence are the building blocks for wellness living.

Although it is popularly believed that risk-taking behavior among teenagers and preteens is most strongly influenced by peer pressure, new research by adolescent medicine specialists concludes that family closeness plays a key role. Young people who have a balance of strong attachment to family and parental encouragement to be independent are least likely to take part in high-risk activities (alcohol and drug use, sexual activities, cigarette experimentation) that could seriously affect their well-being.[9]

Even though the broad concept of wellness is difficult for young children to understand, they can become aware and learn the value of specific wellness choices. Their capacity to understand the cause and effect of certain choices depends on their age and maturity level. Can children learn to habitually fasten their seat belts? Select fruits for snacks? Show respect for others? Appreciate nature? Enjoy vigorous exercise? Of course, they can. Look at Table 14.2 for examples of wellness behaviors that parents are instrumental in developing in their children.

Personal Safety Issues

Throughout this book we have tried to increase your awareness of risks and personal choices that affect your wellness. Injuries and illnesses stemming from accidents and environmental hazards sometimes seem to be beyond the average person's control. Especially accidents—which are the fourth overall cause of death in the United States (and the number one cause of death among teens and young adults)—often appear to be a matter of chance.[10] In fact, you can substantially reduce the risks you are exposed to while driving, traveling, getting around campus, and working around your apartment or house by heeding basic safety precautions. Some of these precautions seem like common sense to most. Yet, for whatever reason, many people fail to follow even common sense precautions. Federal, state, and local regulations have been established to help protect us from a variety of traffic, fire, water, and air travel tragedies. But laws and regulations cannot *make* people act. When you strive for high-level wellness, you must take seriously *all* lifestyle choices. Since the wellness concept is centered on an ongoing personal commitment to positive choices, safety awareness and responsibility cannot be excluded.

We tend to focus solely on the impact an accident has on our physical dimension of wellness. The truth is, such a trauma can equally affect our emotional, social, occupational, and even spiritual dimensions. Consider that one American in six sustains an accident-related injury that results in measurable economic loss.[11] Of these injuries the following is true:

➤ One-fourth occur on the job or during commutes.
➤ One-fourth involve people who work at home.
➤ Thirty percent occur during leisure time.
➤ About 20 percent involve motor vehicles.

The following personal safety issues will focus on choices that can help you control risks in your immediate environment.

Automobile Seat Belts

Motor vehicle crashes are the leading cause of death among people age 40 and younger. In talking about motor vehicle collisions, we deliberately chose not to use the word *accident*, which would imply a luck/fate approach to the topic. Instead, we use *crash* because it is well understood what specific actions you can take to reduce risks. Drunk-driving laws, child car-restraint regulations, seat belt laws, availability of air bags, and designated driver programs have done much to curtail traffic fatalities. Still, approximately 48,000 Americans die annually in car crashes, costing the nation $40 billion per year.[12] Of these casualties, half of the people could have been saved if they had used their seat belts *and* fully half of the serious injuries incurred in collisions could have been

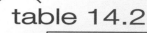

table 14.2

WELLNESS BEHAVIORS THAT CAN BE DEVELOPED BY THE YOUNG CHILD

PHYSICAL DIMENSION

- Forms habits of regular, vigorous exercise
- Establishes healthy eating habits and preferences
- Forms self-care habits (personal hygiene, dental care, etc.)
- Forms safety habits (seat belts, fire, bike riding, etc.)
- Establishes attitudes about smoking, drug use, alcohol

SOCIAL DIMENSION

- Seeks companionship with others
- Senses responsibility for behavior
- Shows concern and respect for others
- Displays willingness to share work responsibilities with others

EMOTIONAL DIMENSION

- Forms feelings of self-worth and self-confidence
- Talks freely about feelings
- Develops appropriate coping behaviors for a variety of situations
- Displays the capacity to give and receive love

SPIRITUAL DIMENSION

- Develops an awareness of life versus death
- Develops a sense of the importance and expanse of life
- Begins establishing a value system; can distinguish right from wrong
- Begins showing compassion and forgiveness

INTELLECTUAL DIMENSION

- Develops creativity and curiosity
- Establishes listening skills
- Learns cause-and-effect concepts
- Recognizes the expanse of the world through a variety of experiences

OCCUPATIONAL DIMENSION

- Identifies a variety of jobs/careers
- Understands the importance of work and effort
- Begins developing work habits
- Begins understanding the importance of money

ENVIRONMENTAL DIMENSION

- Develops habits of recycling bottles, papers, cans, etc.
- Displays habits of energy conservation (water, electricity, etc.)
- Develops an appreciation for nature (plants, wildlife, etc.)
- Learns to maintain a clean environment by not littering

prevented by the use of seat belts.[13] Although drivers initially resisted seat belt use, compliance is growing. The National Transportation Department in Washington, D.C., reports that 67 percent of Americans buckle up (the highest rate ever), and that this growing habit has saved 55,600 lives over the past decade.[14] The importance of using seat belts cannot really be overstated. Even if you practice all the other advice in this book (exercise regularly, eat a nutritious diet, don't smoke, etc.), *one* accident without a seat belt could immediately and irrevocably end your wellness program. It does not make sense, if we care about health and wellness, to not buckle up. Table 14.3 lists the most common excuses people give for choosing not to use their seat belts. We hope you do not use the same flimsy excuses.

To prevent injury, seat belts must not only be worn but must be worn properly every time. You are most likely to survive an automobile crash without injury if you follow these recommendations:

1. *Wear the seat belt low across the pelvis*, not the abdomen. In a crash, a force of 20 to 50 times your body weight is exerted against the belt. The bony pelvis can withstand this load, whereas internal organs would be injured if the belt were higher, across the abdomen.

2. *Keep the belt snug.* A loose belt offers little protection and may compound injuries if you are thrown against it. You can also slide forward under a loose belt and suffer head or neck injuries from the shoulder strap.

3. *Never wear the shoulder strap under your arm or behind your back.* When properly worn, this strap rests on the middle of the collarbone and the upper chest.

4. *Never share a belt.* In a crash, a parent sharing a belt with a child can crush the child. Each passenger must have his or her own belt. Also, know that it is impossible to hold a child in your arms in the event of a collision. In a crash, a 20-pound baby is propelled forward with the force of 400 pounds.[15]

5. *If you are pregnant, wear the seat belt under the abdomen*—across the upper thighs and as low on the hips as possible. The shoulder strap should go across your shoulder and chest. The fetus is at *much greater* risk when the mother does not wear a seat belt. The leading cause of fetal death in a crash is death of the mother.[16]

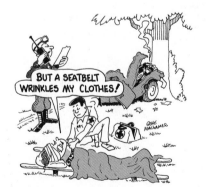

What is your excuse for not wearing a seat belt?

Most new automobile models include two front seat inflatable airbags as standard equipment. These bags will be valuable in preventing thousands of deaths and injuries. But remember, airbags protect only in head-on collisions, not side-impact crashes. Your seat belt is still your first line of defense in all crashes.

Driving Safety

Driving is, on average, approximately 10 times more dangerous than traveling by airplane or train.[17] However, if you are a low-risk driver, you are far less likely to die in a car crash than a high-risk driver is. Statistics define a low-risk driver to be a 40 year old who is sober when driving and who wears a seat belt; a high-risk driver is an 18-year-old, intoxicated male traveling in a lightweight car without wearing a seat belt.[18] The best driver is also a defensive driver—one who can anticipate potential danger and respond appropriately. Attitude is a key ingredient in defensive driving. Speeding, following too closely, and improper lane changing are the most common traffic infractions leading to crashes.[19] Driver inattention is also a major contributor to crashes.

A driving risk causing new concern is *driving while drowsy (DWD)*. DWD has been an underrated risk factor in crashes. DWD accounts for as many as 10,000 traffic fatalities annually in the United States; recent surveys show that 25 percent of drivers have fallen asleep at the wheel, causing one in 10 of them to crash.[20] For a variety of reasons, more Americans (even teenagers) are juggling jobs (sometimes more than one), school, and family responsibilities. Loss of sleep and driving at odd hours have become commonplace. Combining this with the comforts in modern day vehicles (cruise control, automatic climate control, contoured reclining seats), it is easy to lose sight of the fact that driving a powerful automobile carries tremendous responsibility and demands constant attention.

Airplane Safety

Unfortunately, many people take a fatalistic attitude toward airplane crashes. Despite sensational headlines, deaths due to airplane crashes are quite low when compared to those occurring with other modes of transportation. According to statistics collected by the National Transportation Safety Board, passengers who think systematically in advance about their own safety are more likely to survive an airplane accident.[21] Many airplane travelers settle into their seats, bury their heads in a newspaper, and ignore the safety instructions given by the flight attendants. Taking the first few minutes on a plane to review all safety instructions, observe safety features on the plane, and make an escape plan is a responsible wellness behavior. The following steps will help prepare you for an emergency:

➤ Locate the nearest exit and count the number of rows to the exit, so you can find it if the lights are out.
➤ Keep your seat belt fastened throughout the flight.
➤ Study the seat-pocket safety card.
➤ If possible, wear comfortable clothes and shoes.

Contrary to popular belief, where you sit in the plane has not been found to be a significant survival factor; however, sitting in an aisle seat may quicken an escape.

Personal Safety Awareness

Falls, drownings, fires, tornadoes, floods, rape, lightning, thefts, chokings, bicycle accidents, assaults, vandalism—these predicaments don't just happen to *other* people. You may find yourself facing any of these situations at some time. Though chance is one factor, you do have some control over your own fate. You have the capacity to handle a variety of emergencies, possibly minimizing any ill effects. Advanced planning and preparation is the key. Look carefully at Table 14.4 and think seriously about each item as it relates to you. Do you adhere to these common-sense safety precautions?

Crime Prevention

As much as we hate to admit it, crime and violence are a very real part of contemporary U.S. life. Whether you are at school, traveling, at work, or going about daily living

table 14.4

NINE WELLNESS TIPS TO AVOID TROUBLE

1. *Fall-proof your home/apartment.* Falls are the second leading cause of accidental death in the United States.* Stairs, loose carpeting, icy sidewalks, improper lighting, and wet tile help contribute to these statistics. Take charge of your environment to make it safe.

2. *Install smoke detectors throughout your home/apartment.* Test them periodically and replace batteries at least once a year. Plan and rehearse evacuation procedures in preparation for a fire. The heat and toxic gas buildup from a fire can be even more threatening than the flames themselves. In most cases, you only have a few minutes after the smoke detector goes off to safely escape a building.

3. *When checking into a hotel, locate the nearest fire exits to your room.* Count and memorize the number of doorways between your room and these fire exits.

4. *Always wear a helmet when riding a motorcycle or bicycle.*

5. *Learn to swim.* Never swim alone or dive into shallow water (or water of unknown depth).

6. *Always wear a life preserver when boating.*

7. *Find shelter immediately during a lightning storm.* Once inside, stay away from telephones, metal objects, and open doors and windows.

8. *Never use electrical appliances near a sink or tub filled with water.*

9. *When walking, jogging, or cycling at night, always wear light clothing or reflective apparel.*

*"Fall-Proof Your Home." *Safety & Health* 144 (October 1991): 46–48.

routines, you can become a victim. Even in the idyllic setting of a college campus, assaults, sexual attacks, and thefts occur. You can help protect yourself from being a victim with some basic precautions. There is nothing extraordinary about the following personal safety tips. They are simple examples of assuming self-responsibility for your own wellness.

1. *Always lock your house, apartment, residence hall room, and car—even when you are there.*

2. *At night, park in well-lit spots and walk in brightly lit areas.*

3. *Never walk alone at night or in unpopulated areas.* Nearly one in five rapes occur on unfamiliar, darkened, isolated streets. Use a campus escort service if available.

4. *Beware of suspicious persons in buildings, hallways, parking areas, elevators, stairwells, and restrooms.* Note their description and contact the police or security.

5. *Don't let strangers know when you are home alone.*

6. *Glance into your car, checking the seats and floor, before getting in.*

7. *Never hitchhike or pick up hitchhikers.*

8. *If you are being harassed, turn and proceed toward lights and people.*

9. *Watch your alcohol consumption.* Drinking puts you at risk and makes you vulnerable to assault, robbery, and rape.

10. *Secure all valuables and don't flaunt expensive possessions.*

11. *When you are walking alone, walk with your shoulders back and your head held high.* Keep a strong and steady pace. Remain alert and be aware of your surroundings. Muggers and rapists rarely attack those who appear assured and confident. Also, walk facing traffic, even if you're on the sidewalk. This prevents an assailant in a car from sneaking up on you from the rear.

12. *Have a defensive plan in mind should you encounter trouble.*

Not all accidents and injuries are preventable. Some just happen. However, many accidents and personal traumas *are* preventable with some basic precautions. Too often after an accident or tragic event someone says, "I wish I would have . . ." Being careful may seem boring to some, but it *is* the wellness way.

Wellness Trends and Challenges for the Future

Some regard wellness as a passing fad, but we disagree. In his highly acclaimed book, *Megatrends,* John Naisbitt predicted, "The focus of health care is shifting from the short-term treatment of illness to the long-term attainment of wellness. Regarded by some as fad, wellness is a trend that is here to stay."[22] We have already seen the wellness trend give impetus to societal changes. Designated smoking areas, seat belt laws, shopping mall wellness screenings, community walking clubs, and low-fat food choices in groceries and restaurants are all examples of positive wellness changes. What else is down the road for wellness? What other changes and trends will you see in your lifetime? Also, what are the challenges that will continue to demand attention? The remainder of this chapter addresses these questions.

Trend 1: Changing Focus of Health Care

One of the biggest trends is the changing focus in hospitals and the health-care profession. Medical care is shifting from the sickness business to the wellness business. Many community hospitals now offer a variety of wellness programs with the intention of preventing individuals from becoming ill and needing hospitalization. Cholesterol testing, nutrition workshops, family counseling, drug rehabilitation, weight-management classes, and exercise prescription are examples of such programs.

Some health facility administrators have found that a simple name change attracts clients to some of their programs. For example, a *mental health center* renamed a *stress center* has an easier time drawing individuals searching for help in dealing with personal problems. The counseling services of such a center may not be altered at all. But the connotation of learning ways to handle personal stress rather than trying to maintain mental health (often erroneously linked to mental illness) better attracts individuals needing such services.

Another change in medical care deals with the medical education of physicians. Medical schools are expanding their physician training to include studying lifestyle and preventive influences on health and disease, rather than solely learning to identify and cure illness. There is compelling evidence showing that physicians exert a strong influence on their patients' behavior patterns. By incorporating preventive services and counseling into their patient encounters, physicians can dramatically affect the well-being of the nation.[23] In this way, the physician can become a prime force in advocating a wellness lifestyle.

The high cost of medical care and the rising cost of health insurance have initiated another related trend. Insurance companies are beginning to provide incentives for staying well. Insurance benefits are being expanded and costs are being lowered for those who actively strive for optimal well-being by refraining from smoking, participating in periodic health screenings, maintaining a healthy weight, and exercising regularly. Group health benefits at reduced rate will be sought by companies that promote wellness in their workplaces and have predominantly healthy employees.

The underlying theme here is that *preventing* ill health is more efficient and effective than *treating* illness. Prevention saves money, lives, and suffering, and, most important, it enhances human vitality and potential.

Trend 2: Aging America

All demographic studies document that the population of the United States is getting older. In January 1996, the first baby boomer turned 50. Baby boomers (those born after World War II between 1946 and 1964) make up the largest segment of our population—approximately 76 million Americans. It has been more than a decade since the number of Americans over the age of 65 surpassed the number of teenagers. By the year 2000, the "oldest old"—those over age 85—will have increased by about 30 percent to a total of 4.6 million.[24]

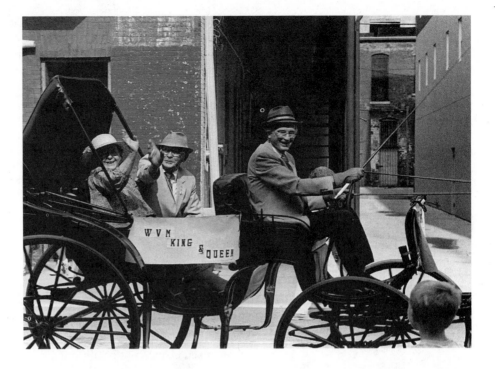

Describing the 50-plus age group is not an easy task. *American Demographics* magazine describes this diverse group as "rich and poor, college-educated and illiterate. Some are vibrant and young; others are sick and elderly. If you think that they are one unified consumer group with similar needs and attitudes, you need a checkup. There are many ways to segment people in this country, and the diversity of segments is growing at a rapid pace."[25] Most of this population is not, as many would think, senile or confined to nursing homes. Many older Americans are healthy, self-sufficient, and physically capable. Many have money to spend and desire to continue as active contributors to society. Some have retired, remarried, and begun second careers. They want and need programs for nutrition education, exercise, personal enrichment, and financial management. This elderly group is one of the top markets perceived by health promotion analysts to be important during the next 10 years.[26] As wellness becomes a way of life, you, too, will want programs as you reach older adulthood, whether they be special exercise classes, social activities, or special living environments.

Trend 3: The Mind-Body Connection

In recent years, there has been an explosion of research in **psychoneuroimmunology (PNI),** the study of how emotions, behavior, and mental attitudes affect the immune system and the onset and course of illness. At one time, physiologists thought the immune system functioned independently from the central nervous and endocrine systems. Now it is clear that emotional states affect us right down to our cells. Researchers have now shown that nerve cells connect directly to organs of the immune system, that hormones responsive to stressful experiences affect the immune response, and that psychological and social factors can affect the immune system's responsiveness.[27] Additional research into the chemicals produced by the brain has shown that the immune system and brain communicate chemically. Mental states such as loneliness, depression, fear, and pessimism alter the responses in the immune system. Experiencing close relationships, hope, compassion, humor, and social support enhance the body's ability to fight diseases. Owning a pet has even been found to have a positive effect on health. The most important and rigorous study in support of psychoneuroimmunology was conducted by Dr. David Spiegel, a psychiatrist at the Stanford University School of Medicine. He and his colleagues found that weekly group therapy sessions dramatically increased the life expectancy of women with advanced breast cancer.[28]

table 14.5

TRAITS THAT CAN HELP BOLSTER RESISTANCE

- *Optimism.* Health can be a self-fulfilling prophecy. Good things happen to people who expect them. Pessimism, fatalism, and resignation are linked to poorer health.
- *An unsinkable spirit.* Belief in the ability to make it through any crisis is essential.
- *Taking charge.* Whereas a fighting spirit provides motivation, a take-charge attitude (also termed *active coping*) puts that spirit into action.
- *Expressing feelings.* Rather than merely describing bodily sensations, honesty in identifying and expressing feelings is important.
- *Altruism.* Giving to others and making the world a better place have physical and mental benefits.
- *A sense of humor.* Being able to laugh at yourself—as opposed to ridiculing others—is very health enhancing.
- *Absence of malice.* Those who have a lot of hostility are especially susceptible to disease.
- *Social connectedness.* How would you answer the question, "Can you count on anyone to provide you with emotional support?" A yes means your relationships with people make a real difference in your health.

This area of research brings a fascinating new approach to health care. Mind-body interventions, including relaxation techniques, meditation, biofeedback, autogenic training, and visualization, are being given new credibility thanks to sophisticated research. Clinical applications of these techniques have shown promise in arresting the development of heart disease, cancer, AIDS, gastrointestinal problems, asthma, and chronic pain.[29] See Table 14.5 for the key emotional traits that have been shown to help boost disease resistance. How many of these traits do you possess?

Challenge 1: Diversity

One of the biggest challenges we face is making wellness information and services available to *everyone*—and making wellness a priority in *all* people's lives, despite our many differences. The racial and ethnic composition of the United States is changing dramatically. In fact, the United States is perhaps one of the most multiracial countries in the world. By the year 2000, whites (not including Hispanic Americans) will decline from 76 to 72 percent of the population. Blacks, presently comprising the largest minority, will increase from 12.4 to 13.1 percent of the population. Hispanics, one of the fastest-growing population groups, will rise from 8.0 to 11.3 percent.[30]

Our diversity should be celebrated and recognized as a basis for national strength; it also presents challenges in meeting the health and wellness needs of everyone. Ideally, wellness has no race, class, or income. However, the gulf is widening between the haves and have-nots, the insured and the uninsured, and whites and minorities. For example, research shows that blue-collar workers, low socioeconomic and low education groups, and persons with the most risk for coronary heart disease (particularly smokers) are the individuals most resistive to public health promotion.[31] These people cannot afford health club memberships and specialized medical screenings. Many of these people are more concerned about maintaining decent housing and feeding their families than about their cholesterol levels.

To better understand the challenges presented by this diversity issue, consider the following facts:[32]

➤ Severe high blood pressure is present four times more often among black men than among white men.
➤ Liver cancer is more than 12 times higher among Southeast-Asian Americans than it is among whites.

- Fifty percent of black women aged 20 and older are overweight (compared to 35 percent for all women). Among Mexican Americans, 40 percent of men and 48 percent of women are obese. Because of this obesity, the rates of diabetes are much higher in these populations.
- Death rates from heart disease and cancer are lower for Hispanic Americans than for non-Hispanics; but homicide, cirrhosis, and AIDS incidences are very high.
- A large portion of American Indians die before age 45—a result of unintentional injuries, cirrhosis, diabetes, suicide, and homicide.
- Homicide is the most frequent cause of death of black men between the ages of 15 and 35.

Generalizations about various subgroups from local studies can be misleading because of the disparities among subgroups living in different geographic locations. Nevertheless, the most striking aspect of all health comparison rates is the tremendous gap between low-income people and all other groups. Nearly one out of every eight Americans lives in a family with an income below the federal poverty level; and for virtually all of the chronic diseases that lead the nation's list of killers, low income is a special risk factor.[33]

Everyone deserves a high level of functioning and well-being. Showing how small lifestyle changes can enhance well-being, providing wellness information, and changing attitudes toward self-responsibility in our diverse population is difficult. Nevertheless, making wellness available to all Americans is in itself a wellness issue. In today's world, television is a common learning environment, especially for the uneducated. While there is a considerable amount of health-related information in television programming and commercials, many times, for our vastly diverse population, the suggestions seem impersonal, impractical, and unrealistic.[34] This presents a considerable challenge to those in health promotion. Perhaps the biggest payoff would be to integrate wellness information, behaviors, and attitudes into all segments of primary and secondary school curricula, reaching all youth before unhealthy life habits develop.

It is not enough to ask or expect every individual to accept responsibility for health and well-being without communities, businesses, health organizations, families, and civic organizations joining with the *government* to bring about national wellness. Dr. Kenneth Pelletier states that "The critical challenges remain to implement established knowledge, to increase awareness and motivation for healthy living, and to provide resources for equitable access to appropriate care. By supporting and reinforcing individual choices with innovations in policy and programs, we *can* achieve health."[35]

Challenge 2: The Environment

Environmental policy has long been an important part of public health. Throughout history, regulations regarding safe food, water, and sewage management have substantially improved our well-being. However, rapid technological changes have resulted in new environmental hazards, many whose effects on the body may remain unrecognized for years. Worldwide consumption has had a tremendous effect on the world's resources and energy supplies. Pogo's insightful quip, "We have met the enemy and he is us," is particularly appropriate in addressing the challenge we all face in saving and protecting the environment. This opens new opportunities for you to make an impact on your wellness—and that of others.

Being apathetic or becoming accustomed to environmental pollution is a very serious matter. The fact that you cannot do everything is no excuse for doing nothing. There is a lot you can do to limit, or at least minimize, the pollution and overconsumption in your "own little world." As in all areas of wellness improvement, form a personal plan to combat environmental hazards. Look at the following list of environmental concerns, and consider ways you could make changes in your daily living in order to make the world a better place in which to live.

1. The earth's protective ozone layer—our shield against the sun's hazardous ultraviolet rays—is being eaten away by human-made chemicals. The result is damaged food crops and ocean plants, increased skin cancer and cataracts, and decreases in human immunities. Aerosol sprays, refrigerants, plastic foam, and cleaning fluids contain chlorofluorocarbons (CFCs)—the chief agents of ozone destruction.
2. Our excessive use of paper, plastic, glass, and aluminum continues to add to our landfills. Recycling can decrease the need for more landfills and cut down on the pollution from the manufacture of new products.
3. Residues of harmful pesticides can be found in the air, on crops, in the ground, and in water supplies. Lawn and garden chemicals are significant contributors to this.
4. Water and air, essentials for life, face increasing contamination. Fish caught in polluted waters may be contaminated.
5. Loud rock music is associated with hearing loss.
6. Traffic sounds, aircraft noise, and noisy industrial areas are associated with stress and stress-related physical symptoms.
7. Radon gas and asbestos have been linked to cancer. Radon is a naturally occurring radioactive gas emitted by soil and rocks. Radon is diluted to safe levels outdoors but can be dangerously concentrated if trapped in poorly ventilated basements, houses, and buildings. Asbestos, a commonly used insulating material, has been linked to a variety of lung diseases. The U.S. government has ordered an end to the production of nearly all asbestos in the country by 1997.
8. Exposure to high levels of lead is toxic to the central nervous system and can be fatal. In our country, nearly three million children are at some risk from elevated lead levels.[36] House paints used before 1980 often contained lead. Also, people who live near airports, battery factories, and landfills are at risk.

It is important to further recognize that the term *environment* does not apply solely to distant wildernesses and ocean floors. A concerned educator states that "For millions of inner-city residents, environment consists chiefly of abandoned or vandalized parks, refuse-filled streets, vacant lots dominated by gangs and drug dealers, gutted factories, and other unsightly effluvia of urban decay."[37]

We often take too many things for granted. Part of your challenge in wellness living will be to assume some individual responsibility for preserving the environment. This personal challenge must then progress to the next level: more social and political action nationwide.

Challenge 3: Cultivating a Wellness Mindset in Everyone

Throughout this book we have addressed many effective strategies that virtually all individuals can utilize to pursue optimal well-being. However, the challenge of wellness extends beyond these commendable personal habits. Wellness goes beyond human physiology; it is also humility, compassion, and true happiness. Complete wellness includes possessing a deep altruistic commitment to the betterment of humankind. **Altruism** means having a regard for the interest of others without concern for oneself. Unfortunately, in this world the residues of self-gratification are very visible—cheating; violence; family breakdown; loss of personal character, integrity, and values; drug use; vanity. Is this the road to happiness? Is this a mindset for personal excellence?

In his book *The Pursuit of Happiness*, social psychologist Dr. David Myers uncovers the underlying recipe for personal happiness and well-being. His recipe includes three ingredients: "Well-being is found in the renewal of *disciplined lifestyles, committed relationships*, and *receiving and giving of acceptance*."[38] Myers' three ingredients intertwine with wellness-living: giving to others, achieving personal excellence, going beyond mediocrity, shaping your environment, seizing life. Wellness is not something to have. Rather it is something to be. The challenge we all face is to achieve a wellness mindset ourselves, as well as creating a wellness mindset in everyone—where just getting by is intolerable.

A Parting Thought

Suppose you are the owner of a very fine show dog. To make this dog a champion, you handle her in very special ways: you make sure she gets proper exercise every day, her coat is brushed and groomed, and her diet is carefully monitored (at the grocery store you walk past the doggie treats and junk food to Be Lean and Win Dog Food). Her living environment is regulated to make her the best show dog possible. Do you treat yourself as you would a champion show dog? Do you walk past the treats and junk food to the "be lean and win" food? Are you managing your environment in such a way that it makes you the best you can be? You have 24 hours a day 365 days a year to make choices. Our society provides you the opportunity to make many positive choices. Our society also allows for choices that are not in your best interest. You now have the knowledge and skills to make choices that enhance your well-being.

Remember, wellness is a journey in which the benefits are gained along the trip. It is not a life of self-sacrifice and delayed gratification. It is being the most you can be every day of your life. It is reveling in the fact that you have considerable control over your own well-being and happiness. Go to it! We wish you well.

SUMMARY

Everyone is born with a genetic blueprint. However, personal lifestyle choices have a great impact on whether you maximize your potential. You, as an educated citizen, know the choices that enhance wellness. You, as an informed consumer, must be able to evaluate wellness products and programs. No doubt your campus offers activities and facilities that can support your quest for wellness. The business world has also discovered the value of wellness in the workplace, in terms of increased productivity, lessened health insurance costs, and enhanced employee morale. Knowing how important a supportive environment is in pursuing wellness, you may want to consider working for a company that supports and values employee wellness. After all, you will spend at least one-third of your life at work.

Wellness is an integral part of a productive family life. Family wellness involves meeting the various physical, psychological, and social needs of all members, regardless of ages, as they strive toward full potential. You, as a parent, will be the master teacher of lifestyle habits to your children. Your example will have a strong influence on your children's ability to make responsible wellness choices.

Accidents are the fourth most common cause of death in the United States, behind heart disease, cancer, and stroke. However, accidents (especially automobile crashes) are the number-one cause of death among young people. All accidents and crime are not just a matter of chance. You can substantially reduce your risks of being a victim by heeding basic precautions. Acting to control risks in your immediate environment is a powerful way to enhance your total wellness.

Wellness is not a passing craze. The wellness trend is revolutionizing medical care and the health insurance system. The broad scope of wellness creates opportunities for life enhancement for everyone: young, old, poor, rich, black, and white. New research in the mind-body relationship, including of how attitudes, beliefs, and emotional states can affect the immune system, is creating increased interest in the *total* wellness concept of health. Wellness becomes a global issue as we work together to protect the environment. The ultimate challenge is to get the word to everyone (especially to those who need wellness the most) and get it to them while they are young. Empowering people to have a mindset of self-responsibility along with an attitude of altruism is the only guaranteed way to perpetuate wellness as the undisputed way of life for everyone.

REFERENCES

1. Sullivan, Louis W., M.D. "Partners in Prevention: A Mobilization Plan for Implementing *Healthy People 2000.*" *American Journal of Health Promotion* 5 (March/April 1991): 291–97.
2. Kime, Robert E. *The Informed Health Consumer.* Guilford, Conn.: The Dushkin Publishing Group, 1992.
3. Schor, Juliet B. *The Overworked American.* New York: Basic Books, 1991.
4. "Businesses Promote Family Health." *The Futurist* 24 (November/December 1990): 48.
5. Zedeck, Sheldon, and Kathleen L. Mosier. "Workplace Wellness: Work in the Family and Employing Organization." *American Psychologist* 45 (February 1990): 240–51.
6. Stucky-Ropp, Renée, and Thomas M. DiLorenzo. "Determinants of Exercise in Children." *Preventive Medicine* 22 (November 1993): 880–89.
7. National Association for Sport and Physical Education. "Shape Up America." *NASPE News* 42 (Spring/Summer 1995): 4.
8. Friedman, Myles I., and George H. Lackey Jr. *The Psychology of Human Control: A General Theory of Purposeful Behavior.* New York: Praeger Publishers, 1991.
9. "Teen Risk-Taking Behavior." *Healthline* 9 (August 1990): 9.
10. University of California, Berkeley. *The Wellness Encyclopedia.* Boston: Houghton Mifflin Co., 1991.
11. Castelli, Jim. "Study Reveals Causes, Costs of Accidents." *Safety & Health* 144 (August 1991): 61–64.
12. Rothman, Howard. *The Employee Handbook for Building a Healthier Lifestyle.* Brookfield, Wis.: International Foundation of Employee Benefit Plans, 1991.
13. Campbell, Sharon Lynn. "Six Reasons Why People Don't Buckle Up." *Safety & Health* 143 (February 1991): 78–80.
14. "Most Americans Are Buckling Up." *Muncie Evening Press* (April 22, 1995), 7A.
15. *The Wellness Encyclopedia.*
16. *The Wellness Encyclopedia.*
17. *The Wellness Encyclopedia.*
18. *The Wellness Encyclopedia.*
19. Sandler, Roberta. "Safe Driving: It's up to You." *Safety & Health* 143 (April 1991): 74–75.
20. "DWD: Driving While Drowsy." *University of California, Berkeley Wellness Letter* 11 (May 1995): 5.
21. *The Wellness Encyclopedia.*
22. Naisbitt, John. *Megatrends.* New York: Warner Books, 1982.
23. "Education for Health: A Role for Physicians and the Efficacy of Health Education Efforts." *The Journal of the American Medical Association* 263 (April 4, 1990): 1816–19.
24. Spencer, G. "Projections of the Population of the United States, by Age, Sex, and Race: 1988 to 2080." *Current Population Reports, Population Estimates and Projections* series p-25, no. 1018. Washington, D.C.: U.S. Department of Commerce, Bureau of the Census, 1989.
25. Market Report—"Mature Americans: Myths and Markets." *American Demographics* (1994), 12.
26. Miller, Cheryl, and Ray Tricker. "Past and Future Priorities in Health Promotion in the United States: A Survey of Experts." *American Journal of Health Promotion* 5 (May/June 1991): 360–67.
27. Dienstfrey, Harris. "The Mind Body Connection." *Healing and the Mind with Bill Moyers: Teacher's Resource Guide.* Kalamazoo, Mich.:, The Fetzer Institute, 1993.
28. Pelletier, Kenneth R. *Sound Mind, Sound Body: A New Model for Lifelong Health.* New York: Simon and Schuster, 1994.
29. Pelletier. *Sound Mind, Sound Body.*
30. Department of Health and Human Services, Public Health Service. *Healthy People 2000: National Health Promotion and Disease Prevention Objectives.* Washington, D.C.: Department of Health and Human Services, 1990.
31. Dishman, Rod K. *Exercise Adherence: Its Impact on Public Health.* Champaign, Ill.: Human Kinetics Publishers, 1988.
32. *Healthy People 2000.*
33. *Healthy People 2000.*
34. Signorielli, Nancy. "Television and Health: Images and Impact." *Mass Communication and Public Health.* Charles Atkin and Lawrence Wallack, eds. Newbury Park, Calif.: Sage Publications, 1990, 96–113.
35. Pelletier. *Sound Mind, Sound Body.*
36. Agency for Toxic Substances and Disease Registry. *The Nature and Extent of Lead Poisoning in Children in the United States: A Report to Congress.* Washington, D.C.: U.S. Department of Health and Human Services, July 1988.
37. Kraus, Richard. "Tomorrow's Leisure: Meeting the Challenges." *The Journal of Physical Education, Recreation, and Dance* 65 (April 1994): 42–47.
38. Myers, David. *The Pursuit of Happiness: Who Is Happy and Why.* New York: Morrow, 1993.

SUGGESTED READINGS

Ardell, Donald B., and John G. Langdon, M.D. *Wellness: The Body Mind and Spirit.* Dubuque, Iowa: Kendall/Hunt Publishing Co., 1989.

Atkin, Charles, and Lawrence Wallack, eds. *Mass Communication and Public Health.* Newbury Park, Calif.: Sage Publications, 1990.

Barrett, Stephen, M.D. *Health Schemes, Scams, and Frauds.* Mount Vernon, N.Y.: Consumer Reports Books, 1990.

Barrett, Stephen, M.D., and William T. Jarvis. *The Health Robbers.* Buffalo, N.Y.: Prometheus Books, 1993.

Brammer, Lawrence M. *How to Cope with Life Transitions: The Challenge of Personal Change.* New York: Hemisphere Publishing Corporation, 1991.

Bricklin, Mark, Mark Golin, Deborah Grandinetti, and Alexis Lieberman. *Positive Living and Health.* Emmaus, Penn.: Rodale Press, 1990.

Bromely, Max L., and Leonard Territo. *College Crime Prevention and Personal Safety Awareness.* Springfield, Ill.: Charles C Thomas, Publisher, 1990.

Cowan, Philip A., and Mavis Hetherington, eds. *Family Transitions.* Hillsdale, N.J.: Lawrence Erlbaum Associates, Publishers, 1991.

Dienstfrey, Harris. *Where the Mind Meets the Body.* New York: HarperCollins Publishers, 1992.

Dychtwald, Ken, and Joe Flower. *Age Wave.* Los Angeles: Jeremey P. Tarcher, Inc., 1989.

Foege, William H. "Closing the Gaps: Ensuring the Application of Available Knowledge in the Promotion of Health and the Prevention of Disease." *Journal of School Health* 60 (April 1990): 130–32.

Gebhardt, Deborah L., and Carolyn E. Crump. "Employee Fitness and Wellness Programs in the Workplace." *American Psychologist* 45 (February 1990): 262–72.

Goleman, Daniel, and Joel Gurin, eds. *Mind/Body Medicine: How to Use Your Mind for Better Health.* Yonkers, N.Y.: Consumer Reports Books, 1993.

Halpern, Charles R. "The Political Economy of Mind-Body Health." *American Journal of Health Promotion* 6 (March/April 1992): 279, 288–91.

Heath, Douglas H., and Harriet E. Heath. *Fulfilling Lives: Paths to Maturity and Success.* San Francisco: Jossey-Bass Publishers, 1991.

Jaffe, Michael. *Understanding Parenting.* Dubuque, Iowa: Wm. C. Brown Publishers, 1991.

Kabat-Zinn, Jon. *Full Catastrophe Living.* New York: Delta Books, 1990.

Kain, Edward L. *The Myth of Family Decline: Understanding Families in a World of Rapid Social Change.* Lexington, Mass.: Lexington Books, 1990.

Kime, Robert E. *The Informed Health Consumer.* Guilford, Conn.: The Dushkin Publishing Group, 1992.

Kuntzleman, Charles T. *Healthy Kids for Life.* New York: Simon and Schuster, Inc., 1988.

Marrone, Robert. *Body of Knowledge: An Introduction to Body/Mind Psychology.* Albany, N.Y.: State University of New York Press, 1990.

Miller, Cheryl, and Ray Tricker. "Past and Future Priorities in Health Promotion in the United States: A Survey of Experts." *American Journal of Health Promotion* 5 (May/June 1991): 360–67.

Miller, Dean F. *Safety: Principles and Issues.* Dubuque, Iowa: Wm. C. Brown Communications, Inc., 1995.

Myers, David G. "Pursuing Happiness: Where to Look, Where Not to Look." *Psychology Today* 26 (July/August 1993): 32–35, 66–67.

Ornstein, Robert, and David Sobel. *Healthy Pleasures.* New York: Addison-Wesley Publishing Co., Inc., 1989.

Ornstein, Robert, and Charles Swencionis. *The Healing Brain: A Scientific Reader.* New York: The Guilford Press, 1990.

Pelletier, Kenneth R. "Mind-Body Health: Research, Clinical, and Policy Applications." *American Journal of Health Promotion* 6 (May/June 1992): 345–58.

Pelletier, Kenneth R. *Sound Mind, Sound Body: A New Model for Lifelong Health.* New York: Simon and Schuster, 1994.

Rothman, Howard. *The Employee Handbook for Building a Healthier Lifestyle.* Brookfield, Wis.: International Foundation of Employee Benefit Plans, 1991.

Schoemaker, Joyce M., and Charity Y. Vitale. *Healthy Homes, Healthy Kids.* Washington, D.C.: Island Press, 1991.

Taylor, Robert L. *Health Fact, Health Fiction.* Dallas, Tex.: Taylor Publishing Co., 1990.

Zedeck, Sheldon, and Kathleen L. Mosier. "Workplace Wellness: Work in the Family and Employing Organization." *American Psychologist* 45 (February 1990): 240–51.

appendix 1

Aerobic Dance
(Including Step Aerobics and Slide Training)

Advantages/Disadvantages

Aerobic dancing is a popular fitness activity. Usually performed under the leadership of an instructor, it combines the cardiovascular benefits of jogging with the joy of dancing. The variety of movements not only strengthens the cardiorespiratory system but also increases flexibility, tones muscles, and enhances body composition. It is a total body workout. The upbeat music tempo creates an atmosphere of excitement; exercising in a group is fun and emotionally stimulating. The popular music and group comraderie help prevent boredom and can keep you motivated. Aerobic dancing can be so much fun, you often forget you are exercising. Because the participants focus on the instructor, aerobic dance classes are good for the beginning or self-conscious exerciser. Aerobic dance allows for individualization of a workout. The same movement sequence or exercise can be done by both a well-conditioned participant and a beginning exerciser with variation in the intensity or number of repetitions. Because aerobic dance is done indoors, the environment provides security and comfort.

Aerobic dance has excellent potential for developing all components of physical fitness, but it can have some drawbacks. Even though participants are urged by instructors to work at their own pace, some exercisers overdo it. These exercisers try to keep up with the group or work as hard as the instructor, even though they may not be ready for this intensity. Many times the result is excessive soreness or fatigue. Performing aerobic dance on a hard, unyielding surface (like cement) or while wearing inappropriate shoes also increases the risk of injury. Some overzealous aerobics participants attend classes one or more times a day, leading to overuse. Excessive impact may cause leg and foot problems. Also, not all aerobic dance instructors have had training in exercise instruction and safety and may teach improper technique. Unless good body mechanics and reasonable progressions are emphasized in a class, the result can be discomfort rather than exhilaration and a desire to continue exercising. Having to join or travel to a fitness facility to take an aerobics class may be viewed as a disadvantage to some exercisers. Others find it motivating to have a set time, to have made a financial investment, and to have a group of friends to exercise with. Aerobic dance videotapes are available for the home exerciser. They allow exercising in private but lack the spontaneity, instruction, and enthusiasm available in a live class.

What to Wear

Even though some aerobic dancers have color-coordinated leotards and fancy exercise apparel, any loose-fitting and comfortable clothing will do. A T-shirt and shorts are fine. More important than the clothing are supportive shoes. Shoes specially designed for the impact and movement of aerobic dance are recommended. A good aerobic shoe has a well-cushioned, resilient midsole to aid in shock dispersion, and a sturdy heel counter to hold the foot in place. The shoe should allow for lateral movement and, as a result, not have a wide heel flair that is often seen in a jogging shoe. Like the jogger, the aerobic participant should replace old shoes when their cushioning ability has decreased.

Techniques and Safety Tips

Many injuries and discomforts can be avoided in aerobic dance with proper shoes, gradual progression, and exercising on a resilient surface. Chapter 5 gives several general suggestions for preventing injury in fitness activities. In aerobic dance, careful attention to technique and body mechanics further eliminates chance for injury and heightens the enjoyment of the activity.

1. *Always warm up with low-intensity, whole body movements.* Your warm-up should include slow, full range-of-motion joint movements. Static stretching should also be included in the warm-up.
2. *Keep abdominals pulled in and buttocks tucked under.*
3. *Avoid twisting the spinal column excessively* (windmill toe touches, elbow-to-knee lunges, etc.).
4. *Limit the hopping on one foot* to a maximum of four consecutive times.
5. *Soften your jumps and bounces by maintaining a slightly bent-knee landing position.*
6. *Try to make your heels go all the way to the floor when landing from jumps.*
7. *Never fling or throw your arms or legs.* Maintain control of limbs throughout movements.
8. *Avoid hyperextending your elbows, knees, or lower back.*
9. *Listen to your body.* If a stretch, exercise, or position causes pain or a burning sensation, do not do it.

The amount of concern for technique and safety in the class depends on your instructor. A wise wellness consumer chooses a knowledgeable, trained instructor. The popularity of aerobic dance has skyrocketed, and the number of qualified instructors has not kept pace. While standards and certification programs have now been established, it is still up to you to select a class. Do not be shy. Check the instructor's qualifications. Is she or he certified by a national fitness organization? Does the instructor have knowledge in anatomy, exercise physiology, kinesiology, and first aid? Is she or he currently certified in CPR (cardiopulmonary resuscitation)? Does the instructor do some health screening or fitness assessment of students? Is the class supervised effectively? Does the instructor monitor the intensity of the workout with periodic heart-rate checks? Does the class begin with a good warm-up and end with a cool-down period? Does the instructor give corrective cues and technique suggestions throughout the workout? Does she or he consider the variances in fitness levels in the class by showing how to modify the intensity of the workout? Is she or he easy to follow? Looking good in a leotard and being a fluid dancer are not requirements for being a quality aerobic dance instructor. Most important is the ability to conduct a safe, yet invigorating, workout from which all participants can benefit.

How to Begin and Progress

As with any other fitness activity, begin slowly. Attend no more than three classes per week for several weeks. Start with 5 to 10 minutes of the aerobic phase and progress gradually. If the aerobic portion of the class is 30 minutes, do low-impact moves or walk in place while the experienced exercisers continue. Monitor your pulse and stay within your target heart-rate range. You should be able to talk or sing with the music throughout the entire workout. Gradually add a few minutes weekly to the aerobic phase until you can exercise aerobically for 20 to 30 minutes.

Some exercisers prefer low-impact aerobics to high-impact aerobics. Low-impact aerobics reduces the strain on knees and ankles by minimizing jumping and bouncing movements. In low-impact aerobics, one foot is in contact with the ground at all times. *Low impact* does not necessarily mean *low intensity*. To maintain a training heart rate, move your arms vigorously and travel along the floor by wide-stride walking, sliding, and sidestepping. Beginners and even well-trained exercisers with joint problems can benefit from low-impact aerobics. You may want to combine low-impact and high-impact moves. Most jumps and steps can be modified to become low-impact steps.

Most aerobic dance classes incorporate in the workout a body toning segment. Once again, use common sense. Do not try to do as many repetitions as the teacher, unless you are equally fit. Stop and stretch if you feel pain or a burning sensation in the muscle. Aerobic dance participants often tend to compare themselves or compete with others in the class. Avoid falling into this trap. Work to be the best you can be without shame or guilt.

Variety

It is easy to add variety to aerobic dance. Vary the music. Use pop, jazz, country, or classical music. Try some holiday or theme music when appropriate. Vary the routines or steps. Aerobics can be taught by using set routines (repetitive movements in a programmed format) or in a freestyle format (participants mimic the instructor and change accordingly). Varying between learned routines and a freestyle approach helps keep interest high. Try circuit aerobic dance. Set up exercise stations around the room. Do different aerobic movements for 1 to 2 minutes per station and then jog to the next station to sustain your training heart rate. There are many other ways to add variety to aerobic dance. One- to 2-pound hand weights can be used during aerobic routines to increase upper body endurance and to maintain a training heart rate. Heavier hand weights are often used during stationary power moves to tone arms and legs. To prevent knee injuries, do not wear ankle weights while doing aerobic dance steps. Weights are, however, an effective way to add resistance while doing floor toning. Thick rubber bands and elastic tubing can also be used to increase the efficiency of body toning exercises.

Step Aerobics

Also known as *bench/step training*, step aerobics is an innovative activity that involves stepping up and down on a 4- to 12-inch platform. Combining a variety of stepping patterns with kicks, turns, and upper body movements results in a brisk workout. Step aerobics appeals to a wide range of exercisers for several reasons: It can be a high-intensity workout with low-impact force; it is adaptable to different fitness levels by adjusting the bench height, adding jumps, varying arm gestures, and adding light hand weights; and it is easy to do. Step aerobics has become especially popular with men, who may be put off by "dance-like" aerobics classes. As with all aerobic exercise activities, proper form and technique are necessary to prevent injury.

To prevent injury while stepping:

1. *As much as possible, keep your shoulders aligned over your hips.*
2. *Step up lightly, making sure the whole foot lands on the platform.*
3. *Keep your knees aligned over your feet when they're pulling your body weight onto the platform.*
4. *At the top, straighten your legs, but don't lock your knees.*
5. *Do not pivot a bent, supporting knee.*
6. *As you step down, stay close to the platform.*

If you are a beginner to step aerobics, start with the lowest bench, and keep your eyes on the bench until you adjust to the activity. Once you learn the stepping patterns, you can add arm movements and light hand weights or challenge yourself by raising the height of the bench. (However, never use a height that flexes your knees to an angle less than 90 degrees.)

Step aerobics is a great workout for the lower body and, when combined with a variety of arm movements, is an exciting new variation in aerobic exercise.

Slide Training

Slide training is a safe, low-impact activity that has gained popularity in recent years. It is offered as a class at many fitness centers or can be performed easily at home. Slide training involves side-to-side sliding, similar to a speed skater's motion, on a slick board. Most boards are 5 to 6 feet in length with small raised ends for pushing off. The slide boards, available at most sports/fitness retail outlets, are lightweight and can be rolled up for easy storage and handling.

While wearing special slippers, the exerciser glides from end to end in a low, crouched position. This exercise improves balance and agility, conditions the lower body, and provides a great cardiovascular workout. Medical and athletic training professionals have used slide training for many years to rehabilitate injured knees, legs, and backs. Arm lifts and various leg lifts can be added to the basic slide motion for a varied workout. To avoid injury and heighten the enjoyment of sliding observe the following guidelines:

1. *Warm up, cool down, and stretch off the slide.*
2. *Keep your weight centered over your feet and slightly bent knees aligned with your toes.*
3. *Contract the abdominals and keep your eyes on the board to start.*
4. *Keep your hips squared and aligned with your torso and shoulders.*
5. *Tuck your shoelaces into the slide socks.*
6. *Control your speed by dragging your trail leg.*
7. *Only add arm movement when you are proficient with the basic slide.*
8. *Maintain the music tempo at 120 to 130 beats per minute (averages to about 30 slides across).*

Common Discomforts

As in most fitness activities, mild soreness can be anticipated by the beginning exerciser. Some discomforts may be avoided by emphasizing stretching and toning the first three to four weeks to condition muscles and connective tissue for the stress of impact and the new movements. Veteran exercisers can suffer pain or injury by increasing frequency, time, or intensity too rapidly. Since most aerobic dance discomfort is found in the legs, be sure to warm up and stretch this area. Refer to Chapter 5 for further information about prevention and treatment of injuries. If you use hand weights, elbow and shoulder strain can be avoided by not flinging the weights. Always move the weights with control. Having a towel or exercise mat with you provides additional comfort and padding for floor exercises.

Resources

Certifying Organizations

Aerobics and Fitness Association of America (AFAA), 15250 Ventura Blvd., Suite 310, Sherman Oaks, CA 91403, (800) 446-2322 or (818) 905-0040.

American College of Sports Medicine, P.O. Box 1440, Indianapolis, IN 46206, (317) 637-9200.

Exer-Safety Association, 10151 University Blvd., Suite 138, Orlando, FL 32817, (407) 677-9501.

International Dance-Exercise Association (IDEA), 6190 Cornerstone Court East, Suite 204, San Diego, CA 92121-3773, (619) 535-8978 or (800) 999-IDEA.

National Dance-Exercise Instructor's Training Association (NDEITA), 1503 S. Washington Ave., Suite 208, Minneapolis, MN 55454, (800) 237-6242.

Books

Bishop, Jan Galen. *Fitness Through Aerobics*. Scottsdale, Ariz.: Gorsuch Scarisbrick, Publishers, 1995.

Casten, Carole, and Peg Jordan. *Aerobics Today*. St. Paul, Minn.: West Publishing Co., 1990.

Francis, Lorna. *Aerobic Dance for Health and Fitness*. Dubuque, Iowa: Brown & Benchmark, 1993.

Francis, Lorna, Peter Francis, and Gin Miller. *Step-Reebok: The First Aerobic Training Workout with Muscle. Instructor Training Manual*. Stoughton, Mass.: Reebok International Ltd., 1990.

Germain, Pam. *Aerobics: Basic and Creative*. Sierra Vista, Ariz.: Body Basics, 1995.

Kennedy, M. S., Carol Legel, and Deb Legel. *Anatomy of an Exercise Class: An Exercise Educator's Handbook*. Champaign, Ill.: Sagamore Publishing Inc., 1992.

Mazzeo, Karen. *Aerobics: The Way to Fitness*. Englewood, Colo.: Morton Publishing Co., 1992.

Mazzeo, Karen. *Fitness Through Aerobics and Step Training*. Englewood, Colo.: Morton Publishing Co., 1993.

McIntosh, Matthew. *Lifetime Aerobics*. Dubuque, Iowa: Wm. C. Brown Publishers, 1990.

National Dance-Exercise Instructors Training Association. *Advanced Fitness Handbook*. Minneapolis, Minn.: NDEITA, 1995.

National Dance-Exercise Instructors Training Association. *Aerobic & Fitness Instructor's Manual*. Minneapolis, Minn.: NDEITA, 1994.

Pryor, Esther, and Minda Goodman Kraines. *Keep Moving! It's Aerobic Dance*, 3d ed. Palo Alto, Calif.: Mayfield Publishing Co., 1996.

Music

Dynamix Music Service, 203 Edgevale Road, Baltimore, MD 21210, (800) 843-6499.

In-Lytes, 9400 Doral Ct., Louisville, KY 40220, (800) 243-7867 (call for a free catalogue) or (502) 495-0222.

Muscle Mixes, 623 N. Hyer Ave., Orlando, FL 32803, (800) 52-MIXES or (407) 872-7576.

Power Productions, P.O. Box 550, Gaitherburg, MD 20884–0550, (301) 926-0707 or (800) 777-BEAT (call for a free catalogue).

The Workout Source, P.O. Box 55278, Sherman Oaks, CA 91413, (800) 552-4552.

Videos

Collage Video Specialists, 5390 Main St. N.E. Dept. 1, Minneapolis, MN 55421, (800) 433-6769.

Creative Instructors Aerobics Educational Videos, 2314 Naudain Street, Philadelphia, PA 19146, (215) 790-9767 or (800) 435-0055.

appendix 2

Bicycling

Advantages/Disadvantages

Cycling is a popular choice for people of all ages. You can fit in a cycling workout while running errands, while going to work, or while at home in front of the TV (on rollers or a stationary bike). You can cycle alone, with family, or with friends. If you have a small child, you can take him or her along in a bike seat instead of having to hire a sitter while you get a workout. It is nonimpact exercise, minimizing stress to the back, shins, and ankles.

Of course, there are a few drawbacks. You must have a bicycle, keep it in good working condition, and store it securely to prevent theft. Cycling in traffic requires alertness and use of defensive driving skills to prevent accidents. Cycling in rain, snow, or icy conditions is uncomfortable and hazardous. Also, bicycles are so efficient that they can do most of the work for you. Most people don't work hard enough to do themselves much good. Cycling to class or short distances is fine for transportation, but if you want to get in shape, you will need to put in more effort. Nevertheless, cycling produces cardiorespiratory benefits without impact, making it the third most popular activity in the United States. It can be enjoyed throughout a lifetime.

What to Wear

In order to be clearly visible to vehicles, wear bright-colored clothing during the day and light-colored clothing at night. Fancy bicycling gear is not necessary, although if you really get into cycling, you might find that a pair of bicycling shorts makes long rides more comfortable. Hard-soled, athletic, or bicycling shoes are fine.

Equipment

There are plenty of bike-pedestrian as well as bike-car accidents on campus, and usually it is the bicyclist who is at fault. Always wear a helmet, one approved by the American National Standards Institute, even if you're just going across campus. The sidewalk is just as hard there as anywhere else. You may lose some skin in a slide or break some bones, but they will heal. Your brain won't. Head injuries account for over 75 percent of deaths and permanent disabilities in cycling crashes. If you hit something and go flying head first, wearing a good helmet is the best way to prevent serious injury.

When you are choosing a helmet, make sure that it has the following characteristics:

Outer shell or cover that is brightly colored (i.e., yellow, white, or red) so that you are easily visible to drivers
Hard shell lined with polystyrene or polystyrene alone
Secure chin strap
Label indicating the helmet is ANSI or Snell approved

Helmets are single-use devices designed to crush and absorb shock upon impact. You should replace a helmet that has been in a significant crash.

A water bottle is essential for workouts, particularly in the heat. Because sweat evaporates so quickly while you are riding, you may not realize how quickly water is lost. Dehydration, leading to heat illness, can easily occur. Drinking regularly from a water bottle to maintain an adequate level of hydration during a workout is a necessity, not a luxury.

It doesn't matter what type of bike you ride—one speed, 10-speed, mountain—but it does matter that it be kept in good working order. If you are not mechanically inclined, your local bicycle shop can help. Most people ride with the bike seat too low, which is inefficient and can make the knees hurt. The bike seat should be high enough that when you sit centered on the seat with your heel on the pedal at its lowest point, your knee is straight. That way, when you move the ball of your foot to its proper position on the pedal, your knee will be almost fully extended at the bottom of the stroke. If the seat is too high, you'll tend to rock side to side with each footstroke and may develop a sore crotch. A sore crotch can also be caused by improper seat tilt. Start with the nose of the seat level. If it bothers you, tilt it down slightly. Pedals, wheels, and steering should turn or spin freely with no binding, catch, or click. The derailleur should shift smoothly. Brakes should close and release easily. Brake shoes should be 1/8 inch or less from and level with the rim of the bike. If they are badly worn, replace them. The air in the tires usually needs to be topped off weekly to keep them hard and rolling smoothly but use caution when filling them. The air pumps at service stations are designed for cars, and it's easy to explode a bicycle tire by overfilling it. If a bike wheel is badly out of true and wobbles, it may hit your brake shoe with each revolution. A bike shop can true a wheel, lubricate sticky brake cables, adjust the derailleur, and show you how to keep your machine running smoothly, which makes riding safe and enjoyable.

Technique and Safety Tips

Shifting

On 10-speeds, the gears overlap slightly and you have to shift by feel. To shift, continue pedaling but ease up on the pedal pressure. Shifting without pedaling can cause a bent or broken chain or gear teeth. As you shift, you should not hear a loud clunk nor a constant rubbing sound, if you are shifting smoothly and getting it into gear correctly.

Most beginners gear too high and pedal too slowly. They feel like they're not getting any exercise unless they're pushing against resistance. This is inefficient and can increase fatigue and cause knees to ache. It is better to pedal quickly against light resistance. An optimal pedal rate is 80 rpm, with a range of 60 to 100 rpm. Racers and experienced tourists often cycle at 90 to 110 rpm.

If your bike has several gears, practice using them. Gearing is a matter of maintaining an even cadence regardless of terrain, weather, or wind conditions. If you're going uphill, shift before you have to slow your cadence so that you can go up smoothly. Also practice downshifting before stop signs so that you don't have to stand on the pedals to get going again.

Pedaling

Ride with the ball of your foot on the pedal. If you have toe clips, you can try ankling—pulling up as well as pushing down on the pedal each stroke—which doubles your efficiency.

Braking

Use your brakes as little as possible. Look ahead, signal, slow down, and learn to anticipate problems instead of simply reacting to them. Be careful not to jam on your brakes too suddenly or you can pitch head-first over the handlebars. The front brake is the most powerful because, as you decelerate, your weight shifts forward, lessening the weight over the back tire. For the most efficient stop, keep the body weight back, gradually increase pressure on the front brake, and hold pressure on the back brake just below the point where the wheel will skid. In wet conditions, brakes lose up to 90 percent of their braking ability. It is good to frequently apply the brakes lightly to wipe water off the rims and to allow extra stopping distance. When going downhill, pump the brakes to avoid overheating the wheel rims or brake shoes. When in doubt, favor the rear brake. It may skid the bike, but at least you won't land on your face.

Bumps

When you come up to bumps, holes, and railroad tracks, don't sit on the seat like a sack of potatoes. Shift your weight to pedals and handlebars to absorb the shock. It's better for you and for your bike.

Safety Tips

1. Wear brightly colored clothing, wear a helmet, and carry water.
2. Keep to the right side of the road and ride in a straight line. Always ride in single file with traffic.
3. Do not make sudden turns or swerves. Signal all turns and stops.
4. Stay alert. Look out for cars pulling out into traffic or turning. Listen constantly for traffic approaching out of your line of vision.
5. Observe all traffic regulations just as if you were driving a car—red and green lights, one-way streets, stop signs. Slow down at all street intersections and look right and left before crossing.
6. Be sure your brakes are operating efficiently and keep your bicycle in perfect running condition. Keep your hands on or near the brakes at all times.
7. Keep speed under control, especially on long downhill runs. Speed should be low enough that you can stop quickly.
8. In rainy weather, allow much more distance for stopping and don't take corners too fast.
9. Watch for sudden door openings from parked cars. Ride at least 3 feet away from them.
10. Avoid sewer grates that parallel your direction.
11. If railroad tracks are rough, walk your bike across them (to prevent blowout or other damage to the bicycle). If you choose to ride over the tracks, cross them at a 90 degree angle.
12. Make sure you are at least 3 feet off the traveled portion of the road when you stop or park.
13. Hug the right-hand shoulder of the road on all curves.
14. Give pedestrians the right-of-way. Avoid sidewalks.
15. Watch out for child cyclists. Children on bicycles usually weave from side to side and turn unpredictably without signaling, and they can run into you even when you are passing them.
16. All dogs are potential adversaries. If a dog is far enough away, you can probably outrun him. Water from your bottle or a bike pump may scare him off. If you stop, keep the bike between you and the dog. Walk slowly away. Generally, a dog will leave you alone, but watch him carefully before you get under way again. You can also buy a small can of "dog repellent," which will shoot a thin stream of chemical about 10 feet. Although the effects are potent, there is no permanent damage done to the animal. Don't try to run down or kick at a dog—this can cause a crash. If you are very scared, you can yell, "Out" at the dog, mimicking a noise made by mother dogs when disciplining their puppies. This will usually startle a dog enough to give you a chance to escape.
17. Don't wear headphones—they block out street sounds that enable you to anticipate traffic.
18. Don't wear a heavy backpack. It can throw off your balance. Carry packages in baskets or bags attached to the cycle.
19. Learn to shift gears while keeping your eyes on the road.

How to Begin and Progress

First, measure your fitness level using the 5-mile timed ride test in Chapter 4. Remember that your *current* fitness level does not indicate your potential. Allow yourself several weeks to show significant improvement. Begin at the step indicated by your current fitness level. If you cannot complete the test, begin at level 1. Exercise three to five days a week at your training pulse. (An appropriate pulse for bicycling appears to be about 5 percent lower than for other exercise, so subtract 5 percent to adjust for this difference.) You may work at one level until you can comfortably handle the recommended distance and intensity; then move to the next step. To develop balanced fitness, add 25 to 30 push-ups, a minute of abdominal curls, and 5 to 15 minutes of stretching to each workout.

Bicycling Program

Fitness Category	Starting Level
Very low	1 or 2
Low	3
Average	4
Good	5
Excellent	6

Level	Cycling	Total Distance
1	20–30 min. (8–10 MPH)	3–5 miles
2	20–30 min. (10–12 MPH)	4–6 miles
3	30–45 min. (12 MPH)	4–8 miles
4	30–60 min. (15 MPH)	7–15 miles
5	40–75 min. (15 MPH)	10–18 miles
6	40–90 min. (15 MPH)	10–22 miles

Variety

Part of the appeal of bicycling is being able to explore an area and see things you wouldn't normally notice as you whizzed past in a car. Try cycling to a park, a lake, or a scenic spot or merely try exploring on a bicycle. Plan an outing with a picnic or refreshment break halfway. Ride to a nearby small town and back. Plan a bike rally, similar to a car rally with checkpoints, or a bike scavenger hunt in which you gather bits of information from certain locations (i.e., what is the name of the store at 21 Oak Street?). If you are interested in more, consult your local bicycle shop for bicycling organizations in your area and find out what rides and tours are planned.

Common Discomforts

Bicyclists beginning a conditioning program often experience a sore crotch the first week or two. As you and your saddle adjust to each other, the syndrome should disappear. Check to see that the seat is not too high. A too-high seat causes you to rock side-to-side with each pedal stroke, and the constant rubbing will prolong soreness. It may help to tilt the nose of the saddle down a bit (not so much you slide off!), to try a different saddle, one with padding under the "sit bones," or to consider padded cycling shorts.

Sore knees? A seat that is too low, so that your knees are excessively bent throughout the pedal stroke is one cause. Riding with excessive resistance at too low a cadence increases pressure on the knees and is another easily remedied cause. A relatively high cadence against light resistance reduces frequency of overuse injuries.

If your fingers feel numb after cycling, you need to change hand position more frequently and ride with elbows slightly bent, not locked. The ulnar nerve runs across the palm, and constant pressure on the hands can temporarily cut off sensation to the area. Wearing padded cycling gloves or cushioning your handlebars with foam grips may also help.

Neck or back soreness usually disappears in a week or so once you grow accustomed to riding. If they do not, try changing hand positions frequently, riding with elbows slightly bent, moving the seat forward a little, or perhaps switching to upright handlebars.

Do your toes tend to go numb on long rides? If you are using toe clips, it may be that pedaling tends to push your foot forward into your shoes until your toes touch the end, reducing blood flow to the area. Try lacing your shoes snugly enough so that they hold your foot back in the heel of the shoe but not so tightly that circulation is hindered. Also, try loosening your toe clips.

References

Alpert, Gerri. *Bike Abroad: 439 Organized Trips with 70 Companies in 49 Countries.* Bedford Hills, N.Y.: New Voyager, 1994

"A Bicycle Built for You." *Women's Sports and Fitness* 16, no. 3 (April 1994): 51–60.

Bicycling Magazine Editors. *Bicycling Magazine's Bike Touring in the 90s.* Emmaus, Penn.: Rodale Press, Inc., 1993.

Bicycling Magazine Editors. *Bicycling Magazine's Training for Fitness & Endurance.* Emmaus, Penn.: Rodale Press, Inc., 1992.

Bicycling Magazine Editors. *Bicycling Magazine's Bicycle Commuting Made Easy.* Emmaus, Penn.: Rodale Press, Inc., 1993.

Burke, Edmund, and Chris Carmichael. *Fitness Cycling.* Champaign, Ill.: Human Kinetics Books, 1994.

Burke, Edmund. *Cycling Health & Physiology: Using Sports Science to Improve Your Riding & Racing.* Battleboro, Vt.: Vitesse Press, 1992.

Erhard, T. "The Best Training Plan . . . Period." *Bicycling Magazine* 35, no. 2 (February 1994): 68–72.

Kennedy, Martha J., et al. *Fat Tire Rider: Everyone's Guide to Mountain Biking.* Battleboro, Vt.: Vitesse Press, 1993.

Matheny, F. "The 10 Simplest Things You Can Do to Improve Your Fitness." *Bicycling Magazine* 35, no. 10 (November 1994): 84–85.

Mellion, Morris B., M.D. "Bicycling." *Sports Medicine Secrets.* Philadelphia, Penn.: Hanley & Belfus, Inc., 1995.

Van der Plas, Rob. *Choosing, Riding, & Maintaining the Off-Road Bicycle,* 34th ed. Mill Valley, Calif.: Bicycle Books, 1993.

Resources

Bicycle Federation of America, 1818 R. St. NW, Washington, DC 20009, (202) 332-6986. (Promotes bicycle transportation, recreation, and programs.)

The Bicycle Institute of America, 1506 21st St., NW, Washington, DC 20036, (800) 251-2453.

Bicycling Magazine, 33 E. Minor Street, Emmaus, PA 18049.

International Mountain Bicycling Association, P.O. Box 412043, Los Angeles, CA 90041, (818) 792–8830. (Promotes bicycle access to public lands and cyclist education.)

League of American Wheelmen, 67 Whitestone Rd., Suite 209, Baltimore, MD 21207, Palatine, IL 60067 (708) 991-1200 (bicyclists and clubs)

National Off-Road Bicycle Association, P.O. Box 1901, Chandler, AZ 85244. (Promotes off-road bicycling.)

Internet Information

For information on biking events, racing, bike guides, general tips, and maintenance, contact Anonymous FTP: Address: draco.acs.uci.edu. Path:/pub/rec.bicycles./*. Address: rtfm.mit.edu. Path: /pub/usenet/news.answers/bicycles-faq/*. Address: ugle.unit.no. Path: /local/biking/*.

Listserve: Bikecommute. Discussion regarding bicycle transportation and improvement of bicycling conditions. To subscribe to the list, send a message requesting a subscription to this URL: Address: Bikecommute-request@bike2work.eng.sun.com.

Basic Bicycle Tool Kit

If you wish to save money and time by doing much of your own maintenance, the following tools are recommended: tire patch kit, tire irons, adjustable wrench or set of crescent wrenches (best), third hand (for brakes), screwdriver, tire gauge, silicone lubricant, tire pump.

How to Fix a Flat Tire

1. *Remove wheel.* Caliper brakes may need to be loosened to permit wheel removal. Loosen axle nuts and remove the wheel from the forks. In the rear, you must also press the tension roller forward to wiggle the wheel out.
2. *Remove the tire.* Push the tire irons between the rim and bead. Pry up the tire carefully so as not to pinch and further damage the tube. Work around the tire.
3. *Push the valve stem into the rim and pull the tube out of the tire.* Locate the source of the puncture and remove it from the tire. Feel the inside of the tire to check for foreign objects. Also check the rim to make sure a spoke is not protruding. Mark the puncture on the tube. If the source of the leak is not readily apparent, slightly inflate the tire and listen for a hiss or put the tube in water and look for bubbles. Dry the tube and mark the hole with chalk. Deflate.
4. *Read and follow the patch kit directions.* Rough around the puncture with a roughing tool. Apply a thin layer of cement and let it dry thoroughly. Apply the patch, pressing out air bubbles.
5. *Replace the tube in the tire, valve first.*
6. *Replace the bead of the tire in the rim,* being careful to avoid pinching the tube between the bead and the tire. Use tire irons to replace the last few inches of the tire bead.
7. *Inflate the tire.* Replace it, center it between the forks, tighten the axle nuts and, if necessary, the brakes.

Bicycle Inspection Checklist

Name _____

Bicycle make & model _____ Serial no. _____

Note: Proper bicycle fit and maintenance are essential for comfort, safety, and riding efficiency. Any problems must be identified and corrected before the first ride.

	OK	FIX

Frame Size
Can you straddle the frame with both feet flat on the ground? You need a 1- to 2-inch space between your crotch and the top bar for road bikes and 3 to 4 inches for all-terrain bikes.   _____ _____

Saddle
Horizontal adjustment: The nose of the saddle should be 1 to 3 inches behind a vertical line drawn through the crank hanger. A cyclist 5 feet 6 inches tall would position the saddle 1 inch back (5 feet 10 inches: 2 inches back; 6 feet 3 inches: 3 inches back).   _____ _____

Vertical adjustment: Sit on the bike with your heel on the pedal at the lowest position. Your knee should be straight.   _____ _____

Tilt: Make sure it is horizontal or slightly downtilted.   _____ _____

Is the saddle tight and in good condition?   _____ _____

Handlebars
Vertical adjustment: The top bar should be level with the nose of the saddle.   _____ _____

Horizontal adjustment: Place your elbow on the nose of the saddle. Your outstretched fingertips should just touch the center of the handlebars. The length of the stem may need to be changed.   _____ _____

The handlebars should be in line with the wheel and symmetrical.   _____ _____

The handlebars should be tight; there should be no horizontal or vertical movement.   _____ _____

The tubing ends should be plugged and the grips tight.   _____ _____

Tire Pressure
The correct pressure (embossed on the side of the tire) for this bike is _____. Check the pressure once a week.   _____ _____

Bolts
Check bolts for looseness monthly.   _____ _____

Hand Brakes
Is there adequate space between the lever and the handlebar when the brakes are engaged? If not, tighten the cable.   _____ _____

The cable should be taut, with no kinks, rust, or frayed ends.   _____ _____

The brake shoes should be tight. The openings should face the rear of the bike.   _____ _____

Are the brake shoes level with and no more than $\frac{1}{8}$ inch from the rim?   _____ _____

Is there at least $\frac{3}{16}$ inch rubber remaining? Replace if needed.   _____ _____

Test the operation of each brake separately. They must hold without catching.

    Front   _____ _____

    Rear   _____ _____

Wheels
Spin each wheel. They should run true, without wobbles.   _____ _____

They should have no bindings or looseness (bearings).   _____ _____

They should be centered between forks (and chain stays in the rear).   _____ _____

Rim: Is it dented or kinked?   _____ _____

Spokes: Are they all intact and tight?   _____ _____

Tire: Is each tire properly seated? Is there at least $\frac{1}{8}$ inch of tread remaining?   _____ _____

Derailleurs
Turn the bike upside down or have a partner lift the rear wheel while you crank the pedal and shift through first the front and then the rear gears. (Shift only while the pedal is turning!) The derailleur should shift the chain smoothly from one sprocket to the next without skipping a gear, catching, or throwing off the chain.   _____ _____

Chain and Sprocket
Is the chain dirty? If so, clean it with silicone spray.   _____ _____

The sprocket teeth should be intact and not bent or broken.   _____ _____

Pedals
The pedals should be intact and tight.   _____ _____

The tread should be intact and tight.   _____ _____

Press down on both pedals at once. Are they tight?   _____ _____

appendix 3

Fitness Swimming

Advantages/Disadvantages

Swimming is a superb form of exercise. It is a total body workout using major muscle groups of both the upper and lower body. Other forms of aerobic exercise, jogging for example, use mainly large muscles of the lower body. In addition, water exercise is a natural form of strength training. Resistance of the water against the body's movements enhances muscle strength. Swimmers are also subject to fewer injuries than are participants in many other activities. Joint and muscle injuries are not common among swimmers because of water buoyancy. Water supports the body, alleviating the jarring effects of weight-bearing exercise such as aerobics or jogging. Swimming is ideal for the overweight, the arthritic, the injured, the elderly, and those prone to joint problems.

Another advantage of swimming is the rare occurrence of heat exhaustion and heat stroke. This can be a concern when exercising in hot, humid weather. If you don't like to sweat, you will probably prefer to exercise in water.

Swimming does have its drawbacks. You must have some swimming ability and have access to a pool at a time convenient for you. That first plunge into the water may be difficult for some, but after a brief warm-up period, the cool water temperature will be invigorating. Warm water quickly becomes uncomfortable during a vigorous workout.

Although the injury rate is very low, you may experience some minor annoyances as you train in water. Eye irritations and "swimmer's ear" are the most common.

The inconvenience of having to redo makeup and hair is minor when you measure the positive outcomes of aquatic exercise. After the workout, an efficient hair and makeup routine develops quickly.

What to Wear

Swimming is an inexpensive sport since the only equipment needed is a comfortable swimming suit. Many swimmers wear goggles to protect their eyes and, for added comfort, you may wish to use ear plugs and a swim cap. Swimmers can exercise indoors or outside, making it a year-round sport.

Technique and Safety Tips

Learn to swim the following five basic strokes efficiently: sidestroke, elementary backstroke, breaststroke, back crawl, and front crawl. Incorporate stroke mechanics sessions on these strokes into each workout. The butterfly stroke is too strenuous for most fitness swimmers.

Learn and practice the front crawl flip turn and the back crawl spin turn. These will make lap swimming more enjoyable. Construct your daily training program to include a water warm-up, conditioning bout, and water cool-down. Monitor your heart rate, and do not allow it to exceed your swimming target zone. Use hand paddles, kickboards, pull buoys, and swim fins to increase muscular strength and stroke efficiency. Hyperextension of the lower back (arching) is natural in water exercise. It is important to strengthen the abdominal muscles and always stretch the lower back area to counteract this tendency.

Here are other safety tips:

1. *Never swim alone.* A lifeguard should be present. Safety equipment, such as a ring buoy and reaching pole, should also be available.
2. *Do not dive into the pool at the shallow end.* The risk is too great. Even experienced swimmers have misjudged the depth of the water and hit the bottom, resulting in serious injuries.
3. *Stay to the right of the lane and make your turns counterclockwise.*
4. *If resting at the pool edge, keep to one side of the lane to allow other swimmers to turn easily.*
5. *Be careful with electrical equipment around the pool* (radios, pace clocks, etc.). Make sure electrical outlets are grounded.
6. *Keep telephone and emergency rescue numbers in the pool area.*
7. *Keep all doors going into the pool area locked unless there is a lifeguard on duty.*

Heart Rate During Swimming

Do not use the same target heart rate range when you swim as when you perform land sports. Weight-bearing activities such as running, aerobic dance, and fitness walking cause the heart to beat faster. Thus, to avoid risk of overtraining and for more comfortable workouts, reduce your swimming THR by approximately *10 percent* (see Chapter 2).

For example, if your THR for land activities is 150 to 170 bpm, your swimming THR would be 135 to 153 bpm:

1. $150 \times 0.10 = 15$ $170 \times 0.10 = 17$
2. $150 - 15 = 135$ $170 - 17 = 153$
3. Swimming THR = 135–153 bpm

How to Begin and Progress

Assess your aerobic swimming fitness on the 500-yard swim as described in Chapter 4. Based on your fitness category, begin at the appropriate starting level. Progress through each level, one step at a time. Do not skip steps and stay on each as long as necessary to adapt to that workload. Remember to monitor your pulse and do not exceed your swimming target heart rate range. When you have completed level M, you may want to swim continuously for distance or time or continue with the routine of four lengths and a brief rest for the measured distance or time. Keep in mind the FITT prescription factors covered in Chapter 2.

Note: In this program, swim the number of lengths suggested, but if the workout feels too hard, rest a few seconds by climbing out of the pool and walking back to the starting point, or rest at the end of the pool for a few seconds before continuing the workout. Swim the front crawl, if possible, or any stroke that allows you to reach the prescribed swimming target heart rate. Consult the pool distance table.

Pool Distance

Most standard pools are 25 yards in length

One length = 25 yards

One lap = two lengths

18 lengths = 1/4 mile	(approx. 450 yds.)
35 lengths = 1/2 mile	(approx. 875 yds.)
53 lengths = 3/4 mile	(approx. 1325 yds.)
70 lengths = 1 mile	(approx. 1750 yds.)

Fitness Swim Program

Fitness category	Starting level
Very low	S
Low	S
Average	W
Good	I
Excellent	M

Level S					Level W			
Lengths		Repeats	Distance		Lengths		Repeats	Distance
1	×	4	=	100 yds.	2	×	4	= 200 yds.
1	×	6	=	150 yds.	2	×	5	= 250 yds.
1	×	8	=	200 yds.	2	×	6	= 300 yds.
1	×	10	=	250 yds.	2	×	7	= 350 yds.
					2	×	8	= 400 yds.
					2	×	9	= 450 yds.
					2	×	10	= 500 yds.
					2	×	11	= 550 yds.

Level I					Level M			
Lengths		Repeats	Distance		Lengths		Repeats	Distance
3	×	7	=	525 yds.	4	×	7	= 700 yds.
3	×	8	=	600 yds.	4	×	8	= 800 yds.
3	×	9	=	675 yds.	4	×	9	= 900 yds.
3	×	10	=	750 yds.	4	×	10	= 1000 yds.
3	×	11	=	825 yds.	4	×	11	= 1100 yds.
3	×	12	=	900 yds.	4	×	12	= 1200 yds.
3	×	13	=	975 yds.				
3	×	14	=	1050 yds.				

Variety

To add variety to your swimming workouts, practice stroke mechanics on the five basic strokes. This will allow you to use a variety of strokes in your workouts instead of being limited to one or two. Swim for time instead of distance for a change or vice versa. Use swim fins, pull buoys, swim trainers, hand paddles, kickboards, webbed gloves, or a tethering system to add interest to your workouts. These devices also improve strength and stroke efficiency. For a complete change of pace, try an aquacircuiting or water running session in shallow water or a deep water jogging workout using some type of flotation device. See Appendix 6.

Discomforts

While swimmers are less susceptible to injuries, they may experience a few minor discomforts. Eye irritations are caused by an imbalance in the pH of the water (balance of acidity and alkalinity) or excessive amounts of chlorine. Wear goggles and you will have no problem. *Swimmer's ear* refers to a rashlike inflammation of the ear canal that is caused by frequent exposure to moisture. Dry your ears thoroughly with a towel to prevent this nuisance. If you have frequent ear infections, it would be wise to purchase a pair of ear plugs. See a specialist to get a good fit; those purchased over the counter do not fit well enough to keep water out of the ear canal. A few swimmers complain of sore shoulders. A certain amount of soreness is normal during the first weeks of training. But if pain persists, you may be developing tendinitis. Shoulder tendinitis may be caused by an inherent structural shoulder problem, use of hand paddles, or improper stroke mechanics. See an orthopedic specialist if shoulder pain persists and use strokes with an underwater recovery (i.e., breaststroke, sidestroke, and elementary backstroke). Some swimmers experience knee pain, especially along the inner borders of the knees when swimming the breaststroke and elementary backstroke. This is caused by the kick used in these strokes. Do not swim the breaststroke or elementary backstroke until the pain subsides or avoid them altogether. It is a common myth that you are more susceptible to colds if you participate in aquatic activities, especially during the winter. Colds and respiratory infections are caused by viruses and are spread by contact with infected individuals. You are more likely to catch a cold in a warm, dry, crowded room than in a swimming pool. Another myth is that swimming during menstruation is prohibited. Minor discomfort during this period may be alleviated by exercise. If cramps are severe, use your judgment.

References

Colwin, Cecil. *Swimming into the 21st Century.* Champaign, Ill.: Human Kinetics Publishers, Inc., 1992 (Box 5076, Champaign, IL 61825-5076).

Costill, David, Ernest Maglischo, and Allen Richardson. *Swimming.* Champaign, Ill.: Human Kinetics Publishers, Inc., 1992 (Box 5076, Champaign, IL 61825-5076).

Thomas, David. *Advanced Swimming.* Champaign, Ill.: Human Kinetics Publishers, Inc., 1990 (Box 5076, Champaign, IL 61825-5076).

Resources

American Red Cross, National Headquarters, 431 18th St. N.W., Washington, DC 20006.

Aquatic Exercise Association (AEA), P.O. Box 1609, Nokomis, FL 34274, (813) 486-8600.

Aquatics International, 6151 Powers Ferry Road, Atlanta, GA 30339-2941.

Council for National Cooperation in Aquatics (CNCA), 901 W. New York Street, Indianapolis, IN 46223, (317) 638-4238.

International Swimming Hall of Fame, 1 Hall of Fame Drive, Ft. Lauderdale, FL 33316, (305) 462-6536.

United States Masters Swimming, 2 Peter Ave., Rutland, MA 01543, (508) 886-6631.

United States Swimming, 1750 E. Boulder St., Colorado Springs, CO 80909, (719) 578-4578.

United States Water Fitness Association (USWFA), John Spannuth, Executive Director, P.O. Box 3279, Boynton Beach, FL 33424.

YMCA of the USA, 101 N. Wacker Dr., 14th fl., Chicago, IL 60606, (312) 977-0031.

appendix 4

Jogging

Advantages/Disadvantages

Running is a simple way to develop cardiorespiratory endurance. You can do it alone, with a partner, or with a group. A good pair of running shoes is the only equipment you need. Finding a place to run is as simple as walking out your front door. Getting a full workout through running takes less time than many other aerobic activities. It can be done in most types of weather, on vacation, or during a lunch break. As a weight-bearing exercise, jogging provides stress to the long bones, which aids in maintenance of bone mineralization and decreases risk of osteoporosis. Like other aerobic activities, jogging has positive benefits in reducing obesity, stress, type II diabetes, and several heart disease risk factors.

Drawbacks to running include traffic, uneven pavement, and, occasionally, an aggressive dog. Trying to progress too quickly may cause impact problems such as shin splints or sore knees. Jogging is not for everyone. For individuals who are prone to musculoskeletal problems, low- or nonimpact activities such as bicycling or water exercise are less likely to precipitate injury. If you are overweight or very out of shape, it may be best to start with a less intense activity, such as walking. Nonetheless, a carefully planned program of progressive activity enables many people to enjoy running as part of their fitness program.

What to Wear

You can run in almost any kind of weather if you dress appropriately. On hot days, wear as little as decently possible—shoes, socks, shirt, and shorts. For cooler weather, add layers: a long-sleeved T-shirt and tights or long pants. In cold weather, add a jacket or a turtleneck sweater and, to protect ears and hands, a stocking cap and mittens. In wet weather, wear a cap with a brim to keep rain out of your eyes and rain-repellent clothing, if desired. Keep in mind that when you are running, you generate a great deal of body heat. When you are warmed up, it will feel about 20 degrees warmer than the actual temperature. A hot day would be 70 degrees or higher, a warm day 50 to 60 degrees, a cool day 30 to 40 degrees, and a cold day below freezing. High humidity on hot days and the windchill factor on cold days also should be considered (see Chapter 8).

A good pair of properly fitted running shoes is important in preventing injuries. When running, your foot strikes the ground with an impact of approximately three times your body weight. A well-made running shoe fitted by a trained salesperson can absorb shock and support the foot. A cheap pair of poor quality shoes is no bargain if it leaves you with blisters or shin splints.

Technique and Safety Tips

Good running form is relaxed and mechanically efficient. Your energy goes into moving you forward and is not dissipated in extraneous movements. Maintain a relaxed, erect posture, head up, eyes looking ahead. Keep your shoulders relaxed and level, arms swinging freely from the shoulder, hands unclenched, traveling between the hips and lower chest. Avoid hunching forward, your eyes watching your feet, your arms held stiffly or swinging across the midline of your body. Knees and feet should aim ahead, not to the center or side. Foot contact should be heel to ball or midfoot, not on the toes like a sprinter. Keep your stride length comfortable and effortless, with your foot landing under your center of gravity. Be careful not to overstride or bounce when you run. Stride length is a product of speed and leg strength. Unless you increase one of these elements, attempts to increase your stride length will waste energy. Breathe through your mouth and nose. It is hard to get enough air breathing through the nose alone.

While you are working on your running form, there are some safety guidelines you need to keep in mind:

1. *Before leaving home, let someone know your route* and when you expect to return. Carry identification.
2. *If you wear a headset, keep the volume low* enough so you can hear approaching traffic.
3. *Keep alert.*
4. *If there is a sidewalk, jog on it.*
5. *If there is no sidewalk, run facing traffic on the extreme left edge or shoulder of the road.*
6. *Respect private property.* Do not run across lawns.
7. *Obey traffic signs and signals.* When crossing a street at the light, cross with the green light only.
8. *Maintain eye contact with motorists* whenever you cross in front of them.
9. *Give the right-of-way to cars.* Don't antagonize drivers, even if they try your patience.
10. *If you run at night, wear light-colored clothing with reflective strips.*
11. *At night, do not run in unfamiliar areas.*
12. *Do not wear a vinyl sweat suit* while exercising, ever!

How to Begin and Progress

Begin at the level indicated by your cardiorespiratory fitness assessment (Chapter 4) and progress slowly. If you cannot complete a mile in 15 minutes, then begin with walking briskly 15 to 30 minutes until your heart rate stays within the target range. When you can comfortably handle 2 miles in 30 minutes, you may begin the jog/walk program. As in all activities, follow the FITT guidelines.

Run/Walk Program

Fitness Category	Starting Level
Very low	1, 2, or 3
Low	4
Average	5 or 6
Good	7 or 8
Excellent	9 or 10

Level	Run	Walk	Repeats
1	——	15–20 min.	1
2	——	20–30 min.	1
3	30 sec.	30 sec.	8–12 plus 10- to 15-min. walk
4	1 min.	30 sec.	6–10 plus 10-min. walk
5	2 min.	30 sec.	4–10 plus 5- to 10-min. walk
6	4 min.	1 min.	4–6
7	6 min.	1 min.	4–5
8	8 min.	1–2 min.	3–4
9	12 min.	2 min.	2
10	20–30 min.	5 min.	1

Start at the level appropriate for your fitness category. Remember that your starting level does not indicate your potential. For each run-walk interval, begin with the lowest number of repeats indicated and, each successive workout, add one repeat. When you can do the maximum number of intervals at one level, move to the next level. A 5-minute warm-up and 5-minute cool-down should accompany each workout. You may stay at one level as long as you need to or even move back a step if the beginning level is too difficult. If the workout has been appropriate, you should feel refreshed and relaxed, not exhausted, after exercise.

Variety

Much of the variety in running comes from running different routes and from observing the changing scenery and seasons. If you run alone, you may wish to occasionally run with a partner or a group. Instead of taking a long run at a continuous pace, you might try *fartlek*, a Swedish term for *speed-play*. Fartlek mixes fast-paced runs, brief all-out sprints, and slow-paced recovery intervals. It is best done on uneven or hilly terrain such as a park or golf course. Interval training done once or no more than twice a week can add a change of pace. This alternates a fast-paced run over a predetermined distance with walking or a slow recovery jog. An example might be running 220 yards, four to six times in 40 to 50 seconds with a 220-yard walk between each. With interval training, you may vary the distance run, recovery interval, number of repetitions, and time or pace of the run. These workouts are usually done on the track but can be done on the road by running and then walking a set amount of time, by running a certain number of telephone pole intervals, or by selecting a long hill on your route and running up it several times. A fitness trail, or parcour, with exercise stations linked by a running trail, may be available at a local park or university or you can make your own. To simulate a parcour on a regular running route, stop every 2 to 4 minutes to do a stretching or toning exercise (i.e., hamstring stretch, run 2 minutes, calf stretch, run 3 minutes, push-ups, run 3 minutes, abdominal curls, . . .).

Some activities are suitable for a small group. You can take a tennis or foam ball along to toss among some friends. You'll get quite a workout because it mixes sprinting and upper body exercise into the run. This is safer if your route has little traffic. Hashing is a popular club sport in the southern United States, Europe, and Russia. The idea is for a group to follow a marked course through an unfamiliar area. Elected group members meet at an earlier time to mark the route, usually with flour. Orienteering is popular in some areas. This is a cross-country type of activity in which participants navigate from point to point utilizing a map and compass, covering distances from 2 to 10 miles. Local fun-runs give you a chance to run with and meet other runners in a noncompetitive atmosphere. If you like competition, you can get information on road races from your local running club or athletic shoe store.

Common Discomforts

Most aches and pains in running do not occur suddenly. They are often from overuse—a long steady erosion that wears down the body. Many general complaints are addressed in Chapter 5. Specific to running, two additional discomforts, easily avoided, occasionally occur. If you run with shoes that are too short or that don't fit well, in addition to developing blisters you could injure a toe. The toenail may turn black and possibly even fall off. While painful, the condition is not permanent. The nail will grow back. If your thighs rub together when you run, you may suffer an abrasion. The solution is to apply vaseline to the area and to wear tights or shorts that cover your thighs.

References

Boyer, Brian, M.D., et al. "Preventing Common Runners' Injuries." *Patient Care* 28, no. 2 (July 1994): 72–81.

Brown, Dick, and Joe Henderson. *Fitness Running*. Champaign, Ill.: Human Kinetics, 1994.

"Conditioning for the Beginning Runner." *Patient Care* 28, no. 2 (July 1994): 85.

Ellis, Joe, and Joe Henderson. *Running Injury Free: How to Prevent, Treat and Recover from Dozens of Painful Problems*. Emmaus, Penn.: Rodale Press, Inc., 1994.

Lebow, Fred. *New York Road Runners Club Complete Book of Running*. New York: Random House Press, 1994.

Newsholme, Eric, et al. *Keep on Running: The Science of Training and Performance*. New York: Wiley, 1994.

"Running for Health and Fitness: Tips for Beginners." *Patient Care* 28, no. 2 (July 1994): 85.

"Select a Shoe That Fits, and Wear It." *Patient Care* 28, no. 2 (July 1994): 85.

Sheehan, George. *George Sheehan on Running to Win: How to Achieve the Physical, Mental and Spiritual Victories of Running*. Emmaus, Penn.: Rodale Press, Inc., 1994.

Silva Orienteering Services. "Learn Orienteering," "Orienteering," "So You Want to Know About Orienteering," and "Teaching Orienteering." Binghamton, N.Y.: Silva, 1994.

"Stretch Before You Run." *Patient Care* 28, no. 2 (July 1994): 85.

Resources

American Running and Fitness Association, 9310 Old Georgetown Road, Bethesda, MD 20814-1111, (301) 897-0197.

The Runner, Ziff-Davis Publishing Co., P.O. Box 2702, Boulder, CO 80321.

Runner's World Magazine, Box 366, Mountain View, CA 94042.

Silva Orienteering Services USA, P.O. Box 1604, Binghamton, NY 13902.

Internet Addresses

The Dead Runners Society is a mailing list for runners who like to talk about the mental and personal aspects of running. To subscribe to the list, send an e-mail message requesting a subscription to Mailto:dead-runners-request@unix.sas.com.

Fitness Walking

Walking is man's best medicine.

Hippocrates

Advantages/Disadvantages

Walking is simple, enjoyable, and probably the safest form of aerobic exercise known. It is inexpensive and can be done by almost anyone, any place, any time. There is no need to join a club or to find partners or opponents. It is a wise exercise choice for the overweight, the older adult, the very out-of-shape, the postsurgical patient, and the individual in a cardiac rehabilitation program. Appropriate shoes and comfortable clothes are the only equipment you need. Walking is excellent for weight control. In fact, you use as many calories walking a mile as you would jogging the same distance. The difference is that walking takes longer. Even though the injury rate is very low, some walkers who try to increase distance and pace too quickly may experience sore muscles and knees or other discomforts. Another disadvantage to walking is that the already physically fit may not be able to elevate the heart rate into the target zone. In this case, try one of the advanced forms of fitness walking, such as power walking (with hand weights) or race walking. Dogs and inclement weather present other problems to the walker. Many shopping malls have opened their doors for early morning walking and also to provide a safe, weather-controlled environment year-round.

What to Wear

You don't have to buy special clothes; anything loose and comfortable will do. It is a good idea to have a pocket for carrying identification, keys, and a handkerchief. For suggestions on dealing with weather, read the tips for hot and cold weather dressing provided in Appendix 4.

Studies show that walking generates a downward force of about one and one-half times your body weight, so wearing appropriate shoes is important in helping you progress smoothly and injury free. You may save a few dollars on inexpensive shoes, but a good pair of shoes will help protect your feet, legs, and back. When purchasing new shoes, go to a reputable store and ask for a trained salesperson. Look for shoes with a cushioned heel, flexible sole, firm heel support, and arch supports that fit your feet. The toe box must provide room for the toes to work to prevent blisters. Several companies manufacture shoes designed for the sport of walking. Try one of these or one made for crosstraining or jogging but be sure it fits your foot. The shoe should never feel like it needs to be broken in. It should feel comfortable from day one.

Do you replace your worn-out shoes soon enough? A study at Tulane University found that all shoes, regardless of brand, price, or type of construction, lose most of their shock absorbency after 500 miles of use. This is a good reason for keeping records of your mileage. Take your old shoes with you when shopping for a new pair so that a knowledgeable salesperson can evaluate the wear pattern to help you choose a suitable shoe.

Technique and Safety Tips

Walking posture is erect but relaxed. To alleviate tension, the abdomen should be pulled in, the rib cage lifted, and the shoulders pulled down. This will help you keep relaxed and increase your endurance. Your arms should be bent at about a 90 degree angle, and your hands (loose fist) should swing slightly above your waist. Your arms counterbalance your leg motion. You may discover during your walk that your arms have dropped, resulting in a slower pace. Visualize that you are walking in a straight line. Hold your head up with eyes focused ahead, watching the ground but not your feet. Your foot contact should be a heel roll to the ball of the foot and toes for pushing off. Resist the tendency to lean forward at the waist.

While you are walking, keep in mind these simple tips for a safe workout:

1. *Always carry some form of identification* (include pertinent medical information).
2. *Choose a safe time and place to exercise.* Take keys with you and lock the car and/or house.
3. *Plan your route carefully.* Use well-populated, well-lighted areas. Avoid areas that are dark and have dense shrubs and alleys.
4. *Know where you can get help along your route.*
5. *Use sidewalks or walk facing oncoming traffic* and walk in single file.
6. *Obey traffic signals and signs.* Do not jaywalk.
7. *Keep alert at all times.* Give the right-of-way to cars. Don't assume the driver sees you.
8. *Wear bright, reflective clothing at dusk or night.*
9. *Tell someone where you are going and when you think you will return.* Better yet, use the buddy system. It's more fun to walk with someone.
10. *Avoid dogs by selecting routes that are free of them.* The best advice is to ignore a barking dog, and never walk between a barking dog and its human, especially if the human is a child.
11. *For the cleanest air, walk in the morning.* The air is more polluted at midday, and pollution drops after rush hour in the evening.
12. *Don't wear a headset;* you would be losing one of your most valuable sensory aids. If you wear a headset, keep volume low so you can hear traffic or approaching strangers.
13. *Avoid walking on snow/ice-covered roads and walks.*
14. *Avoid peak traffic hours* unless you can use a jogging path or a sidewalk.

Tips for Increasing Walking Pace

If you would like to increase your fitness walking pace try these techniques:

1. *Increase foot flexion.* This helps to increase the power of your pushing off from the ground as your foot extends. Mentally concentrate on forcing your foot to flex (as much as possible)

with each step. When attention to foot form relaxes, quickly return your awareness to proper form.

2. *Pump your arms*. When your arms drag, the tendency is to slow down. Resist this. Keep your arms pumping and your legs will be forced to keep pace.

3. *Set "walk-to" targets*. Set a "walk-to" target a short distance in front of you (about 30 yards). Walk quickly to the target, reset the target, and walk fast to the new target. Keep resetting the walk-to targets throughout the route. Use mailboxes, driveways, road signs, and trees for targets. This technique helps to keep you mentally involved in your fitness walking workout and helps you resist the tendency to stroll.

How to Begin and Progress

Test your fitness using the 1-mile walk test described in Chapter 4 (Fitness Assessment). Then follow the appropriate level on the W.A.L.K.S. Program. After completing the "S" level, continue on the W.A.L.K.S. Maintenance Program for a lifetime of fitness.

Warm up for 5 to 10 minutes before starting the conditioning segment of your workout. The warm-up should be activity specific, so for fitness walking begin gradually increasing the pace to that at your conditioning level. During the conditioning bout, always check your heart rate to be sure it stays within the target zone. Listen to your body and progress slowly for optimal results.

Cool down for 5 to 10 minutes following the conditioning bout. As in the warm-up, the cool-down should be activity specific. Thus, reduce your pace, finishing with 5 to 10 minutes of slow walking.

For total fitness, it is important to stretch for flexibility. Improved flexibility is best achieved if it occurs at the end of the cool-down when the muscles and joints are thoroughly warmed and pliable. Use the flexibility exercises found on pages 73–74 for your stretching routine.

Take each step on the chart and don't skip ahead. If the increase is too difficult, go back to the preceding level for awhile. You should feel energized after your workout, not exhausted.

W.A.L.K.S. Program

Fitness category	Starting program
Very low	W Level
Low	A Level
Average	L Level
Good	K Level
Excellent	S Level

W level

Week	1–2	3–4	5–6	7–8	9–10	11–12	13–14
Warm-up (min.)	5–10	5–10	5–10	5–10	5–10	5–10	5–10
Conditioning bout (mileage)	1.00	1.25	1.50	1.75	2.00	2.25	2.50
Intensity % (target heart rate)	60–75	60–75	60–75	60–75	60–75	60–75	60–75
Cool-down (min.)	5–10	5–10	5–10	5–10	5–10	5–10	5–10
Frequency	3	3	3	3	4	4	4

A level

Week	1–2	3–4	5–6	7–8	9–10	11–12	13–14
Warm-up (min.)	5–10	5–10	5–10	5–10	5–10	5–10	5–10
Conditioning bout (mileage)	2.00	2.25	2.50	2.75	3.00	3.25	3.50
Intensity % (target heart rate)	60–75	60–75	60–75	60–75	60–75	60–75	60–75
Cool-down (min.)	5–10	5–10	5–10	5–10	5–10	5–10	5–10
Frequency	3	3	3	4	4	4	4

L level

Week	1–2	3–4	5–6	7–8	9–10	11–12	13–14
Warm-up (min.)	5–10	5–10	5–10	5–10	5–10	5–10	5–10
Conditioning bout (mileage)	3.00	3.25	3.25	3.50	3.75	3.75	4.00
Intensity % (target heart rate)	60–75	60–75	60–75	60–75	60–75	60–75	60–75
Cool-down (min.)	5–10	5–10	5–10	5–10	5–10	5–10	5–10
Frequency	3	3	4	4	4	4	4

K level

Week	1–2	3–4	5–6	7–8	9–10	11–12	13–14
Warm-up (min.)	5–10	5–10	5–10	5–10	5–10	5–10	5–10
Conditioning bout (mileage)	3.50	3.75	3.75	4.00	4.00	4.00	4.00
Intensity % (target heart rate)	60–75	60–75	60–75	60–75	60–75	60–75	60–75
Cool-down (min.)	5–10	5–10	5–10	5–10	5–10	5–10	5–10
Frequency	4	4	4	4	5	5	5

	S level						
Week	1–2	3–4	5–6	7–8	9–10	11–12	13–14
Warm-up (min.)							
	5–10	5–10	5–10	5–10	5–10	5–10	5–10
Conditioning bout (mileage)							
	4.00	4.00	4.00	4.25	4.25	4.50	4.50
Intensity % (target heart rate)							
	60–75	60–75	60–75	60–75	60–75	60–75	60–75
Cool-down (min.)							
	5–10	5–10	5–10	5–10	5–10	5–10	5–10
Frequency							
	5	5	5	5	5	5	5

W.A.L.K.S. Maintenance Program (for a lifetime of fitness)

Warm-up:	5–10 min.
Conditioning bout:	3–5 miles per workout
Intensity %:	60–75
Cool-down:	5–10 min.
Frequency:	3–5 times per week
Weekly mileage:	9–25 miles

Variety

Adding variety to your walking workouts can keep you enthused about the sport for many years. Varying your walking routes gives you a change of scenery. Drive the car to a new area, park, and explore the surroundings during your workout. Mailing a letter, walking an errand, taking window shopping walks, and doing shopping mall workouts can be fun. Walk with a friend, in a group, or by yourself for a change. Get a dog; they make excellent walking companions. For a challenge, try an advanced exercise walking technique such as race walking, power walking, hill walking, or walking a fitness trail. Participate in a volksmarch, a competitive walking event, or join a Hashing Club (described in Appendix 4). Water walking (walking in waist-deep water) is popular in many areas; give it a try. Some people enjoy listening to music while exercising in a traffic-free area. You won't become stale or bored with exercise if you vary your workouts.

Common Discomforts

As in running, most aches, pains, and injuries from walking occur from overuse. Listen to your body. Don't attempt to work through an injury. It will only aggravate the condition. The two most common walking complaints are shin splints and back-of-the-knee soreness. Refer to Chapter 5 for information about shin splints. Cut back on pace and distance until all soreness subsides. Comfortable, well-fitting shoes will help prevent blisters. Consult a sports podiatrist if you suffer from foot problems such as calluses, bunions, heel spurs, ingrown toenails, high arches, flat feet, or an overly pronated foot. These conditions can be remedied but, if not corrected, may prevent you from fully enjoying your walking program.

References

Decker, June. *Y's Way to Fitness Walking*. Champaign, Ill.: Human Kinetics Publishers, Inc., 1989.

Ford, Normal. *Walk to Your Hearts Content: The Way to Fitness, Health and Adventure*. Woodstock, Vt.: The Countryman Press, Inc., 1992.

Hawkins, Jerald, and Sandra Weigle. *Walking for Fun and Fitness*. Englewood, Colo.: Morton Publishing Co., 1992.

Iknoian, Therese. *Fitness Walking*. Champaign, Ill.: Humans Kinetics Publishers, 1995.

Least Heat-Moon, William. *Prairyerth*. Boston: Houghton Mifflin, 1991.

Rose, Jessica, and James Gamble, eds. *Human Walking*, 2d ed. Williams and Wilkins, 1994.

Seiger, Lon, and James Hesson. *Walking for Fitness*, 2d ed. Dubuque, Iowa: Brown & Benchmark, 1994.

Sweetgall, Robert, James Rippe, and Frank Katch. *Fitness Walking*. New York: The Putnam Publishing, 1990.

Thoreau, Henry David. *Walking*. San Francisco: Harper, 1994.

Walking: A Complete Guide to the Complete Exercise. New York: Random, 1992.

Yanker, Gary. *Walking Medicine*. New York: McGraw Hill, 1990.

Resources

American Heart Association Walking Program, American Heart Association National Center, 7320 Greenville Ave., Dallas, TX 75231.

Heart and Sole Newsletter, National Organization of Mall Walkers, P.O. Box 191, Hermann, MO 65041.

North American Race-Walking Foundation (NARF), Box 50312, Pasadena, CA 91105-0312, (818) 577-2264.

Reebok Walking Program, Reebok International Ltd., 100 Technology Center Dr., P.O. Box 9116, Stoughton, MA 02072-9801.

The Rockport Walking Institute, P.O. Box 480, Marlboro, MA 01752.

Walkers Club of America, 445 E. 86th, New York, NY 10028.

The Walking Magazine, 11 Harcourt St., Boston, MA 02116, (617) 266-3322.

Walk Ways, Walk Ways Center, 733 15th St., NW, Washington, DC 20005.

W.A.L.K.S Fitness Walking Log

(make extra copies of this form as needed)

Week _____   Level _____

Date	Time of walk	Distance of walk	Exercise HR	Location of walk

Totals: _____   _____   _____   _____

Comments/goals: _____

_____

_____

Water Exercise/Aqua Aerobics

Advantages/Disadvantages

You don't have to know how to swim to get a vigorous workout in the water. You don't even have to get your head wet! As more and more people are discovering, exercising against water resistance in shallow water is a fine workout and great fun, especially with a group. Water exercise can be a social activity because you can carry on a conversation while working out. It is low impact, so joint problems are rare. The supportive effect of water buoyancy makes water exercise enjoyable and relaxing for individuals who have concerns about other forms of exercise. In chest-deep water, a person weighs only about 1/10th what he or she does on land. People who have arthritis or joint problems find that this buoyancy decreases stress to the joints, allowing a fuller range of motion than on land. It is easy to individualize intensity levels so that you get a good workout, whatever your level of fitness. Inclement weather is a not a problem. Water exercise is cool, even on the hottest summer days, so heat stress is eliminated. It is also a comfortable indoor workout for rainy or cold winter days. If you are overweight and sensitive about exercising in public, the water covers you up so that you don't feel so self-conscious. Water exercise is also beneficial during pregnancy because of both decreased joint stress and decreased heat stress as compared to other forms of exercise.

The drawbacks are few. You need access to a pool at a time when you can have a lane separate from lap swimmers. It is probably best to first join a class to learn the exercises and activities. Then you can work out on your own.

What to Wear

A comfortable swimsuit is all that is required. Some people also like to wear pool shoes to protect their feet when doing water running and walking workouts.

Technique and Safety Tips

Workouts may have a muscle toning emphasis or an aerobic emphasis or combine the two. In constructing workouts, maintain muscle balance by exercising all major muscle groups. Particularly emphasize stretching tight muscle groups (i.e., lower back, hamstrings, calves) and toning weak areas (i.e., abdominals, upper body). To overload, keep in mind that, as in weight training, water adds resistance. The harder you push and pull, the more resistance you create and the more benefit you receive. In any activity, it is important to limit back hyperextension by keeping abdominals firm while exercises are being performed. In the water, as on land, workouts must maintain a training heart rate for 20 to 30 minutes to produce aerobic benefit. Training heart rates for swimmers appear to be about 10 percent lower than for land exercisers. This may also be true for other cardiorespiratory water exercise. In order to calculate an appropriate exercise intensity for water exercise, subtract ` percent from your training pulse on land. Jogging in the water, aqua

aerobics, and other vigorous activities can all provide aerobic benefit if an adequate overload occurs. Several books that give examples of water exercises are available and are listed at the end of this appendix.

Whenever you exercise in the water, a few safety guidelines must be followed:

1. *Never work out in the water alone.* A lifeguard or workout partner, preferably one who can swim, should be present. Safety equipment, such as a life ring or reaching pole, should also be available.
2. *Shower before entering the pool.*
3. *Do not go into the deep water unless you can swim.*
4. *Don't mix water and electricity.* If you like to exercise to music, keep electrical equipment away from the water and make sure that all electric outlets have ground-fault circuit interrupters that shut off the electricity if it contacts water. Better yet, use battery-powered equipment.
5. *Do not enter the pool if you have an open sore, infection, or rash.*
6. *Do all exercises through a full range of motion with slow, controlled movements.* Swinging or flinging movements can injure joints.
7. *Maintain good body alignment in walking and jogging.* Keep abdominals tight and hips tucked under and avoid excessive forward lean.

How to Begin and Progress

Water exercise workouts, like other aerobic programs, should incorporate a warm-up, conditioning period, and cool-down. The warm-up may be started on deck or in the water and may include a musculoskeletal (thermal) warm-up, stretching, and cardiorespiratory warm-up, transitioning smoothly into the conditioning bout. A thermal warm-up includes controlled movements using a gradually increasing range of motion and is designed to gradually increase muscle temperature. Prestretching exercises are designed to prepare muscles for activity and are generally held 5 to 10 seconds. A cardiorespiratory warm-up follows to transition the heart, lungs, and muscles gradually to an increased intensity level. Water exercise may involve many different activities—aerobic, muscle toning, and stretching. Recommendations on how to progress are given for the aerobic portion of the workout (i.e., water running) in terms of length of time at a training heart rate.

Water Exercise Program

Fitness category	Starting level
Very low	1
Low	2
Average	3
Good	4
Excellent	5 or 6

Level	Vigorous	Easy	Sets	Total time
1	1 min.	30 secs.	8–12	10–18 mins.
2	2 mins.	30 secs.	6–8	15–20 mins.
3	4 mins.	30 secs.	4–6	18–27 mins.
4	6 mins.	30 secs.	3–4	19–26 mins.
5	8–10 mins.	1 min.	3	26–32 mins.
6	continuous		1	30 min.

Follow the conditioning bout with a 5 to 10 minute cool-down combining a period of gradually decreasing intensity exercise with stretching for flexibility.

Variety

Exercise with friends or with music. After mastering the exercises with only water resistance, you may wish to add kickboards, pull buoys, or other water exercise equipment to increase resistance. Vary the exercises and activities so that you don't do the same workout two days in a row. For example, an aerobic workout may involve, on different days, running or walking widths, aqua-aerobics, step aerobics, water games, deep water running, treading and kicking drills, or circuit training. There are so many different things to do in the water it is easy to add variety. Some examples of different types of workouts follow.

Muscular strength and endurance are built by performing repeats of exercises against resistance: side leg swings to tone inner thigh and outer hip, straight arm raises to tone deltoids, back leg swings to strengthen hamstrings and gluteus. A series of 8 to 12 exercises covering all major muscle groups can be performed 1 minute each and repeated two to three times for a thorough muscular workout.

Water walking involves walking in waist- to chest-deep water fast enough to produce a target heart rate. Good body alignment during walking and jogging is important. Walk tall with abdominals pulled in and buttocks tucked in to avoid leaning forward. It is also essential, for muscle balance, to vary the walking movements. Variations include walking forward, backward, or sideways and adding different arm variations such as forward pulls, breaststroke, or backstroke.

Shallow-water jogging is similar to water walking but is more intense, using a faster, bounding stride. A common error here is running too much on the balls of the feet, which causes excessive calf tightness. Try to press your heel down to the pool bottom before pushing off on your toes.

Deep-water jogging is a nonimpact workout. Exercisers wear a flotation vest or belt and run, varying directions and arm movements.

Interval training alternates high- and low-intensity workout segments. This can allow even the most athletic exerciser to get a vigorous workout. For example, you might alternate four laps of shallow-water running with two laps of water walking.

Water aerobics, like land aerobics, puts exercise to music. Workouts may be either choreographed or freestyle. Bench step workouts have also made the transition into the aquatic environment, with similar benefits as in land workouts.

Plyometrics are vigorous jumping and bounding exercises that increase muscle strength and power. They are also very aerobic. Examples include high jumps in place, bounding across the pool, and a series of high two-foot hops. Because these are impact exercises, they can cause injury, are only for well-conditioned exercisers, and should be avoided if you have ankle, knee, or back problems.

In circuit training, a series of exercises are performed for a certain number of repetitions or a given amount of time (i.e., 1 minute each of side leg circles, jumping jacks, push-ups, forward kicks, etc.).

Exercises may be written on numbered cards placed around the pool edge, and as each exercise is completed, participants move quickly to the next exercise station. Exercises may stress one fitness component or several. A set of 8 to 12 exercises can be repeated, or time at each station can be increased to produce overload.

Flexibility exercises are often used as a part of a water exercise program. A static stretch is held 20 to 30 seconds or more for each major muscle group in order to increase range of motion. Occasionally, it is fun to try a water game for variety. Examples include shallow-water polo, inner-tube water polo, water baseball, freeze tag, sharks and minnows, water basketball, or volleyball.

Common Discomforts

The most common discomforts water exercisers encounter are tight calves and blisters from running barefoot on the pool bottom. Blisters can be avoided by starting with only a few minutes of running in the pool and giving the feet time to toughen as you gradually progress in workouts. You could also wear pool shoes or clean sneakers during workouts. Calves tend to get tight because, due to buoyancy, most running and walking in the pool is done on the ball of the foot. Simply take care to stretch calves before and after the workout to maintain flexibility.

References

Casten, Carole M. *Aqua Aerobics Today.* St. Paul, Minn.: West Publishing Co., 1993.

Katz, Jane. *Water Fitness During Your Pregnancy.* Champaign, Ill.: Human Kinetics Publishers, 1994.

Kinder, Tom, and Julie See. *Aqua Aerobics: A Scientific Approach.* Dubuque, Iowa: Eddie Bowers Publishing, Inc., 1992.

Mehale, G. A. "Deep Water Exercise—A New Approach to Fitness." *Journal of Strength and Conditioning Research* 16, no. 3 (June 1994).

Rettig, Sam, and Drucie French. *Training for Fabulous People of Every Kind.* McLean, Va.: DFC Seminars, 1993.

Roitman, V. "Water Exercise." in Corbin, D. E. and J. Metal-Corbin, eds. *Reach for It: A Handbook for Health, Exercise and Dance Activities for Older Adults,* 2d ed. Dubuque, Iowa: Eddie Bowers, 1990.

Sova, Ruth. *Aquatics: The Complete Reference Guide for Aquatic Fitness Professionals.*

Sova, Ruth. *Aquatics Activities Handbook.* Boston: Jones and Bartlett, 1993.

Spitzer, Terry-Ann, and Werner Hoeger. *Physical Fitness the Water Aerobics Way.* Englewood, Colo.: Morton Publishing Company, 1990.

Whitelock, Helen. *Water Exercise for Better Health.* New York: Lothian Publishing, 1993.

Resources

The Aquatic Exercise Association, Inc., P.O. Box 1609, Nokomis, FL 34274, (813) 486-8600.

IDEA Resource Library: Aqua Exercise, IDEA: The Association for Fitness Professionals, 6190 Cornerstone Court E., Suite 204, San Diego, CA 92121-3773.

U.S. Water Fitness Association, John Spannuth, Executive Director, P.O. Box 3219, Boynton Beach, FL 33424-3279.

Equipment Companies

AFA/Aquarobics, Inc., Box 5752, Greenville, SC 29606.

Aqua-Circuit, U.S. Games, Inc., P.O. Box 117028, Carrolton, TX 75011-7028, (800) 327-0484.

Dynamix Music Services, 711 W. 40th St., Suite 428, Baltimore, MD 21211, (800) 843-6499.

Fitness Wholesale, 895 Hampshire Rd., Stowe, OH 44224, (800) 537-5512.

Hydro-Tone Fitness Systems Inc., 16691 Gothard St., Suite M, Huntington Beach, CA 92647, (800) 622-TONE.

appendix 7

Indoor Exercise Equipment

Advantages/Disadvantages

When winter's plummeting temperatures, ice, snow, and chill winds make outdoor exercise difficult, indoor exercise equipment may be for you. If it is too rainy, too hot, too dark, or unsafe to exercise outside, you can work out in the relative comfort and safety of a health club or your own home. Indoor exercise equipment allows you to alternate indoor and outdoor workouts according to weather, your schedule, and your mood.

Indoor workouts can be done either on your own equipment at home or in a health club. If you like working out with others, don't want to deal with equipment maintenance, and enjoy a variety of different types of exercise, a health club is a good place to start. At a club, you can try different types of equipment: steppers, treadmills, bicycles, rowers, and skiers and see what you like best. If, on the other hand, you can't seem to make time to get to the health club, with exercise equipment at home, you don't have to go anywhere. You can exercise before or after work, be with your family, read or watch TV at the same time. If you have children, you can keep an eye on them and won't have to hire a baby-sitter while you work out.

Advantages of working out at a health club include the fact that you can switch from one type of equipment to another to avoid boredom or work different muscle groups; you can meet a lot of people; professionals are readily available to answer your questions; you don't have to buy, maintain, and repair the equipment; and you don't have to make space at home for it year-round. The main advantage to working out at home is the convenience.

Disadvantages of working out at a health club to keep in mind include that you will have to pay membership fees, schedule it in your day, have transportation, and at popular workout times may have to wait to get on some equipment. Disadvantages of home exercise equipment are that you have to decide what type of equipment and features you want, purchase it, make room for it in your house, perform your own maintenance, find someone to repair it (or fix it yourself) if it breaks, will likely be working out alone, and may get bored with the same workout day after day. Also, if your enthusiasm wanes, the equipment may become a constant reminder of failed resolutions. However, working out in private is very appealing to many people. You know who used the equipment last, and, for what you pay for a one-year club membership, you can have your own equipment at home.

What to Wear

Since you are working out inside, any comfortable workout gear will be fine with a T-shirt and shorts, supportive shoes, a water bottle, and a towel to wipe off sweat and you are ready to go.

Equipment

Equipment comes in two main types: aerobic and strength machines. Strength training information is covered in Chapter 3. This section will focus on aerobic equipment. Equipment ranges in price from a couple hundred to several thousand dollars, depending on quality and options desired, but indoor exercise equipment need not be expensive. A jump rope, an exercise mat, elastic resistance bands, a step or a slide mat, and an aerobics video are low budget. More costly exercise machines include steppers, cross-country ski simulators, climbers, treadmills, exercise bicycles, and rowers.

If you would like to work out at home and are not familiar with the variety of equipment available, it is important to join a health club for a one- to three-month trial period to try out and compare the different types. Then you will know what type of equipment you want to purchase and will be more familiar with features available. Do not, however, expect a $200 home unit to function like a $2,000 health club model. Shop informed. Ask friends and family about equipment and features they like.

Be choosy. Avoid cheap equipment, which may be flimsy, noisy, unstable, or jerky and which can make the whole workout experience so unpleasant that you'll soon use the machine as a coat rack. Shop for well-designed exercise equipment from a specialty retailer rather than from a TV infomercial or chain department store. The quality and durability will be worth the cost in terms of ease of use and maintenance. Think compact. Unless you have a lot of space, you probably will not want equipment that takes up a whole room. Steppers and exercise bicycles have the smallest "footprint" and are easily moved to the side when not being used. Think simple. Not much can go wrong with a jump rope, but plenty can go wrong with a flimsy treadmill. The more complicated a piece of equipment is to use and adjust, the more maintenance it needs. Many devices have timers, heart rate monitors, and ergometers that calculate your work output in calories.

Before you invest in home exercise equipment, try out several models and ask these questions:

1. How much will I use this? Do I enjoy this type of exercise?
2. Does the sales staff ask about my needs and fitness goals before helping me select equipment rather than automatically recommending the most expensive machine?
3. Does it have the features I want?
4. Is it easy to assemble?
5. If it breaks, how will I get it repaired? Can it be fixed locally?
6. What kind of warranty comes with it? What is the store's return policy?
7. Is it well-constructed of steel or alloy to last 10 or more years?
8. What kind of maintenance is needed, according to the manual?
9. Are the seats and grips comfortable, durable, and easily adjustable?
10. Does it work smoothly? How stable is it? Is it relatively quiet? Is it safe?
11. Where will I put it? How much space does it require?
12. Does the manual show how to use the equipment correctly and how to reach my target heart rate?
13. Do I need all the fancy gadgets or will a more simple model do?
14. Can I get a workout with this machine that is intense enough for my current and future fitness levels?

Stationary Bikes

Advantages/Disadvantages

Most models work the lower body—primarily legs, hips, and buttocks—but some models have handlebars for exercising arms and shoulders. Some of the more expensive electronic models have programmed workouts such as interval training or hills to add variety. Upright models make efficient use of space, and you can read or watch TV as you exercise. They give you a good nonimpact workout, easier on the joints than treadmills. They are particularly good for overweight people who need to avoid extra stress on the back, knees, and ankles. Both upright and recumbent models are effective. Recumbent bikes, in which you sit back on a seat and pedal in front of the body tend to be more expensive and need at least 6 to 7 feet of space but are easier on the back. Bicycle trainers, which put your regular bicycle on a stand with resistance to the rear wheel, require balance but are less expensive than stationary bicycles. Another model, popularized by Health Rider, does not involved pedaling; rather, you push on both pedals simultaneously as you pull on handlebars, exercising both upper and lower body muscles.

How to Select

A good machine is easy to adjust, moves smoothly, and feels stable. The seat should be comfortable and should adjust to your height. In many models, handlebars are also adjustable. The controls should be within easy reach, and the workload should adjust smoothly and easily. Look for a smooth, quiet ride; a sturdy frame; a wide, comfortable, adjustable seat; and an easy-to-read instrument panel. Cheaper models are made of flimsier metal; the resistance mechanism may be grabby, the seat less comfortable, and the whole device more "tippy."

Technique and Safety Tips

Proper seat height and pedaling cadence are the keys to avoiding knee problems. Seat height should be adjusted so that when you sit on the seat, your knee is almost fully extended on the downstroke. Also, keep the resistance moderate so that you maintain a cadence of about 60 to 80 rpm.

Steppers

Advantages/Disadvantages

Steppers work out primarily legs, hips, and buttocks and do not work the upper body. They take relatively little space and allow you to read or watch TV as you exercise. They may aggravate some knee problems. They tend to work the calves more than other types of equipment do.

How to Select

Steppers come with either dependent or independent pedals. With dependent pedals, as one goes down, the other goes up. The machine does some of the work for you because you are exercising one foot at a time. Independent pedal models, in which both feet have to be working at the same time, take a little more work to get the rhythm and coordination but give a better workout. Hydraulic resistance mechanisms provide a fluid feel at an affordable price. High-end models have computerized interval resistance programs that can increase and decrease the workload through the exercise bout. Self-leveling pedals are a nice feature. Make sure pedals are big enough for you to balance on them comfortably. Some also come with poles for working the arms. Less expensive models are manually adjustable, so if you want to change resistance in the middle of a workout, you will have to get off and turn knobs or slide levers. They still give you a good workout, however, so the lower price may be worth some minor inconvenience.

Technique and Safety Tips

Rest your hands lightly on the handlebars or railings for balance and take small steps at first. Stand tall and gradually begin to take deeper steps after you warm up. Do not lean on the railings or you will decrease the effectiveness of the workout.

Treadmills

Advantages/Disadvantages

Treadmills are very popular and easy to use, giving a good cardiovascular and lower body workout. They also tend to be used more than other types of equipment. However, they are noisy and more prone to breakdowns than other types of equipment. They also require a large space, about 6 by 4 feet.

How to Select

A motorized treadmill should have at least a 1.5 continuous-duty horsepower to be strong enough to maintain even speed. Walkers need a speed of at least 5 MPH and joggers a speed faster than your normal pace. Ability to simulate at least a 10 percent incline is important for you to always be able to reach your target pulse. Look for a safety lock so a child cannot accidentally start the treadmill and an emergency shut-off button to cut power immediately. You need at least one handrail, preferably two for balance, and wide footrails. Also look for a wide two-ply rubber belt for durability on the running surface, some flexibility so that it gives a little with each stride, and a belt long enough so that you can maintain a comfortable stride. Decide if you want a motorized or hand-crank incline and what other computerized features you desire, such as heart rate or calorie counting. Less expensive machines tend to have a shorter, narrower bed; lower horsepower; a faster starting speed; a lower top speed; a less durable one-ply belt; and fewer computerized features. They are also noisier, wear out faster, and may not keep the belt speed as consistent as the higher-end models do.

Nonmotorized treadmills are cheaper but move only with the pull of your feet on the belt, and they slow down if you do. They are better for walking than running and may be harder on the joints than motorized treadmills which move continuously at a preset speed.

Technique and Safety Tips

Start the machine at a slow pace. Straddle the belt, step with one foot a few times to get a feel for the speed, and then begin. Increase to normal speed as you warm up. Keep near the front of the belt at all times.

Ski Machines

Advantages/Disadvantages

Ski simulators can work both upper and lower body muscles and give a smooth, nonimpact workout. They do require a lot of space, up to 9 by 3 feet, but some models fold for storage when not in use. They are not suitable for people with balance problems that lead to dizziness or difficulty coordinating movements when standing. You can listen to music or watch TV, but you cannot read while you ski. Ski machines do require practice to master the coordination, but they reward the effort with an excellent workout.

How to Select

Ski machines come in two basic types. One type, popularized by NordicTrack, has skilike rails onto which you place your feet. These glide back and forth on a track, and your hands alternately pull a cable. The other type has small platforms that slide back and forth on a track, and your hands usually pull on poles rather than cables. Cables are usually better than poles because they exercise your arms through a fuller range of motion, giving the muscles a better workout.

Like steppers, ski machines come in independent and dependent pedal models. Dependent pedal models are connected so that, as one foot slides backward, the other automatically comes forward, producing a stiff-legged gait. Independent pedal models require more learning, but the gait is more natural. The muscles in both legs have to work with each stride, and you get a fuller workout. Look for skis that move smoothly, have a base long enough for your stride, and offer adjustable leg and arm resistance.

Technique and Safety Tips

Be forewarned that with a skier it may take several weeks to master the coordination, and that they are not for anyone who has balance problems.

Rowing Machines

Advantages/Disadvantages

Rowers provide an excellent upper as well as lower body workout, toning shoulders, back, arms, and legs. They do, however, require a lot of space, up to 8 feet by 3 feet. They can also be noisy, and you cannot read while working out.

How to Select

They come in piston and flywheel models. The piston models are cheaper and more compact, but flywheel models have smoother action. Some models give strokes per minute, total distance, time, and power output per stroke.

Technique and Safety Tips

Correct rowing technique takes practice to master and is important to avoid back injury. Do not lean into the pull, but keep upright throughout the range of motion. Your legs, arms, and shoulders, not your back, should do much of the work, and your arms should move forward before you bend your knees. With a flywheel model, pull the bar into your abdomen, not your chin. The workout can be very intense.

How to Begin and Progress

Consult the owner's manual for guidelines specific to your exercise equipment regarding how to begin and progress. In general, treadmills and stationary bikes have the quickest learning curves, steppers run third, with ski machines and rowers requiring more balance and skill. However, for the time invested in the latter two, you can get a better upper body workout along with aerobic fitness, so the time is well spent. Also keep in mind that the rule of specificity applies, so if you are in great running shape but begin working out on a stepper or cycle, give yourself some time to build up to the same level of intensity and duration. If you are a beginner, start with 5 to 10 minutes, low intensity, three days the first week to get a feel for correct mechanics and how to use the equipment. Increase the workout by a couple of minutes each week. Pace your progress according to how you feel during and after the workout. If you feel tired and washed out, you are trying to progress too quickly and need to move back or maintain the same level until your endurance increases. If you feel good, then you can continue to add a couple of minutes a week to each workout until you reach 20 to 30 minutes of continuous activity. To increase frequency, add an additional day each month until you are exercising up to five days a week at your target pulse. A suggested workout schedule follows:

Sample Beginning Program

Week	1–2	3–4	5–6	7–8	9–10	11–15
Warm-up (min.)	5–10	5–10	5–10	5–10	5–10	5–10
Conditioning bout (min.)	5–10	8–14	12–18	17–22	21–26	25–30
Intensity (target heart rate)	50–60	60–75	60–75	60–75	60–75	60–75
Cool-down (min.)	5–10	5–10	5–10	5–10	5–10	5–10
Frequency	3	3	3	3–4	3–4	3–5

How to Select a Health Club

1. Ask friends and family about local clubs, equipment, and advantages and disadvantages.
2. Visit several clubs at times you would be going, such as after work, to see how crowded they are. Check out the bathrooms, locker room, pool, weight room. All should be clean and well-maintained. Equipment should be in good repair. Talk to the regulars to see how they judge it. See that it has all the features and types of equipment you want to use.
3. Professionals should be available to show you how to use the equipment correctly for the most effective workout and to avoid injury. Ask about instructor qualifications. Certification by a professional group demonstrates a commitment to quality instruction. There are many national certifying organizations that certify instructors in different activities. Some of these are the American College of Sports Medicine, YMCA, YWCA, International Dance-Exercise Association, Aerobics and Fitness Association of America, and National Strength and Conditioning Association.
4. Look for a health club with at least three years of continuous operation. Call your local Better Business Bureau or your state or local consumer protection agency to check if any negative reports have been filed. Ask to see evidence of bonding from the club (this protects you if the club goes out of business).
5. Membership fees are negotiable, so no matter what is printed on the brochure, negotiate!
6. Start with a short-term membership. Only 10 percent of members are still working out after three months, so either pay on a monthly basis, or sign up for a three-month trial membership.
7. Read the contract carefully before signing, making sure it covers everything you have discussed with the club employees. If you change your mind, most states have a three-day cooling-off period during which you can void the contract and get a full refund.

Resources

Aerobics Inc. (treadmills), (201) 256-9700.

Bodyguard, (800) 665-3407.

Concept II (rowers), (800) 245-5676.

LifeFitness (Lifecycle stationary bikes, Lifestep climbers, Lifestride treadmills, Life rowers), (800) 877-3867 and (800) 735-3867.

NordicTrack (ski simulators, walkfit, treadmills), (800) 228-6635 and (800) 445-2360.

Parabody, (800) 352-2719.

Precor (climbers, ski simulators, stationary bikes, treadmills), (800) 477-3267 and (800) 786-8404.

StairMaster, (800) 635-2936.

StarTrac (treadmills, climbers), (800) 228-6635.

Tectrix (climbers, stationary bikes), (800) 767-8082.

Tunturi (stationary bikes, climbers, ski simulators, treadmills, rowers), (800) 827-8717.

Nutritive Value of the Edible Part of Food
(Tr indicates nutrient present in trace amount.)

NUTRIENTS IN INDICATED QUANTITY

Foods, Approximate Measures, Units, and Weight (Weight of Edible Portion Only)		Water		Food Energy	Protein	Fat	Fatty Acids			Choles-terol	Carbo-hy-drate	Cal-cium	Iron	Potas-sium	So-dium
							Satu-rated	Mono-unsatu-rated	Polyun-satu-rated						
		(g)	(%)	(Kcals)	(g)	(g)	(g)	(g)	(g)	(mg)	(g)	(mg)	(mg)	(mg)	(mg)
Beverages															
Alcoholic:															
Beer:															
Regular	12 fl oz	360	92	150	1	0	0.0	0.0	0.0	0	13	14	0.1	115	18
Light	12 fl oz	355	95	95	1	0	0.0	0.0	0.0	0	5	14	0.1	64	11
Gin, rum, vodka, whiskey:															
80-proof	1 1/2 fl oz	42	67	95	0	0	0.0	0.0	0.0	0	Tr	Tr	Tr	1	Tr
Wines:															
Table:															
Red	3 1/2 fl oz	102	88	75	Tr	0	0.0	0.0	0.0	0	3	8	0.4	113	5
White	3 1/2 fl oz	102	87	80	Tr	0	0.0	0.0	0.0	0	3	9	0.3	83	5
Carbonated[1]															
Club soda	12 fl oz	355	100	0	0	0	0.0	0.0	0.0	0	0	18	Tr	0	78
Cola type:															
Regular	12 fl oz	369	89	160	0	0	0.0	0.0	0.0	0	41	11	0.2	7	18
Diet, artificially sweetened	12 fl oz	355	100	Tr	0	0	0.0	0.0	0.0	0	Tr	14	0.2	7	32[2]
Ginger ale	12 fl oz	366	91	125	0	0	0.0	0.0	0.0	0	32	11	0.1	4	29
Lemon-lime	12 fl oz	372	89	155	0	0	0.0	0.0	0.0	0	39	7	0.4	4	33
Orange	12 fl oz	372	88	180	0	0	0.0	0.0	0.0	0	46	15	0.3	7	52
Pepper type	12 fl oz	369	89	160	0	0	0.0	0.0	0.0	0	41	11	0.1	4	37
Root beer	12 fl oz	370	89	165	0	0	0.0	0.0	0.0	0	42	15	0.2	4	48
Coffee															
Brewed	6 fl oz	180	100	Tr	Tr	Tr	Tr	Tr	Tr	0	Tr	4	Tr	124	2
Instant, prepared (2 tsp powder plus 6 fl oz water)	6 fl oz	182	99	Tr	Tr	Tr	Tr	Tr	Tr	0	1	2	0.1	71	Tr

Source: Adapted from U.S. Department of Agriculture. *House and Garden Bulletin* no. 72 (revised 1985). Washington, D.C.: Superintendent of Documents, U.S. Government Printing Office, 1985.

1. Mineral content varies depending on water source.
2. Blend of aspartame and saccharin; if only sodium saccharin is used, sodium is 75 mg; if only aspartame is used, sodium is 23 mg.

Dairy Products

Food	Measure	Grams	Water (%)	Food energy (cal)	Protein (g)	Fat (g)	Saturated (g)	Monounsaturated (g)	Polyunsaturated (g)	Cholesterol (mg)	Carbohydrate (g)	Calcium (mg)	Iron (mg)	Potassium (mg)	Sodium (mg)
Fruit drinks, noncarbonated:															
Canned:															
Fruit punch drink	6 fl oz	190	88	85	Tr	0	0.0	0.0	0.0	0	22	15	0.4	48	15
Grape drink	6 fl oz	187	86	100	Tr	0	0.0	0.0	0.0	0	26	2	0.3	9	11
Frozen:															
Lemonade concentrate:															
Diluted with 4 1/3 parts water by volume	6 fl oz	185	89	80	Tr	Tr	Tr	Tr	Tr	0	21	2	0.1	30	1
Tea:															
Brewed	8 fl oz	240	100	Tr	Tr	Tr	Tr	Tr	Tr	0	Tr	0	Tr	36	1
Instant, powder, prepared:															
Unsweetened (1 tsp powder plus 8 fl oz water)	8 fl oz	241	100	Tr	Tr	Tr	Tr	Tr	Tr	0	1	1	Tr	61	1
Sweetened (3 tsp powder plus 8 fl oz water)	8 fl oz	262	91	85	Tr	Tr	Tr	Tr	Tr	0	22	1	Tr	49	Tr
Dairy Products															
Cheese:															
Cheddar:															
Cut pieces	1 oz	28	37	115	7	9	6.0	2.7	0.3	30	Tr	204	0.2	28	176
Shredded	1 cup	113	37	455	28	37	23.8	10.6	1.1	119	1	815	0.8	111	701
Creamed (cottage cheese, 4% fat):															
Large curd	1 cup	225	79	235	28	10	6.4	2.9	0.3	34	6	135	0.3	190	911
Small curd	1 cup	210	79	215	26	9	6.0	2.7	0.3	31	6	126	0.3	177	850
Lowfat (2%)	1 cup	226	79	205	31	4	2.8	1.2	0.1	19	8	155	0.4	217	918
Cream	1 oz	28	54	100	2	10	6.2	2.8	0.4	31	1	23	0.3	34	84
Mozzarella, made with:															
Whole milk	1 oz	28	54	80	6	6	3.7	1.9	0.2	22	1	147	0.1	19	106
Part skim milk (low moisture)	1 oz	28	49	80	8	5	3.1	1.4	0.1	15	1	207	0.1	27	150
Muenster	1 oz	28	42	105	7	9	5.4	2.5	0.2	27	Tr	203	0.1	38	178
Parmesan, grated	1 oz	28	18	130	12	9	5.4	2.5	0.2	22	1	390	0.3	30	528
Parmesan, grated	1 tbsp	5	18	25	2	2	1.0	0.4	Tr	4	Tr	69	Tr	5	93
Ricotta, made with:															
Whole milk	1 cup	246	72	430	28	32	20.4	8.9	0.9	124	7	509	0.9	257	207
Part skim milk	1 cup	246	74	340	28	19	12.1	5.7	0.6	76	13	669	1.1	307	307
Swiss	1 oz	28	37	105	8	8	5.0	2.1	0.3	26	1	272	Tr	31	74
Pasteurized process cheese:															
American	1 oz	28	39	105	6	9	5.6	2.5	0.3	27	Tr	174	0.1	46	406
Swiss	1 oz	28	42	95	7	7	4.5	2.0	0.2	24	1	219	0.2	61	388
Pasteurized process cheese spread, American	1 oz	28	48	80	5	6	3.8	1.8	0.2	16	2	159	0.1	69	381
Cream, sweet:															
Half-and-half (cream and milk)	1 cup	242	81	315	7	28	17.3	8.0	1.0	89	10	254	0.2	314	98
Half-and-half (cream and milk)	1 tbsp	15	81	20	Tr	2	1.1	0.5	0.1	6	1	16	Tr	19	6
Whipped topping, (pressurized)	1 cup	60	61	155	2	13	8.3	3.9	0.5	46	7	61	Tr	88	78
Whipped topping, (pressurized)	1 tbsp	3	61	10	Tr	1	0.4	0.2	Tr	2	Tr	3	Tr	4	4

Foods, Approximate Measures, Units, and Weight (Weight of Edible Portion Only)

NUTRIENTS IN INDICATED QUANTITY

| Foods, Approximate Measures | | Water (%) | Food Energy (Kcals) | Protein (g) | Fat (g) | Fatty Acids | | | Cholesterol (mg) | Carbohydrate (g) | Calcium (mg) | Iron (mg) | Potassium (mg) | Sodium (mg) |
	Weight (g)					Saturated (g)	Monounsaturated (g)	Polyunsaturated (g)						
Cream, sour	1 cup / 230	71	495	7	48	30.0	13.9	1.8	102	10	268	0.1	331	123
	1 tbsp / 12	71	25	Tr	3	1.6	0.7	0.1	5	1	14	Tr	17	6
Whipped topping:														
Frozen	1 cup / 75	50	240	1	19	16.3	1.2	0.4	0	17	5	0.1	14	19
	1 tbsp / 4	50	15	Tr	1	0.9	0.1	Tr	0	1	Tr	Tr	1	1
Milk:														
Fluid:														
Whole (3.3% fat)	1 cup / 244	88	150	8	8	5.1	2.4	0.3	33	11	291	0.1	370	120
Lowfat (2%), no milk solids added	1 cup / 244	89	120	8	5	2.9	1.4	0.2	18	12	297	0.1	377	122
Lowfat (1%), no milk solids added	1 cup / 244	90	100	8	3	1.6	0.7	0.1	10	12	300	0.1	381	123
Nonfat (skim), no milk solids added	1 cup / 245	91	85	8	Tr	0.3	0.1	Tr	4	12	302	0.1	406	126
Buttermilk	1 cup / 245	90	100	8	2	1.3	0.6	0.1	9	12	285	0.1	371	257
Canned:														
Condensed, sweetened	1 cup / 306	27	980	24	27	16.8	7.4	1.0	104	166	868	0.6	1,136	389
Evaporated:														
Whole milk	1 cup / 252	74	340	17	19	11.6	5.9	0.6	74	25	657	0.5	764	267
Milk beverages:														
Chocolate milk (commercial):														
Regular	1 cup / 250	82	210	8	8	5.3	2.5	0.3	31	26	280	0.6	417	149
Lowfat (2%)	1 cup / 250	84	180	8	5	3.1	1.5	0.2	17	26	284	0.6	422	151
Shakes, thick:														
Chocolate	10-oz container / 283	72	335	9	8	4.8	2.2	0.3	30	60	374	0.9	634	314
Vanilla	10-oz container / 283	74	315	11	9	5.3	2.5	0.3	33	50	413	0.3	517	270
Milk desserts, frozen:														
Ice cream, vanilla:														
Regular (about 11% fat), hardened	1/2 gal / 1,064	61	2,155	38	115	71.3	33.1	4.3	476	254	1,406	1.0	2,052	929
	1 cup / 133	61	270	5	14	8.9	4.1	0.5	59	32	176	0.1	257	116
Soft serve (frozen custard)	1 cup / 173	60	375	7	23	13.5	6.7	1.0	153	38	236	0.4	338	153
Ice milk, vanilla:														
Hardened (about 4% fat)	1/2 gal / 1,048	69	1,470	41	45	28.1	13.0	1.7	146	232	1,409	1.5	2,117	836
	1 cup / 131	69	185	5	6	3.5	1.6	0.2	18	29	176	0.2	265	105
Soft serve (about 3% fat)	1 cup / 175	70	225	8	5	2.9	1.3	0.2	13	38	274	0.3	412	163
Sherbert (about 2% fat)	1/2 gal / 1,542	66	2,160	17	31	19.0	8.8	1.1	113	469	827	2.5	1,585	706
	1 cup / 193	66	270	2	4	2.4	1.1	0.1	14	59	103	0.3	198	88

Fats and Oils

Food	Measure	Grams	Water (%)	Food energy (cal)	Protein (g)	Fat (g)	Saturated (g)	Monounsaturated (g)	Polyunsaturated (g)	Cholesterol (mg)	Carbohydrate (g)	Calcium (mg)	Iron (mg)	Potassium (mg)	Sodium (mg)
Yogurt,															
With added milk solids:															
Made with lowfat milk:															
Fruit-flavored[3]	8-oz container	227	74	230	10	2	1.6	0.7	0.1	10	43	345	0.2	442	133
Plain	8-oz container	227	85	145	12	4	2.3	1.0	0.1	14	16	415	0.2	531	159
Made with nonfat milk	8-oz container	227	85	125	13	Tr	0.3	0.1	Tr	4	17	452	0.2	579	174
Eggs, large (24 oz per dozen):															
Raw:															
Whole, without shell	1 egg	50	75	80	6	6	1.7	2.2	0.7	274	1	28	1.0	65	69
White	1 white	33	88	15	3	Tr	0.0	0.0	0.0	0	Tr	4	Tr	45	50
Yolk	1 yolk	17	49	65	3	6	1.7	2.2	0.7	272	Tr	26	0.9	15	8
Cooked:															
Fried in butter	1 egg	46	68	95	6	7	2.7	2.7	0.8	278	1	29	1.1	66	162
Hard-cooked, shell removed	1 egg	50	75	80	6	6	1.7	2.2	0.7	274	1	28	1.0	65	69
Poached	1 egg	50	74	80	6	6	1.7	2.2	0.7	273	1	28	1.0	65	146
Scrambled (milk added) in butter or omelet	1 egg	64	73	110	7	8	3.2	2.9	0.8	282	2	54	1.0	97	176
Fats and Oils															
Butter (4 sticks per lb):															
Tablespoon (1/8 stick)	1 tbsp	14	16	100	Tr	11	7.1	3.3	0.4	31	Tr	3	Tr	4	116[4]
Pat (1 in square, 1/3 in high; 90 per lb)	1 pat	5	16	35	Tr	4	2.5	1.2	0.2	11	Tr	1	Tr	1	41[5]
Margarine:															
Regular (about 80% fat):															
Hard (4 sticks per lb)	1 tbsp	14	16	100	Tr	11	2.2	5.0	3.6	0	Tr	4	Tr	6	132[5]
Soft	8-oz container	227	16	1,625	2	183	31.3	64.7	78.5	0	1	60	1	86	2,449[5]
	1 tbsp	14	16	100	Tr	11	1.9	4.0	4.8	0	Tr	4	Tr	5	151[4]
Spread (about 60% fat):															
Hard (4 sticks per lb)	1 tbsp	14	37	75	Tr	9	2.0	3.6	2.5	0	0	3	0	4	139[5]
Soft	8-oz container	227	37	1,225	1	138	29.1	71.5	31.3	0	0	47	0	68	2,256[5]
	1 tbsp	14	37	75	Tr	9	1.8	4.4	1.9	0	0	3	0	4	139[5]
Oils, salad or cooking:															
Corn	1 cup	218	0	1,925	0	218	27.7	52.8	128.0	0	0	0	0.0	0	0
	1 tbsp	14	0	125	0	14	1.8	3.4	8.2	0	0	0	0.0	0	0
Olive	1 cup	216	0	1,910	0	216	29.2	159.2	18.1	0	0	0	0.0	0	0
	1 tbsp	14	0	125	0	14	1.9	10.3	1.2	0	0	0	0.0	0	0
Peanut	1 cup	216	0	1,910	0	216	36.5	99.8	69.1	0	0	0	0.0	0	0
	1 tbsp	14	0	125	0	14	2.4	6.5	4.5	0	0	0	0.0	0	0
Safflower	1 cup	218	0	1,925	0	218	19.8	26.4	162.4	0	0	0	0.0	0	0
	1 tbsp	14	0	125	0	14	1.3	1.7	10.4	0	0	0	0.0	0	0

3. Carbohydrate content varies widely because of amount of sugar added and amount and solids content of added flavoring. Consult the label if more precise values for carbohydrate and calories are needed.
4. For salted butter; unsalted butter contains 2 mg per tbsp, or 1 mg per pat.
5. For salted margarine.

NUTRIENTS IN INDICATED QUANTITY

Foods, Approximate Measures, Units, and Weight (Weight of Edible Portion Only)

		Water		Food Energy	Protein	Fat	Fatty Acids Satu-rated	Mono-unsatu-rated	Polyun-satu-rated	Choles-terol	Carbo-hy-drate	Cal-cium	Iron	Potas-sium	So-dium
		(g)	(%)	(Kcals)	(g)	(g)	(g)	(g)	(g)	(mg)	(g)	(mg)	(mg)	(mg)	(mg)
Soybean oil, hydrogenated (partially hardened)	1 cup	218	0	1,925	0	218	32.5	93.7	82.0	0	0	0	0.0	0	0
	1 tbsp	14	0	125	0	14	2.1	6.0	5.3	0	0	0	0.0	0	0
Sunflower	1 cup	218	0	1,925	0	218	22.5	42.5	143.2	0	0	0	0.0	0	0
	1 tbsp	14	0	125	0	14	1.4	2.7	9.2	0	0	0	0.0	0	0
Salad dressings:															
French:															
Regular	1 tbsp	16	35	85	Tr	9	1.4	4.0	3.5	0	1	2	Tr	2	188
Italian:															
Regular	1 tbsp	15	34	80	Tr	9	1.3	3.7	3.2	0	1	1	Tr	5	162
Low calorie	1 tbsp	15	86	5	Tr	Tr	Tr	Tr	Tr	0	2	1	Tr	4	136
Mayonnaise:															
Regular	1 tbsp	14	15	100	Tr	11	1.7	3.2	5.8	8	Tr	3	0.1	5	80
Imitation	1 tbsp	15	63	35	Tr	3	0.5	0.7	1.6	4	2	Tr	0.0	2	75
Mayonnaise type	1 tbsp	15	40	60	Tr	5	0.7	1.4	2.7	4	4	2	Tr	1	107
Tartar sauce	1 tbsp	14	34	75	Tr	8	1.2	2.6	3.9	4	1	3	0.1	11	182
Fish and Shellfish															
Crabmeat, canned	1 cup	135	77	135	23	3	0.5	0.8	1.4	135	1	61	1.1	149	1,350
Fish sticks, frozen, reheated (stick, 4 by 1 by 1/2 in)	1 fish stick	28	52	70	6	3	0.8	1.4	0.8	26	4	11	0.3	94	53
Flounder or Sole, baked, with lemon juice:															
With margarine	3 oz	85	73	120	16	6	1.2	2.3	1.9	55	Tr	14	0.3	273	151
Without added fat	3 oz	85	78	80	17	1	0.3	0.2	0.4	59	Tr	13	0.3	286	101
Haddock, breaded, fried[6]	3 oz	85	61	175	17	9	2.4	3.9	2.4	75	7	34	1.0	270	123
Salmon:															
Canned (pink), solids and liquid	3 oz	85	71	120	17	5	0.9	1.5	2.1	34	0	167[7]	0.7	307	443
Shrimp:															
French fried (7 medium)[8]	3 oz	85	55	200	16	10	2.5	4.1	2.6	168	11	61	2.0	189	384

6. Dipped in egg, milk, and breadcrumbs; fried in vegetable shortening.
7. If bones are discarded, value for calcium will be greatly reduced.
8. Dipped in egg, breadcrumbs, and flour; fried in vegetable shortening.

Food (approximate measure)	Measure	Grams	Water (%)	Food energy (cal)	Protein (g)	Fat (g)	Saturated (g)	Mono-unsaturated (g)	Poly-unsaturated (g)	Cholesterol (mg)	Carbohydrate (g)	Calcium (mg)	Iron (mg)	Potassium (mg)	Sodium (mg)
Tuna, canned, drained solids:															
Oil pack, chunk light	3 oz	85	61	165	24	7	1.4	1.9	3.1	55	0	7	1.6	298	303
Water pack, solid white[9]	3 oz	85	63	135	30	1	0.3	0.2	0.3	48	0	17	0.6	255	468
Tuna salad[9]	1 cup	205	63	375	33	19	3.3	4.9	9.2	80	19	31	2.5	531	877
Fruits and Fruit Juices															
Apples, raw, unpeeled, without cores, 3 1/4-in diam. (about 2 per lb with cores)	1 apple	212	84	125	Tr	1	0.1	Tr	0.2	0	32	15	0.4	244	Tr
Apple juice, bottled or canned[10]	1 cup	248	88	115	Tr	Tr	Tr	Tr	0.1	0	29	17	0.9	295	7
Applesauce, canned:															
Sweetened	1 cup	255	80	195	Tr	Tr	0.1	Tr	0.1	0	51	10	0.9	156	8
Unsweetened	1 cup	244	88	105	Tr	Tr	Tr	Tr	Tr	0	28	7	0.3	183	5
Avocados, raw, whole, without skin and seed, California (about 2 per lb with skin and seed)	1 avocado	173	73	305	4	30	4.5	19.4	3.5	0	12	19	2.0	1,097	21
Bananas, raw, without peel, whole (about 2 1/2 per lb with peel)	1 banana	114	74	105	1	1	0.2	Tr	0.1	0	27	7	0.4	451	1
Blueberries, raw	1 cup	145	85	80	1	1	Tr	0.1	0.3	0	20	9	0.2	129	9
Fruit cocktail, canned, fruit and liquid:															
Heavy syrup pack	1 cup	255	80	185	1	Tr	Tr	Tr	0.1	0	48	15	0.7	224	15
Juice pack	1 cup	248	87	115	1	Tr	Tr	Tr	Tr	0	29	20	0.5	236	10
Grapefruit: Raw, without peel, membrane and seeds (3 3/4-in diam., 1 lb 1 oz, whole, with refuse)	1/2 grapefruit	120	91	40	1	Tr	Tr	Tr	Tr	0	10	14	0.1	167	Tr
Grapes, European type (adherent skin), raw, Thompson seedless	10 grapes	50	81	35	Tr	Tr	0.1	Tr	0.1	0	9	6	0.1	93	1
Cantaloupe, orange-fleshed (5-in diam., 2 1/3 lb, whole, with rind and cavity contents)	1/2 melon	267	90	95	2	1	0.1	0.1	0.3	0	22	29	0.6	825	24
Oranges, raw, whole, without peel and seeds (2 5/8-in diam., about 2 1/2 per lb, with peel and seeds)	1 orange	131	87	60	1	Tr	Tr	Tr	Tr	0	15	52	0.1	237	Tr

9. Made with drained chunk light tuna, celery, onion, pickle relish, and mayonnaise-type salad dressing.
10. Also applies to pasteurized apple cider.

Foods, Approximate Measures, Units, and Weight (Weight of Edible Portion Only)

Food	Measure	Water (g)	Water (%)	Food Energy (Kcals)	Protein (g)	Fat (g)	Fatty Acids: Saturated (g)	Mono-unsaturated (g)	Polyun-saturated (g)	Choles-terol (mg)	Carbo-hydrate (g)	Cal-cium (mg)	Iron (mg)	Potas-sium (mg)	So-dium (mg)
Orange juice:															
Raw, all varieties	1 cup	248	88	110	2	Tr	0.1	0.1	0.1	0	26	27	0.5	496	2
Canned, unsweetened	1 cup	249	89	105	1	Tr	Tr	0.1	0.1	0	25	20	1.1	436	5
Frozen concentrate Diluted with 3 parts water by volume	1 cup	249	88	110	2	Tr	Tr	Tr	Tr	0	27	22	0.2	473	2
Peaches:															
Raw, sliced	1 cup	170	88	75	1	Tr	Tr	0.1	0.1	0	19	9	0.2	335	Tr
Canned, fruit and liquid:															
Heavy syrup pack	1 cup	256	79	190	1	Tr	Tr	0.1	0.1	0	51	8	0.7	236	15
	1 half	81	79	60	Tr	Tr	Tr	Tr	Tr	0	16	2	0.2	75	5
Juice pack	1 cup	248	87	110	2	Tr	Tr	Tr	Tr	0	29	15	0.7	317	10
	1 half	77	87	35	Tr	Tr	Tr	Tr	Tr	0	9	5	0.2	99	3
Pears:															
Raw, with skin, cored, Bartlett, 2 1/2-in diam. (about 2 1/2 per lb with cores and stems)	1 pear	166	84	100	1	1	Tr	0.1	0.2	0	25	18	0.4	208	Tr
Canned, fruit and liquid:															
Heavy syrup pack	1 cup	255	80	190	1	Tr	Tr	0.1	0.1	0	49	13	0.6	166	13
	1 half	79	80	60	Tr	Tr	Tr	Tr	Tr	0	15	4	0.2	51	4
Juice pack	1 cup	248	86	125	1	Tr	Tr	Tr	Tr	0	32	22	0.7	238	10
	1 half	77	86	40	Tr	Tr	Tr	Tr	Tr	0	10	7	0.2	74	3
Pineapple, canned, fruit and liquid:															
Heavy syrup pack, crushed, chunks, tidbits	1 cup	255	79	200	1	Tr	Tr	Tr	0.1	0	52	36	1.0	265	3
Juice pack, chunks or tidbits	1 cup	250	84	150	1	Tr	Tr	Tr	0.1	0	39	35	0.7	305	3
Raisins, seedless, not pressed down	1 cup	145	15	435	5	1	0.2	Tr	0.2	0	115	71	3.0	1,089	17
Strawberries, raw, capped, whole	1 cup	149	92	45	1	1	Tr	0.1	0.3	0	10	21	0.6	247	1
Watermelon, raw, without rind and seeds, diced	1 cup	160	92	50	1	1	0.1	0.1	0.3	0	11	13	0.3	186	3

Grain Products

Food	Measure	g	%	cal	g	g	g	g	g	mg	g	mg	mg	mg	mg
Bagels, plain or water, enriched, 3 1/2-in diam.[10]	1 bagel	68	29	200	7	2	0.3	0.5	0.7	0	38	29	1.8	50	245
Biscuits, baking powder, from mix	1 biscuit	28	29	95	2	3	0.8	1.4	0.9	Tr	14	58	0.7	56	262
Breads:															
White bread, enriched[11]	1 slice	25	37	65	2	1	0.3	0.4	0.2	0	12	32	0.7	28	129
Whole-wheat bread[11]	1 slice	28	38	70	3	1	0.4	0.4	0.3	0	13	20	1.0	50	180
Breakfast cereals:															
Oatmeal or rolled oats, regular, quick, instant, nonfortified	1 cup	234	85	145	6	2	0.4	0.8	1.0	0	25	19	1.6	131	2[12]
Ready to eat:															
Cap'n Crunch® (about 3/4 cup)	1 oz	28	3	120	1	3	1.7	0.3	0.4	0	23	5	7.5[13]	37	213
Cheerios® (about 1 1/4 cup)	1 oz	28	5	110	2	2	0.3	0.6	0.7	0	20	48	4.5[14]	101	307
Corn Flakes (about 1 1/4 cup, Kellogg's®)	1 oz	28	3	110	2	Tr	Tr	Tr	Tr	0	24	1	1.8[14]	26	351
Honey Nut Cheerios® (about 3/4 cup)	1 oz	28	3	105	3	1	0.1	0.3	0.3	0	23	20	4.5[14]	99	257
100% Natural Cereal (about 1/4 cup)	1 oz	28	2	135	3	6	4.1	1.2	0.5	Tr	18	49	0.8	140	12
Raisin Bran, Kellogg's® (about 3/4 cup)	1 oz	28	8	90	3	1	0.1	0.1	0.3	0	21	10	3.5[14]	147	207
Rice Krispies® (about 1 cup)	1 oz	28	2	110	2	Tr	Tr	Tr	0.1	0	25	4	1.8[14]	29	340
Shredded Wheat (about 2/3 cup)	1 oz	28	5	100	3	1	0.1	0.1	0.3	0	23	11	1.2	102	3
Sugar Smacks® (about 3/4 cup)	1 oz	28	3	105	2	1	0.1	0.1	0.2	0	25	3	1.8[14]	42	75
Total® (about 1 cup)	1 oz	28	4	100	3	1	0.1	0.1	0.3	0	22	48	18.0[14]	106	352
Wheaties® (about 1 cup)	1 oz	28	5	100	3	Tr	Tr	Tr	0.2	0	23	43	4.5[14]	106	354
Cakes prepared from cake mixes with enriched flour:[15]															
Devil's food with chocolate frosting:															
Piece, 1/16 of cake	1 piece	69	24	235	3	8	3.5	3.2	1.2	37	40	41	1.4	90	181
Cupcake, 2 1/2-in diam.	1 cupcake	35	24	120	2	4	1.8	1.6	0.6	19	20	21	0.7	46	92

10. Also applies to pasteurized apple cider.
11. Made with vegetable shortening.
12. Cooked without salt. If salt is added according to label recommendations, sodium content is 374 mg.
13. Nutrient added.
14. Value based on label declaration for added nutrients.
15. Excepting angel food cake, cakes were made from mixes containing vegetable shortening and frostings were made with margarine.

Foods, Approximate Measures, Units, and Weight (Weight of Edible Portion Only)

Foods, Approximate Measures, Units, and Weight (Weight of Edible Portion Only)		Water (g)	Water (%)	Food Energy (Kcals)	Protein (g)	Fat (g)	Fatty Acids			Choles-terol (mg)	Carbo-hy-drate (g)	Cal-cium (mg)	Iron (mg)	Potas-sium (mg)	So-dium (mg)
							Satu-rated (g)	Mono-unsatu-rated (g)	Polyun-satu-rated (g)						
Carrot, with cream cheese frosting,[16] piece, 1/16 of cake	1 piece	96	23	385	4	21	4.1	8.4	6.7	74	48	44	1.3	108	279
Plain sheet cake,[17] piece, 1/9 of cake	1 piece	121	21	445	4	14	4.6	5.6	2.9	70	77	61	1.2	74	275
Snack cakes: Devil's food with creme filling (2 small cakes per pkg)	1 small cake	28	20	105	1	4	1.7	1.5	0.6	15	17	21	1.0	34	105
Sponge with creme filling (2 small cakes per pkg)	1 small cake	42	19	155	1	5	2.3	2.1	0.5	7	27	14	0.6	37	155
Cheesecake: Piece, 1/12 of cake	1 piece	92	46	280	5	18	9.9	5.4	1.2	170	26	52	0.4	90	204
Chocolate chip, commercial, 2 1/4-in diam., 3/8 in thick	4 cookies	42	4	180	2	9	2.9	3.1	2.6	5	28	13	0.8	68	140
Cookies made with enriched flour: Chocolate chip, from refrigerated dough, 2 1/4-in diam., 3/8 in thick	4 cookies	48	5	225	2	11	4.0	4.4	2.0	22	32	13	1.0	62	173
Peanut butter cookie, from home recipe, 2 5/8-in diam.[11]	4 cookies	48	3	245	4	14	4.0	5.8	2.8	22	28	21	1.1	110	142
Sandwich type (chocolate or vanilla), 1 3/4-in diam., 3/8 in thick	4 cookies	40	2	195	2	8	2.0	3.6	2.2	0	29	12	1.4	66	189
Corn chips	1-oz pack-age	28	1	155	2	9	1.4	2.4	3.7	0	16	35	0.5	52	233

16. Made with vegetable oil.
17. Cake made with vegetable shortening; frosting with margarine.

Food	Measure	Grams	Water (%)	Food energy (cal)	Protein (g)	Fat (g)	Saturated (g)	Mono-unsat. (g)	Poly-unsat. (g)	Cholesterol (mg)	Carbohydrate (g)	Calcium (mg)	Iron (mg)	Potassium (mg)	Sodium (mg)
Crackers:[18]															
Cheese, Sandwich type (peanut butter)	1 sandwich	8	3	40	1	2	0.4	0.8	0.3	1	5	7	0.3	17	90
Saltines[19]	4 crackers	12	4	50	1	1	0.5	0.4	0.2	4	9	3	0.5	17	165
Wheat, thin	4 crackers	8	3	35	1	1	0.5	0.5	0.4	0	5	3	0.3	17	69
Croissants, made with enriched flour, 4 1/2 by 4 by 1 3/4 in	1 croissant	57	22	235	5	12	3.5	6.7	1.4	13	27	20	2.1	68	452
Danish pastry, round piece, about 4 1/4-in diam., 1 in high	1 pastry	57	27	220	4	12	3.6	4.8	2.6	49	26	60	1.1	53	218
Doughnuts, made with enriched flour:															
Cake type, plain, 3 1/4-in diam., 1 in high	1 doughnut	50	21	210	3	12	2.8	5.0	3.0	20	24	22	1.0	58	192
Yeast-leavened, glazed, 3 3/4-in diam., 1 1/4 in high	1 doughnut	60	27	235	4	13	5.2	5.5	0.9	21	26	17	1.4	64	222
English muffins, plain, enriched	1 muffin	57	42	140	5	1	0.3	0.2	0.3	0	27	96	1.7	331	378
Macaroni, enriched, cooked (cut lengths, elbows, shells), hot	1 cup	140	72	155	5	1	0.1	0.1	0.2	0	32	11	1.7	85	1
Muffins made with enriched flour, 2 1/2-in diam., 1 1/2 in high:															
Blueberry	1 muffin	45	33	140	3	5	1.4	2.0	1.2	45	22	15	0.9	54	225
Bran	1 muffin	45	28	140	3	4	1.3	1.6	1.0	28	24	27	1.7	50	385
Pancakes, 4-in diam., from mix (with enriched flour), egg, milk, and oil added	1 pancake	27	54	60	2	2	0.5	0.9	0.5	16	8	36	0.7	43	160
Pies, piecrust made with enriched flour, vegetable shortening, 9-in diam.:															
Apple (1/6 of pie)	1 piece	158	48	405	3	18	4.6	7.4	4.4	0	60	13	1.6	126	476
Cherry (1/6 of pie)	1 piece	158	47	410	4	18	4.7	7.7	4.6	0	61	22	1.6	166	480
Creme (1/6 of pie)	1 piece	152	43	455	3	23	15.0	4.0	1.1	8	59	46	1.1	133	369
Lemon meringue (1/6 of pie)	1 piece	140	47	355	5	14	4.3	5.7	2.9	143	53	20	1.4	70	395
Pecan (1/6 of pie)	1 piece	138	20	575	7	32	4.7	17.0	7.9	95	71	65	4.6	170	305
Pumpkin (1/6 of pie)	1 piece	152	59	320	6	17	6.4	6.7	3.0	109	37	78	1.4	243	325
Pies, fried, cherry	1 pie	85	42	250	2	14	5.8	6.7	0.6	13	32	11	0.7	61	371
Popcorn, air-popped, unsalted	1 cup	8	4	30	1	Tr	Tr	0.1	0.2	0	6	1	0.2	20	Tr

18. Crackers made with enriched flour except for rye wafers and whole-wheat wafers.
19. Made with lard.

Foods, Approximate Measures, Units, and Weight (Weight of Edible Portion Only)

			Water	Food Energy	Protein	Fat	Fatty Acids			Choles-terol	Carbo-hy-drate	Cal-cium	Iron	Potas-sium	So-dium
							Satu-rated	Mono-unsatu-rated	Polyun-satu-rated						
		(g)	(%)	(Kcals)	(g)	(g)	(g)	(g)	(g)	(mg)	(g)	(mg)	(mg)	(mg)	(mg)
Pretzels, made with enriched flour, twisted, dutch, 2 3/4 by 2 5/8 in	1 pretzel	16	3	65	2	1	0.1	0.2	0.2	0	13	4	0.3	16	258
Rice:															
Brown, cooked, served hot	1 cup	195	70	230	5	1	0.3	0.3	0.4	0	50	23	1.0	137	0
White, enriched, commercial varieties, all types, cooked, served hot	1 cup	205	73	225	4	Tr	0.1	0.1	0.1	0	50	21	1.8	57	0
Rolls, enriched, commercial:															
Frankfurter and hamburger (8 per 11 1/2-oz pkg.)	1 roll	40	34	115	3	2	0.5	0.8	0.6	Tr	20	54	1.2	56	241
Hoagie or submarine, 11 1/2 by 3 by 2 1/2 in	1 roll	135	31	400	11	8	1.8	3.0	2.2	Tr	72	100	3.8	128	683
Spaghetti, enriched, cooked, tender stage, served hot	1 cup	140	73	155	5	1	0.1	0.1	0.2	0	32	11	1.7	85	1
Toaster pastries	1 pastry	54	13	210	2	6	1.7	3.6	0.4	0	38	104	2.2	91	248
Tortillas, corn	1 tortilla	30	45	65	2	1	0.1	0.3	0.6	0	13	42	0.6	43	1
Legumes, Nuts, and Seeds															
Beans															
Pea (navy)	1 cup	190	69	225	15	1	0.1	0.1	0.7	0	40	95	5.1	790	13
Red kidney	1 cup	255	76	230	15	1	0.1	0.1	0.6	0	42	74	4.6	673	968
Chickpeas, cooked, drained	1 cup	163	60	270	15	4	0.4	0.9	1.9	0	45	80	4.9	475	11
Mixed nuts, with peanuts, salted:															
Dry roasted	1 oz	28	2	170	5	15	2.0	8.9	3.1	0	7	20	1.0	169	190[20]
Roasted in oil	1 oz	28	2	175	5	16	2.5	9.0	3.8	0	6	31	0.9	165	185[20]
Peanut butter	1 tbsp	16	1	95	5	8	1.4	4.0	2.5	0	3	5	0.3	110	75
Pecans, halves	1 cup	108	5	720	8	73	5.9	45.5	18.1	0	20	39	2.3	423	1
	1 oz	28	5	190	2	19	1.5	12.0	4.7	0	5	10	0.6	111	Tr
Refried beans, canned	1 cup	290	72	295	18	3	0.4	0.6	1.4	0	51	141	5.1	1,141	1,228
Walnuts, black, chopped	1 cup	125	4	760	30	71	4.5	15.9	46.9	0	15	73	3.8	655	1
	1 oz	28	4	170	7	16	1.0	3.6	10.6	0	3	16	0.9	149	Tr

20. Mixed nuts without salt contain 3 mg sodium per oz.

Meat and Meat Products

Beef, cooked:[21]

Food	Measure														
Cuts braised, simmered, or pot roasted, lean and fat, piece, 4 1/8 by 2 1/4 by 1/2 in	3 oz	85	54	220	25	13	4.8	5.7	0.5	81	0	5	2.8	248	43
Ground beef, broiled, patty, 3 by 5/8 in., regular	3 oz	85	54	245	20	18	6.9	7.7	0.7	76	0	9	2.1	248	70
Roast, oven cooked, no liquid added, lean and fat, 2 pieces, 4 1/8 by 2 1/4 by 1/4 in	3 oz	85	46	315	19	26	10.8	11.4	0.9	72	0	8	2.0	246	54
Steak, sirloin, broiled, lean and fat, piece, 2 1/2 by 2 1/2 by 3/4 in	3 oz	85	53	240	23	15	6.4	6.9	0.6	77	0	9	2.6	306	53
Pork, cured, cooked:															
Bacon, regular	3 medium slices	19	13	110	6	9	3.3	4.5	1.1	16	Tr	2	0.3	92	303
Ham, canned, roasted, 2 pieces, 4 1/8 by 2 1/4 by 1/4 in, luncheon meat: Cooked ham (8 slices per 8-oz pkg), regular	3 oz	85	67	140	18	7	2.4	3.5	0.8	35	Tr	6	0.9	298	908
Cooked ham (8 slices per 8-oz pkg), regular	2 slices	57	65	105	10	6	1.9	2.8	0.7	32	2	4	0.6	189	751
Pork, fresh, cooked:															
Chop, loin (cut 3 per lb with bone), pan fried, lean and fat	3.1 oz	89	45	335	21	27	9.8	12.5	3.1	92	0	4	0.7	323	64
Bologna, slice (8 per 8-oz pkg)	2 slices	57	54	180	7	16	6.1	7.6	1.4	31	2	7	0.9	103	581
Frankfurter (10 per 1-lb pkg), cooked (reheated)	1 frankfurter	45	54	145	5	13	4.8	6.2	1.2	23	1	5	0.5	75	504
Pork link (16 per 1-lb pkg), cooked[22]	1 link	13	45	50	3	4	1.4	1.8	0.5	11	Tr	4	0.2	47	168
Salami,[22] cooked type, slice (8 per 8-oz pkg)	2 slices	57	60	145	8	11	4.6	5.2	1.2	37	1	7	1.5	113	607

Mixed Dishes and Fast Foods

Mixed dishes:

Food	Measure														
Beef and vegetable stew, from home recipe	1 cup	245	82	220	16	11	4.4	4.5	0.5	71	15	29	2.9	613	292

21. Outer layer of fat was removed to within approximately 1/2 inch of the lean. Deposits of fat within the cut were not removed.
22. One patty (8 per pound) of bulk sausage is equivalent to 2 links.

Foods, Approximate Measures, Units, and Weight (Weight of Edible Portion Only)

Foods, Approximate Measures, Units, and Weight (Weight of Edible Portion Only)		Water	Food Energy	Protein	Fat	Fatty Acids			Choles-terol	Carbo-hy-drate	Cal-cium	Iron	Potas-sium	So-dium
						Satu-rated	Mono-unsatu-rated	Polyun-satu-rated						
	(g)	(%)	(Kcals)	(g)	(g)	(g)	(g)	(g)	(mg)	(g)	(mg)	(mg)	(mg)	(mg)
Beef potpie, from home recipe, baked, piece, 1/3 of 9-in. diam. pie[23] 1 piece	210	55	515	21	30	7.9	12.9	7.4	42	39	29	3.8	334	596
Chicken and noodles, cooked, from home recipe 1 cup	240	71	365	22	18	5.1	7.1	3.9	103	26	26	2.2	149	600
Chicken potpie, from home recipe, baked, piece, 1/3 of 9-in diam. pie[23] 1 piece	232	57	545	23	31	10.3	15.5	6.6	56	42	70	3.0	343	594
Chili con carne with beans, canned 1 cup	255	72	340	19	16	5.8	7.2	1.0	28	31	82	4.3	594	1,354
Macaroni (enriched) and cheese, canned[24] 1 cup	240	80	230	9	10	4.7	2.9	1.3	24	26	199	1.0	139	730
Spaghetti (enriched) in tomato sauce with cheese, canned 1 cup	250	80	190	6	2	0.4	0.4	0.5	3	39	40	2.8	303	955
Spaghetti (enriched) with meatballs and tomato sauce, canned 1 cup	250	78	260	12	10	2.4	3.9	3.1	23	29	53	3.3	245	1,220
Fast food entrees:														
Cheeseburger:														
Regular 1 sandwich	112	46	300	15	15	7.3	5.6	1.0	44	28	135	2.3	219	672
4 oz patty 1 sandwich	194	46	525	30	31	15.1	12.2	1.4	104	40	236	4.5	407	1,224
Enchilada 1 enchilada	230	72	235	20	16	7.7	6.7	0.6	19	24	97	3.3	653	1,332
English muffin, egg, cheese, and bacon 1 sandwich	138	49	360	18	18	8.0	8.0	0.7	213	31	197	3.1	201	832
Fish sandwich, regular, with cheese 1 sandwich	140	43	420	16	23	6.3	6.9	7.7	56	39	132	1.8	274	667
Hamburger:														
Regular 1 sandwich	98	46	245	12	11	4.4	5.3	0.5	32	28	56	2.2	202	463
4 oz patty 1 sandwich	174	50	445	25	21	7.1	11.7	0.6	71	38	75	4.8	404	763
Pizza, cheese, 1/8 of 15-in diam. pizza[23] 1 slice	120	46	290	15	9	4.1	2.6	1.3	56	39	220	1.6	230	699
Roast beef sandwich 1 sandwich	150	52	345	22	13	3.5	6.9	1.8	55	34	60	4.0	338	757
Taco 1 taco	81	55	195	9	11	4.1	5.5	0.8	21	15	109	1.2	263	456

23. Crust made with vegetable shortening and enriched flour.
24. Made with corn oil.

Poultry and Poultry Products

Food	Measure														
Poultry and Poultry Products															
Chicken:															
Fried, flesh, with skin,[25] batter dipped:															
Breast, 1/2 breast (5.6 oz with bones)	4.9 oz	140	52	365	35	18	4.9	7.6	4.3	119	13	28	1.8	281	385
Drumstick (3.4 oz with bones)	2.5 oz	72	53	195	16	11	3.0	4.6	2.7	62	6	12	1.0	134	194
Roasted, flesh only:															
Breast, 1/2 breast (4.2 oz with bones and skin)	3.0 oz	86	65	140	27	3	0.9	1.1	0.7	73	0	13	0.9	220	64
Drumstick, (2.9 oz with bones and skin)	1.6 oz	44	67	75	12	2	0.7	0.8	0.6	41	0	5	0.6	108	42
Turkey, roasted, flesh only:															
Dark meat, piece, 2 1/2 by 1 5/8 by 1/4 in	4 pieces	85	63	160	24	6	2.1	1.4	1.8	72	0	27	2.0	246	67
Light meat, piece, 4 by 2 by 1/4 in	2 pieces	85	66	135	25	3	0.9	0.5	0.7	59	0	16	1.1	259	54
Soups, Sauces, and Gravies															
Soups, canned, condensed:															
Prepared with equal volume of milk:															
Clam chowder, New England	1 cup	248	85	165	9	7	3.0	2.3	1.1	22	17	186	1.5	300	992
Cream of mushroom	1 cup	248	85	205	6	14	5.1	3.0	4.6	20	15	179	0.6	270	1,076
Tomato	1 cup	248	85	160	6	6	2.9	1.6	1.1	17	22	159	1.8	449	932
Prepared with equal volume of water:															
Bean with bacon	1 cup	253	84	170	8	6	1.5	2.2	1.8	3	23	81	2.0	402	951
Chicken noodle	1 cup	241	92	75	4	2	0.7	1.1	0.6	7	9	17	0.8	55	1,106
Minestrone	1 cup	241	91	80	4	3	0.6	0.7	1.1	2	11	34	0.9	313	911
Pea, green	1 cup	250	83	165	9	3	1.4	1.0	0.4	0	27	28	2.0	190	988
Tomato	1 cup	244	90	85	2	2	0.4	0.4	1.0	0	17	12	1.8	264	871
Vegetable beef	1 cup	244	92	80	6	2	0.9	0.8	0.1	5	10	17	1.1	173	956
Gravies, from dry mix:															
Brown	1 cup	261	91	80	3	2	0.9	0.8	0.1	2	14	66	0.2	61	1,147
Chicken	1 cup	260	91	85	3	2	0.5	0.9	0.4	3	14	39	0.3	62	1,134
Sugars and Sweets															
Candy:															
Caramels, plain or chocolate	1 oz	28	8	115	1	3	2.2	0.3	0.1	1	22	42	0.4	54	64

25. Fried in vegetable shortening.

Foods, Approximate Measures, Units, and Weight (Weight of Edible Portion Only)

Food	Measure	(g)	Water (%)	Food Energy (Kcals)	Protein (g)	Fat (g)	Fatty Acids Saturated (g)	Mono-unsaturated (g)	Polyun-saturated (g)	Cholesterol (mg)	Carbohydrate (g)	Calcium (mg)	Iron (mg)	Potassium (mg)	Sodium (mg)
Chocolate:															
Milk, plain	1 oz	28	1	145	2	9	5.4	3.0	0.3	6	16	50	0.4	96	23
Milk, with almonds	1 oz	28	2	150	3	10	4.8	4.1	0.7	5	15	65	0.5	125	23
Milk, with rice cereal	1 oz	28	2	140	2	7	4.4	2.5	0.2	6	18	48	0.2	100	46
Hard	1 oz	28	1	110	0	0	0.0	0.0	0.0	0	28	Tr	0.1	1	7
Gelatin dessert prepared with gelatin dessert powder and water	1/2 cup	120	84	70	2	0	0.0	0.0	0.0	0	17	2	Tr	Tr	55
Jellies	1 tbsp	18	28	50	Tr	Tr	Tr	Tr	Tr	0	13	2	0.1	16	5
Popsicle, 3-fl-oz size	1 popsicle	95	80	70	0	0	0.0	0.0	0.0	0	18	0	Tr	4	11
Puddings:															
Chocolate	5-oz can	142	68	205	3	11	9.5	0.5	0.1	1	30	74	1.2	254	285
Tapioca	5-oz can	142	74	160	3	5	4.8	Tr	Tr	Tr	28	119	0.3	212	252
Syrups:															
Chocolate-flavored syrup or topping, thin type	2 tbsp	38	37	85	1	Tr	0.2	0.1	0.1	0	22	6	0.8	85	36
Table syrup (corn or maple)	2 tbsp	42	25	122	0	0	0.0	0.0	0.0	0	32	1	Tr	7	19
Vegetables and Vegetable Products															
Beans:															
Lima, immature seeds, frozen, cooked, drained, thin-seeded types (baby limas)	1 cup	180	72	190	12	1	0.1	Tr	0.3	0	35	50	3.5	740	52
Snap, canned, drained solids (cut)	1 cup	135	93	25	2	Tr	Tr	Tr	0.1	0	6	35	1.2	147	339[26]
Broccoli, cooked, drained:															
From raw, spears, cut into 1/2-in pieces	1 cup	155	90	45	5	Tr	0.1	Tr	0.2	0	9	177	1.8	253	17
From frozen, chopped	1 cup	185	91	50	6	Tr	Tr	Tr	0.1	0	10	94	1.1	333	44
Cabbage, common varieties, cooked, drained	1 cup	150	94	30	1	Tr	Tr	Tr	0.2	0	7	50	0.6	308	29
Carrots, Raw without crowns and tips, scraped, whole 7 1/2 by 1 1/8 in, or strips, 2 1/2 to 3 in long	1 carrot or 18 strips	72	88	30	1	Tr	Tr	Tr	0.1	0	7	19	0.4	233	25

26. For regular pack; special dietary pack contains 3 mg sodium.

Food	Measure	(g)	(%)												
Cauliflower, cooked, drained, from raw (flowerets)	1 cup	125	93	30	2	Tr	Tr	Tr	0.1	0	6	34	0.5	404	8
Celery, pascal type, raw, stalk, large outer, 8 by 1 1/2 in (at root end)	1 stalk	40	95	5	Tr	Tr	Tr	Tr	Tr	0	1	14	0.2	114	35
Corn, sweet, cooked, drained, canned:															
Cream style	1 cup	256	79	185	4	1	0.2	0.3	0.5	0	46	8	1.0	343	730[27]
Whole kernel, vacuum pack	1 cup	210	77	165	5	1	0.2	0.3	0.5	0	41	11	0.9	391	571[28]
Cucumber, with peel, slices, 1/8 in thick (large, 2 1/8-in diam.; small, 1 3/4-in diam.)	6 large or 8 small slices	28	96	5	Tr	Tr	Tr	Tr	Tr	0	1	4	0.1	42	1
Lettuce, raw, crisphead, as iceberg, pieces, chopped or shredded	1 cup	55	96	5	1	Tr	Tr	Tr	0.1	0	1	10	0.3	87	5
Mushrooms, raw, sliced or chopped	1 cup	70	92	20	1	Tr	Tr	Tr	0.1	0	3	4	0.9	259	3
Onions, raw, chopped	1 cup	160	91	55	2	Tr	0.1	0.1	0.2	0	12	40	0.6	248	3
Peas, green, frozen, cooked, drained	1 cup	160	80	125	8	Tr	0.1	Tr	0.2	0	23	38	2.5	269	139
Potatoes, cooked:															
Baked (about 2 per lb, raw, with skin	1 potato	202	71	220	5	Tr	0.1	Tr	0.1	0	51	20	2.7	844	16
French fried, strip, 2 to 3 1/2 in long, frozen fried in vegetable oil	10 strips	50	38	160	2	8	2.5	1.6	3.8	0	20	10	0.4	366	108
Potato products, prepared:															
Hashed brown	1 cup	156	56	340	5	18	7.0	8.0	2.1	0	44	23	2.4	680	53
Mashed, from home recipe, milk added	1 cup	210	78	160	4	1	0.7	0.3	0.1	4	37	55	0.6	628	636
Potato salad, made with mayonnaise	1 cup	250	76	360	7	21	3.6	6.2	9.3	170	28	48	1.6	635	1,323
Scalloped, from home recipe	1 cup	245	81	210	7	9	5.5	2.5	0.4	29	26	140	1.4	926	821
Potato chips	10 chips	20	3	105	1	7	1.8	1.2	3.6	0	10	5	0.2	260	94

27. For regular pack; special dietary pack contains 8 mg sodium.
28. For regular pack; special dietary pack contains 6 mg sodium.

Foods, Approximate Measures, Units, and Weight (Weight of Edible Portion Only)

			Water	Food Energy	Protein	Fat	Fatty Acids			Choles-terol	Carbo-hy-drate	Cal-cium	Iron	Potas-sium	So-dium
							Satu-rated	Mono-unsatu-rated	Polyun-satu-rated						
		(g)	(%)	(Kcals)	(g)	(g)	(g)	(g)	(g)	(mg)	(g)	(mg)	(mg)	(mg)	(mg)
Spinach, canned, drained solids	1 cup	214	92	50	6	1	0.2	Tr	0.4	0	7	272	4.9	740	683[29]
Tomatoes, raw, 2 3/5-in diam. (3 per 12 oz pkg.)	1 tomato	123	94	25	1	Tr	Tr	Tr	0.1	0	5	9	0.6	255	10
Tomato juice, canned	1 cup	244	94	40	2	Tr	Tr	Tr	0.1	0	10	22	1.4	537	881[30]
Miscellaneous Items															
Catsup	1 tbsp	15	69	15	Tr	Tr	Tr	Tr	Tr	0	4	3	0.1	54	156
Mustard, prepared, yellow	1 tsp or individual packet	5	80	5	Tr	Tr	Tr	0.2	Tr	0	Tr	4	0.1	7	63
Olives:															
Green	4 medium or 3 extra large	13	78	15	Tr	2	0.2	1.2	0.1	0	Tr	8	0.2	7	312
Ripe	3 small or 2 large	9	73	15	Tr	2	0.3	1.3	0.2	0	Tr	10	0.2	2	68
Pickles, cucumber:															
Dill, medium, whole, 3 3/4 in long, 1 1/4-in diam.	1 pickle	65	93	5	Tr	Tr	Tr	Tr	0.1	0	1	17	0.7	130	928
Sweet, gherkin, small, whole, about 2 1/2 in long, 3/4-in diam.	1 pickle	15	61	20	Tr	Tr	Tr	Tr	Tr	0	5	2	0.2	30	107

29. With added salt; if none is added, sodium content is 50 mg.
30. With added salt; if none is added, sodium content is 24 mg.

Name_____

Class/Activity Section_____

Evaluation of *Healthy Lifestyle: A Self-Assessment*

After completing *Healthy Lifestyle: A Self-Assessment,* answer the following questions:

1. What lifestyle strengths have you identified with this test?

2. Describe your life choices that have helped to establish these strengths.

3. What are the weak areas that you have identified in the test?

4. Describe what benefits you would receive if you were to change your lifestyle in the weak areas.

5. List obstacles that stand in your way (in the event that you choose to change).

6. Identify what support you will be able to enlist to help you change (if you desire to do so).

Name_____

Class/Activity Section_____

Assessing Your Wellness

Read each statement carefully and respond honestly by using the following scoring:

Almost always = 2 points
Sometimes/occasionally = 1 point
Very seldom = 0 points

Physical Dimension

_____ 1. I exercise aerobically (vigorous, continuous) for 20 to 30 minutes at least three times per week.

_____ 2. I eat fruits, vegetables, and whole grains every day.

_____ 3. I avoid tobacco products.

_____ 4. I wear a seat belt while riding in and driving a car.

_____ 5. I deliberately minimize my intake of cholesterol, dietary fats, and oils.

_____ 6. I avoid drinking alcoholic beverages *or* I consume no more than one drink per day.

_____ 7. I get an adequate amount of sleep.

_____ 8. I have adequate coping mechanisms for dealing with stress.

_____ 9. I maintain a regular schedule of immunizations, physical and dental checkups (including Pap smears and blood pressure and cholesterol checks), and monthly self-exams of breasts or testicles.

_____10. I maintain a reasonable weight, avoiding extremes of overweight and underweight.

_____Physical total

Social Dimension

_____ 1. I contribute time and/or money to social and community projects.

_____ 2. I am committed to a lifetime of volunteerism.

_____ 3. I exhibit fairness and justice in dealing with people.

_____ 4. I have a network of close friends and/or family.

_____ 5. I am interested in others, including those from different backgrounds than my own.

_____ 6. I am able to balance my own needs with the needs of others.

_____ 7. I am able to communicate with and get along with a wide variety of people.

_____ 8. I obey the laws and rules of our society.

_____ 9. I am a compassionate person and try to help others when I can.

_____10. I support and help with family, neighborhood, and work social gatherings.

_____Social total

Spiritual Dimension

_____ 1. I feel comfortable and at ease with my spiritual life.

_____ 2. There is a direct relationship between my personal values and daily actions.

_____ 3. When I get depressed or frustrated by problems, my spiritual beliefs and values give me direction.

_____ 4. Prayer, meditation, and/or quiet personal reflection is/are important in my life.

_____ 5. Life is meaningful for me, and I feel a purpose in life.

_____ 6. I am able to speak comfortably about my personal values and beliefs.

_____ 7. I am consistently striving to grow spiritually and I see it as a lifelong process.

_____ 8. I am tolerant of and try to learn about others' beliefs and values.

_____ 9. I have a strong sense of hope and optimism in my life and use my thoughts and attitudes in life-affirming ways.

_____10. I appreciate the natural forces that exist in the universe.

_____Spiritual total

Intellectual Dimension

_____ 1. I am interested in learning new things.

_____ 2. I try to keep abreast of current affairs—locally, nationally, and internationally.

_____ 3. I enjoy attending special lectures, plays, musical performances, museums, galleries, and/or libraries.

_____ 4. I carefully select movies and television programs.

_____ 5. I enjoy creative and stimulating mental activities/games.

_____ 6. I am happy with the amount and variety that I read.

_____ 7. I make an effort to improve my verbal, writing, and expression skills.

_____ 8. A continuing education program is/will be important to me in my career.

_____ 9. I am able to analyze, synthesize, and see more than one side of an issue.

_____10. I enjoy engaging in intellectual discussions.

_____Intellectual total

Occupational Dimension

_____ 1. I am happy with my career choice.

_____ 2. I look forward to work.

_____ 3. My job responsibilities/duties are consistent with my values.

_____ 4. The payoffs/advantages in my career field choice are consistent with my values.

_____ 5. I am happy with the balance between my work time and leisure time.

_____ 6. I am happy with the amount of control I have in my work.

_____ 7. My work gives me personal satisfaction and stimulation.

_____ 8. I am happy with the professional/personal growth provided by my job.

_____ 9. I feel my job allows me to make a difference in the world.

_____10. My job contributes positively to my overall well-being.

_____Occupational total

Emotional Dimension

_____ 1. I am able to develop and maintain close relationships.

_____ 2. I accept the responsibility for my actions.

_____ 3. I see challenges and change as opportunities for growth.

_____ 4. I feel I have considerable control over my life.

_____ 5. I am able to laugh at life and myself.

_____ 6. I feel good about myself.

_____ 7. I am able to appropriately cope with stress and tension and make time for leisure pursuits.

_____ 8. I am able to recognize my personal shortcomings and learn from my mistakes.

_____ 9. I am able to recognize and express my feelings.

_____ 10. I enjoy life.

_____ Emotional total

Environmental Dimension

_2_ 1. I consciously conserve energy (electricity, heat, light, water, etc.) in my place of residence.

_0_ 2. I practice recycling (glass, paper, plastic, etc.).

_0_ 3. I am committed to cleaning up the environment (air, soil, water, etc.).

_2_ 4. I consciously carpool, ride a bicycle, walk, etc. in order to conserve fuel energy and to lessen the pollution in the atmosphere.

_1_ 5. I limit the use of fertilizers and chemicals when managing my yard/lawn/outdoor living space.

_0_ 6. I do not use aerosol sprays.

_1_ 7. I do not litter.

_0_ 8. I volunteer my time for environmental conservation projects.

_1_ 9. I purchase recycled items when possible, even if they cost more.

_0_ 10. I feel very strongly about doing _my_ part to preserve the environment.

_7_ Environmental total

Scoring

Add your total score for each dimension of wellness.

Scores of 15 to 20 Points
Excellent strength in this dimension.

Scores of 9 to 14 Points
There is room for improvement. Look again at the items in which you scored 1 or 0. What changes can you make to improve your score?

Scores of 0 to 8 Points
This dimension needs a lot of work. Look again at this dimension and challenge yourself to begin making small steps toward growth here. Remember: The goal is balanced wellness.

Take your score in each dimension of wellness and shade it in on Figure A.1. How smoothly will your wellness wheel roll? A smooth ride indicates _balanced_ wellness, and the LARGER the wheel, the better!

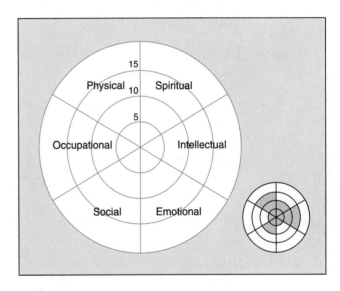

FIGURE A.1 ➤
Wellness wheel.

Name_____

Class/Activity Section_____

Is Your Campus/Community Supportive of Wellness?

List ways your campus and/or community supports or promotes wellness living in each dimension of wellness. List as many resources as you can.

Can you think of *improvements* that could be made?

Social Dimension

Emotional Dimension

Environmental Dimension

Occupational Dimension

1

Physical Dimension

Intellectual Dimension

Spiritual Dimension

Chapter 1 Activities

chapter **2**
activities

Calculate Your Target Heart Rate Range (THR)

The target heart rate represents the intensity level at which you should exercise to produce cardiorespiratory benefits. This amount of exercise (overload) is enough to condition the heart, lungs, and muscles but is not overly strenuous. Monitoring intensity during a workout is done by measuring the heart rate. For fitness to occur, your heart rate must be raised to approximately 60 percent of the difference between the resting and maximal heart rates. An increase in heart rate equal to 75 percent of the difference between resting and maximal rates is a reasonable upper intensity level for most exercisers. This is the target heart rate range (or training heart range). The Karvonen formula for calculating your target heart rate is as follows:

THR = (maximal HR* − resting HR) × Intensity % + Resting HR**
> ***Maximal HR = 220 minus age**
> ****Resting HR = count your pulse at rest for 60 seconds**

When estimating your target heart rate range, two factors are involved:

➤ Your age: _____.
➤ Your resting heart rate (RHR): _____.

Use these numbers in the formula that follows:

1. 220 − _____ = _____
     (your age)   (estimated maximal heart rate (MHR))

2. _____ − _____ = _____
   (MHR)   (resting HR)   (HR reserve)

3. _____ ×   0.60   + _____ = _____
   (HR reserve) (lower intensity) (resting HR) (lower target heart rate)

   _____ ×   0.75   + _____ = _____
   (HR reserve) (higher intensity) (resting HR) (higher target heart rate)

4. Target heart rate range is _____ to _____ beats per minute.

Example: Jeff is 22 years old and has a resting heart rate of 78 beats per minute.

1. 220 − 22 = 198 MHR

2. 198 − 78 = 120 heart rate reserve

3. 120 × 0.60 = 72 + 78 = 150

   120 × 0.75 = 90 + 78 = 168

4. THR range is 150 to 168 beats per minute.

Name_____

Class/Activity Section_____

Exercise/Activity Log Sheet

(make extra copies of this form as needed)

	S	M	T	W	Th	F	Sa
Week 1							
Week 2							
Week 3							
Week 4							

Goals: _____

_____

_____

_____

Comments: _____

_____

_____

Name_____

Class/Activity Section_____

Strength Training Log

Exercise											

Name_____

Class/Activity Section_____

Health-Related Fitness Analysis Chart

After completing your *Personal Fitness Profile,* use norms in Chapter 4 to determine your fitness level on each of the tests. Use Figure A.2 to graph the results. Match fitness levels on the left with the norm ratings for each of the following tests: cardiorespiratory endurance, abdominal curls, push-ups, and sit and reach. Use the descriptors on the right for body fat norms. Place a dot in the center of the space that indicates your rating on each of the health-related fitness norms. Use straight lines to connect the dots.

FIGURE A.2 ➤

source: From Assmann, N. Muncie, Ind.: Ball State University. Used by permission.

Fitness level						Body fat descriptors
						Very low fat
Excellent						Low fat
Good						Average fat
Average						Above average fat
Low						High fat
Very low						Obese
	CR endur.	Curls	Push-ups	Sit & reach	Body fat	

1. In which fitness components did you score average or higher? Why?

2. In which fitness components did you score below average? Why?

3. What are your fitness goals for the next 8 to 12 weeks, six months to a year, five years or more?

Name_____

Class/Activity Section_____

Understanding Health-Related Fitness Assessments

This exercise allows you to check your understanding of which assessments correspond to which fitness components and of how to interpret fitness test results based on age-adjusted norms. It also gives you practice in applying fitness test results to an appropriate workout in Appendices 1 to 7.

Jenny, age 23, completed her fitness assessments and the results follow. Using norms given in Chapter 4, evaluate her fitness levels and, for each assessment, determine what fitness component was being tested.

Assessment	Results	Fitness Level	Fitness Component Tested
1.5-mile run	16:30	_____	_____
Abdominal curls	45	} Percent fat_____	_____
Push-ups	45	_____	_____
Skinfolds:			
Tricep	20 mm		_____
Iliac	10 mm		_____
Sit and reach	3 inches	_____	_____

Using the *Run/Walk Program* chart in Appendix 4, what is her starting workout level? _____

From this *Run/Walk Program* chart, what is prescribed for her initial workout?

Name_____

Class/Activity Section_____

Plan for Cardiorespiratory Fitness

Using the following chart and a sample cardiorespiratory fitness program given in Appendices 1 to 7, develop a three-week individualized workout plan based on results of your cardiorespiratory fitness assessment. Include frequency, intensity, time, and type of activity.

Type of activity: _____

CR fitness level: _____

Program starting level: _____

Frequency: _____

Target heart rate: _____

Sunday	Monday	Tuesday	Wednesday	Thursday	Friday	Saturday

Describe your warm-up activities:

Describe your cool-down activities:

Name_____

Class/Activity Section_____

Waist-to-Hip Ratio

Recent investigations have begun pointing to the location of excess fat as a risk factor for heart disease and certain cancers. Fat distributed in the abdominal area is linked to increased health risks; hip/thigh fat is not as risky. As a result, the waist-to-hip ratio has become a common assessment used for health-risk identification. To compute this ratio, divide the waist measurement by the hip measurement. Some experts feel that weight-related health problems are increased for women whose ratio is 0.80 or higher and for men whose ratio is 0.95 or higher.

Beth's waist is 29 inches and her hips are 38 inches.

$$\frac{29 \text{ in. (waist)}}{38 \text{ in. (hip)}} = 0.76 \quad \text{Waist-to-hip ratio does not indicate increased risk.}$$

Steve's waist is 42 inches and his hips measure 36 inches.

$$\frac{42 \text{ in. (waist)}}{36 \text{ in. (hip)}} = 1.17 \quad \text{Waist-to-hip ratio indicated increased risk.}$$

Calculate your waist-to-hip ratio:

Your waist measurement:_____ in.

Your hip measurement:_____ in.

Waist-to-hip ratio:_____

Evaluation:_____

_____

_____

Phil A. Case Study

Phil is 20 years old and is a student at State College. He has kept himself in good shape and has been running road races for the past four years. This morning, while running on White River Road, he stepped into a chuck hole and sprained his ankle. He was able to limp home. You are one of his best friends, and he has come to you for advice. He asks, "Should I go to a doctor?"

1. List four questions you would ask Phil to determine whether you should recommend a doctor:

   a.

   b.

   c.

   d.

2. Phil answers "No" to all of your questions. He asks, "What do you think I should do to keep it from swelling?" List and describe four treatments you would prescribe for Phil's injury:

   a.

   b.

   c.

   d.

3. Phil wants to keep in shape and plans to start running again as soon as possible. He asks, "Do you think I should try to run tomorrow?" List three steps in the progression of getting back into action. Also, tell him how he might keep in shape while his injury heals:

   a.

   b.

   c.

   d.

Name_____

Class/Activity Section_____

Action Plan for the Back

Back Exercises

Complete the series of back exercises that are described in Figure 5.3 in Chapter 5.

1. Describe how your lower back area felt at the completion of the exercise session.

2. Explain how you will fit this exercise regimen into your daily schedule.

Back Care

Explain how you will perform the following tasks utilizing proper body mechanics/alignment:

1. Lifting a garage door to open it:

2. Lifting a heavy box to put in the back of a station wagon:

3. Sitting several hours at a desk studying:

4. Driving a car for five hours:

5. Standing/working at a checkout counter for five hours:

6. Sleeping:

Name_____

Class/Activity Section_____

Are You at Risk?

Read the question, and circle the most appropriate response as it relates to your lifestyle. Finally, add the points associated with your response to get your total score and your risk of developing heart disease.

1. Do you smoke cigarettes?	YES	12
	NO	0
2. Do you use other tobacco products (pipe, cigars, chewing, snuff)?	YES	3
	NO	0
3. Do you usually exercise vigorously at least three times per week for 20 to 30 minutes?	YES	0
	NO	10
4. How would you describe your lifestyle?	Sedentary (inactive)	6
	Somewhat active	2
	Very active	0
5. What is your blood pressure?	High 140/90+	9
	Normal or low	0
	Don't know	2
6. What is your total cholesterol?	High 240mg/dl+	9
	Normal	0
	Don't know	2
7. Has anyone in your family ever been told they had any form of heart disease (parents or siblings ≤55 years)?	YES	5
	NO	0
8. Have you ever had any of the following?		
a. Pain or discomfort in chest and surrounding areas?	YES	2
	NO	0
b. Unaccustomed shortness of breath with mild exertion?	YES	2
	NO	0
9. What is your gender?	Female	0
	Male	4
10. Have you ever been told you have diabetes?	YES	4
	NO	0
11. Have you suffered a personal loss or misfortune in the past year that had a serious impact on your life? (i.e., job loss, disability, separation/divorce, jail term, or the death of someone close to you)	NO	0
	YES, 1 serious loss or misfortune	1
	YES, 2 or more	2
12. Do you feel you handle everyday stress well?	YES	0
	NO	2
13. Would you describe yourself as a Type A person (i.e., aggressive, competitive, time-conscious)?	YES	4
	NO	2
14. If you are male, what is your age?	Under 40	1
	40+	3
If you are female, what is your age?	Under 50	0
	50+	3

15. What is your race?	White	0
	Black	3
	Hispanic	1
	Other	1
16. How would you describe your weight?	Normal/below	0
	Normal to +30 lbs.	1
	+30 lbs. or more	2
17. Do you consume meat, eggs, cheese, butter, whole milk, and fried foods?	0 to 5 times/week to 10 times/week	0
	daily	2
	2 to 3 servings/day	3
	over 3 servings/day	6

Your Total Score _____

Scoring

Scores of 0 to 16

Your risk is **low** for developing heart disease at this time. Evaluate your risk every year since risk factors such as blood pressure, cholesterol levels, and age change from year to year. If you have any uncontrollable risk factors, you would be wise to modify other risk factors to protect your cardiorespiratory system.

Scores of 17 to 29

Your risk is **average** or moderate. Your score indicates there is room for improvement on some risk factors. If you have any uncontrollable risk factors, it is imperative that you modify other risk factors to protect your cardiorespiratory system.

Scores of 30+

You have a **high** risk of developing heart disease. You should take action **immediately** to modify all controllable risk factors.

Name_____

Class/Activity Section_____

Evaluation of *Are You at Risk?*

After completing the *Are You at Risk?* assessment, answer the following questions:

1. List at least five personal lifestyle changes you can make to lower your risk for heart disease. Be specific; don't simply say, "Eat better," for example.

2. Take the *Are You At Risk?* assessment for a parent or friend. What is his or her score? What advice would you give to help to lower his or her score?

3. List your personal controllable risk factors.

4. List your personal uncontrollable risk factors.

5. Some physicians are refusing to treat people when they discover that they smoke or don't exercise or have diets high in fat. Discuss how you feel about this decision.

Name_____

Class/Activity Section_____

How to Mend a Broken Heart

Read the opening scenario concerning Rob on page 2 in your text. You were the physician on call when he was brought in. Complete a medical history on this patient and answer his wife's questions.

1. List Rob's three primary risk factors for heart disease given in the scenario.

2. List Rob's five secondary risk factors for heart disease.

3. What three lifestyle changes will you tell Rob to make to reduce his heart disease risk?

Rob's wife has read the chart. She is distraught and has several questions for you. Please respond.

4. "Doctor, I really don't understand some of the words used on the chart. What is angina? Myocardial infarction? What is atherosclerosis, and will it ever go away?"

5. "I saw that his cholesterol was 280 and his HDL level was 28. What does that mean? What is normal?"

6. "Rob doesn't want to quit smoking—since he's smoked for 20 years. Why is smoking bad for his heart?"

7. "A nurse said Rob needs a special exercise program to aid in recovery. Won't exercise strain his heart? What good will it do?" (Give three benefits.)

8. "Rob enjoys having an occasional beer. Will he have to give this up?"

Life Event Scale for the College Student

Determine which of the following events you have experienced within the past year. (G. E. Anderson "College Schedule of Recent Experience." Unpublished Masters Thesis, 1972. Department of Education, North Dakota State University, Fargo, North Dakota.)

Mean value	Life event
(87)	Death of a spouse
(77)	Death of a close family member
(77)	Marriage
(76)	Divorce
(74)	Marital separation from your mate
(68)	Pregnancy or fathering a child
(68)	Death of a close friend
(65)	Major personal injury or illness
(62)	Being fired from work
(60)	Going broke or breaking off a marital engagement or a steady relationship
(58)	Sexual difficulties
(58)	Marital reconciliation with your mate
(57)	Major change in self-concept or self-awareness
(57)	Major change in usual type and/or amount of recreation
(56)	Major change in the health or behavior of a family member
(54)	Becoming engaged to be married
(53)	Major change in financial state (a lot worse or a lot better off than usual)
(52)	Taking a mortgage or loan less than $10,000 (such as purchase of a car, TV, school loan)
(50)	Change to a different line of work
(50)	Major change in the number of arguments with spouse (either a lot more or a lot less than usual)
(50)	Entering college
(50)	Change to a new school
(50)	Gaining a new family member (through birth, adoption, older person moving in, etc.)
(50)	Major conflict in or change in values
(49)	Major change in the amount of independence and responsibility (for example, for budgeting time)
(48)	Major change in social activities
(47)	Major change in responsibilities at work (promotion, demotion, lateral transfer)
(46)	Major change in the use of alcohol (a lot more or a lot less)
(45)	Revision of personal habits (friends, dress, manners, associations, etc.)
(44)	Trouble with school administration (instructors, advisors, class scheduling)
(43)	Holding a job while attending school
(42)	Trouble with in-laws
(42)	Change of residence or living conditions
(41)	Spouse beginning or ceasing work outside the home
(41)	Change in choice of a major field of study
(41)	Change in dating habits
(40)	Outstanding personal achievement
(38)	Major change in the amount of participation in school activities
(36)	Major change in church activities (a lot more or a lot less than usual)
(34)	Major change in sleeping habits (sleeping a lot more or a lot less or sleeping during a different part of the day)
(33)	Taking a trip or vacation
(30)	Major change in eating habits (a lot more or a lot less food intake or very different meal hours or surroundings)
(26)	Major change in the number of family get-togethers (a lot more or a lot less)
(22)	Being found guilty of minor violations of the law (traffic tickets, jaywalking, etc.)

Scoring . . . Your score is _____.

To obtain your score, multiply the number of times an event occurred by its mean value. Then total all of the scores. Your score is termed your **life change units (LCU).** This is a measure of the amount of significant changes in your life to which you have had to adjust. In other words, your LCU is a measure of the stressors you have encountered this past year.

Rating	Score	Implications for Illness
Low stress	150 or less	This indicates that a person has a 37 percent chance of getting a stress-related disease in the next year or two.
Moderate	151 to 300	This indicates that a person has a 51 percent chance of getting a stress illness in the next year.
High stress	301 or more	This indicates that a person has an 80 percent chance of getting a stress illness in the next year.

7

Name_____

Class/Activity Section_____

Evaluation of the *Life Event Scale for the College Student*

After completing the *Life Event Scale for the College Student* or the Holmes-Rahe scale (p. 147), answer the following questions:

1. What was your score?_____

2. What was your rating?_____

3. Discuss the results of this test in terms of its implication for you having a stress illness this year. List at least four or five factors that influence this implication.

4. Describe *one* of the relaxation techniques (Strategy #2) you would enjoy practicing on a regular basis.

5. List and discuss *three* stress management strategies you could incorporate into your current lifestyle.

Name_____

Class /Activity Section_____

How to Meditate and Experience the Relaxation Response

Meditation is recognized as a valuable antidote for stress. This powerful mind/body approach is the natural, non-chemical, inexpensive method to help you calm down and gain greater control over your life. Meditation relieves stress by lowering the level of powerful stress hormones that inhibits immune function and interferes with our natural healing processes. Meditation increases body-mind relaxation by calming feelings of panic, fear, and pain. Learning to meditate is a do-it-yourself, self-help project. You do not need a guru, special lessons, an expensive club membership, or an expert to help you learn how to meditate. You can't simply wish to be a more relaxed person; meditation is a skill that takes commitment and practice. Plan now to incorporate meditation into your daily schedule so that you, too, may profit from its numerous benefits.

Read the following helpful meditation guidelines before you begin:

1. The best times to meditate are before breakfast and before dinner. Do not meditate directly after a meal. After eating, the blood is diverted toward the stomach area, aiding the digestive process. This diversion inhibits complete relaxation.

2. Find a quiet room and sit in a comfortable chair. A straight-back chair is best because you do not want to be so comfortable that you fall asleep. Rest your arms on the arms of the chair or in your lap.

3. Wear nonrestrictive clothing while meditating or loosen the clothes you happen to be wearing at the time.

4. Relax all your muscles as best you can, without forcing it. Focus on your breathing.

5. The goal is to meditate for 20 minutes but don't worry about meditating for a full 20 minutes at first. As you become more comfortable with the process, you will be able to progress up to 20 minutes or more, twice a day.

6. Do not smoke cigarettes or drink coffee, tea, or colas before meditating. These substances are stimulants and will not promote relaxation.

7. It would be helpful to disconnect the telephone. Also, do *not* set the alarm clock for 20 minutes.

8. Relax and enjoy this time. Your problems will be there when you're finished. They will seem less distressing to you after meditation if you commit yourself to the time necessary to do it.

9. Don't come out of the meditative state too abruptly.

10. Practice regularly. It takes practice to learn to sit still, meditate, relax, and calm the mind. Be patient. You won't discover the benefits unless you practice every day.

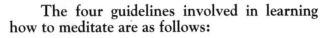

The four guidelines involved in learning how to meditate are as follows:

1. *Find a quiet environment.* Find a quiet room and sit in a comfortable chair. A straight-back chair is best because you don't want to be so comfortable that you fall asleep.

2. *Choose a comfortable position.* It is best to close your eyes (unless you are using a mental device). There should be no tension in your forehead or eyes. Breathe easily and naturally through your nose. Rest your arms on the arms of the chair or in your lap.

3. *Identify a word, phrase, sound, image, thought, or prayer (a mantra) on which to focus your attention.* For starters you can keep it simple by focusing on your breathing, feeling it as it moves in and out. Use the breath as an anchor to bring you back when your attention is disrupted. As you gain experience you may wish to select a mantra that you can focus on silently. The mantra should be easy to pronounce and short enough to repeat silently as you exhale. A fixed gazing at an unchanging object, a mental device, may also be used. The silently repeated mantra or the unchanging mental device merely helps to break the train of distracting thoughts and sounds that will interfere with the meditative process. Relax all your muscles as best you can, without forcing it. *Focus on your breathing.* Now silently repeat the mantra very, very slowly, without a break. Many meditators like to use as a mantra a word, such as *one, love, calm,* or *peace,* as they slowly exhale.

4. *Maintain a calm, relaxed attitude.* Keep a calm, relaxed mindset. Do not force yourself to relax or watch yourself relax; the rhythm of the mantra (or the fixed gazing) will be interrupted and so will your relaxation period. It is normal for distracting thoughts to occur; do not worry about them—let them pass on when this happens. Return your focus to the repetition of the mantra or the mental device.

Continue to meditate for approximately 20 minutes. It is recommended that you meditate twice a day for 20 minutes each time.

When you stop meditating, give your body time to adjust. Keep your eyes closed for 1 minute and let regular thoughts return. Next, open your eyes and focus on the objects in the room. Take several deep breaths. Stretch while seated. When you feel ready, stand and stretch.

Meditation Log Sheet

Practice meditating for one week. Use the following log to record the time of day, the location, the length of time, and comments about the meditative session. Make copies of this log form as needed.

Week:

	Time of day	Location	Length of meditation	Comments
Sunday				
Monday				
Tuesday				
Wednesday				
Thursday				
Friday				
Saturday				

Name_____

Class/Activity Section_____

Becoming Stress Resistant and Hardy

List two ways your "hardiness" can be strengthened in each of the following categories:

1. *Control:* Do you feel you are in control of your life? List at least two ways you gain more control. (Example: Plot out all the courses you need to complete your degree, semester by semester.)

2. *Commitment (task involvement):* How can you build commitment in your life (i.e., family, friends, studies, work, community)? List at least two ways to improve commitment. (Example: I will complete my nursing degree by 19__.)

3. *Challenge:* Do you see change and/or setbacks as challenges instead of stumbling blocks? Give at least two examples that have occurred recently or list two strategies you can use in the future. (Example: So I didn't do very well on this anatomy pop quiz. . . . Now I know that I need to study daily for this course.)

4. *Choices in lifestyle:* How healthy is your current lifestyle? List at least two improvements you can make in your lifestyle. (Example: I will get at least eight hours of sleep every night for two weeks.)

5. *Connectedness:* Do you have anyone you can count on for emotional support? Do you feel *connected* with at least one other person or group? Do you have close friends and family? List at least two ways to improve connectedness. (Example: Twice a week I will either telephone or write a note to a friend to keep in touch with friends I rarely get to see.)

Name_____

Class/Activity Section_____

Relaxation

There are many ways to relax. Meditation, progressive relaxation, autogenic training, and imagery. Hatha yoga, massage, abdominal breathing, and floatation tanks are all excellent tension relievers. You cannot simply wish to become a more relaxed person. Becoming relaxed is a **skill** that takes *commitment* and *practice!* Make the commitment now!

    Choose any relaxation technique on pages 156–60 in Chapter 7 and practice it for 20 minutes every day for one week. Then respond to the following questions. Before you begin, rate your current ability to relax. How good are you at relaxing? Mark the line where you would rate your current skill:

Very poor	Poor	Average	Good	Excellent

1. How often do you practice relaxation now? Circle one: . . . never . . . once in a while . . . every day

    Explain: (i.e., why don't you practice relaxation, what method do you use, how often do you practice?)

2. Do you believe you could benefit by improving your ability to relax? Explain your response.

3. Which relaxation technique did you choose to practice? Why did you select this technique? Describe your experience with this technique (i.e., how you felt before and after).

4. Did this technique help you feel relaxed? Why or why not?

5. Is this a skill you feel you can use to manage the stress in your daily life? Explain.

6. Would you like to try any of the other techniques? If so, which and why?

7. Do you think relaxation is important in the management of your stress? Why or why not?

8. Take the Holmes-Rahe life event scale or the *Life Event Scale for the College Student*. What was your score?_____
   What was your implication for illness?_____

9. What role does diet play in the total stress picture of your life? List *three* ways you can improve the diet-stress connection in your everyday life.

10. List the top *three* daily hassles and top *three* daily uplifts in your life.

Name_____

Class/Activity Section_____

Measuring Your Stress and Coping Skills

This is a four-part test. The first three parts are designed to give you an indication of how vulnerable you might be to certain types of stress and to make you aware of how they might affect you. The last part of the test will provide you with information on how to cope with stressful situations. (Daniel Girdano/George S. Everly, *Controlling Stress and Tension: A Holistic Approach*, © 1979, pp. 62, 67, 108–109. Adapted by permission of Prentice Hall, Englewood Cliffs, New Jersey.)

Part I

Choose the most appropriate answer for each of the 10 questions.

	a. Almost always true	b. Usually true	c. Usually false	d. Almost always false
1. When I can't do something "my way," I simply adjust and do it the easiest way.	___	___	___	___
2. I get upset when someone in front of me drives slowly.	___	___	___	___
3. It bothers me when my plans are dependent upon others.	___	___	___	___
4. Whenever possible, I tend to avoid large crowds.	___	___	___	___
5. I am uncomfortable when I have to stand in long lines.	___	___	___	___
6. Arguments upset me.	___	___	___	___
7. When my plans don't flow smoothly, I become anxious.	___	___	___	___
8. I require a lot of space in which to live and work.	___	___	___	___
9. When I am busy at some task, I hate to be disturbed.	___	___	___	___
10. I believe that it is worth waiting for all good things.	___	___	___	___

Total score _____

Scoring
For 1 and 10, a=1, b=2, c=3, d=4; for 2 through 9, a=4, b=3, c=2, d=2. This test measures your vulnerability to stress from being frustrated or inhibited. Scores in excess of 25 seem to suggest some vulnerability to this source of stress.

Part II

Check or mark the letter of the response that best answers the following 10 questions. How often do you . . .

	a. Almost always	b. Very often	c. Seldom	d. Never
1. find yourself with insufficient time to complete your work?	___	___	___	___
2. find yourself becoming confused and unable to think clearly because too many things are happening at once?	___	___	___	___
3. wish you had help to get everything done?	___	___	___	___
4. feel your boss/professor expects too much from you?	___	___	___	___
5. feel your family and friends expect too much from you?	___	___	___	___
6. find your work infringing on your leisure hours?	___	___	___	___
7. find yourself doing extra work to set an example to those around you?	___	___	___	___
8. find yourself doing extra work to impress your superiors?	___	___	___	___
9. have to skip a meal so that you can get work completed?	___	___	___	___
10. feel that you have too much responsibility?	___	___	___	___

Total score _____

Scoring
a=4, b=3, c=2, d=1. This test measures your vulnerability to overload; that is, to having too much to do. Scores in excess of 25 seem to indicate vulnerability to this source of stress.

Part III

Answer each question as it is generally true for you.

	a. Almost always true	b. Usually true	c. Usually false	d. Almost always false
1. I hate to wait in lines.	____	____	____	____
2. I often find myself racing against the clock to save time.	____	____	____	____
3. I become upset if I think something is taking too long.	____	____	____	____
4. When under pressure I tend to lose my temper.	____	____	____	____
5. My friends tell me that I tend to get irritated easily.	____	____	____	____
6. I seldom like to do anything unless I can make it competitive.	____	____	____	____
7. When something must be done, I'm the first to begin even though the details may still need to be worked out.	____	____	____	____
8. When I make a mistake it is usually because I've rushed into something without giving it enough thought and planning.	____	____	____	____
9. Whenever possible, I try to do two things at once, such as eating while working or planning while driving or bathing.	____	____	____	____
10. When I go on a vacation, I usually take along some work to do just in case I get a chance.	____	____	____	____

Total score _____

Scoring

a=4, b=3, c=2, d=1. This test measures the presence of compulsive, time-urgent, and excessively aggressive behavioral traits. Scores in excess of 25 suggest the presence of one or more of these traits.

Part IV

This scale was created largely on the basis of results compiled by clinicians and researchers who sought to identify how individuals effectively cope with stress. This scale is an educational tool, not a clinical instrument. Its purpose, therefore, is to inform you of ways in which you can effectively and healthfully cope with the stress in your life. At the same time, through a point system, it will give you some indication of the relative desirability of the coping strategies you are currently using. Simply follow the instructions given for each of the 14 items listed. Total your points when you have completed all of the items.

1. Give yourself 10 points if you feel that you have a supportive family. _____
2. Give yourself 10 points if you actively pursue a hobby. _____
3. Give yourself 10 points if you belong to some social or activity group (other than your family) that meets at least once a month. _____
4. Give yourself 15 points if you are within 5 pounds of your ideal body weight, considering your height and bone structure. _____
5. Give yourself 15 points if you practice some form of deep relaxation at least three times a week. Deep relaxation exercises include meditation, imagery, and yoga. _____
6. Give yourself 5 points for each time you exercise 30 minutes or longer during one average week. _____
7. Give yourself 5 points for each nutritionally balanced and wholesome meal you consume during one average day. _____
8. Give yourself 5 points if you do something just for yourself that you really enjoy during an average week. _____
9. Give yourself 10 points if you have some place in your home that you can go in order to relax and/or be alone. _____
10. Give yourself 10 points if you practice time management techniques in your daily life. _____
11. Subtract 10 points for each pack of cigarettes you smoke during one average day. _____
12. Subtract 5 points for each evening during an average week that you take any form of medication or chemical (including alcohol) to help you sleep. _____
13. Subtract 10 points for each day during an average week that you consume any form of medication or chemical substance (including alcohol) to reduce your anxiety or to calm you down. _____
14. Subtract 5 points for each evening during an average week that you bring work home—work that was meant to be done at your place of employment. _____

Total score _____

Scoring

Now calculate your total score. A perfect score would be 115 points or more. If you scored in the 50 to 60 range, you probably have an adequate collection of coping strategies for most common sources of stress. You should keep in mind, however, that the higher your score, the greater your ability to cope with stress in an effective and healthful manner.

Name_____

Class/Activity Section_____

Time Management

I. Yearly and Lifetime Goals

Read the time management strategies in Chapter 7 on page 160. Complete sections A and B before proceeding to parts II and III.

A. *Setting lifetime goals*. List three to five goals you wish to accomplish in your lifetime. Next, prioritize them by numbering them from 1 to 5:

-
-
-
-
-

B. *Prioritizing lifetime goals*. List three to five goals you wish to accomplish this year. Next, prioritize them by numbering them from 1 to 5:

-
-
-
-
-

Keep Part I to review at a later date.

II. Daily Time Study Log

Analyze how you spend your time by keeping a daily log for one week. Record at half-hour intervals the activities you do. At the end of each day, use a highlighter to identify the times of the day you feel were wasted. Then plan for tomorrow about how to correct the wasted time and how to be more productive. Make copies of this form as needed.

7:00 A.M.	7:00 P.M.
7:30 A.M.	7:30 P.M.
8:00 A.M.	8:00 P.M.
8:30 A.M.	8:30 P.M.
9:00 A.M.	9:00 P.M.
9:30 A.M.	9:30 P.M.
10:00 A.M.	10:00 P.M.
10:30 A.M.	10:30 P.M.
11:00 A.M.	11:00 P.M.
11:30 A.M.	11:30 P.M.
Noon	Midnight
12:30 P.M.	12:30 A.M.
1:00 P.M.	1:00 A.M.
1:30 P.M.	1:30 A.M.
2:00 P.M.	2:00 A.M.
2:30 P.M.	2:30 A.M.
3:00 P.M.	3:00 A.M.
3:30 P.M.	3:30 A.M.
4:00 P.M.	4:00 A.M.
4:30 P.M.	4:30 A.M.
5:00 P.M.	5:00 A.M.
5:30 P.M.	5:30 A.M.
6:00 P.M.	6:00 A.M.
6:30 P.M.	6:30 A.M.

III. Weekly Goals

A. *Set goals:* Think through the entire week and list the specific goals you wish to accomplish (or tasks you wish to complete) this week. Schedule into the week your appointments, obligations, and other responsibilities. Be sure to leave time for work projects, schoolwork, exercise, time with family and friends, and play/recreation/time for you (i.e., watching TV, socializing).

-
-
-
-
-

B. *Prioritize:* To beat the negative effects of stress, you have to learn to prioritize. Not everything on your list can be number one. Prioritize the week's tasks now by numbering them from 1 to 5.

C. *Complete a weekly evaluation:* After completing the *Daily Time Study Log* in Part II, evaluate how successfully you managed your time this week. Explain in a few sentences how you did. What goals/tasks did not get completed? Should these be eliminated or reestablished on next week's list? Explain.

IV. Daily Planning

The goal of time management is not to eliminate leisure time (time for self, family, friends, etc.); it is to eliminate life's real time wasters and redundancies.

A. *Analyze your time and set goals.* After completing a week of the *Daily Time Study Log* in Part II (analyzing how you actually spend your time) and establishing *Weekly Goals* in Part III, you are ready to begin daily planning. Look over the goals and tasks you have prioritized for the week. Include any of these you want to check off today. Write the goals/tasks that must get done today on the *must do* list (no more than five items on this list). This way you are more likely to get all the things done, and you will feel a greater sense of accomplishment and control. The ones you would like to take care of today put on the *maybe* list; and those you would like to complete if all items are completed on the first and second list put on the *if possible* list. Be sure to schedule into the day appointments, meetings, study time, exercise, recreation (and/or time to just do nothing), and errands. Make extra copies of this form as needed.

B. *Prioritize and schedule priorities into your day.*

Must do:
-
-
-
-
-

Maybe:
-
-
-
-
-

If possible:
-
-
-
-
-

C. *Evaluation.* A good time manager takes 5 to 10 minutes each day to evaluate how he or she did.

1. How did you do today? Explain in a few sentences.

2. Did you check off everything on the *must do* list? List what did not get checked off. Will it be added to tomorrow's list?

3. How did you do on the *maybe* and *if possible* lists?

4. How many hours today did you feel were unproductive or wasted? Why? Explain in a few sentences.

5. Were you able to say "no" or to "delegate" any chores that would have made too great a demand on your time? Describe.

Special Exercise Considerations Challenge

1. Your sister's gynecologist just told her she is pregnant. Knowing you are taking a college fitness/wellness course, she asks you for advice concerning the fitness walking program she began two months ago to help her get back into shape and lose a few pounds. Give her three or four tips.

2. At dinner, two of your friends were debating whether to use a popular sports drink to replace all the sweat they expected to lose in the July 4th 12-mile run, which they estimated would take *more* than one hour to complete. The July 4th festivities are tomorrow with the race beginning at noon in Old Town and ending at the top of Heartbreak Hill. What advice would you give them?

3. Your grandparents (age 65) were advised by their neighbor to stop all that "foolish" exercising, to slow down, and to start acting their age. They ask you your opinion of this advice. What can you tell them about the benefits of staying physically active?

4. In Speech 101, your topic for the final exam speech is "The Difference Between Men's and Women's Exercise Performance Levels. Are They More Alike Than Different?" List three similarities and differences you want to highlight in your speech.

5. Your friend signed up for a fitness class, and, while he was demonstrating one of the workouts, you noticed he was doing standing toe-touches with his legs crossed and double leg lifts. Explain to your friend why those two exercises are contraindicated (not advisable) and give him safe alternatives for them.

Name_____

Class /Activity Section_____

Food Log

Write down everything you eat and drink for three to five full days. Make copies of the log as needed. Be sure to note the approximate quantity of food and assess combination foods (e.g., pizza, casseroles, tacos, salads) to list the foods in them. Keep track of the number of servings in each food group. Use the columns at the right to record calories, sodium milligrams, fat grams, cholesterol milligrams, and so on, as desired.

Date _____
(12:01 A.M. to 12:00 midnight)

			Major Food Groups—Servings						Other: calories, calcium, cholesterol, fat, etc.			
Time	Food	Amount	Bread, cereal, rice, pasta	Vegetable	Fruit	Meat, poultry, fish, beans, eggs, nuts	Milk, yogurt, cheese	Fats, oils, sweets				
Totals =												

Vitamin supplements:

9

| Time | Food | Amount | Major Food Groups—Servings | | | | | | Other: calories, calcium, cholesterol, fat, etc. | | | |
			Bread, cereal, rice, pasta	Vegetable	Fruit	Meat, poultry, fish, beans, eggs, nuts	Milk, yogurt, cheese	Fats, oils, sweets				
Totals =												

Vitamin supplements:

Name_____

Class /Activity Section_____

Analyze Your Diet

After completing the *Food Log*, analyze your diet as follows.

1. Looking at the seven *Dietary Guidelines for Americans*, how does your diet measure up with *each* guideline?

   a.   e.

   b.   f.

   c.   g.

   d.

2. Look at the Food Guide Pyramid. Do you meet the daily criteria for recommended servings in each food group? Explain.

   a. Bread, cereal, rice, and pasta group: d. Milk, yogurt, and cheese group:

   b. Vegetable group: e. Meat, poultry, fish, dry beans, eggs, and nuts
                                                        group:

   c. Fruit group:

9

3. Identify three positive dietary changes that you could implement that would enhance your nutritional wellness. Include *what* you would do and a *specific strategy* of how you would do it.

   a.

   b.

   c.

Name_____

Class/Activity Section_____

How Much Fat?

1. Lisa consumes 1,500 calories per day. To keep her percentage of fat right at 30 percent of her calories, figure how many *grams* of fat she can consume per day. _____ (Show your work.)

   If Lisa wants to eat even *healthier* and limit her fat percentage to 20 percent of her daily calories, how many fat grams per day can she consume? _____ (Show your work.)

2. Robert consumes 2,700 calories per day. To keep his percentage of fat right at 30 percent of his calories, how many *grams* of fat can he consume per day? _____ (Show your work.)

   If Robert wants to eat even *healthier* and limit his fat percentage to 20 percent of his daily calories, how many fat grams per day can he consume? _____ (Show your work.)

What About You?

Goal = _____ calories per day.

Number of daily fat grams at 30 percent of calories = _____ (Show your work.)

Number of daily fat grams at 20 percent of calories = _____ (Show your work.)

Name_____

Class/Activity Section_____

Label Reading Assignment

FIGURE A.3 ➤
Honey wheat muffin mix.

Simply combine mix with
1/3 c. milk
1 T. oil
1 egg
Bake 15 min. at 400°.

Nutrition Facts

Serving Size 1 muffin (from 31g mix)
Servings Per Container 6

Amount Per Serving	Mix	Prepared
Calories	120	160
Calories from Fat	25	60

	% Daily Value**	
Total Fat 3g*	4%	10%
Saturated Fat 0.5g	3%	7%
Cholesterol 0mg	0%	12%
Sodium 210mg	9%	9%
Potassium 15mg	<1%	1%
Total Carbohydrate 23g	8%	8%
Dietary Fiber <1g	2%	2%
Sugars 12g		
Other Carbohydrate 11g		
Protein 1g		
Calcium	0%	2%
Iron	2%	2%

Not a significant source of vitamin A and vitamin C.

*Amount in mix. As prepared, one serving provides 6g fat (1.5g saturated fat), 35mg cholesterol, 220mg sodium, 45mg potassium, 24g total carbohydrate (12g sugars) and 3g protein.

**Percent Daily Values are based on a 2,000 calorie diet. Your daily values may be higher or lower depending on your calorie needs:

	Calories:	2,000	2,500
Total Fat	Less than	65g	80g
Sat Fat	Less than	20g	25g
Cholesterol	Less than	300mg	300mg
Sodium	Less than	2,400mg	2,400mg
Potassium		3,500mg	3,500mg
Total Carbohydrate		300g	375g
Dietary Fiber		25g	30g

Calories per gram:
Fat 9 • Carbohydrate 4 • Protein 4

Ingredients: Enriched Flour, Sugar, Hydrogenated Vegetable Oil (Coconut and/or Palm Kernel) Corn Syrup, Salt, Cellulose Gum, Dextrose, Rice Flour, Artificial Flavor

Look at the muffin mix label in Figure A.3 and complete the following:

1. What constitutes one serving?

2. Why are there two columns (mix, prepared)?

3. How many grams of fat are there in two prepared muffins? _____

4. In one prepared muffin, figure the

   a. percent of calories from fat: _____

   b. percent of calories from carbohydrates: _____

   c. percent of calories from protein: _____

5. Give one source of complex carbohydrate: _____

6. Give one source of simple carbohydrate: _____

7. Name the source of cholesterol in this prepared product: _____

8. Name and comment on the sources of fat in this prepared product:

9. What is your overall assessment of this food (i.e., nutritional density; sodium, fat, cholesterol content; types of carbohydrates; fiber content)?

Name_____

Class/Activity Section_____

Select and Analyze a Food Label

Select a label from a food that you commonly eat. Make sure the ingredients are listed on the label. Attach the label to this form. Analyze the food as follows:

Food:_____   Manufacturer:_____

Serving size:_____   In your opinion, is this an appropriate portion size? Why or
why not?

_____

_____

_____

Total calories per serving:_____

Total fat grams per serving:_____   Percentage of calories from fat: _____

Total carbohydrate grams per serving:_____   Percentage of calories from carbohydrates: _____

Total protein grams per serving:_____   Percentage of calories from protein: _____

Comment on the amount of cholesterol in this food: _____

_____

_____

Comment on the amount of sodium in this food: _____

_____

_____

Comment on the type of carbohydrates in this food (i.e., complex or simple). Is this food a good source of fiber?_____

_____

_____

List any source(s) of added sugar: _____

_____

What is your overall assessment of this food (i.e., nutritional value, nutritional density, etc.)?_____

_____

_____

Why Do You Eat? (An Eating Diary)

Use the following eating diary to analyze the reasons you eat. Knowing the cues and factors that affect eating can help you manage your eating behavior.

Date: _____

Time of day	Location	Companion(s) (if any)	Food consumed	Quantity	Total time	Mood/psychological state during meal	Activity during meal

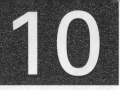

Observations:

Strategies for Change:

Name_____

Class/Activity Section_____

How Active Are You?

Finding the time to exercise can be a challenge. However, there are several times during a day that you can weave activity into your life (i.e., walking rather than driving; riding a stationary bike while watching TV; taking the stairs rather than the elevator; getting up 45 minutes earlier in the morning to jog). Use the following log to keep track of your activity during the day. Then, analyze *when* and *how* you could adapt your lifestyle to include more activity.

Date: _____

Activity	Time of day	Location	Duration	Positive outcomes	Negative outcomes (if any)

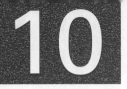

10

Assess your activity level today:

Describe ways you could fit more activity into your day:

What obstacles do you face in trying to be active?

What are your strategies for combatting these obstacles and for adhering to a lifetime of activity/exercise?

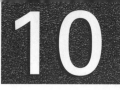

Name_____

Class/Activity Section_____

Behavior-Change Contract
(for Weight Management)

Goal: _____

Date: _____

Motivation (What's in it for me?):

Identify the stage of change you are currently in:

_____ Precontemplation   _____ Contemplation   _____ Preparation   _____ Action   _____ Maintenance

Processes and Techniques

1. Consciousness raising

   a.

   b.

   c.

2. Social liberation

   a.

   b.

   c.

3. Emotional arousal

   a.

   b.

   c.

4. Self-reevaluation

   a.

   b.

   c.

10

5. Commitment

   a.

   b.

   c.

6. Reward

   a.

   b.

   c.

7. Countering

   a.

   b.

   c.

8. Environment control

   a.

   b.

   c.

9. Helping relationships

   a.

   b.

   c.

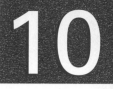

Name_____

Class /Activity Section_____

Weight-Management Plan

Date: _____

Weight: _____

  Goal weight: _____

Body fat percentage: _____

  Goal body fat: _____

Body mass index (BMI): _____

  Goal BMI: _____

Waist-to-hip ratio: _____

  Goal ratio: _____

I. Nutrition

➤ Fat grams per day: _____ (goal)

➤ Calories per day: _____ (goal)

➤ Food Guide Pyramid Compliance (Strategies)

➤ Snacks:

➤ Food Preparation Adjustments:

II. Eating Management

Behavior modification strategies:

1.

2.

3.

4.

5.

6.

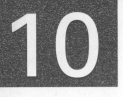

III. Exercise

Physical activity strategies:

Sunday	Monday	Tuesday	Wednesday	Thursday	Friday	Saturday

Cancer-Risk Reduction

Cancer-risk reduction is as simple as choosing your next meal. Use the guidelines in Chapter 11 to complete the following items:

1. From the menu that follows, select four foods that reduce cancer risk and tell why you chose each.

2. From the menu that follows, list four foods that increase cancer risk and tell why.

Lunch Box
Residence Hall Dining Service

Lunch

Cream of Chicken Soup, Lentil Soup, Toasted Bacon Sandwich, Tuna in Lettuce Cup, Hardcooked Eggs, Yogurt, Sliced American Cheese, Luncheon Meats and Cheeses on Deli Line, Dill Pickles, Potato Chips, Buttered Whole Kernel Corn, Bread and Butter

Salad Bar includes: Shredded Lettuce, Chopped Broccoli and Cauliflower, Fresh Spinach, Grape Gelatin, Apple Sauce, Canned Onion Rings, Alfalfa Sprouts, Tomato Slices, Cottage Cheese, Shredded Cheddar Cheese, Shredded Carrots

For dessert: Strawberries, Soft Serve Frozen Yogurt, Ice Cream Cone

Dinner

Baked Lasagna, Turkey Breast Fillet, Broiled Fish, Beans and Corn Bread, Cooked Spinach, Corn on the Cob, Mashed Potatoes, Turkey Gravy, Parsley Buttered Potatoes, Broccoli Spears, Honey Glazed Baby Carrots, Whole Grain Roll and Butter

Salad Bar includes: Combination Salad, Alfalfa Sprouts, Fresh Spinach, Pea Peanut and Cheese Salad, Croutons, Tomato Slices, Cauliflower Buds, Bacon Bits, Shredded Cheddar Cheese, Cubed Ham, Cottage Cheese, Parmesan Cheese

For dessert: Peaches, Soft Serve Frozen Yogurt, Ice Cream Cone

Substance Abuse

1. Complete each of the following value clarification statements according to your feelings. Discuss each response in a few sentences:

   a. I view substance abuse as . . .

   b. The thought that alcohol, tobacco, and caffeine are drugs . . .

   c. If my sister continued to smoke while pregnant I would . . .

   d. If my 16-year-old brother asked me to get him some beer, I would . . .

   e. If the police picked me up for driving while intoxicated, I would . . .

   f. The next time my roommate comes in drunk and disturbs my study time (or sleep), I'm going to . . .

   g. How serious is substance abuse (on a scale of 1 to 5, 5 being most serious)?
      ➤ in the United States:_____
      ➤ at this university:_____
      ➤ in my residence hall (fraternity/sorority house, apartment):_____
      ➤ in my home:_____
      ➤ Defend your ratings. What substances are being abused; what can/should be done to curb the abuse?

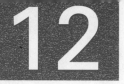

2. Discuss the pros and cons of each of the following statements:

   a. A mother should be charged with murder if she takes illegal drugs during pregnancy and her baby dies of addiction at birth.

   b. A nursing mother should be charged with child abuse if she uses illegal drugs.

3. a. Do the following lyrics reflect society's values? Do they reflect your values? Explain your responses to both questions.

   ➤ Do cocaine to get over the blues. ("Cocaine," by Eric Clapton)

   ➤ Alcohol counteracts loneliness, as a lover does. ("The Piano Man," by Billy Joel)

   ➤ Look to drugs for help. ("With a Little Help from My Friends," by the Beatles)

   b. What current music depicts substance use? List three examples and tell how.

   ➤

   ➤

   ➤

   c. How do music/videos/TV influence the use of drugs in our society?

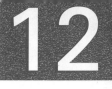

Name_____

Class/Activity Section_____

Substance Abuse

Use the text (Chapter 12) to respond to the following:

1. Leaving a party, you see a girl passed out on the lawn. What should you do? List six actions you should take.

2. Use five factors that affect alcohol absorption to give a profile of a person who will get drunk fastest.

3. How does alcohol change people's behavior? Give five examples from your observations.

4. You want to plan a safe party. List five ways you can help those attempting to reduce their use of or abstain from using alcohol (or drugs).

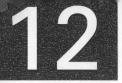

5. Any pregnant woman has a right to drink alcohol as much as she wants. Argue for and then against.

For:

Against:

6. Describe eight strategies to avoid irresponsible use of alcohol.

7. George can drink two six-packs before he feels drunk. Susan feels tipsy after two drinks. Should both be considered legally drunk at the same BAC? Discuss the reasons for your response.

STD Information

1. List three new facts you learned about STDs:

2. List the five most common sexually transmitted diseases and two symptoms of each:

3. List two incurable STDs other than AIDS:

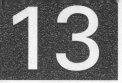

4. List three ways HIV is transmitted:

5. List three steps you can take to prevent transmission of STDs:

6. List three places you could go for advice or treatment concerning an STD in this community:

7. Describe two strategies for preventing unwanted sexual pressure:

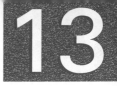

Name_____

Class/Activity Section_____

Values Clarification Statements

Complete or respond to the following statements. They may be used for class discussion.

1. AIDS is _____.

2. STDs are _____.

3. If I found out I had an STD, I would _____.

4. If I found out my partner had an STD, I would _____.

5. Five ways to show someone you care about them without having sex are

_____

_____

_____

_____

_____

6. Money for AIDS research should be cut because people get AIDS due to immoral lifestyles. Agree or disagree? Explain.

_____

_____

_____

_____

_____

7. HIV infection is not a significant risk for college students. Agree or disagree? Explain. _____

_____

_____

_____

_____

8. My peers are changing their sexual behavior because of AIDS. Agree or disagree? Explain. _____

_____

_____

_____

_____

9. Condoms are not used much to prevent STDs on this campus. Agree or disagree? Explain._____

_____

_____

_____

_____

13

10. Because of the AIDs crisis, it is easier to talk to my peers about sex. Agree or disagree? Explain. _____

_____

_____

_____

_____

11. Both men and women should share responsibility for safer sex. Agree or disagree? Explain. _____

_____

_____

_____

_____

12. "Just Say No" is the right message to give young people about how to prevent STDs. Agree or disagree? Explain. ____

_____

_____

_____

_____

13. Schools should distribute condoms to students. Agree or disagree? Explain. _____

_____

_____

_____

_____

14. Sexual intercourse improves a relationship. Agree or disagree? Explain. _____

_____

_____

_____

15. Condom ads should be allowed on television. Agree or disagree? Explain. _____

_____

_____

16. The media responsibly portray sex. Agree or disagree? Explain. _____

_____

_____

_____

Quackery Detection

Doctors Accidentally Discover "Lazy Way" to Remove Cellulite

Discovery Astounds Scientific Community

Swedish researchers at the University of Pelento have discovered (accidentally) a secret formula that ACTUALLY SHRINKS CELLULITE! This astounding discovery has virtually *eliminated the need for dieting or torturous exercise!* This miracle formula is being marketed exclusively under the trade name SHRINK-IT 5000.

Clinically Tested

Exhaustive medical tests at a world famous medical center in Burgess, Australia, have proven that **SHRINK-IT 5000** has no harmful side effects and is the most effective cellulite-reducing formula of all time. Like a magnet, the chemical molecules in **SHRINK-IT 5000** tie up and trap undigested fat particles many times their size. And it begins happening almost instantly! In fact, it is so effective that some people tend to overdo it and become too thin—within days!!

6 Week Supply (Was $79.90) NOW ONLY

$59.90 SAVE $20!!

Eat All You Want and Keep Losing Cellulite

This amazing formula was discovered by scientists searching for a compound to shrink varicose veins. Researchers were amazed to find the test group actually lost a considerable amount of cellulite fat—all while eating anything they wanted! Dr. Garth Robbins stated in the *Universal Journal of Clinical Science:* "This formula will virtually revolutionize the way people typically try to lose fat (with deprivating diets and exhaustive exercise)."

Act Now

This is a limited time offer. Since news of this product is sweeping the country, send in your order today. Don't let this golden opportunity get away. Imagine being the thin, attractive person you've dreamed about! **SHRINK-IT 5000** is only available from Powers Pharmaceuticals, which holds exclusive North American rights. Call now. Orders accepted by phone only.

1-800-987-6543 ALL CREDIT CARDS ACCEPTED

Answer the following questions:

1. List signs of quackery in the advertisement for SHRINK-IT 5000.

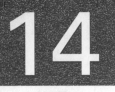

2. What makes this advertisement attractive or seem legitimate to the uninformed consumer?

3. If your sister were ready to send away for this product with the hope of reducing fat thighs, what would you tell her? How would you advise anyone wanting to reduce the fat on his or her thighs?

Name_____

Class/Activity Section_____

Look to the Future

Imagine that you are 10 years older, married with two children, and working in your chosen field.

1. Describe the wellness programs that you want your employer/company to offer. (If you plan to be self-employed or involved in a small business, describe the wellness programs you would want your hospital or community to offer.)

2. What family activities are important to you in order to promote family wellness?

14

3. Describe how you manage a regular fitness program. (Where? When? What type of activity? etc.)

4. Not including fitness, what other lifestyle and wellness habits are you committed to for your lifetime? (Your answer may involve the entire wellness spectrum.)

Name_____

Class/Activity Section_____

The Environment

Steve and Jane Brown have a 3-month-old baby and a 9-year-old Oldsmobile with a leaky air conditioner. They live in a 45-year-old house (with a basement) near a large shopping mall. The battery factory where they both work is about 1 mile from their home.

Steve has not had a lawn grub or mole problem since he hired Chemlawn to take care of his lawn. He is considering buying a lawn tractor.

For recreation, the Browns like to fish in the nearby White River. They also enjoy working in their large garden and taking long drives in the country.

1. Using the information in Chapter 14 of your text, list six or more environmental concerns that affect the Browns' wellness.

   a.   d.

   b.   e.

   c.   f.

2. For each concern, list at least two steps they can take to protect the environment and, in turn, enhance their wellness.

   a.   d.

   b.   e.

   c.   f.

3. List three ways you consciously protect the environment. Explain why you choose to do so.

   a.   d.

   b.   e.

   c.   f.

4. Name some actions you are not taking now but could begin to take to contribute to a better environment.

   a.   d.

   b.   e.

   c.   f.

Glosssary

a

Acquired Immune Deficiency Syndrome (AIDS) is the final stage in a Human Immunodeficiency Virus (HIV) infection and a group of symptoms resulting from infections due to a weakened immune system. These may include pneumocystis carinii pneumonia, Kaposi's sarcoma, persistent infections, and damage to the brain and spinal cord. AIDS is spread through sexual intercourse, sharing infected needles, and, rarely, through tainted blood products. It can be spread from a pregnant woman to her fetus.

Addiction is a pathological or abnormal relationship with an object or event. It is an illness that progresses from a definite, though often unclear, beginning toward an end point. Beginning as a voluntary, pleasurable act, it then becomes a reflective and compulsive behavior.

Aerobic literally means "with oxygen." Aerobic activities are those that demand large amounts of oxygen, follow the FITT prescription, and improve cardiorespiratory endurance.

Agonist is a muscle primarily responsible for producing a movement. For example, in a biceps curl, the biceps muscle is the agonist.

Alcohol (ethyl alcohol/ethanol) is a beverage and a CNS depressant. Alcohol slows reaction time, dulls alertness, and impairs body coordination. It intensifies emotions, lowers inhibitions, and increases risk-taking behaviors. Alcohol is the most abused legal drug in our society.

Alcoholism is a chemical dependence on (an addiction to) alcohol that causes physical, mental, emotional, social, and economical damage to the alcoholic's life and to the lives of those close to him or her.

Altruism is having an unselfish interest in the welfare of others.

Amenorrhea is a menstrual abnormality that results in absent menses.

Amotivational syndrome is characterized by low energy, apathy, and little drive to do anything. It is linked to marijuana use which, after time, results in changes in brain cell membranes.

Amphetamines (speed, uppers, crank, bennies, meth, or crystal) are powerful CNS stimulants. They are controlled substances legitimately used for short-term diet control in obesity and for narcolepsy. They have the ability to relieve sleepiness and fatigue and to increase alertness, confidence, and short-term performance. Truck drivers, pilots, entertainers, and athletes may use amphetamines nonmedically to enhance their performance.

Anabolic steroids are artificial forms of the male hormone testosterone. They are used legitimately in the treatment of anemia, hormone disorders, and multiple sclerosis. They are also used to increase muscle mass by both male and female athletes at all levels of competition, and they have numerous adverse side effects.

Anaerobic means "without oxygen." This type of activity demands more oxygen than the body can supply while exercising, causing an oxygen debt. Start and stop activities, such as sprinting, are examples of anaerobic exercise.

Angina pectoris is chest pain and is primarily caused by atherosclerosis.

Anorexia nervosa is an eating disorder characterized by self-inflicted starvation and dramatic weight loss. The anorexic is obsessed with achieving thinness.

Antagonist is a muscle opposing a movement. For example, in a biceps curl, the triceps muscle is the antagonist.

Antioxidants are compounds that help protect the body's cells from the damaging effects of the normal oxygenation process. Vitamin C, vitamin E, beta-carotene, and selenium are antioxidants.

Arteriosclerosis is thickening and hardening of the arteries.

Atherosclerosis is a type of arteriosclerosis and is a progressive condition that results in a buildup of plaque in the blood vessels.

Atrophy is the condition of diminished muscle size and strength due to lack of use.

Autogenic training and imagery is a self-generating or self-induced relaxation technique. This method uses mental concentration exercises to bring about sensations of warmth and heaviness in the limbs and torso and then uses relaxing images (i.e., clouds drifting by) to expand the relaxed state.

b

Ballistic stretching involves jerking and bouncing movements and is not the recommended type of stretching.

Basal metabolic rate (BMR) is the amount of energy (calories) expended by the body at rest to sustain vital functions.

Behavior modification is the utilization of techniques to enhance awareness or consciousness about a behavior and to subsequently alter the behavior. For example, a behavior modification technique for weight management would be refraining from grocery shopping while hungry.

Benign tumors are lumps of cells that are usually nonthreatening and seldom cause death. They usually resemble surrounding tissue, remain localized, and spread by expansion, like a wart or mole. They do not spread to other parts of the body.

Beta-carotene is a plant substance that the body uses to make vitamin A, an antioxidant that helps prevent cellular damage from free radicals.

Biofeedback training is a technique in which machines measure certain physiological processes of the body. The machines convert this information to an understandable form and feed it back to the individual. This process allows a person access to biological information not usually available through consciousness alone.

Blackout, an inability to remember a period of time, may result after a night of abusive alcohol consumption.

Blister is an inflamed burn caused by the friction of skin against a fabric or surface (like a shoe).

Blood alcohol concentration (BAC), or blood alcohol level (BAL), is the amount of alcohol in the blood and is expressed as a percentage. Most states have defined drunk driving as driving with a BAC of 0.10 percent or greater.

Body composition refers to the amount of body fat in proportion to fat-free weight.

Body fat is tissue made up of billions of cells that are filled with varying amounts of triglyceride. If triglyceride is added to or removed from a fat cell, the cell will increase or shrink in size accordingly.

Body image is the mental picture a person has of his or her body, and the associated attitudes and feelings toward it.

Body mass index (BMI) is a ratio between weight and height. It is calculated as weight (in kg) divided by the square of height (in m). The BMI is used by many health professionals as a measure of obesity.

Bulimia is an eating disorder characterized by alternating bouts of eating large quantities of food (binging), followed by purging through vomiting, use of laxatives, or fasting.

C

Caffeine is a powerful CNS stimulant. In healthy, rested people, a dose of 100 milligrams (about one cup of coffee) increases alertness, banishes drowsiness, quickens reaction time, enhances intellectual and muscular effort, increases heart and respiratory rates, and stimulates urinary output. It occurs naturally in coffee, tea, colas, cocoa, and chocolate and is added to some drugs. It is probably the most common drug used by adults and children in our society.

Calorie (kcal) is a measure of food energy. One pound of body fat equals 3,500 calories.

Cancer is a group of over 100 different diseases, all characterized by abnormal cell growth and replication. It has a lethal tendency to invade and destroy normal tissues and spread to other parts of the body. While cancer is the second leading cause of death in the United States, about half of all cancers can be cured.

Carbohydrates are the major source of energy for the body. Starches (such as potatoes, rice, and grains) and sugars are the main sources of carbohydrates in our diet.

Carcinogen is a substance that causes cancer, such as tobacco, UV radiation from sunlight, and certain chemicals.

Cardiovascular disease is a condition in which blood flow through the heart is impeded.

Cardiorespiratory endurance is the ability to deliver essential nutrients, especially oxygen, to the working muscles of the body and to remove waste products during prolonged physical exertion. It involves efficient functioning of the heart, blood vessels, and lungs.

Catecholamines are powerful, adrenalinelike chemicals that are pumped into the bloodstream during stressful situations. These stress chemicals are damaging to the cardiovascular system.

CD4+ or **T-cells** are lymphocytes (white blood cells) that are important in immune system response. They are destroyed by the AIDS virus, weakening a person's immunity to disease.

Cellulite is a slang term used to describe dimpled fat found primarily on the buttocks and thighs of women. It is no different from any other body fat.

Chancre is a small painless sore that appears at the site of infection within 1 to 12 weeks of infection with syphilis.

Chlamydia is the most common bacterial STD, causing inflammation of the urethra. Symptoms include burning during urination, painful scrotal swelling, and pelvic inflammatory disease.

Cholesterol is a fatlike waxy substance found in animal tissue. Even though it plays a vital role as a structural component of cell membranes, too much cholesterol has been linked to coronary artery disease.

Chondromalacia is knee pain caused by the irritation or wearing away of the cartilage on the underside of the patella.

Circuit is a group of exercises, each performed a certain number of reps or for a given amount of time, generally at different exercise stations.

Cocaine is a euphoriant and a CNS stimulant whose effects last from 20 minutes to several hours, depending on the drug's purity. It is a fine, opalescent, white, fluffy, odorless, and bitter-tasting drug that is sold for illegal, recreational use. It is the second most widely used illegal drug in the United States. Cocaine may be snorted, injected, swallowed, or smoked.

Collateral circulation is a process in which new blood vessels develop to nourish the areas of the heart muscle that are starved of oxygen and other nutrients.

Complex carbohydrates are nutritionally dense foods (grains, rice, pasta, potatoes, fruits, and vegetables) that are a rich source of vitamins and minerals and provide a steady amount of energy for many hours. Complex carbohydrates are an important source of fiber.

Concentric contraction occurs when a muscle shortens as it overcomes resistance. For example, the biceps muscle contracts concentrically during arm flexion in a biceps curl.

Conditioning bout is the middle part of a three-segment workout. It contains vigorous aerobic exercise that stimulates the cardiorespiratory system and should follow the FITT formula.

Contraindicated exercises are exercises indicated to be injurious to some people.

Cool-down is the final segment of the three-segment workout. The purpose of the cool-down is to safely ease your body back to its resting state.

Crack is crystallized, freebase cocaine sold in the form of ready-to-smoke "rocks." The rocks are nicknamed *crack* because of the crackling sound they make as they are smoked. The drug is an illegal CNS stimulant. Because crack is such a pure drug (about 90 percent pure cocaine) and approximately five times more potent than cocaine, smoking crack gives the user a far more intense and rapid euphoria than does snorting cocaine.

Cramp is a sharp, painful, involuntary muscle contraction.

Crank is a powerful CNS stimulant. It is odorless, yellow or off-white in color, and sold in capsules, chunks, or crystals. The drug is methamphetamine (a synthetic form of amphetamine) and is often sniffed, inhaled, or injected.

Cross training involves developing all five health-related components of fitness.

Cruciferous vegetables are members of the mustard family, such as broccoli and cabbage, and contain powerful phytochemicals that help prevent certain cancers.

d

Daily hassles are the events or interactions in daily life that are bothersome, annoying, or negative in some way. Examples are losing things, having too many things to do, and filling-out paperwork.

Daily uplift is the counterpart to daily hassles. These are the positive events that make us feel good. Examples are payday; being visited, phoned, or sent a letter; being complimented; having fun with a friend.

Delta-9-tetrahydrocannabinol (THC) is the principle psychoactive ingredient in marijuana.

Diabetes mellitus is a condition characterized by the body's inability to produce insulin or to use the hormone properly.

Diastolic blood pressure is the resting blood pressure and is the force of blood against the artery wall when the heart relaxes between beats. It is recorded as the lower number.

Distress refers to unpleasant or harmful stress under which health and performance begin to decline.

Diuretics cause the body to pass water by increasing urine output. They are used in treating edema and mild hypertension.

Drug is a chemical that alters a person's physical or mental condition.

Dynamic flexibility is the range of motion achieved by quickly moving a limb to its limits as in a bouncing hamstring stretch.

Dysmenorrhea is painful menstruation.

e

Eating disorder is a disturbance in eating behavior that jeopardizes a person's physical or psychosocial health.

Eccentric contraction occurs when a muscle lengthens and contracts at the same time, gradually allowing a force to overcome muscular resistance. For example, the biceps contracts eccentrically during the lowering phase of a biceps curl.

Emotional dimension is the dimension of wellness that deals with the ability to control or cope with the vast array of human feelings/emotions. Adjusting to life's ongoing changes is one sign of emotional wellness.

Endorphins are pain-relieving chemicals that are produced by the brain. Some individuals report experiencing their effects during aerobic exercise.

Environmental dimension is the dimension of wellness that deals with the preservation of natural resources and the protection of plant and animal wildlife, as well as the defining of your relationship with the environment. Practicing recycling shows evidence of environmental wellness.

Essential fat is the body fat required for normal functioning. This fat is stored in major body organs and tissues such as the heart, muscles, intestines, the nervous system, and breasts.

Estrogen is a female sex hormone.

Eustress refers to happy or pleasant events under which health and performance improve even as stress increases.

Exercise tolerance test is a test of aerobic capacity in which a person exercises while heart rate and oxygen consumption are measured. A maximal effort on a treadmill or bicycle ergometer is an example. This test gives an excellent measure of overall physiological functioning.

f

Fat cell (adipose cell) is a storage site for energy. This type of cell shrinks and enlarges depending on the amount of excess calories (energy) in storage.

Fat-free tissue is all body tissue except fat (muscle, bones, etc.).

Fats are the most concentrated form of food energy, providing 9 calories per gram—more than twice the energy provided by carbohydrates and proteins. Diets high in fat have been linked to coronary heart disease, some cancers, and obesity.

Fat soluble vitamins are vitamins that are stored in the fatty tissues of the body. Vitamins A, D, E, and K are fat soluble.

Fetal alcohol effect (FAE) is a less severe manifestation of fetal alcohol syndrome and is a condition acquired by the fetus. It is caused by the mother drinking alcohol during pregnancy.

Fetal alcohol syndrome (FAS) is a condition acquired by the fetus and is caused by the mother drinking alcohol during pregnancy. Alcohol irreversibly damages the developing brain. The damage can range from severe physical deformity, clumsiness, behavioral problems, and stunted growth to mental retardation.

Fiber is the part of plant food that is not digested in the small intestine. It helps the movement of solid waste through the digestive tract.

Fight-or-flight response (alarm) is the first stage in the Stress Response, in which the body prepares to cope with a stressor. Physiological and psychological responses appear. It is a basic survival mechanism.

FITT prescription factors should be followed to develop cardiorespiratory endurance. The factors include recommendations about frequency, intensity, time, and type of exercise.

Flashbacks are recurrences of certain aspects of a person's drug use without the user having repeated the use of the drug. They are experienced by many LSD users.

Flexibility refers to the movement of a joint through a full range of motion.

Free radicals are oxygen molecules that can produce precancerous cellular damage.

g

General adaptation syndrome (GAS) was described by Hans Selye and is today known as the Stress Response. It is the body's reaction or adaptation to stress and includes three stages: the fight-or-flight response, the stage of resistance, and the stage of exhaustion.

Genital herpes is an STD that produces small painful genital sores or blisters that break open and crust over, causing intense itching and pain. Active herpes may also be accompanied by fever, swollen glands, and flulike feelings. Symptoms usually occur within 2 to 30 days of having sex with an infected person, last from one to three weeks, and then subside, only to recur later.

Genital warts are flat or rounded bumps with a cauliflowerlike appearance resulting from a human papilloma virus infection. They are highly contagious and take one to eight months to appear after exposure. They may appear on the genitals, mouth, throat, or anus.

Glycogen is the storage form of carbohydrates, found in the muscles and liver.

Gonorrhea is a bacterial STD that can cause inflammation in the cervix, mouth, rectum, or urinary tract. Symptoms include burning during urination, penile discharge, swollen lymph glands in the groin, abnormal vaginal discharge, and abdominal pain.

h

Hatha yoga, or physical yoga, is the most familiar form of yoga. It is a discipline that involves the use of various exercises or postures (called *asanas*) in combination with proper breathing rhythm to remove tension and inflexibility in the body.

Health, in a simplistic view, is a state of not being ill. If you show no signs or symptoms of illness, you are considered healthy.

Health promotion involves the systematic efforts made by organizations to help people change their lifestyles toward a state of optimal well-being. Smoking cessation workshops, stress management classes, low-fat cooking demonstrations, and bulletin boards with cholesterol information are examples of health promotion activities.

Heel spur is a bony growth found on the underside of the heel.

Hemoglobin is the oxygen-carrying component of red blood cells.

Hepatitis B, formerly called *serum hepatitis*, is an inflammatory disease that can be spread through sexual contact and that destroys liver tissue.

Heroin (sometimes called *smack, junk, H,* and *hard stuff*) is a psychoactive drug and a CNS depressant. Pure heroin is a white powder with a bitter taste. It is a semisynthetic drug made by treating morphine with acetic anhydride to yield diacitylmorphine. Heroin is an illegal and highly addictive narcotic.

Herpes simplex virus type I is the virus that produces cold sores. Type II produces genital herpes. Both may be spread through sexual contact.

High-density lipoprotein (HDL) is considered to be the good form of cholesterol because of its dense structure. It cleans out plaque and debris (i.e., athersclerotic buildup) from the blood vessel walls.

Hot reactors are apparently healthy individuals who are prime candidates for stress-related heart attack or stroke because of the extreme reactions they demonstrate in response to daily stress.

Human immunodeficiency virus (HIV) attacks white blood cells (T-cells), weakening the immune system. It has an incubation period of up to 12 years during which a person feels fine and may have no symptoms. When enough of the immune system is destroyed, symptoms may include chronic fatigue, swollen lymph glands, weight loss, fevers or night sweats, poor appetite, and diarrhea.

Human papilloma virus (HPV) is a group of viruses that may produce genital warts and genital tract cancers.

Hydrogenation is a manufacturing process in which hydrogen atoms are added to unsaturated fats, making them more saturated. Manufacturers use hydrogenated oils to extend the shelf life of products. Consumption of hydrogenated oils has been shown to increase blood cholesterol levels.

Hypercholesterolemia is the term for high cholesterol levels in the blood.

Hypertension is high blood pressure that is acknowledged to be equal to or greater than 140/90.

Hyperthermia is a life-threatening condition in which the body temperature rises to a dangerously high level.

Hypertrophy is an increase in muscle size due to enlargement of existing muscle fibers. Muscles hypertrophy when exercised.

Hypokinetic diseases are lifestyle diseases resulting from inadequate physical fitness. Examples are heart disease, diabetes, osteoporosis, stroke, back pain, and cancer.

Hypothermia is a life-threatening condition in which the body temperature drops to a dangerously low level.

i

Ice is the street name for the crystallized (and smokable) form of crank. It is sometimes called *crystal meth*. The drug is more addictive than crack cocaine.

Insoluble fiber absorbs water as it passes through the digestive tract, increasing fecal bulk. By quickening the passage of food through the system, insoluble fiber is a good deterrent to digestive disorders, including cancer.

Intellectual dimension is the dimension of wellness that involves ongoing curiosity and the pursuance of knowledge. Attending lectures, reading newspapers, discussing new ideas with people, and visiting museums are just a few practices that reflect intellectual wellness.

Intervertebral disc is a fluid-filled cushion that separates each bony vertebra in the back.

Ischemia means "insufficient oxygen." It is used in reference to conditions in which cells are deprived of oxygen, resulting in pain or discomfort (heart angina, side stitch, etc.).

Isokinetic muscle contraction occurs when speed of movement is controlled as force is applied through a range of motion. Cybex or Orthotron equipment employs isokinetic contraction to strengthen muscles.

Isometric muscle contractions are those in which the muscle does not change length and no movement occurs. If you pushed your palms together hard, your pectoral muscles would contract and try to shorten, but your arms would not move.

Isotonic muscle contractions are those in which the muscle tension or force of contraction is controlled throughout the motion, as in a bench press.

k

Karvonen Equation is used to determine the target heart rate range (THR) for exercise. It takes into account the current fitness level of the exerciser by using his or her resting heart rate. (Karvonen was a Finnish researcher.) The formula is THR = MAX HR − RHR × IF + RHR.

Kegel exercises strengthen the pelvic floor muscles and may prevent or cure stress incontinence. They are done by contracting the perineal muscles, which surround the bladder and vagina. The exercises are named after the physician who invented them.

Ketone bodies is a toxic waste product that builds up in the body if fats are burned for energy in the absence of carbohydrates. This build-up, or *Ketosis*, can result in fatigue, nausea, and even nerve and brain damage.

l

Lacto-ovo-vegetarian is the type of vegetarian who will consume plant foods, dairy products, and eggs.

Lactovegetarian is the type of vegetarian who will consume plant foods and dairy products.

LDL cholesterol receptors, primarily in the liver cells, bind and remove cholesterol from the blood.

Lean-body mass (muscle mass) is specifically the *muscle* part of the fat-free body mass.

Ligament is the fibrous connective tissue that binds bones together to form a joint.

Liposuction is a surgical procedure in which fat is removed/suctioned from selected parts of the body.

Low-density lipoprotein (LDL) is considered to be the bad form of cholesterol because it more easily attaches to the blood vessel wall, thereby increasing the atherosclerotic process.

LSD (lysergic acid diethylamide) is a controlled substance and a dangerous and unpredictable hallucinogenic drug. This illegal drug is manufactured from lysergic acid which is found in ergot, a fungus that grows on rye or other grains. It is commonly referred to as *acid* on the street and is sold in many forms, including tablets, gelatin chips, and thin squares of absorbent paper soaked in liquid LSD.

Lymphocytes are white blood cells that are an important part of the body's immune system.

m

Macrominerals are minerals needed in large doses (more than 100 mg daily). Examples are calcium, magnesium, and potassium.

Malignant (cancerous) cells tend to spread from their origin to other sites in the body where they continue to grow, invade, and destroy normal tissue.

Marijuana (sometimes called *pot* or *grass*) is a CNS depressant. It is a psychoactive drug (i.e., mind-affecting) made from the leaves and flowers of the cannabis sativa plant. The principle psychoactive ingredient is delta-99-tetrahydrocannabinol (THC).

Maximal heart rate is the highest possible heart rate. Maximal heart rate can be estimated by subtracting age from 220 bpm.

Maximal oxygen uptake (max VO$_2$) is the greatest amount of oxygen that can be utilized by the body during intense exercise.

Meditation is a mental exercise that elicits the body's relaxation response. The purpose of meditation is to gain control over one's attention—to internally quiet down, allowing the individual to choose what to focus upon and to block out distracting thoughts.

Melanoma is a type of skin cancer that usually starts out as a dark wart or mole, has a deadly tendency to metastasize, and may be fatal.

Menarche is the start of a young female's mentrual cycle. Menarche is usually experienced between 11 and 12 years of age.

Metastasis is a process by which cancer cells break away from the primary tumor and migrate to other tissues through the lymph or blood systems where they continue to grow.

Mindfulness meditation involves focusing on whatever a person happens to be experiencing at the time and learning to experience anything calmly, whether it is pleasant or unpleasant. This type of meditation was popularized by Dr. Jon Kabat-Zinn. Traditional meditation involves training the mind on a single point of focus, such as a word or phrase.

Minerals are inorganic substances critical to many enzyme functions in the body.

Monounsaturated fat is a fatty acid that has one double bond between carbon atoms, thus reducing the number of hydrogen atoms attached. Monounsaturated fats are better for the heart than are saturated fats. Olive oil and peanut oil are monounsaturated.

Muscular endurance is the ability of the muscle to exert a submaximal force repeatedly against resistance or to sustain muscular contraction.

Muscular power, a function of strength and speed, is the ability to apply force rapidly. Jumping requires muscular power.

Muscular strength is the ability of the muscle to exert one maximal force against resistance.

Myocardial infarction is a heart attack.

n

Narcolepsy is a condition involving uncontrollable attacks of deep sleep.

Nitrosamines are highly carcinogenic ingredients found in tobacco products.

o

Obesity is an excessive accumulation of body fat. A woman over 30 percent body fat or a man over 25 percent body fat is considered obese. Having a body mass index (BMI) over 27 is generally classified as obesity.

Occupational dimension is the dimension of wellness that entails the ability to integrate skills, interests, and values that will heighten job satisfaction. Being able to identify a well work environment and balancing work time and personal leisure time are important skills in the occupational dimension.

Oligomenorrhea is a menstrual abnormality that results in infrequent or irregular menses.

Omega-3 is a polyunsaturated fat that is prevalent in fish. Omega-3 fatty acids inhibit atherosclerosis and can reduce blood cholesterol levels.

Opportunistic diseases are produced by common bacteria, viruses, parasites, and fungi that surround but do not usually have the opportunity to infect people with healthy immune systems. If a person is infected with HIV and enough of the immune system is destroyed, he or she will be more susceptible to unusual infections such as pneumocystis carinii pneumonia, an uncommon parasitic lung infection.

Optimal stress is the point at which stress is intense enough to motivate and physically prepare us to perform optimally yet not intense enough to cause the body to overreact or to sustain harmful effects.

Orthotics are shoe inserts that are specially molded to the foot to correct foot, arch, or leg abnormalities.

Osteoporosis is an age-related condition in which the formation of bone fails to keep pace with lost bone tissue. The result is brittle, porous bone that is susceptible to fracture.

Overpronation is a condition in which the foot rolls inward excessively upon contact with the ground during walking, jogging, or running.

Overuse is a condition of excessive overloading of fitness activities, resulting in nagging injuries. It often means doing too much, too soon—before the body is ready. The body and muscles must be given time to gradually adapt to new demands with *gradual* overloading.

Overweight is a term that refers to body weight greater than that which is considered normal. Normal weight is most often considered the average weight for a specific height (according to a standard height-weight chart).

p

Passive smoking occurs when nonsmokers breathe air polluted by tobacco smoke.

Pelvic inflammatory disease (PID) is an inflammation of the sexual organs that may cause fever and pain in the lower abdomen and scarring and blockage of the fallopian tubes and leave a woman unable to bear children. PID is sometimes a result of an untreated infection of chlamydia or gonorrhea.

Physical dimension is the dimension of wellness that deals with the functional operation of the body. Committing to a regular exercise program, not smoking, and low-fat eating are signs of physical wellness.

Physical fitness is the capacity of the heart, lungs, blood vessels, and muscles to function at optimal efficiency.

Phytochemicals are plant chemicals that we consume when we eat vegetables.

Plaque is an accumulation of cholesterol on the inner walls of coronary arteries.

Plantar fasciitis is an inflammation of the plantar fascia—the long thick band of connective tissue on the undersurface of the foot.

Plyometrics are bounding and jumping drills designed to increase explosive power (strength and speed).

Polyunsaturated fat is a fatty acid that has two double bonds between carbon atoms, thus reducing the number of hydrogen atoms attached. Corn oil, soybean oil, and safflower oil are examples.

Precancerous cells exhibit potentially cancerous changes such as abnormal growth.

Primary prevention refers to behaviors that reduce the risk of acquiring cancer, such as avoiding excessive sun exposure or not using tobacco.

Primary risk factors are linked directly to the development of CHD; they increase the possibility of having a heart attack more so than do the secondary risk factors. All primary risk factors are controllable.

Principle of overload is the gradual increase in physical activity to stress a muscle group or body system beyond accustomed levels. Gradual adaptation occurs, resulting in improved physiological functioning. The FTI order of overload and 10 percent increase per week rules should be followed to overload correctly.

Principle of specificity means that only the muscles or body systems being exercised will show beneficial change.

Progressive overload is a gradual increase in a workload, such as in strength training, either in the number of lifts performed or in the amount of weight lifted.

Progressive relaxation is a series of exercises designed by physician Edmund Jacobson for his tense patients. The method emphasizes the relaxation of the voluntary skeletal muscles by contracting a muscle group and then relaxing it, progressing from one muscle group to another until the total body is relaxed. Individuals eventually learn to recognize tenseness and to consciously relax whenever needed.

Pronation is the slight inward roll of the foot as it contacts the ground. It is natural for the foot to pronate slightly.

Proprioceptive neuromuscular facilitation (PNF) is a type of flexibility exercise in which you perform a static stretch, contract the muscle to produce fatigue, and then relax while a partner stretches your limb.

Proteins build and repair tissue, maintain chemical balance, and regulate the formation of hormones, antibodies, and enzymes. Good sources of protein are found in both animal sources (meat, dairy) and plant sources (beans, nuts, grains).

Psychedelic drugs have mind-expanding or mind-affecting capabilities and include hallucinogens such as LSD.

Psychoneuroimmunology is the study of the effects of emotions, behavior, and mental attitudes on the immune system and the onset/course of illness.

Psychosomatic disease is a physical ailment that is mentally induced. *Psycho* refers to the mind and *somatic* refers to the body. This type of disease is frequently called a *stress disease*.

q

Quackery is the promotion of a misleading and fraudulent health claim that is unproven. Most quackery products are foods, drugs, gadgets, or cosmetics that promote physical change.

r

Rate of perceived exertion (RPE) is a method of measuring exercise intensity developed by Gunnar Borg. Using this method, exercisers are able to accurately sense (or perceive) their own exercise intensity levels.

Recommended dietary allowances (RDA) is the amount of a nutrient considered to be adequate to meet the nutritional needs of most healthy Americans.

Reframing is a way of looking at life in a positive manner. For example, seeing the glass half full is a reframing of seeing it as half empty.

Relaxation response is the body's built-in defense mechanism against the harmful effects of the inappropriate elicitation of the fight-or-flight response caused by everyday living. Dr. Herbert Benson of Harvard University discovered that, with training, the healing mechanism can be summoned at will.

Repetition (rep) is the performing of an exercise one time, such as lifting a weight once.

Repetition maximum (1 RM) is the heaviest weight you can lift once with correct form.

R.I.C.E., an acronym for Rest, Ice, Compression, and Elevation, is the recommended treatment for many injuries.

Risk factors are the conditions, situations, and behaviors that increase the likelihood that an undesirable outcome (injury, illness, or death) will occur.

'roid rage is uncontrollable, aggressive behavior and can be a side effect of anabolic steroid use.

S

Saturated fat is a fatty acid that has hydrogen atoms attached to every carbon atom. Consumption of saturated fats has been shown to increase blood cholesterol levels. Coconut oil, butter, cheese, bacon, and meats are high in saturated fat.

Secondary hypertension is high blood pressure caused by a specific condition, such as kidney disease, tumor of the adrenal gland, or a defect of the aorta.

Secondary prevention refers to early detection of cancer, such as by knowing cancer's warning signals and performing a monthly self-exam.

Secondary risk factor contributes to the development of CHD but not as directly as a primary risk factor.

Self-management involves having a systematic, personal strategy for change or self-improvement. It means taking charge of one's daily choices by linking knowledge with action.

Semi-vegetarian is the type of vegetarian who only excludes red meat from his or her diet.

Set is a group of several repetitions of an exercise. For example, lifting a weight eight times might be one set.

Set point is a fat amount or weight level that the body physiologically works to maintain. It is thought that the brain regulates a "weight thermostat" for the body's metabolism. The set point can be altered, especially by engaging in regular exercise.

Sexually transmitted diseases (STDs) are diseases spread primarily through sexual intercourse but also through other intimate behavior and sex play and, occasionally, nonsexually.

Shin splint is a condition of pain along the front of the lower leg (shin). Involving the anterior tibialis muscle, the pain may range from mild discomfort to acute burning.

Side stitch is pain that sometimes occurs on the side of the body just below the ribs during vigorous exercise. A variety of conditions may contribute to this spasm

of the diaphragm— poor conditioning, shallow breathing, inadequate warm-up, exercising too soon after eating.

Simple carbohydrates are sugars that provide energy but lack much nutritional value. Honey, corn syrup, sucrose, fructose, dextrose, and brown sugar are examples.

Skinfold calipers are devices that measure skinfold thickness in order to determine body fat percentage.

Social dimension is the dimension of wellness that deals with the ability to get along with other people—regardless of race, ethnic background, or beliefs. It involves appreciating the uniqueness of others, as well as demonstrating a sensitivity to the needs of others. Regular community volunteerism demonstrates social wellness.

Societal norms are those behaviors or practices that are expected in a culture and that are accepted and supported by its members. The practice of giving candy in heart-shaped boxes on Valentine's Day is an example of an American cultural norm.

Soluble fiber travels through the digestive tract in a gel-like form, pacing the absorption of carbohydrates. This prevents dramatic shifts in blood sugar levels.

Sprain is a partial or complete tear of a ligament. Both ankles and knees are vulnerable to sprains because of the sudden force or twisting motion that these joints often endure.

Spiritual dimension is the dimension of wellness that involves looking within and exploring one's values and beliefs to discover a source of inner strength and serenity. It includes the ongoing search for personal meaning and purpose in life. Exhibiting honesty and having a clear sense of right and wrong are signs of spiritual wellness.

Stage of exhaustion is the third stage of the General Adaption Syndrome (GAS), which is now known as the Stress Response. During this stage, adaptation energy is exhausted and the organ system involved in the repeated stress response breaks down. Disease or malfunction of the organ system or even death may occur.

Stage of resistance is the second stage of the General Adaptation Syndrome (GAS), which is now known as the Stress Response. During this stage, the body actively resists and attempts to cope with the stressor.

Static flexibility refers to the range of motion you can achieve through a slow controlled stretch, as in a sitting hamstring stretch that you hold for 15 to 30 seconds.

Static stretching is the recommended method of stretching for flexibility. Each stretch is held for 15 to 30 seconds with no bouncing or jerking movements.

Storage fat is the extra fat that accumulates in fat (adipose) cells around internal organs and beneath the skin surface to insulate, pad, and protect the body from trauma and extreme cold.

Strain is a partial or complete tear of muscle fibers and/or a tendon. Sometimes referred to as a *pull*, a strain is often a result of a violent contraction of a muscle.

Stress is the response of the body to any type of change and to any new, threatening, or exciting situation. Dr. Hans Selye, one of the foremost authorities on stress, defined stress as the "nonspecific response of the human organism to any demand made upon it." *Nonspecific* means that the body reacts the same regardless of the cause.

Stress fracture is a microscopic break in a bone caused by overuse. Rather than a result of a distinct traumatic event, a stress fracture results from cumulative overload on a bone (typically the lower leg and foot) that has not been able to adjust to the repeated force.

Stress incontinence is an involuntary leakage of urine when laughing, coughing, sneezing, or exercising. It is a common problem particularly in women over 30 who have given birth.

Stress response, once known as the General Adaptation Syndrome (GAS), is the body's adaptation (reaction) to stress. Regardless of the cause, the reaction to stress is both psychological and physiological.

Stressors are factors causing stress. They may be pleasant or unpleasant, real or imagined, and physical, psychological, or emotional in nature.

Stretch reflex is a reflex tightening of a muscle (to protect it from injury) when it is quickly stretched. For example, when you do a bouncy stretch, the muscle reflexively tightens as you reach the limits of your range of motion to prevent muscle strain.

Strict vegetarian (vegan) is the type of vegetarian who consumes only plant foods.

Stroke occurs when blood flow to the brain is blocked. It is primarily caused by atherosclerosis.

Subcutaneous fat is fat that underlies the skin.

Supination is the rolling outward of the foot upon contact with the ground.

Synergistic reaction is a phenomenon that occurs when various drugs are taken in combination, so the cumulative effect is greater than the effects of the drugs when taken separately.

Syphilis is a bacterial STD that has four stages. The primary stage is a chancre, the secondary may produce skin rash, fever, headache, sore throat, swollen lymph glands, flulike symptoms, and patchy hair loss.

Systolic blood pressure is the pumping pressure of the heart as it pushes the blood out of the heart. It is recorded as the upper number.

t

Target heart rate range (THR) is the recommended heart rate range (or intensity level) for exercise. It is the range of intensity that assures adequate stimulation of the cardiorespiratory system yet is not so strenuous that symptoms of overtraining develop.

Task specific activity is an exercise (or activity) using the same muscles that will be used in the conditioning bout. Warm-up and cool-down should be task specific. For example, if you jog during the conditioning bout, a period of jogging at a lower intensity should precede (warm-up) and follow (cool-down).

T-cells are a type of lymphocyte (white blood cell) destroyed by HIV.

Tendinitis is the inflammation of a tendon from repeated stress.

Tendon is the fibrous cord that connects a muscle to a bone. The most familiar tendon in the body is the Achilles tendon, which connects the calf muscle to the heel.

Testosterone is a male hormone secreted by the testes.

Three-segment workout is the recommended pattern for exercise workouts. It should include a warm-up, conditioning bout, and cool-down.

Tolerance is the body's physical adjustment to the habitual use of a chemical.

Trace minerals are minerals needed in small amounts. Examples are iron, zinc, copper, iodine, and fluoride.

Training effect is the total beneficial change or physiological adaptation that results from regular aerobic exercise.

Transcendental meditation (TM) is a form of meditation that originated in the Eastern cultures of India and Tibet. It was exported to the Western world by the Maharishi Mahesh Yogi. It involves training the mind on a single point of focus, such as a word or phrase.

Triglycerides are known as *free fatty acids* and contribute to the atherosclerotic process. They are manufactured in the body and stored as excess fats.

Tumor is a lump of cells. It can be either benign or malignant.

Type A emotional behavior is described as competitive, ambitious, driven, impatient, and workaholic and demonstrates a high degree of time urgency. Type As put big demands on themselves to accomplish more and more in less and less time. These demands may lead to angry, cynical, and hostile behavior, which is a risk factor of CHD.

Type B emotional behavior is relaxed, noncompetitive, patient, and slow to anger, the opposite of Type A emotional behavior.

Type C emotional behavior is actually Type A emotional behavior in individuals who demonstrate stress-resistant, "hardiness" traits and who are thus not prone to the deleterious effects of stress, even though they live highly stressed lives. These traits are called the *Five Cs* (control, commitment, challenge, choices in lifestyle, and connectedness).

Type A personality is described as competitive, ambitious, driven, impatient, workaholic, and always rushed. Type As put big demands on themselves to accomplish more and more in less and less time. They have little time for or interest in hobbies or leisure pursuits and have few intimate friends. The key problem with Type A behavior is stress. Type As put themselves under constant pressure and their bodies react by producing extra amounts of stress hormones which can be harmful.

Type B personality is the opposite of Type A personality. Type Bs are relaxed, casual, unaggressive, and patient. Most Type Bs build in time in the day for absorbing activities such as exercise, hobbies, and friendship. They speak more softly, are less obsessed with success, and tend to deal more effectively with stressful situations.

Type C personality is actually a Type A personality who has stress-resistant, "hardiness" traits and who thus are not prone to the deleterious effects of stress, even though they live highly stressed lives. Type Cs have five common traits called the *Five Cs* (control, commitment, challenge, choices in lifestyle, and connectedness).

V–Z

Valsalva maneuver involves holding your breath while you strain against a closed epiglottis, as in holding your breath while lifting a weight. You should avoid doing this because it can cause a dangerous elevation of blood pressure. When you lift weights, exhale on the exertion.

Vitamins are the organic catalysts necessary to initiate the body's complex metabolic functions.

Warm-up is the first part of the three-segment workout. It prepares the body physically and mentally for the conditioning bout.

Water soluble vitamins are vitamins that remain in the body tissues for a short time. Excesses are excreted out of the body.

Wellness is an integrated and dynamic level of functioning oriented toward maximizing potential, dependent on self-responsibility. It is a mindset of self-empowerment and lifelong growth in the emotional, spiritual, physical, occupational, intellectual, environmental, and social dimensions.

Yo-yo syndrome (weight cycling) is the repetitive cycle of weight loss and weight gain. Off and on fad dieters typically experience weight cycling.

index